D1145951

Encephal- (G) *brain:* encephalitis, inflammation
End- (G) *within:* endothelium, layer of cells lini
Entero- (G) *intestine:* enterosis, falling of intesti
Epi- (G) *above or upon:* epidermis, outermost la
Erythro- (G) *red:* erythrocyte, red blood cell.
Eu- (G) *well:* euphoria, well feeling, feeling of g
Ex- or **E-** (L) *out:* excretion, material thrown out of the body or the organ.
Exo- (G) *outside:* exocrine, excreting outwardly (opposite of endocrine).
Extra- (G) *outside:* extramural, situated or occurring outside a wall.

Febri- (L) *fever:* febrile, feverish.

Galacto- (G) *milk:* galactose, a milk-sugar.
Gastr- (G) *stomach:* gastrectomy, excision of the stomach.
Gloss- (G) *tongue:* glossectomy, surgical removal of tongue.
Glyco- (G) *sugar:* glycosuria, sugar in the urine.
Gynec- (G) *woman:* gynecology, science of diseases pertaining to women.

Hem- or **hemat-** (G) *blood:* hemopoiesis, forming blood.
Hemi- (G) *half:* heminephrectomy, excision of half the kidney.
Hepat- (G) *liver:* hepatitis, inflammation of the liver.
Hetero- (G) *other* (opposite of homo): heterotransplant, using skin from a member of another species.
Hist- (G) *tissue:* histology, science of minute structure and function of tissues.
Homo- (G) *same:* homotransplant, skin grafting by using skin from a member of the same species.
Hydr- (G) *water:* hydrocephalus, abnormal accumulation of fluid in cranium.
Hyper- (G) *above, excess of:* hyperglycemia, excess of sugar in blood.
Hypo- (G) *under, deficiency of:* hypoglycemia, deficiency of sugar in blood.
Hyster- (G) *uterus:* hysterectomy, excision of uterus.

Idio- (G) *self, or separate:* idiopathic, a disease self-originated (of unknown cause).
Im- or **In-** (L) *in:* infiltration, accumulation in tissue of abnormal substances.
Im- or **In-** (L) *not:* immature, not mature.
Infra- (L) *below:* infra-orbital, below the orbit.
Inter- (L) *between:* intermuscular, between the muscles.
Intra- (L) *within:* intramuscular, within the muscle.

Kerat- (G) *horn, cornea:* keratitis, inflammation of cornea.

Lact- (L) *milk:* lactation, secretion of milk.
Leuk- (G) *white:* leukocyte, while cell.

Macro- (G) *large:* macroblast, abnormally large red cell.
Mast- (G) *breast:* mastectomy, excision of the breast.
Meg- or **Megal-** (G) *great:* megacolon, abnormally large colon.
Ment- (L) *mind:* dementia, deterioration of the mind.
Mer- (G) *part:* merotomy, division into segments.
Mesa- (G) *middle:* mesaortitis, inflammation of middle coat of the aorta.
Meta- (G) *beyond, over, change:* metastasis, change in seat of a disease.
Micro- (G) *small:* microplasia, dwarfism.
My- (G) *muscle:* myoma, tumor made of muscular elements.
Myc- (G) *fungi:* mycology, science and study of fungi.

Necro- (G) *corpse, dead:* necrosis, death of cells adjoining living tissue.
Neo- (G) *new:* neoplasm, any new growth or formation.
Neph- (G) *kidney:* nephrectomy, surgical excision of kidney.
Neuro- (G) *nerve:* neuron, nerve cell.

Continued on back end paper

Surgical Nursing

Surgical

ELDRIDGE L. ELIASON, A.B., M.D., SC.D., F.A.C.S.

Late Emeritus John Rhea Barton Professor of Surgery, University of Pennsylvania School of Medicine; Emeritus Professor of Surgery, University of Pennsylvania Graduate School of Medicine; Consulting Surgeon, Hospital of the University of Pennsylvania, Presbyterian and Philadelphia General Hospitals

L. KRAEER FERGUSON, A.B., M.D., F.A.C.S.

Professor of Surgery, Graduate School of Medicine of the University of Pennsylvania and Woman's Medical College of Pennsylvania; Surgeon, Graduate Hospital of the University of Pennsylvania, Hospital of the Woman's Medical College of Pennsylvania, Philadelphia General Hospital and Doctors Hospital; Consulting Surgeon, U.S. Naval Hospital, Philadelphia; Consultant in Surgery, Veterans Administration Hospital, Philadelphia

LILLIAN A. SHOLTIS, R.N., B.S., M.S.

Consultant in Medical and Surgical Nursing, Bryn Mawr Hospital School of Nursing; formerly Assistant Professor of Surgical Nursing, Yale University School of Nursing; Supervisor of Operating Rooms, Hospital of the University of Pennsylvania

Dardanella De Good
Box 17 Neil Hall
Ohio State Univ.

Nursing

TENTH EDITION

337 Illustrations, Including 9 Subjects in Color

J. B. LIPPINCOTT COMPANY

Philadelphia • Montreal

Tenth Edition, Fifth Impression

COPYRIGHT, 1955, BY J. B. LIPPINCOTT COMPANY

This book is fully protected by copyright and, with the exception of brief excerpts for review, no part of it may be reproduced in any form without the written permission of the publishers.

First to fifth editions by E. L. Eliason, L. Kraeer Ferguson and Elizabeth K. Lewis. Copyright, 1929, 1930, 1931, 1934, 1936 by J. B. Lippincott Company.
Sixth to eighth editions by E. L. Eliason, L. Kraeer Ferguson and Evelyn M. Farrand. Copyright, 1940, 1945, 1947 by J. B. Lippincott Company.
Ninth edition by E. L. Eliason, L. Kraeer Ferguson and Lillian A. Sholtis. Copyright, 1950, by J. B. Lippincott Company.

Surgical Nursing
has been translated into the
French and the Portugese languages

Distributed in Great Britain by
Pitman Medical Publishing Co., Limited
London

Library of Congress
Catalog Card Number
54-11530

PRINTED IN THE UNITED STATES OF AMERICA

Preface to the Tenth Edition

In this tenth edition of our book, *Surgical Nursing*, we have continued to emphasize the nursing care of the individual surgical patient and, as before, have described not only the "how" but also the "why" of the methods that the nurse must know. In addition, we recognize the necessity of teaching the nurse to look upon the patient as a person with a surgical disease, and we have pointed out the social, economic, psychological and public health factors that affect the patient and his disease. New material has been introduced not only to help the student give better nursing care but also to help her in the teaching and the rehabilitation of her surgical patient.

There has been a major revamping of the material presented, as to both form and substance. Those who have been familiar with previous editions will note that some chapters dealing with methods have been deleted completely, and others have been combined in a more logical fashion for teaching. New chapters include one on the nursing care of the surgical geriatric patient. New material has been introduced throughout to keep pace with the rapid progress of present-day surgery.

Sterilization methods have been brought up to date in line with the latest research in this field. An appendix includes helpful charts on the sterilization of various articles. The recovery room and its importance in the care of the postoperative patient is described, and its various functions are emphasized. A chapter on "Special Therapy" has been added to include fluid therapy and oxygen therapy. The newer trends in the field of anesthesia are presented.

It is understandable that radical revision was necessary to present to the nurse the present status of the ever-changing field of chemotherapy and antibiotic therapy. The section on wound care has been amplified to include the newer trends in the preparation and the utilization of surgical dressings.

Considerable emphasis has been placed upon the psychological aspects of preoperative and postoperative care, and suggestions are made concerning the nurse's role in this part of patient care. Cancer nursing care has been amplified, and here again stress has been placed on the psychological, social, economic and rehabilitation aspects. Material also has been added concerning terminal nursing care.

In the part of the book that deals with the special nursing care of individual surgical lesions, changes have been made to keep apace with the latest surgical technics. The section on the "Respiratory System" has been divided into two chapters, one on "Surgery of the Nose and the Throat" and a second on "Chest Surgery." The latter chapter is almost entirely new, reflecting the importance of this branch of surgery today. An effort has been made to acquaint the nurse with the operative procedures and to place emphasis on the specific nursing care involved. Water-seal and chest drainage is described in detail. The newer concepts in the surgical care of the patient with tuberculosis are expressed.

A new chapter on "Surgery of the Heart and the Great Vessels" has been added to keep the nurse abreast of the latest developments in this field. Included are discussions of such subjects as commissurotomy for mitral stenosis, the treatment of aortic aneurysms, congenital cardiac and vascular defects, vessel grafts, vascular shunts, etc. The chapters on gastro-intestinal surgery have been brought up to date, with amplification of the section on hernia. The chapters on urology and the text on burns have been reorganized, and new material has been incorporated.

In the chapter on "Surgery of the Eye," much new material has been added on glaucoma and cataract. More information has been provided to help the nurse in teaching eye and ear patients, with helpful suggestions in the active and psychological care of the newly blind and the hard of hearing.

The newer methods in orthopedic care have been introduced into the chapter on "Surgery of the Musculoskeletal System." Included in this chapter is a section on the use of the intramedullary pin in fracture treatment.

The chapters on the operating room now reflect the effect of streamlined equipment, a greater trend toward standardization in sterilization methods and the wider use of auxiliary personnel. A section on operating-room hazards and safety measures is included.

Throughout the book, teaching aids have been used. Many new charts and illustrations have been added. Newly defined words are placed in italics. At the end of chapters in the clinical areas, clinical situations with related questions have been used to assist the student in directing her learning experiences to the care of a patient. An up-to-date bibliography is found at the end of each unit to aid the student in reference reading. Cross references for edition 17 of *Essentials of Medicine*, by Charles P. Emerson and Jane S. Bragdon, now are located in these bibliographies.

We are indebted to many consultants and advisers concerning their specialties: Dr. Robert Dripps, Jr., Professor of Surgery (Anesthesiology) and Gas Therapy, University of Pennsylvania Medical School; Dr. Louis E. Silcox, Professor of Clinical Otolaryngology, Graduate School of Medicine, University of Pennsylvania; Miss Emily C. Cardew, Acting Director of Nursing, University of Illinois School of Nursing; Miss Juanita A. Booth, Assistant Professor of Nursing, School of Nursing, Medical Center, University of California, Los Angeles; Miss Mary E. Quinlan, Public Health Supervisor, Massachusetts General Hospital School of Nursing. Mr. Wayne Comer, Director, Nursing Education Program, Johnson and Johnson, kindly gave us permission to draw freely upon their postoperative wound-care study. Many others, including our families, have aided and encouraged us in the preparation of this tenth edition. Finally, a grateful acknowledgment should be made to the various members of the staff of the J. B. Lippincott Company for their patient co-operation.

L. Kraeer Ferguson
Lillian A. Sholtis

Preface to the First Edition

One of our most eminent surgeons has said that to "cut well and sew well" means to "get well." This is not enough, for we must "nurse well" also. How important good nursing is in surgery is fully appreciated only by the surgeon. He recognizes how essential to his success is a nurse well trained in bedside nursing technic. Not only must the nurse be adept in this important phase of her work, but she must also be keenly alive to the observation of signs and symptoms that arise from time to time under her eye. Further, she must have some knowledge as to the cause and the seriousness of these same changes in order that she may know their relative value with reference to reporting them to the surgeon. These accomplishments can be obtained only by long-continued practice at the bedside. Didactic teaching in the classroom has its place, but it should be made to occupy a very minor role when compared to the actual knowledge learned from real contact with the patient.

Cyanosis as described in the class makes little impression upon the pupil, but the bedside picture of the cyanotic patient, with the associated dyspnea and anxious expression, makes a lasting impression. The classroom may show a pupil how to find acetone in the urine, but how much more important that she recognize the fruity odor of the breath, the pulse hurry and restlessness of the actual condition under her charge! How much better that she should recognize audible peristalsis rather than to be able to define glibly the term borborygmi!

Higher nursing education is an excellent ideal and should be advocated and commended, but not at the expense of real actual care of the patient as a human individual, rather than as a pathologic specimen.

Experience has shown that less mistakes are made, and more efficient nursing is obtained, when the nurse understands not only what to do, but also why a procedure must be carried out in a certain way. In so far as possible, an effort has been made to explain the reason, as well as the method, for each procedure. To accomplish this purpose, sections on anatomy and physiology have been inserted where deemed advisable.

The authors have drawn freely upon their own experience as a senior surgeon, a junior surgeon, and a nurse who has been both an operating-room head nurse as well as an instructress of nurses at the University of Pennsylvania Hospital Training School. All three authors have been instructing nurses for many years, both in the lecture hall and in the practical work in the sickroom.

The teaching value of thoughtfully made pictures cannot be overemphasized, and these illustrations represent many hours of careful posing to present through the eye a helpful adjunct to the text.

Much thanks and appreciation are due Dr. Rachel Winlock for her excellent hand-drawn illustrations.

THE AUTHORS

Contents

UNIT ONE

INTRODUCTION TO SURGICAL NURSING

UNIT TWO

NURSING IN CONDITIONS OF THE UPPER RESPIRATORY TRACT

UNIT THREE

NURSING IN CONDITIONS OF THE CIRCULATORY SYSTEM, THE BLOOD AND THE BLOOD-FORMING ORGANS

UNIT FIVE

NURSING IN CONDITIONS OF THE URINARY TRACT—MALE UROLOGY

UNIT SIX

NURSING IN CONDITIONS OF THE INTEGUMENTARY SYSTEM (INCLUDING THE SUBCUTANEOUS AND THE AREOLAR TISSUE AND THE BREASTS)

UNIT EIGHT

NURSING CONDITIONS OF THE ENDOCRINE GLANDS

UNIT TEN

NURSING IN CONDITIONS OF THE MUSCULOSKELETAL SYSTEM

UNIT ELEVEN

NURSING IN CONDITIONS OF THE REPRODUCTIVE SYSTEM

UNIT TWELVE

NURSING IN SURGICAL COMMUNICABLE DISEASES

UNIT THIRTEEN

OPERATIVE ASEPTIC TECHNIC

UNIT ONE

Introduction to Surgical Nursing

CHAPTER ONE

The Surgical Nurse and Her Patient

SURGERY IN THE PAST

Surgery was performed long before the dawn of civilization with the aid of a sharpened flint. Neolithic skulls with trephined holes show evidence of bony repair and prove that patients did survive major operations. Surgery developed remarkably in ancient India: a clear-cut and logical classification of surgical operations is given in the famous writing, the Samhita. It is recorded also that women who helped with the sick had to have clean hands and nails cut short. In Greece (400 B.C.) Hippocrates knew and described surgical conditions varying from a clubfoot to a fracture of the vertebra. Prostheses, such as false limbs and dentures, were made for patients. Plastic operations were performed, and bladder stones were removed. Surgery advanced more rapidly than medicine, probably because its results were more dramatic. Surgical nursing as such is not mentioned in these early histories, but it must have existed.

One of the many stories in the Bible at the beginning of the Christian era is:

> And he went to him, and bound up his wounds, pouring in oil and wine, and set him on his own beast, and brought him to an inn, and took care of him.
>
> LUKE 10:34

The good Samaritan gave nursing care. He found a man who had been beaten cruelly by thieves. After he had cared for his wounds, the Samaritan took his patient to an inn and continued to care for him. One realizes that the emphasis of his care was on the person with the wound and not the wound alone.

There were no remarkable developments in surgery or in nursing for many centuries after the beginning of the Christian era. Through these years there is reference to two groups of nurses: those associated with some religious group and those of the Sairey Gamp type who nursed for hire. Little mention is made of nurses who cared specifically for surgical patients. At the time of Lister's introduction of carbolic acid as an antiseptic in the nineteenth century, one is made aware that nurses assisted in the operating room. About this time the seeds of present-day nursing were planted by Florence Nightingale as she cared for the wounded soldiers in the Crimean War. In particular, she emphasized the significance of good hygiene and she was a strong advocate of planned instruction for nurses.

Up to the nineteenth century tradition had a strong influence and a restricting effect on progress. The general practitioner treated all ills. There were few who limited their practice to surgery and almost none who limited their field to specialized types of surgery. However, following the industrial revolution, tradition relaxed, and the more highly skilled tasks necessary to operate machinery introduced specialization. A parallel in the medical field was the rise of the specialist. If a person had difficulty with his ear, he went to an ear specialist. Now we are living in an age in which we are seeing a return in the professions to the more desirable middle course. Our emphasis today is not on the ear as such, but on the person who has an ear problem. And so, in surgical nursing, our concern is not the appendectomy, but the patient who has undergone surgery for appendicitis.

SURGERY AT PRESENT

The greatest progress in the care of the surgical patient has taken place since the beginning of the present century. An increasing knowledge of disease as a result of research has permitted the development of many diagnostic aids. Some of these depend upon roentgenograms and others upon various laboratory procedures: chemical, bacteriologic, pathologic and so forth. The result is that the diagnosis of surgical disease is made with more exactness and certainty than was possible from the simple clinical examinations of previous days. It became apparent that the nutritional condition of the patient was an important factor in the outcome of a surgical procedure. The surgeon recognized the value to the patient of a normal fluid and electrolyte balance. In addition, he realized that good nutrition depended upon the maintenance of normal vitamin intake and a replacement of vitamins if there had been a loss of them. The significance of protein in the body nutrition has led to increasing attention to its intake in the surgical patient, both before and after operation. When this food element cannot be taken by mouth, water-soluble protein may be given intravenously. In addition, replacement of protein and hemoglobin now is achieved commonly by plasma and blood transfusions. Blood also is used

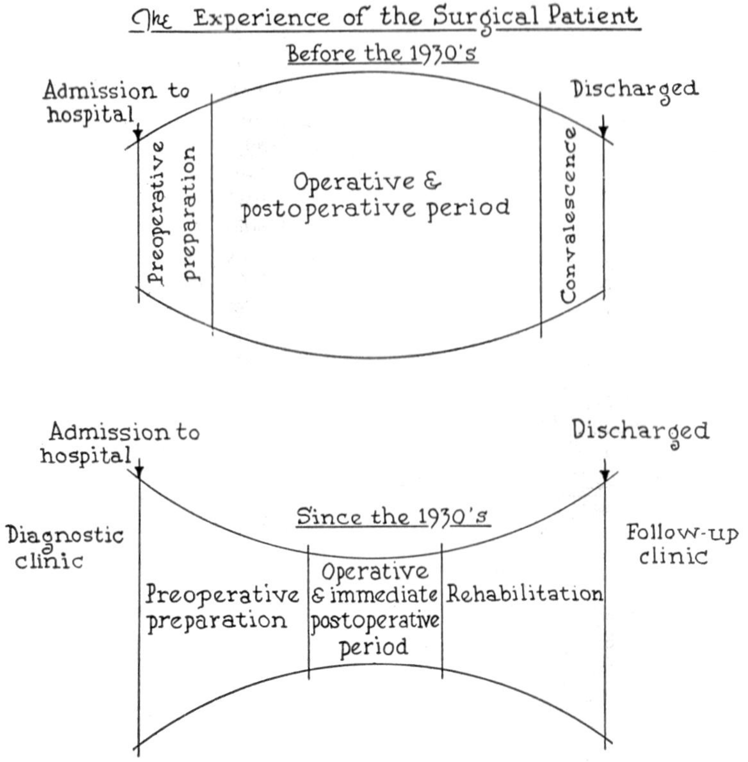

FIGURE 1

extensively during and after operation to replace blood loss and to prevent shock.

In the operating room the surgeon has been aided by a progressive improvement in instruments, equipment and conveniences in construction. Improvement in the understanding and the practice of asepsis and various technical procedures has made it possible to perform operations that would not have been possible before. Not the least of these improvements has been the development of the anesthesiologist, and with him have come many advances in the technic of the administration of anesthesia. These advances have made it possible to deal surgically with lesions in the chest, the brain, the heart and the great vessels and with extensive malignancies in many parts of the body—something unheard of before.

One of the most striking developments has been the result of research in the control of infection. The discovery of the sulfonamides and the production of more effective and less toxic drugs were followed by the advent of the antibiotics, so that many infections that led previously to surgery now can be treated conservatively. These drugs are used to prevent infections after operations and, should they arise, to treat them, and this has reduced greatly the operative hazard.

Many new fields of therapy have opened for the surgical patient. To mention them all would be impossible, but the therapeutic use of radiant energy, such as radium, x-rays and radioactive materials, may be used as an example.

A final advance in the care of the surgical patient is the change in attitude of all those who have a part in his care. It is recognized that the care of the surgical lesion is only a part of the care of the patient as a person: the important thing is to rehabilitate the patient and to return him to his home a healthy, happy, economically competent member of society. This concept has many aspects. It may be concerned with the psychosomatic cause of the surgical disease, such as the influence of mental stress and overfatigue upon the production of peptic ulcer, or it may deal with the development of a mental attitude toward the acceptance of a colostomy or an amputation. In this rehabilitation, the patient, and even his family, frequently requires training and instruction. Realizing that the best rehabilitation is a return to normal activities at an early date, there has been a gradual trend toward getting the patient out of bed as soon as possible after operation. Experience has proved that wounds heal well, that complications are decreased and that the general metabolism and the morale of the patient are improved by early ambulation. Prosthetic appliances that permit a more normal life for patients who have deformities have helped a great deal. Along with these important contributions to the rehabilitation of patients has come an increasing interest in the prevention of disease. Periodic health examinations, cancer detection clinics and industrial and public health education are playing an increasingly important part in the prevention of disease and the early detection of what would lead to serious surgical lesions if neglected.

With this improvement in the care of the surgical patient has come a change in the attitude, the functions and the responsibilities of the surgical nurse. Although she still is expected to understand and carry out the bedside duties required in the care of the surgical patient, she also is expected to understand and take an important part in all phases of the patient's care.

The nurse, from her daily contact with the patient and the opportunity it affords her to observe him, can begin the rehabilitation of the patient even before operation. She must be able to carry out the immediate details of treatment while maintaining the over-all purpose of surgical care as related to the patient as a whole. This demands increasing knowledge and, therefore, increasing study. But it is important that with this increasing knowledge and responsibility she should not lose the human attribute that the connotation of the word "nurse" implies. The highly educated nurse

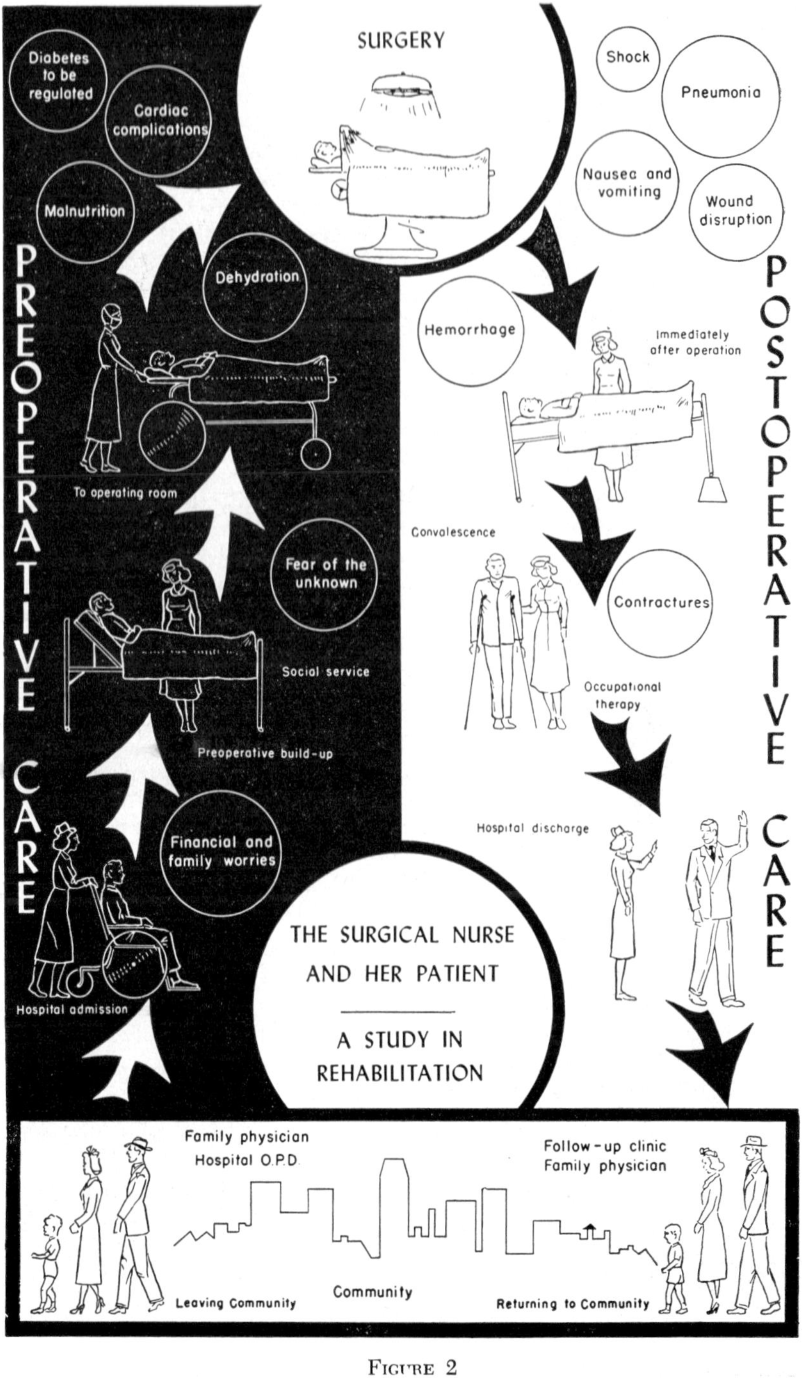
SURGERY
Diabetes to be regulated
Cardiac complications
Malnutrition
Dehydration
PREOPERATIVE CARE
To operating room
Fear of the unknown
Social service
Preoperative build-up
Financial and family worries
Hospital admission
THE SURGICAL NURSE AND HER PATIENT
A STUDY IN REHABILITATION
Shock
Pneumonia
Nausea and vomiting
Wound disruption
POSTOPERATIVE CARE
Hemorrhage
Immediately after operation
Convalescence
Contractures
Occupational therapy
Hospital discharge
Family physician
Hospital O.P.D.
Follow-up clinic
Family physician
Leaving Community
Community
Returning to Community

FIGURE 2

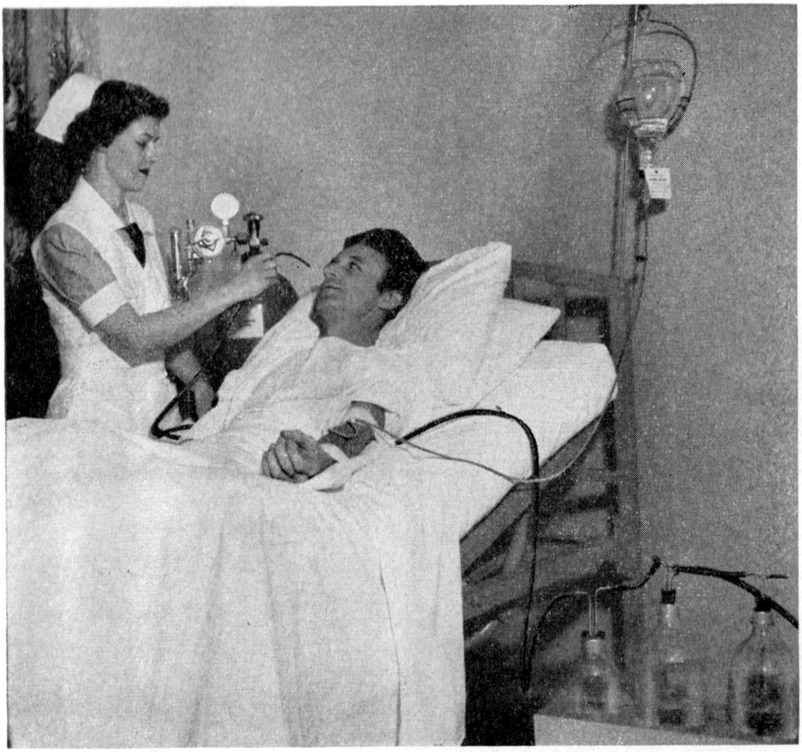

FIG. 3. The nurse and her patient. Multiple bottle chest suction and an intravenous infusion can be seen. The nurse is about to pass a nasal catheter for oxygen therapy. (Taken at the Grace-New Haven Hospital)

with a scientific knowledge does not help the patient unless this knowledge is directed toward making the patient a more comfortable, healthy and contented individual. In present-day practice, less highly trained individuals may be given responsibility for certain types of care that do not demand extensive preparation. Thus nurses' aides and practical nurses now are being employed more widely to take over some of the less responsible duties. However, the professional nurse must realize that her responsibility to her patient entails careful supervision of her aide who has less training.

THE NURSE AND HER PATIENT BEFORE SURGERY

The girl who is studying and practicing surgical nursing learns that essentially she is caring for a person with a surgical condition. She becomes cognizant of the fact that mind, body and soul should be in a healthy condition. From the psychological point of view, she will learn that a mind that is not at peace influences directly the proper functioning of the body. Fear of the unknown, fear of death, fear of anesthesia and fear of cancer may be apparent immediately, but other fears may be more tangible: about the probable loss of a job, about the support of a family or about permanent incapacity. Not infrequently one sees a sick body that has resulted wholly from emotional insecurity, such as is evident many times in patients with a stomach ulcer or an inflamed, ulcerating colon. Emotional upsets are more apparent in illness. Consequently, the nurse who learns this early in her career will be more tolerant and understanding. Unfortunately, all adults are not mature persons. They may be adult physically but not emotionally.

An essential part of this preoperative phase of patient care is the diagnostic study. The nurse should understand the purpose of each test and help to keep the patient informed. Too many times, a patient feels that he is a guinea pig. There need be no such reaction if the nurse assumes her full role. The summation of diagnostic tests serves as a road map for the physician in directing him to his goal—the cure of illness.

Increasing emphasis is placed on achieving nutritional, fluid and electrolyte balance in the body. It has been learned that a person who has been eating an adequate diet and is not undernourished or dehydrated is able to tolerate surgery much better. Here again, the nurse will recognize why it is important to produce tempting trays at mealtime. She will make sure that the environment is conducive esthetically to the stimulation of a healthy appetite. She will encourage a patient to take fluids and food, but she will recognize that when a patient does not desire to eat or to drink there usually is a reason for it. If a patient is unable to eat, perhaps the essential ingredients for tissue growth and repair can be given by intravenous methods.

It is important for the nurse to observe the patient's reactions, both physical and mental. Even more important is her ability to report and chart her most pertinent observations in a clear and concise manner. Some observations of the reactions of a patient have to be reported immediately, so that treatment may be initiated promptly. These will be dealt with in the different units of study.

The ideal situation is for the nurse who has cared for the patient to prepare him for operation and accompany him to the operating room. It means a great deal to a patient who is approaching a new experience with some degree of apprehension to have someone that he knows with him.

THE NURSE AND HER PATIENT AFTER SURGERY

Immediately after operation the nurse is concerned with lifesaving measures. It is here that intelligent bedside nursing is most important. The patient's life, in many cases, depends upon the accurate noting, recording and interpreting of vital signs, the administration of drugs and intravenous fluids and the efficient working of such apparatus as gastric or intestinal suction, oxygen therapy and so forth. After the immediate danger from the operative procedure, postoperative care is directed primarily toward helping the patient to help himself so that he can be a happy and useful member of society. The nurse must be understanding and tactful as she encourages her patient to become increasingly more independent. Throughout this period, she will employ many principles of surgical care in an attempt to prevent postoperative complications. All treatments and medications, as well as general directives for patient care, are ordered specifically by the surgeon.

The trend is to get the patient up and about at an early date after surgery. Correct bed and walking posture must be maintained for comfort and to prevent deformities. Rehabilitation is achieved by means of a team of workers whose efforts are directed toward a definite goal. This team is made up primarily of the patient, the physician, the nurse and the physical and occupational therapists. The most effective teaching and learning situation is one that is practical; therefore, the activities of daily living should serve as the focus of concentration in this rehabilitative phase.

When the patient is to be discharged from the hospital, he should be well on the road to recovery. He should know what his immediate range of activity should include and exclude. To be effective, the instructions given to him must be clear. The physician, the nurse, the nutritionist, as well as the medical social worker, can give invaluable assistance at this time.

THE OVER-ALL RESPONSIBILITY OF THE SURGICAL NURSE

So far we have limited our remarks to the patient with a surgical problem. Just as in all other phases of illness, there are preventive aspects that must be recognized by the nurse and emphasized over and over again in her teaching of patients if she is to assume her rightful place as a health teacher in society. Much radical surgery can be avoided if precautions are taken early enough. For example, the proper control of diabetes may eliminate the necessity of amputating a leg, and the early reporting to a physician of rectal bleeding may prevent extensive intestinal surgery. True, everything that leads to surgical intervention cannot be prevented, but the nurse can help to teach that in some conditions surgery can be avoided, or that minor surgery often will eliminate major surgery at a later time.

To give comprehensive nursing care is the aim of every surgical nurse. The fundamentals learned in her preclinical experience are not replaced but are amplified with more specialized technics. She should continue to promote good general health and prevent complications. She is in a position to sustain the morale of the patient, for she has more contact with him than any other person. Consequently, she can keep the prospect continually before her patient that he can overcome his handicap. This can be accomplished only if her attitude toward disease is an optimistic one. Quite unconsciously, she transmits this to her patient. It is important that the family regard disease or deformity as an obstacle that can be overcome. The nurse can gather reinforcement for optimistic thinking by observing the constructive work that is being done along these lines and by studying statistical reports.

All through her care it is the aim of the nurse to maintain the comfort of her patient. She must have a working knowledge of the principles of good body mechanics. When a patient complains of discomfort, it is the nurse's responsibility to seek the cause of it and not alleviate it with a drug unless it is justified.

By utilizing her powers of observation, she is able to acquire a wealth of information to relay to the physician; negative, as well as positive, responses often are important. By showing a personal interest in her patient, she reaps a double harvest: first, such an interest may be the key to securing the patient's confidence in those who are caring for him; second, it gives her an opportunity to recognize individual differences. She learns that the "real misery" of the Negro is meaningful, that some people have lower pain thresholds, that the overly protected child has greater insecurities, that there is a male as well as a female psychology, and that the care of the older-age group is quite different from that of the middle-age group.

To summarize, the responsibilities of the surgical nurse are many. No longer is the team limited to the surgeon, the nurse and the patient; it includes the patient's family, the medical social worker, the clergyman and the physical and diversional therapists. The nurse functions as an active member of such a group. Her personality, integrity and initiative are significant factors in her make-up. She must be honest and dependable. Her ability to think logically and act promptly may save lives. With such personal qualifications and a substantial reservoir of usable knowledge any nurse should be able to handle any surgical problem.

A SUGGESTED PATTERN OF STUDY FOR THE STUDENT

The ability to organize one's activity, whether it is study, nursing care or extraprofessional responsibilities, often determines whether a person is successful or not. Time, energy and money are saved when work is organized. With this premise in mind, how can a student nurse develop a comprehensive plan that can be used as she studies each unit? How can this be related to what she studied in her preclinical period? Does it apply to other clinical experiences? How can it be applied in giving the most effective nursing care?

The outline on the following page is offered as a flexible guide:

The unit of study on the left may be a functional system of the body, such as the genito-urinary system, or it may be one part of such a system, such as the prostate gland. The related background and associated courses that are listed on the right present a wide gamut of source material. Often a student begins experience in a clinical field feeling oversaturated with basic courses. Here she will find innumerable applications of the many facts and principles that she learned earlier.

Although this outline has many uses, when a student is assigned to the care of a surgical patient her immediate plan of care should stem from the answers to three questions: (1) why is this person in the hospi-

UNIT OF STUDY	ORDER OF STUDY	RELATED BACK-GROUND AND ASSOCIATED COURSES
EXAMPLE: Conditions of the Genito-urinary System	ASSUMPTION: One can learn deviations from the normal only if one knows the normal.	Anatomy Physiology Chemistry Physics
	What is the normal function?	Nutrition
	What is the relation to the whole?	
	What are the deviations from normal?	
	1. Congenital anomalies 3. Disease	Pathology
	2. Trauma 4. Tumors	Microbiology
	What are preventive aspects? Causative factors?	Community nursing
	What care is essential in an emergency situation?	Sociology (Economics)
	What is necessary to treat this patient? Why?	First aid
	1. Establishment of a diagnosis A. How can I help the physician in this function? B. Have I been complete and concise in charting? 2. Achievement of optimal physical and mental health.	Psychology
	A. How can I help the patient to achieve this level so that he can tolerate surgery with the least difficulty and accept the results as a means of getting well? B. What factors affect the degree of illness? C. How can I care best for my patient, utilizing nursing principles? (a) Comfort and safety.	Psychology Nutrition Nursing arts Pharmacology Professional ethics
	(b) Conservation of time, energy and equipment. D. In charting, how can I be of most help to the physician? E. How can I help my patient best to avoid postoperative complications?	Medicolegal aspects Nursing arts
	F. How can I help my patient to help himself? Have the patient's family and future been taken into consideration? G. Has my attitude been a healthy one?	Rehabilitation Personal and professional development

tal?; (2) how can I be of most help to him?; and (3) what is my time restriction? The student must learn to evaluate a situation, develop a sense of proportion and use her judgment in determining how she can give that care best within an allotted time. The factor of time cannot be ignored; nor can the patient's mental reaction be overlooked. The nurse may have ample time, but the patient may not be able to tolerate a prolonged treatment. Many times a complete bed bath is given and no time is left to do a special treatment, such as a colostomy irrigation. Often a patient may have a complete bath but no mouth care, which in many instances may be more important than the complete bath. Nursing care is effective if it is planned so that the most essential care is given first. Plans may have to be shifted as emergency situations arise; nevertheless, a logical method of approach still can be achieved.

Finally, surgical nursing can be studied in more than one way. The approach may be made by studying independently each of the obvious divisions of the body, such as the head, the neck and so forth. On the other hand, a study can be made according to degrees of illness, such as minor surgery or major surgery, local affections or systemic disturbances. In this book, the method of presentation is according to the functional divisions of the body, such as the respiratory, the circulatory and so forth. These areas are prefaced by a unit of introduction in which the basic principles in the care of the patient before and after surgery are presented. A selected bibliography follows each unit.

CHAPTER TWO

Inflammation—Nursing Care

HOW BACTERIA CAUSE DISEASE

Since infections are associated intimately with the great majority of surgical lesions, it is essential that we know something about the small organisms which invade our bodies and understand how they cause these diseases. These small, single-celled organisms, the lowest form of plant life, are called *bacteria.* They may enter the body through any break in its protective layer of cells or through the piercing of the lining membranes of the systems that connect with the outside; viz., the alimentary, the respiratory and the genito-urinary systems. Once they have entered the body tissues, they may remain at the site of their entrance or they may be carried by the blood or the lymphatic systems to distant parts. The bacteria with which we are concerned in surgery fall into two main groups: (1) spheroidal or ball-shaped organisms called cocci and (2) rod-shaped organisms called bacilli. They are divided into many subdivisions, each of which causes a distinctive type of disease.

Cocci. The ball-shaped group contains many of the bacteria that are characterized by the formation of pus (pyogenic bacteria). The chief members of the group are (1) staphylococci, (2) streptococci and (3) gonococci.

STAPHYLOCOCCI are cocci that grow in groups. They are the chief organisms that form thick, yellowish or white pus.

STREPTOCOCCI are cocci that are arranged in chains. They frequently cause widespread inflammation with a thin, watery type of pus.

GONOCOCCI are cocci that are arranged in pairs. They cause an inflammation which produces copious pus in the genital tract, the eyes and elsewhere.

Bacilli. The rod-shaped organisms likewise are divided into groups:

BACILLUS COLI COMMUNIS (*Escherichia coli*), a large group in itself. It is a normal habitant of the intestinal tract and is responsible for a large group of abdominal diseases.

Bacillus pyocyaneus (*Pseudomonas aeruginosa*), an organism that is characterized by the production of a greenish pus with a distinctive musty odor.

Bacillus tuberculosis (*Mycobacterium tuberculosis*), an organism that does not produce pus primarily. It is met with surgically when it attacks bones, joints and the abdominal cavity.

Bacillus tetani (*Clostridium tetani*), a non-pus-producing bacillus that causes tetanus (lockjaw). This organism may live during part of its life in what appears to be a dense envelope at one end of the rod. This is called spore formation. Spores are very resistant to deleterious agencies. In comparison with other bacteria, they are much harder to kill by heat and chemicals. When spores enter the body, they develop into the vegetative or growing form of the bacillus. *Clostridium tetani* has another characteristic that is of importance surgically: being an anaerobe, it cannot live in the presence of oxygen. Therefore, it is found characteristically in deep wounds having small external openings, puncture wounds—for example, those made with a nail or a bullet.

Bacillus welchii (*Clostridium welchii*), the gas bacillus, an organism that infects dead or dying tissues. It is characterized by the formation of gas in them. It is also an anaerobe, i.e., an organism that cannot live in the presence of oxygen.

How Bacteria Cause Disease. Bacteria are present constantly in the air we breathe, the water we drink and the food we eat. Any break in the protective covering of our bodies permits the entrance of these minute organisms. Finding warmth, moisture and food, they multiply rapidly.

Exotoxins. As they grow, certain bacteria excrete highly toxic substances that are absorbed by the body and cause disease. Such toxins are called exotoxins. *Clostridium tetani,* the tetanus bacillus, is an example of an organism forming this type of poison.

Endotoxins. Other bacteria store up toxic substances in their bodies. These are liberated only as they die and disintegrate. Such substances, called endotoxins, are formed by harmful bacteria, such as the staphylococcus and the streptococcus. When absorbed by the body, these poisonous substances, toxins, cause disease.

BODY DEFENSE MECHANISMS

To combat the actions of these toxins, we possess several natural means: phagocytosis and immune substances (sera and antitoxins).

Phagocytosis

Many cells, especially the white blood cells, may attack and destroy the offending organisms.

Immune Substances (Sera and Antitoxins)

Immunity. Immune substances are those found in the blood plasma that act against the bacteria or neutralize their toxins. The most important of these are called *antitoxins,* which are produced when exotoxins are formed, and *antibodies,* which are developed when endotoxins appear.

These substances combine with the toxins formed by the bacteria to render the bacteria harmless. In a normal case of a moderate infection, the body forms increasing amounts of these substances, and we say that an immunity has developed when the immune substances are sufficient to neutralize all the toxins formed.

The antitoxins and the antibodies can be formed in the blood of animals by injecting into them the organisms or toxins. Thus we can obtain sera containing these protective substances that can be given to patients before their powers of protection have developed or when they are insufficient to combat the disease. The sera produced by injection of toxins are called *antitoxins;* those formed by injection of dead or living bacteria are called *antisera.* Those used most often in surgery are the tetanus antitoxin, the gas-gangrene antitoxin, the antistreptococcic serum and the antierysipeloid serum.

Serum Reaction and Treatment

Anaphylaxis. The antitoxins and the antisera derived from the blood of animals or other individuals contain substances of a protein nature that may cause a reaction, called *anaphylaxis,* when they are injected into a patient. The picture is one of typical shock, with cyanosis, fall of blood pressure, rapid thready pulse and even death. Adrenalin hydrochloride (epinephrine) injections are the best therapeutic measures. The nurse should have epinephrine on hand when the biologic product is injected and from 0.3 to 0.1 cc. of it in a syringe should be ready for immediate use.

Many individuals are sensitive to foreign protein, especially if they have had previous serum injections, or if they are subject to such allergic diseases (those caused by the introduction of foreign protein into the body) as asthma, hay fever, strawberry rash and urticaria (hives).

Desensitization. Sera must be given cautiously to such persons. Usually, an attempt is made to desensitize the patient by the administration of the serum in graduated doses, beginning with minute amounts of the serum diluted with saline. The first injections are made intradermally and, if the patient shows no reaction, large doses are injected subcutaneously and intramuscularly. Many physicians test all patients before giving serum by injecting a very small amount of the serum into the skin of the forearm. A similar injection of normal saline should be given on the opposite arm as a control. A reaction to the serum is indicated by the appearance, in from 5 to 15 minutes, of a reddened, itching wheal (hive) about the site of the serum injection. Such a reaction indicates that the patient is sensitive to serum and, therefore, must be desensitized.

Serum Sickness. Frequently, when an antitoxin or other serum is given without previous desensitization, and even when the patient has been desensitized, a marked reaction may occur in from 5 to 9 days after the injection. This so-called "serum sickness" is characterized by marked and diffuse urticaria, itching, joint pains and sometimes even by edema of the glottis. Epinephrine injections, followed by ephedrine, by calcium

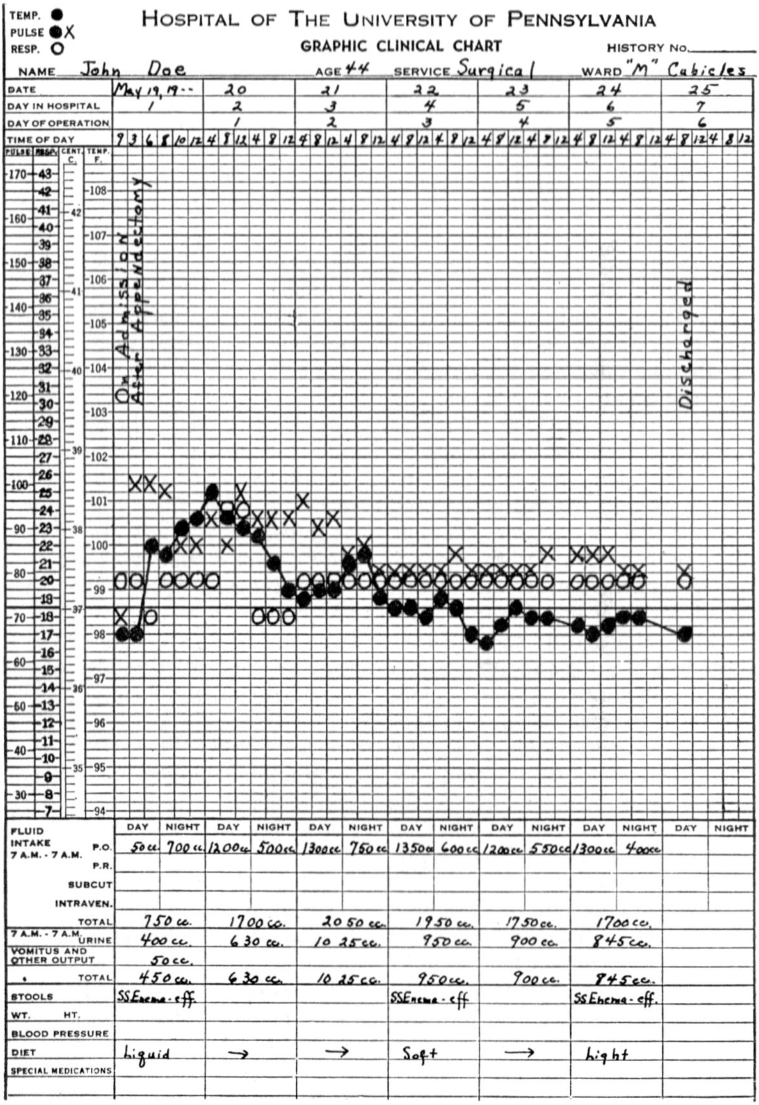

FIG. 4. Chart showing temperature, pulse and respiratory rate in a mild inflammation. Crosses indicate pulse; dots indicate temperature; circles indicate respirations.

lactate and by salicylates for the relief of joint pains, all by mouth, usually produce good results. The reaction may not last more than from 24 to 48 hours.

It is wise to warn patients that such a reaction may occur.

Asepsis. Our knowledge concerning bacteria and the diseases caused by them would be of little use if it did not tell us how we can avoid them. The history of present-day surgery begins really with the time when it was discovered that wounds could be made without the entrance of bacteria into them. At first an effort was made to kill the bacteria by using a solution poisonous to them. The skin, the wound, the instruments and the materials used were washed with this solution, called an *antiseptic.* With the advance of knowledge, it was learned that all bacterial life, the organisms and even the hardy spore forms, were killed by subjecting them for a time to a high temperature. Thus, today we sterilize all instruments used in wounds by boiling or autoclaving, and all other materials are sterilized by subjecting them to the high temperatures formed by steam under pressure. This is the *aseptic* method of operating.

Ultraviolet light rays also are used to kill bacteria. The direct rays of the sun are known to kill bacteria, and lights now are being made that produce the same rays and they can be used to treat infected wounds and to kill bacteria in the air of operating rooms. These questions are discussed more fully in Chapter 3

INFLAMMATION

By *inflammation* we mean the reaction of the body tissues to an injury. The reactions may be rapid in appearance, producing marked and significant signs and symptoms that often require early surgical intervention. Such an inflammation is spoken of as *acute;* for example, a sudden inflammation of the appendix is spoken of as acute appendicitis. When the tissue reaction is insidious and continues over a long period of time, the inflammation is said to be *chronic.*

The Injuring Agent. This may be any one of several kinds. Physical agents, such as a blow, or even a surgeon's sterile knife, excite a typical inflammation. Chemicals, especially acids and caustic alkalies, electricity, heat and cold—all cause reactions when they are applied to body tissues. Bacteria are by far the most common and the most serious of the injuring agents; they invade and become a secondary factor in a large majority of inflammations that may have been begun by physical, chemical or thermal causes.

Tissue Reactions

Minute Pathology of Inflammation. Each of the agents just mentioned produces an injury or trauma to tissues that excites a tissue reaction that differs only in degree.

Local Symptoms of Inflammation. Perhaps the simplest kind of inflammation may be found in an injury inflicted by the sterile knife of a surgeon. However sharp the knife, millions of tiny cells are damaged, blood vessels are cut, and lymphatics are crushed. Even if the wound is sutured accurately, the tissues show their resentment by progressing through all the stages of a mild inflammation. In a very short time the edges of the wound will be found to be redder than the surrounding skin, and the tissues will feel somewhat more tense and slightly warmer near the wound. The area about the wound will appear to be somewhat raised, it will be painful, and movement of the cut tissues will increase the pain. From these observations we discover the *cardinal signs of an inflammation:* redness, swelling, heat, pain and loss of function.

Blood Supply. In order to understand the cause of the appearance of these signs, we must examine these tissues microscopically. The first reaction of the injured tissues is to increase their blood supply. The capillaries and the veins dilate widely, and the blood, flowing rapidly at first, slows gradually because it is flowing from a smaller to a larger area. This increase in the blood supply accounts for the redness and the heat associated with an inflammation.

As the capillaries dilate, their walls become permeable, so that serum and white blood cells—and red blood cells to a lesser degree—escape into the surrounding tissues. This increase of fluid and blood cells extending into the tissues accounts for the swelling observed above, and, by causing pressure on the delicate nerve endings, pain is produced.

If the wound is sterile, the inflammation goes no farther. The white blood corpuscles, called leukocytes, having the power of independent movement, seek out and literally devour all fragments of dead cells, while the serum is being reabsorbed into the blood vessels and the lymphatics. Soon the wound edges are united by delicate long cells (fibroblasts) that are the forerunners of the strong fibrous network called connective tissue. The hemorrhage is absorbed, and the superficial layers of cells bridge the gap to close the wound. Such healing is called *healing by primary union, per primam* or *by first intention.* Every surgeon strives for this type of union. When primary union does not take place because of infection or loss of tissue for any reason, healing occurs by *secondary intention* or by *granulation* (discussed in detail on page 20).

Acute Inflammation. Most forms of acute inflammation with which we deal surgically are caused by bacteria. The reaction of the tissues to these minute organisms is of the same character as described above but to a more marked degree. The bacteria that make their way into the tissues find food, moisture and warmth—an environment in which they can multiply very rapidly. Substances toxic to the tissues about them are formed, and an inflammation occurs. The increased blood supply produces a redness and an increased temperature of the tissues for some distance about the area of infection, and the fluid that leaks out of the dilated capillaries causes a swelling. This hot area of red, swollen tissue about an area of inflammation is called a *cellulitis.* The white blood cells reaching the area attempt to devour and kill the offending organisms. The blood serum that has escaped contains antitoxins and other immune substances that are believed to make the bacterial toxins harmless and inert or to make the bacteria more easily digested by the phagocytes. If these defensive measures are sufficient, the bacteria are killed and the inflammation subsides. However, more often the rapidly forming toxins are too much at

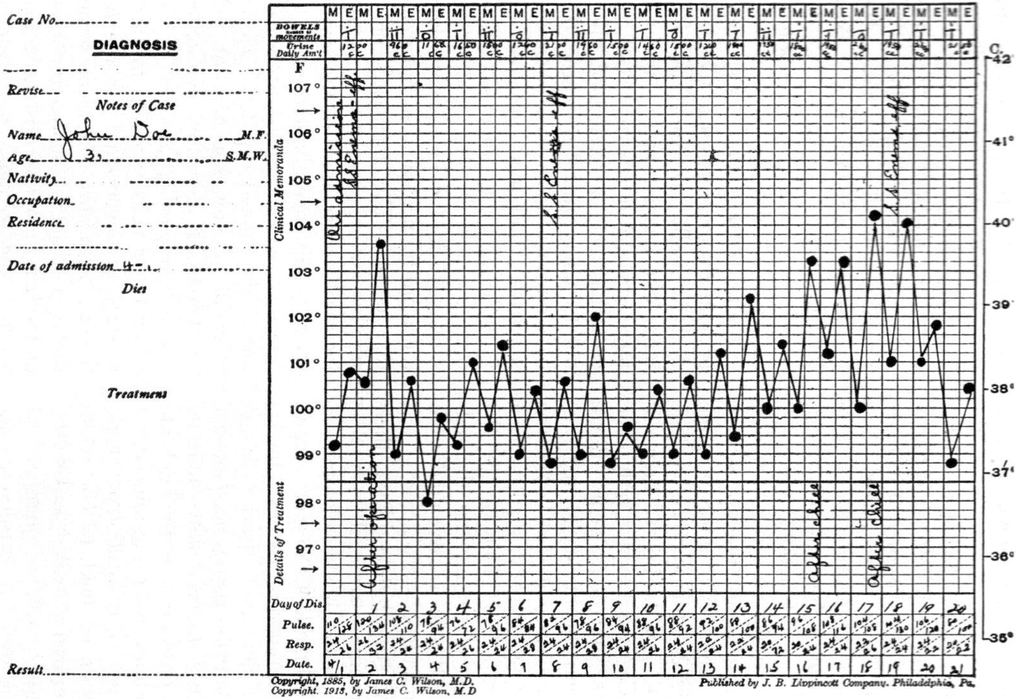

FIG. 5. Illustrates another type of clinical chart of the same character case; i.e., a septic one due to peritonitis. Note that on this chart only 1 A.M. and 1 P.M. graphic record is made of the temperature; the pulse and the respiration are noted below.

first for the early defense measures with the result that many white blood cells are killed, along with the cells of the tissue in which the inflammation is taking place. These dead leukocytes and tissue cells and dead and living bacteria, with the blood and tissue fluids round them, form what is called *pus*. As a result of the action of bacterial toxins, tissue cells are killed. These cells lose their characteristics and separate from the living tissue, becoming a yellow mass of soft dead tissue called *slough*. Through the action of enzymes the dead tissue undergoes a gradual liquefaction. This process is called *necrosis*, and the tissue is said to be *necrotic*.

Round this area of dead cells the body attempts to build a protective wall composed of tissue and white blood cells, firmly packed together by the coagulation of the blood and tissue fluids about them. When pus is enclosed by such a wall, an *abscess* is formed. The abscess, which at first is small, grows larger gradually and advances in the direction in which there is the least resistance to its progress.

If the abscess approaches the skin, its outer wall grows weaker because the pressure of the abscess closes the tiny capillaries that bring the cells to strengthen it. The weakest point appears often as a small, raised yellow dot on the skin surface, and the abscess then is said to "point" or to "come to a head." As these skin cells die and disintegrate, the pressure inside the abscess pushes them out and they are followed by the pus from its cavity. Often the surgeon must aid nature, save many cells from death and relieve the patient of much pain and discomfort by making an incision in the abscess wall and allowing the pus to escape.

SYMPTOMS OF ACUTE INFLAMMATION. These usually are constitutional as well as local. We have already mentioned the local symptoms (redness, swelling, heat, pain and loss of function), and an effort was made to correlate them with the tissue reactions that caused them.

The Constitutional Symptoms. These are caused by the absorption of toxic substances by the blood from the inflamed area. Their severity depends upon the amount and the degree of toxicity of the absorbed substances. Some bacteria—for example, streptococci—form pus that is much more toxic than other varieties.

The usual symptoms are fever, increase in pulse and respiratory rates, headache and general malaise, hot dry skin, flushed cheeks, loss of appetite, thirst, coated tongue, constipation and highly colored, scanty urine. When the toxic absorption is rapid, there may be chills, followed by sweating, and even delirium. An examination of the blood usually shows an increase in the number of white cells (leukocytes), and there is said to be *leukocytosis*.

When the inflammation is mild or when the resistance of the individual is low, the leukocyte count may have changed little. Hence, we may regard the variation of the number of white cells in the blood as somewhat of an indication of the patient's natural resistance to disease and of the severity of the inflammation. There are some inflammations, one of which is due to the tubercle bacillus, that cause a lowering of the number of leukocytes and produce a *leukopenia*.

The constitutional symptoms of an inflammation may be much more marked in children than in adults. Besides the symptoms mentioned above, nausea and vomiting are frequent, even with moderately severe inflammation. The child often may show distressing nervous symptoms, such as convulsions or delirium. These reactions are not so pronounced in the aged. The patient does not complain very much, often he is listless and indifferent, the temperature is lower, the pulse has increased only slightly, and the leukocyte count is lower or shows no increase. Frequently he will not swallow even water, and often he is incontinent. The whole picture is that of an acutely sick patient apparently without acute symptoms.

Reparative Processes

Healing by First Intention. Wounds made aseptically and with a minimum of tissue destruction heal with very little tissue reaction "by first intention."

Healing by Granulation. In cases in which pus formation (suppuration) has occurred, the process of repair is less simple and delayed longer. When an abscess is incised, it collapses partly, but the dead and the dying cells forming its walls are still being thrown out into the cavity. For this reason rubber tubes, rubber tissue or gauze packing often is inserted into the abscess pocket to allow the pus to escape easily. Gradually the necrotic material disintegrates and escapes, and the abscess cavity fills with a red, soft, insensitive tissue that bleeds very easily. It is composed of minute thin-walled capillaries, growing off from the parent vessels, each bud surrounded by cells that later form connective tissue. These buds, called granulations, enlarge until they fill the area of the tissue destroyed. The cells surrounding the capillaries change their round shape; they become long and thin, intertwining with each other to form a *scar or cicatrix*. Healing is complete when skin cells (epithelium) grow over these granulations. This method of repair is called *healing by granulation,* and it takes place whenever pus is formed or when loss of tissue has occurred for any reason.

Complications

The body makes every effort to localize an inflammation and to prevent the absorption of its toxic products. When the patient is in good physical condition, his natural powers to resist inflammation are great. His blood rapidly supplies increasing numbers of vigorous leukocytes, immune substances are added quickly to those present naturally in his blood, and the protective wall forms fast and strong about the area of inflammation.

Occasionally, the defensive measures are inadequate to cope with the virulent organism causing the inflammation. The process of walling-off is incomplete or the formation of immune substances is slow, with a consequent absorption into the blood of a large amount of very poisonous products.

Toxemia, Septicemia and Pyemia. If only the toxins are absorbed, the condition is called a *toxemia*. When the bacteria and their toxins are absorbed into the blood, we have a *septicemia* and, if pus is discharged into the blood stream, a *pyemia* has occurred. Such complications are often called *blood poisoning*.

These conditions are somewhat similar in their symptoms. There is an increasing severity of the constitutional symptoms, associated with an inflammation. To these are added chills, sweats, a temperature that shows abrupt rises and rapid falls once or oftener daily, a very rapid pulse and a very high leukocyte count. A toxic delirium often occurs.

When a smear of the white cells is examined under the microscope, it is noted often that some of the cells are immature. This is the result of the action of the toxic substances upon the bone marrow. Frequently, the severity of the toxemia may be judged by noting the number of immature leukocytes in relation to the number of mature cells. When the number of immature cells is high, the infection is severe and the prognosis is more grave. This method of estimation is called the Schilling count.

In septicemia, and especially in pyemia, the bacteria floating in the blood stream lodge often at points far distant from the original inflammation and there set up secondary or metastatic abscesses.

Chronic Inflammation. This differs from an acute inflammation in that the injuring agent is weak, but its action continues over a long period of time. Consequently, the reaction of the tissues is less, and the cardinal symptoms of an inflammation may be hard to demonstrate. Swelling usually is present, pain often is moderate or slight, redness usually is indistinct, and heat may be absent. The process may go on to pus formation. The most common organisms causing chronic inflammation are those of tuberculosis and syphilis. The treatment indicated is that for acute inflammation plus the specific measures for the diseases mentioned. Chronic diseases usually require prolonged care.

Principles of Nursing Care of a Local Inflammation

The nursing care of a local inflammation consists of the following: (1) rest of the inflamed part, (2) elevation of it and (3) the application of heat or cold.

These measures all are directed toward the relief of the local pain and the hastening of the termination of the inflammation.

Often it may be necessary to add to the above (4) incision and drainage of the inflamed area, which procedure is a duty of the surgeon.

Rest of the Inflamed Part

Rest of the inflamed part is indicated for two reasons: first, because it allows all the forces of nature to be directed to combating the inflammation, which tends to hasten the walling-off process and thereby lessen the absorption of toxin; second, because any movement of the inflamed part is painful to the patient. The painful smile of the patient with cracked lips is a common example of the discomfort caused by even a slight movement in the case of a mild inflammation. The delayed healing of a wound over a finger joint is an illustration of how movement hinders the delicate healing processes. To ensure absolute rest, splints, bandages, plaster casts or plaster

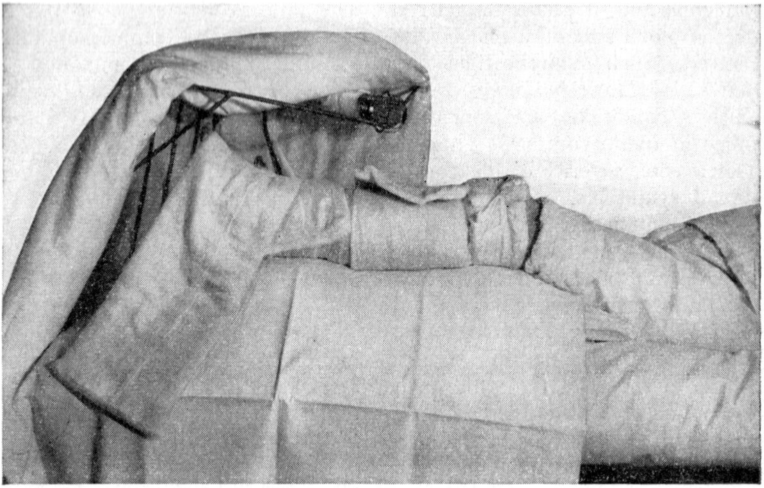

FIG. 6 A. Application of hot moist dressings to lower extremity. The leg is elevated, and the entire foot and leg are swathed in gauze compresses, lint or commercial pads in 3-foot lengths. A folded pad is tied round the upper part of the dressing to prevent leakage of the solution.

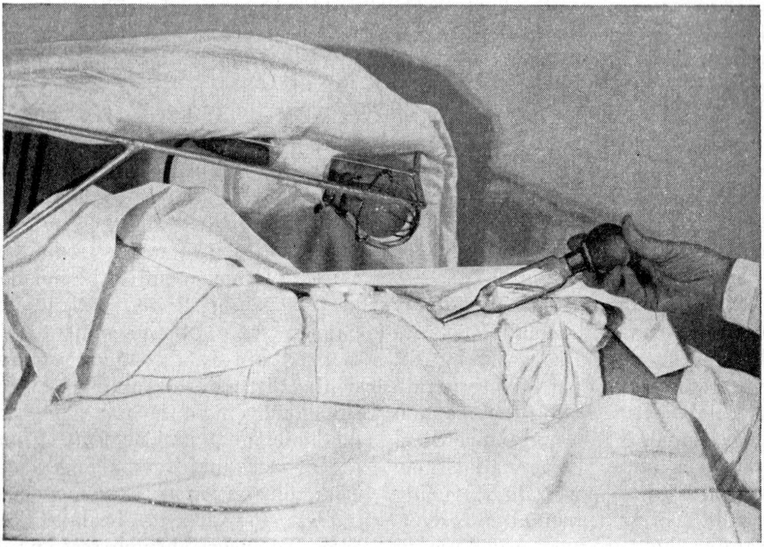

FIG. 6 B. The compresses are moistened with warm solution.

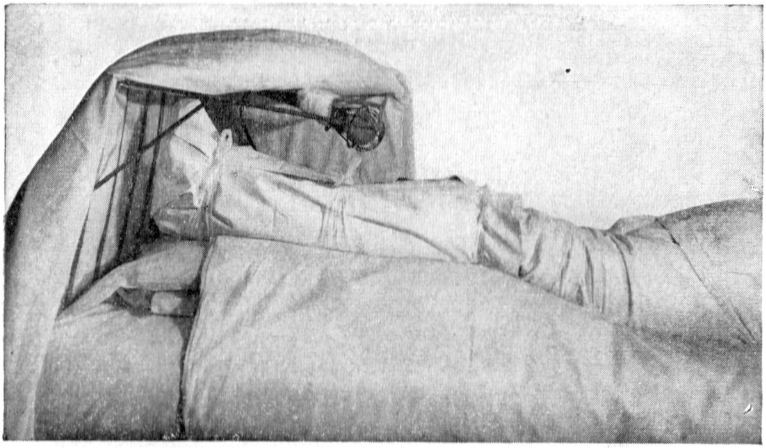

FIG. 6 C. The entire leg then is enclosed in a light mackintosh, oiled silk, waxed paper or Pliofilm. This waterproof dressing should be held in place by bandage ties. If it is desired to apply heat externally by hot-water bottles or an electric pad, these are placed outside the mackintosh and are held in position by pinning a towel round them. Note elevation of the extremity with protection of bed and pillows by a mackintosh covered with a sheet. Heat is applied in this case by a guarded electric light attached to the bed cradle.

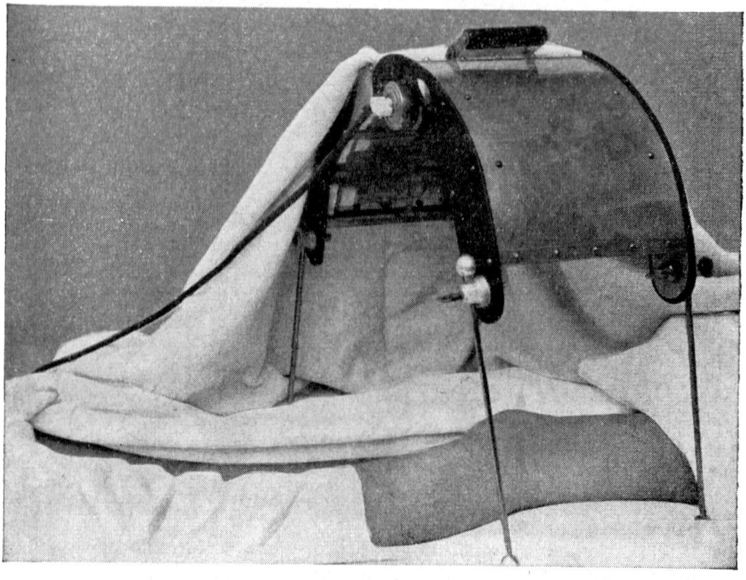

FIG. 7. Dry heat being applied in traumatic arthritis of the knee. Position for heat cabinet.

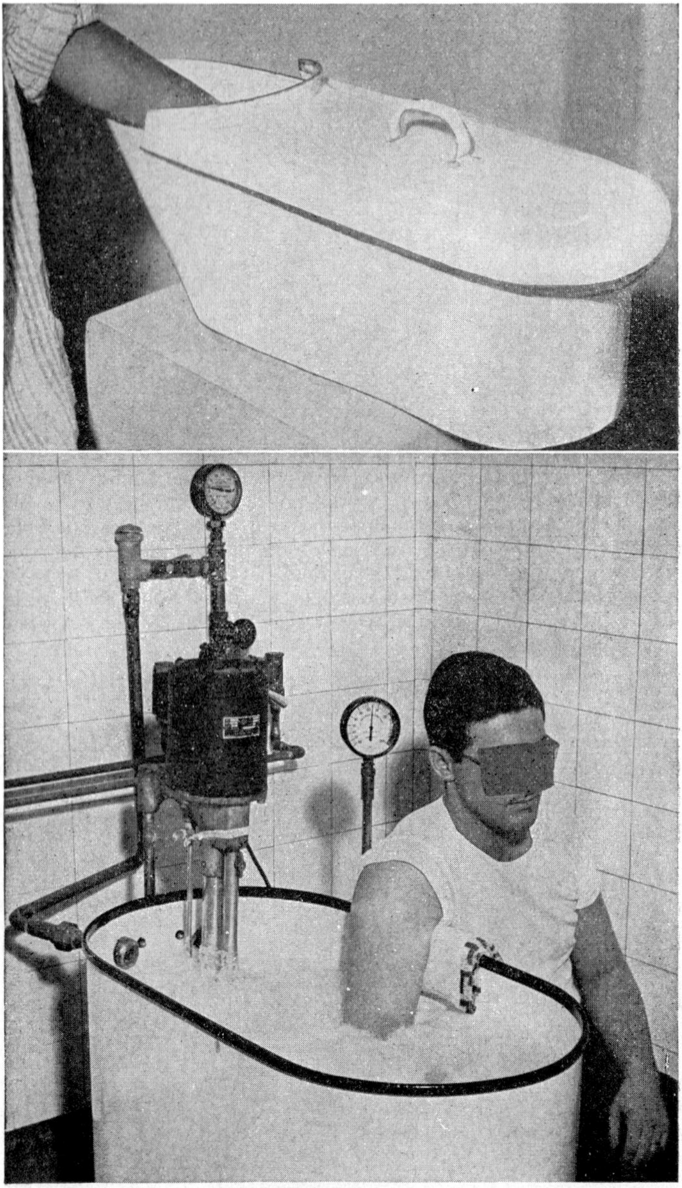

FIG. 8. Methods of application of heat to the extremity. (*Top*) Arm baths are used for treatment of inflammation in the hand and the arm. (*Bottom*) Whirlpool baths may be used for both extremities. *Note:* The temperature of the fluid in the bath never should be more than 110° F.

splints are applied when possible. In inflammations of the head, the trunk and the lower extremities, rest in bed often is a necessity.

Elevation of the Inflamed Part

Elevation of the inflamed part is one of the procedures for which the patient will be most grateful. In this manner the throbbing pain and the swelling may be relieved greatly; the force of gravity helps to drain the engorged blood vessels and tissue spaces and at the same time permits an increased arterial circulation that brings new forces in greater numbers to combat the inflammation. The almost immediate relief obtained by elevation of the hand in cases of fingertip infection is a familiar example of this.

This procedure cannot be practiced when the inflammation is of the chest or the abdomen, but it can be used to advantage in inflammation of the head, the neck and the extremities The degree of elevation (above the heart level) will vary according to the site of the inflammation. In cases of the extremities, it is better to elevate the whole part. Thus, in elevating the arm, the hand should be higher than the elbow and the elbow higher than the shoulder. The same would apply to the leg.

Elevation can be accomplished best by pillows when the patient is in bed or by a sling when the patient is ambulatory. The pillows should be protected with rubber or plastic pillowcases or sheeting and should support the extremities completely. The areas which do not come in contact with the pillow—for example, the knee joint—can be made more comfortable by placing small pillows or cotton pads underneath them. A bed cradle should be used to relieve pressure of the bedclothes on the elevated part.

Application of Heat

Very frequently applications of heat are valuable aids in the treatment of surgical diseases. The heat causes a local hyperemia (increased blood supply), a function that may be used to advantage in the treatment of inflammation, especially after the stage of extravasation of cells and serum has taken place. Heat often relaxes the spasm of involuntary muscle, especially that occurring in cases of renal, biliary or intestinal colic.

Pain often is completely relieved by heat applications, especially in cases of acute infective inflammations and in the later stages of many traumatic conditions. However, at times heat actually increases the amount of pain. In such cases cold applications usually give some measure of relief.

Heat may be applied in the dry or the moist form.

DRY HEAT

Dry heat may be applied in the following ways:

Hot-water Bottle. This probably is the form in most common use by the laity. The bottle always should be covered with a layer of flannel cloth before being applied to skin surfaces, and the temperature never should exceed 130° F. Heat may be applied in this manner (1) to relieve "deep" pain; (2) to supply heat when the temperature of the patient becomes subnormal in cases of shock and hemorrhage and after operations;

and (3) to retain heat in various forms of moist dressings. Special care is necessary to prevent burns from hot-water bottles when they are used to supply heat to unconscious patients, those under treatment for shock or those still under the effect of an anesthetic.

Electric Pad. This appliance is a source of great comfort to patients when heat is to be applied over large surfaces for a long time. The pad should not be allowed to get wet, because of the danger of causing a short circuit. Therefore, unless it is covered with rubber or very well protected by oiled silk or waxed paper, the electric pad should not be used with moist dressings.

Bake Oven. This apparatus is made in many shapes and sizes adaptable for the application of heat to various parts of the body. The heat usually is generated by electric-light bulbs. The part to be baked is wrapped well in cotton or flannel to prevent blistering. This method of heat application is useful in the treatment of the more chronic inflammation of bones and joints—for example, arthritis, after fractures and bursitis. (Fig. 7, p. 23.)

The chief hazard associated with the application of dry heat is the danger of burning the patient. For this reason the nurse should keep under observation the area to which the heat is being applied, and at the first signs of burning—pain to the patient or marked redness of the part—the application must be discontinued. The pain sense in extremely ill, toxic, shocked or aged patients often is markedly dull, so that these patients, and also those who are unconscious, must be watched with extreme care.

Diathermy. Heat may be induced in the tissues by the passage through them of high-frequency electric currents. The resistance offered by the tissues to the passage of the current generates heat in the same way that the filament of a light bulb becomes hot when the electricity is turned on. The current is applied to the part to be treated through two metal electrodes fixed firmly in place. Usually either the electrodes or the skin is moistened to give a better contact to the skin surface. The amount of heat generated in the tissues is regulated by the amount of current used, and the greatest intensity of heat is in the area between the electrodes, through which the current passes. By this method of application, heat may be induced deep in the tissues and directly at the site of the lesion to be treated. Diathermy is valuable especially in the treatment of traumatic inflammations of soft tissues, such as sprains and bruises, and of low-grade or chronic inflammations of muscles, joints and bursae.

Electric Warmers with Controlled Circulation of Warm Air. Electric warmers made to furnish controlled circulation of warm air are available. These are very convenient for drying plaster-of-Paris casts, for warming beds for shocked patients and for taking the place of hot-water bottles and heat lamps in other treatments.

MOIST HEAT

Moist heat probably is the most valuable application that can be made to an acute inflammation, especially inflammation at or near the skin surface. Other uses of moist heat are indicated below with descriptions of the various methods of application.

Hot Compresses–Hot Wet Dressings. These dressings may be applied by frequent changing of gauze compresses wrung out of hot solutions, or by application of hot solutions to dressings already bandaged to a part. The solutions in common use are physiologic salt solution and antiseptic solutions (such as boric acid) or hypertonic salt solutions (such as saturated magnesium sulfate solution or Wright's solution).

These dressings are most comforting to the patient suffering from superficial infective or traumatic inflammations—for example, hand and finger infections, burns and sprains. In the case of a hot solution, especially when the compress is bandaged in place, care should be taken that the solution is not too hot. If there is no thermometer at hand, the nurse should draw the solution into a dressing syringe and expel a little on the back of her hand or arm to test its temperature before she applies it slowly to the dressings. (See Fig. 6 A, B and C.)

The moisture will be retained if the dressings are covered with waxed paper, thin rubber, heavy toweling or oiled silk. The heat can be kept fairly constant if hot-water bottles are applied; however, the weight of the hot-water bottles should be considered in placing them. A much more constant heat can be applied by the use of rubber-covered electric pads. A cradle with electric lights also may be placed over the dressings to keep a constant elevated temperature about the part (Fig. 6 B). If the solution is used from about 105° to 110° F. and the hot-water bottles from 115° to 120° F., there is little chance of burning the patient. Because moist heat burns more readily than dry heat, the area should be inspected frequently.

The nurse should not forget that hot solutions applied to compresses on a bandaged part are more likely to burn the patient than when applied to the open skin because of the fact that evaporation cannot take place and cool the dressings. Therefore, extreme care should be taken that burning does not occur. This is especially important in treating aged and debilitated or paralyzed patients. Excessive heat in extremities with disturbed metabolism, such as exists in arteriosclerosis or diabetic gangrene, does more harm than good. Moist heat in the form of hot baths is frequently used in the treatment of infections of the hands and the feet.

Douches. The application of heat by a current of warm solution is a valuable method of treatment in inflammations of the ear, the vagina and the pelvis. The solutions should be as warm as the patient can tolerate with comfort. Those employed most commonly are saline for the ear and various other antiseptic solutions for the vagina.

Baths. SITZ BATH. The patient sits for from 15 to 20 minutes in a bath of water heated to a temperature of from 105° to 110° F. There should be just enough water to cover the patient's hips. The bath is useful for treating acute pelvic inflammatory disease and for producing relaxation of the bladder sphincters in cases of urinary retention. It may be tried at times as a means of producing sufficient relaxation to permit the reduction of a strangulated hernia. It is of special value in the postoperative treatment of lesions about the anus and the perineum, such as hemorrhoids, fissure in ano and ischiorectal abscess.

WARM BATHS FOR PARTS OF THE BODY often are indicated in the treatment of acute infections, sprains and severely traumatized wounds when there is a threat of sloughing. The part is placed in the solution at the ordered temperature—usually as warm as the patient can stand comfortably—and is kept there the specified length of time. If there is an open wound, the basin and the solution should be sterile. The temperature of the solution must be kept constant by adding warmer solution as necessary, but this must be done with care to avoid burning (Fig. 8).

WARM BATH, ENTIRE BODY. The body is submerged in a tub of warm solution, preferably physiologic saline solution at from 95° to 100° F. This is useful in cases of severe superficial burns.

The Application of Cold

Cold is used in the treatment of recent inflammations. It causes a constriction of the vessels in the inflamed zone. This results in a lessening of serum and cellular leakage into the tissues. There is also an inhibition of bacterial growth. If the application is continued for a sufficient time, a paralysis of the vessels occurs, so that, when the cold is removed, it increases the hyperemia. The result, therefore, is an inhibition of the inflammatory process. In addition, cold causes a sensation of comfort to an inflamed part and, if continued, produces an anesthesia of the skin.

DRY COLD

Icebags. Dry cold is applied best in the form of icebags (rubberized bags filled with cracked ice). These are made in several forms for ease of application to different parts of the body. Care should be taken that the cap is watertight, and a layer of fabric should be interposed between the skin and the icebag to prevent too great cooling of the skin.

MOIST COLD

Moist cold is used most logically in the treatment of recent traumatic inflammation.

Moist Cold Compresses. These may be applied best in the form of moist compresses wet with saline or boric acid solution. The solutions are kept cool by placing the vessel containing them in a basin of ice and water or by placing the compresses on a block of ice. The compresses require changing every 3 or 4 minutes, and they should not be applied for more than 10 minutes at a time. If bluish discoloration of the skin appears, the compresses should be discontinued, and the circulation stimulated by rubbing.

Cold compresses are especially useful in the prevention of swelling and inflammation after operations on the eye, and in the treatment of other traumatic inflammation—for example, sprains, bruises and contusions.

Refrigeration. This means the chilling of tissues. It is not freezing. Freezing damages tissues; refrigeration does not. Water freezes at 32° F. Blood and tissues freeze at a slightly lower level. Refrigerating a limb with cracked-ice packs lowers the temperature to between 0.5° and 5° above freezing. Mechanically, this can be controlled with a margin of safety. This procedure is being used on extremities for complete operative anesthesia.

Therapeutically, refrigeration is of great value in the treatment of severe infections, including *Bacillus welchii* (*Clostridium welchii*), and of severe crushes. It is used also as a palliative procedure when pain is an enervating factor. It can be applied safely for days. (For technic, see Chap. 5, Anesthesia, p. 79.)

Evaporating Lotions. Evaporating lotions are of special value in the treatment of sprains and other injuries of joints. Several layers of gauze are bandaged to the part and kept moist with solution. Evaporation is allowed to take place; therefore, no effort should be made to cover the dressing with waxed paper or oiled silk.

Solutions of normal salt, boric acid, epsom salts (1 tablespoonful to a pint of water) and alcohol (50 per cent) are in common use.

Dangers

Tissue below par, due to poor blood supply from arteriosclerosis, diabetes, trauma and senility, does not tolerate either prolonged or excessive heat or cold. Any increase in discomfort or extreme color change should be reported at once.

Incision and Drainage

Incision and drainage always are necessary when the inflammation has gone on to pus formation. It is of advantage also in certain inflammations, even before suppuration has occurred. By the relief of tension and the reduction of tissue swelling the pain is relieved, and tissue destruction is decreased.

Principles of Nursing Care of a General Inflammation

The nursing care of a general inflammation often is as important as the measures used locally. This consists of: constitutional rest (of heart, lungs, alimentary tract and the mind); promoting elimination (encouraging the intake of fluids and giving laxatives); increasing the patient's resistance (by sera, antitoxins, vaccines, transfusions, chemotherapy and antibiotics); and the relief of pain.

Constitutional Rest

Rest of Heart and Lungs. Constitutional rest is imperative in most inflammations of more than a mild nature, and this is especially the case in inflammations of the abdominal organs. By keeping the patient in bed, the least possible strain is placed upon the heart and the lungs, and all the body activities may be turned toward overcoming the inflammation. In desperate cases, a daily bath often is too exhausting.

Rest of the Alimentary Tract. The diet usually should be soft or liquid and easily assimilated. Milk, fruit juices, broths and so forth may be given while fever is present, and soft foods (eggs, milk toast, junket, chicken, baked potatoes and so forth) may be added as the temperature decreases.

Mental Rest. Finally, it should not

be forgotten that rest of the mind, as well as of the body, is necessary. Every effort should be made to prevent undue disturbance and mental anxiety in a patient who is very ill.

Promoting Elimination

Administration of Fluids. The elimination of the toxic materials absorbed during the course of an inflammation is largely the function of the kidney. This organ often shows the effects of this work in the form of a nephritis. It is believed that we can dilute the circulating toxins, lessen their effect upon the kidneys and increase their elimination by administering fluids to the patient. Fluids may be given in any form by mouth in all cases of inflammation, except those involving the abdominal organs, when often it is best to give the fluid by rectum, under the skin or by vein. In order to increase elimination via the urine, the patient should receive between 3,000 and 5,000 cc. of fluid daily.

Laxatives may be of use in the early stages of inflammations, except those of the abdomen. This treatment overcomes the constipation and promotes elimination by the bowel. Enemas may be used thereafter.

Increasing the Patient's Resistance

Body Defense Forces. Every measure employed in the treatment of an inflammation is, or should be, simply an effort to aid nature. Some inflammations could be cared for by body defense forces with no treatment at all; others are combated with more difficulty. A great deal can be known about the severity of the inflammation if we identify the infecting organism. This can be done easily by culture, by staining smears and by the symptoms which they produce. Thus, when a patient develops stiffness of the jaw several days after a rusty nail has punctured his foot, we recognize the tetanus organism by its symptoms. Or, if we culture the blood in a septicemia, we can identify the infecting bacteria as a staphylococcus or a streptococcus. Knowing the organism, we know whether the body needs aid in combating the infection, because we know the usual course of that disease. So we know that inflammations caused by the tetanus bacillus are nearly always fatal, and that those caused by the streptococcus of erysipelas produce an intense toxemia that often leads to death.

Conferred Immunity. We are fortunate in the knowledge that present-day science has given us ways of combating these infections. We can supply immune substances in the form of antitoxins and antisera until the body is able to develop an immunity. Thus, we give tetanus antitoxin to patients with tetanus.

The earlier these sera are given in the course of the disease, the more beneficial they are. Knowing this, we often try to steal a march on certain diseases. Thus, tetanus antitoxin is given to every patient who has received a contaminated wound, because we know that *Clostridium tetani*, the tetanus bacillus, often infects such wounds. This treatment has reduced the incidence of tetanus to a comparatively few cases and, when it does develop, usually it is of very moderate severity. Such measures used to anticipate infection and prevent disease are called *prophylaxis*.

Induced Immunity. By the hypodermic injection of toxins which have been treated to reduce the toxic effects, the body may be forced to develop an active immunity. This is used most commonly in the prevention of tetanus. An injection of the combination of attenuated toxin and antitoxin toxoid is made on 3 occasions in increasing doses. The toxin and the antitoxin induce in the patient gradually increasing immunity to tetanus. Immunity may be elevated further by the injection of a small "booster" dose if a wound occurs in which tetanus may be a contaminating organism. This method of preventing tetanus was used during World War II so successfully that even though many of the wounds were wide and deep, the appearance of tetanus was relatively rare.

Chemotherapy–Antibiotic Therapy. We have at our command, in addition to the various defense mechanisms of the body, a group of sulfanilamide drugs which have proved to be of value in the treatment of infection. These drugs, frequently called the sulfa drugs, are used perhaps less frequently since the appearance of antibiotics but they still offer considerable help in the treatment of infection.

The antibiotics are a group of drugs which have been developed during and since World War II. They are powerful bactericidal agents producing rapid results which are much superior to those that are obtained by any other form of treatment. These drugs will be discussed fully in the following chapter.

Relief of Pain

Sedatives often are necessary to relieve the pain associated with an inflammation. The salicylates and other coal-tar drugs frequently are adequate, but for pain that cannot be relieved otherwise, to quiet the patient and to allow sleep, morphine, Dilaudid or Demerol should be used. Since opium so easily becomes an addiction, it is best to withhold it until other measures are given a fair trial. However, its benefits far outweigh its disadvantages, and a suffering patient is most grateful for its effects.

CHAPTER THREE

Antisepsis and Asepsis

DEVELOPMENT OF ANTISEPSIS
DEVELOPMENT OF ASEPSIS
PRINCIPLES OF ASEPTIC SURGERY
METHODS OF STERILIZATION
CHEMOTHERAPY
ANTIBIOTICS

DEVELOPMENT OF ANTISEPSIS

Surgery as practiced up to the nineteenth century was a discouraging and distressing branch of medicine. Pus formed in a majority of all open wounds, whether accidental or as a result of operation. Many patients developed more serious complications, such as septicemia (blood poisoning), hemorrhage and gangrene. As a consequence, amputations were frequent, prolonged illness with crippling disability often resulted and, only too often, death occurred.

The first advance toward the present-day practice of surgery was made by a chemist, Louis Pasteur. In 1857, while studying the phenomena of fermentation, he demonstrated the presence and the activity of micro-organisms or bacteria. Later, he showed that "putrefaction was a fermentation caused by the growth of microbes." These organisms, he found, were killed by heat, and putrefaction could be avoided by preventing further entrance of the germs, the present-day concept of prophylaxis in surgery.

A short time later, an English surgeon, Joseph Lister, directed his attention to Pasteur's work. He attempted first to prevent putrefaction and pus formation in wounds infected with microbes by destroying the germs with carbolic acid, a solution of which, he had found, would kill bacteria. Later, he developed an elaborate technic for operation on clean wounds, with the carbolization of the patient's skin and wound, the surgeon's hands and all the materials used at the operation. He even attempted to destroy the germs in the surrounding air by the use of a carbolic acid spray.

DEVELOPMENT OF ASEPSIS

Surgery has made great strides since Lister's time. The principles that he laid down are still adhered to, but with fuller knowledge and added experience his methods have been modified. It is known now that the materials used in the treatment of wounds may be freed from living organisms by heat, thus largely replacing chemical sterilization. It has been found unnecessary to attempt to rid the air of bacteria because, when germs are excluded from entrance to the wound by other paths, healing occurs usually without infection. Experience has shown that tissues have a natural power of self-protection against the action of bacteria. This power is lessened markedly by the application of strong antiseptics but, in most cases of clean wounds, is sufficient in itself to kill organisms that gain entrance to the wound during an operation.

For these reasons, surgical procedures have been changed largely from the *antiseptic* (against putrefaction) methods of Lister to the *aseptic* (without infection) technic of today. An effort is made to operate without any initial entrance of bacteria into the wounds. This object is gained by *sterilizing* (killing the bacteria in) all materials used in the operation.

PRINCIPLES OF ASEPTIC SURGERY

"The successful practice of aseptic surgery requires a strict observance of preoperative sterilization of surgical materials, of rigid precautions against infection during the course of the operation, and of guarding the wound from infection afterwards until such time as it is healed."

Preoperative Treatment. This comprises sterilizing and keeping sterile (free from micro-organisms) all surgical materials that are to come in contact with the wound and exposed tissues or that are to be handled by the surgeon or his assistants. These include all instruments, needles, sutures, dressings, gloves, covers and so forth. In addition, the surgeon and his assistants and nurses must prepare themselves before touching any of these materials. While their hands and arms cannot be rendered absolutely sterile, they must be made as clean as possible by the use of soap, water and chemicals, and then covered with sterile rubber gloves. A cap is used to cover the head and enclose the hair. Masks covering the nose and the mouth are employed to prevent bacteria from the upper respiratory system from entering the wound. A long-sleeved sterile gown must be worn over the clothing. The patient's skin, over an area considerably larger than that requiring exposure during the course of operation, also demands the highest possible degree of cleanliness and the application of some chemical agent. The rest of the patient's body is covered with sterile drapes.

During Operation. During the operation neither the surgeon nor his sterile nurses or assistants touch anything that has not been rendered and kept sterile. Nonsterile assistants refrain from touching or infecting anything that is sterile.

After Operation. After the operation the wound is protected from possible infection by means of sterile dressings and by an occasional sterilization of the surrounding skin with chemical agents. Particular care is taken to prevent contact of anything that is not sterile with the unhealed wound. In most cases not previously infected, this aseptic regimen is all that is necessary to ensure rapid aseptic healing. In recently infected wounds, it is necessary to remove and destroy such micro-organisms as are already in the tissues, and also to prevent subsequent infection from without. The first condition is effected by the removal of foreign bodies and devitalized tissues from the wounds (*débridement*). The second condition is fulfilled by the use of a rigid aseptic technic during the course of the treatment.

When infection already has developed in the tissues, the chief indication is to help the body to eliminate the organisms by incision and prevent the entrance of further infection from without.

It must be recognized then that, although the surgical technic of today is said to be aseptic, there are still many uses for chemical disinfection in the treatment of infected, and even of aseptic, wounds.

METHODS OF STERILIZATION AND DISINFECTION

Knowledge of the general methods of sterilization is necessary in the intelligent nursing of surgical cases. It will be well to define some of the terms used generally in this connection:

Sterilization, in surgery, means the destruction of all organisms, including spores.

Disinfection is the act of destroying all non-spore-bearing pathogenic organisms, i.e., those responsible for the communicable diseases. This method would be applicable for the disinfection of clothing, bedding, bedpans and so forth.

Disinfectants are agents, usually a chemical, that destroy disease-producing organisms.

Antiseptics are agents that prevent the growth of micro-organisms without necessarily destroying them.

Germicides or **bactericides** are agents that kill micro-organisms.

Deodorizers or deodorants are agents employed to destroy or prevent offensive odors.

Mechanical Disinfection

When a physician or a nurse "scrubs" or prepares the skin of the operative site, it is an effort to cleanse mechanically the skin surfaces that may be exposed during the operation. This means removal of the surface dirt and fat and the organisms that are found normally on the skin. This usually is accomplished by the use of warm water and a soap that produces an abundant lather. Some surgeons prefer soaps containing antiseptics that appear to be more efficient in reducing the bacterial habitants of the skin surface. Others use detergents containing antiseptics for the same purpose.

A further method of mechanical disinfection is utilized in recently infected traumatic wounds. Under sterile conditions an effort is made to cut away all the devitalized tissue, so as to remove foreign materials and contaminating bacteria. This procedure is known as *débridement.*

Sterilization

The methods of sterilization are physical and chemical. Physical sterilization can be subdivided further into (1) thermal and (2) radiant energy.

Physical Methods of Sterilization—Heat

Sterilization by heat applied to surgical materials ensures the destruction of micro-organisms and their spores. It is the method to be chosen for all materials, except those that suffer damage from repeated exposure to heat. Before subjecting a material to sterilization by heat, it

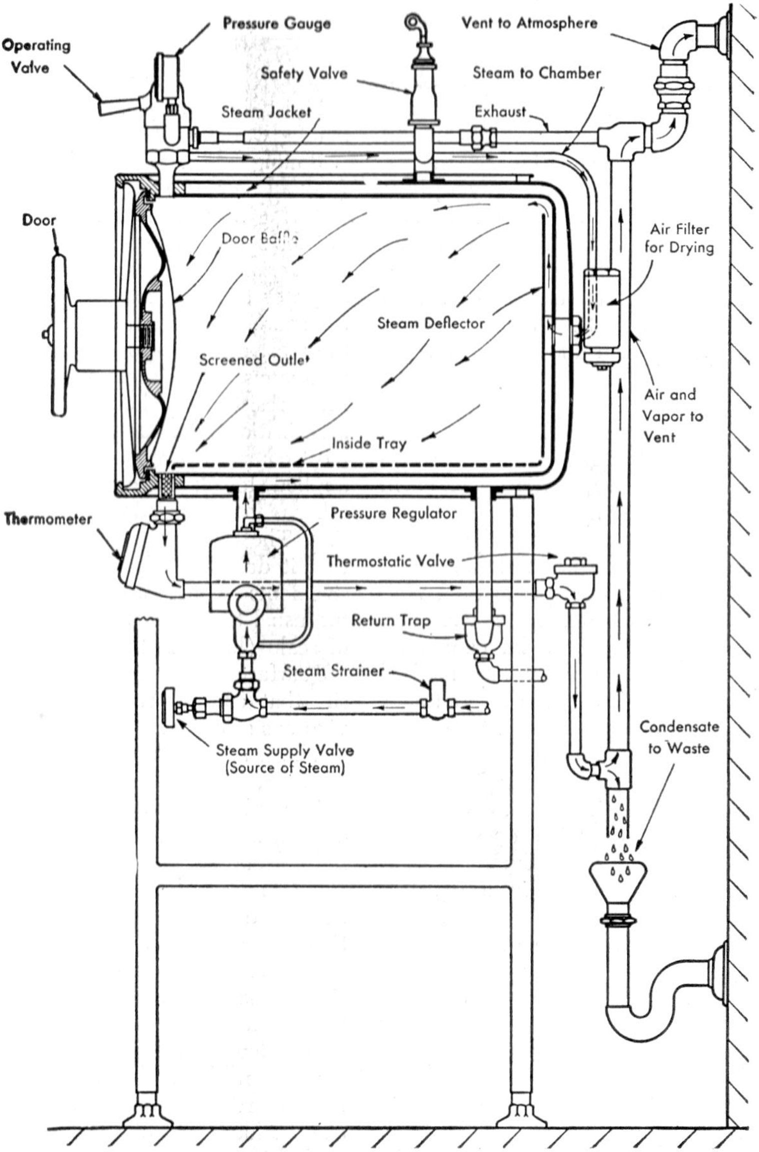

FIG. 9. Longitudinal cross section of steam-heated pressure steam sterilizer. Steam is delivered from source to steam jacket through a pressure regulator that maintains automatically the desired range. The same principle applies for steam heat (as shown) or for sterilizers heated by gas or electricity. Jacket steam then is admitted through operating valve to chamber at back end behind a deflector. Arrows indicate passage of air and steam through chamber to screened outlet drain at front end. Drainage system includes thermometer and thermostatic valve. All discharge flows to the vertical riser, which drains water through the open air break to the waste system. Steam or vapors are exhausted to atmospheric vent. (The Surgical Supervisor, American Sterilizer Co., Erie, Pa.)

is essential that it ordinarily be clean and free from any dirt, threads, ravelings and so forth that might remain as foreign bodies in the wound. The mode of applying heat varies with the nature of the material to be sterilized and with the circumstances under which the sterilization is to be carried out. Two main forms of heat are used commonly: dry heat and moist heat.

DRY HEAT

Actual Cautery. This is used to sterilize cut tissue surfaces—for example, the base of the appendix in an appendectomy.

Hot Air. Some surgical supplies, such as petrolatum in bulk, gauze strips covered with petrolatum, various forms of oil, bone wax and talcum powder in bulk, cannot be sterilized properly by any method other than prolonged exposure to dry heat in the hot-air oven. The moist heat of the autoclave, to be discussed later, is inadequate because the moisture factor of the steam, essential to autoclave sterilization, does not permeate such masses. Such materials should be sterilized in a dry-heat sterilizer at a temperature of 320° F. (160° C.) for 1 hour or at 250° F. (121° C.) for 4 hours. Usually it is not advisable to attempt sterilization of such materials except in relatively small quantities; that is to say, in small jars or containers.

A hot-air oven can be created in the ordinary autoclave. Steam is allowed to enter the jacket but not the chamber; in this way, syringes, needles, sharp-edged instruments, etc., can be adequately sterilized overnight or for a minimum of 4 hours at 250° F. (121° C.).

MOIST HEAT

Moist heat may be applied as boiling water or as steam.

Boiling Water. Boiling water (212° F. or 100° C.) will destroy all living bacteria in a few seconds, but the spores of some organisms are very resistant and require boiling for a longer time (at least 20 minutes) to ensure their destruction. Some of the most difficult spores to kill, such as tetanus and gas gangrene organisms, resist many hours of boiling. Sterilization by boiling water is the most common of all methods and is applied to all instruments and to other materials not damaged by wetting. The disadvantage of boiling is that it dulls the edge of cutting instruments—scalpels and so forth; also, the usual tap water leaves a deposit of scale (lime) in the joints and on the surfaces of instruments and utensils that can be removed only by vigorous scouring.

The usual technic for sterilization of instruments requires that they boil in plain water for 30 minutes or in water containing 2 per cent of sodium carbonate (from 3 to 4 teaspoonfuls to the quart of water) for not less than 15 minutes. The addition of sodium carbonate brings about the destruction of the more resistant spores in a shorter period of time than is possible in plain water. The following are important points for the nurse to remember when boiling articles: *The article must be clean.* Blood, pus, oils, grease and so forth hinder the sterilizing process. The timing of sterilization is started when the water begins to boil. *All articles must be submerged* completely. The speed at which the water boils does not change the time element; therefore, it is better to have the water boiling quietly.

Steam Under Pressure. This is the most useful method of sterilizing nearly all surgical supplies. The sterilizer or autoclave (Fig. 9) is built in such a manner that steam enters the sterilizing chamber under pressure for the purpose of attaining high temperatures. Materials thus sterilized are subjected to a temperature of from 115° to 123° C. (240° to 254° F.). The steam of the autoclave at these temperatures destroys all vegetative bacteria, and even the most resistant pathogenic spores, in a relatively brief interval of time. Tests have proved that the spores of *Cl. oedematiens*, *Cl. tetani* and *Cl. welchii* are destroyed in direct contact with steam at 121° C. (250° F.) in one minute, at 115° C. (240° F.) in four minutes and at 110° C. (230° F.) in 10 minutes. Since these are the absolute minimum requirements, a considerably longer period of time is necessary in order to provide for the steam to permeate the mass, whatever it is. (For recommended periods of exposure, see Appendix.) Surrounding the sterilizing chamber is a steam jacket, where from 15 to 17 pounds of pressure is maintained before, during and after the sterilization period. One purpose of the jacket is to prevent condensation of the water vapor, with consequent wetting of the supplies.

Principles of Sterilization by Steam Under Pressure. The principle of sterilization by the use of steam is the same as in other methods of sterilization—the coagulation of the proteins in the bacterial body, which destroys the bacteria. It has been found by experiment that coagulation occurs at a much lower temperature with moist heat than with dry heat, which is the reason for the use of boiling water and of steam under pressure as sterilizing agents. Steam at atmospheric pressure can transmit a temperature of only 212° F. (100° C.). This temperature is able to kill all living or vegetative forms of bacterial life, but many spores are resistant to this temperature and are not killed.

Removal of Air. In order to reach such high temperatures, it is necessary that the air be removed as completely as possible from the sterilizing chamber. The temperature can be gauged by the pressure indicator only when the pressure represents that of steam and not that of steam plus air in the sterilizing chamber. Therefore, an attempt is made in all types of sterilizers to remove the air from the sterilizing chamber. This is accomplished best by permitting the air to escape through a drain controlled thermostatically from the bottom of the chamber, including an accurate mercury thermometer that indicates consequently the temperature of the coolest medium surrounding the load, since air or steam mixed with air will gravitate unfailingly below pure steam in the chamber. The thermostatic valve remains open and permits air and condensate to escape freely. It closes only after the air has been driven out, and relatively pure steam follows. This thermometer thus becomes the one gauge (rather than the pressure indication) under which all sterilization is controlled. Every performance is timed when the thermometer indicates 240° F. (115° C.) in its advance toward the regulated maximum of 254° F. (123° C.).

The importance of withdrawing the air is due to the fact that the presence of air reduces the ultimate temperature of the steam at any given pressure, because steam and air do not mix; therefore, the materials at the top of the sterilizer, heated by pure steam, become sterilized easily and rapidly, and those at the bottom of the sterilizer, where most of the air accumulates, are heated by a mixture of warm air and steam, and the temperature does not rise to the point which will produce sterilization for a considerable period of time. Furthermore, the presence of air in the sterilizer reduces very materially the power of the steam to penetrate and sterilize large packages of materials, because the penetration of steam into these packages depends upon the displacement of air due to gravity. If the chamber is two thirds filled with air, there is no displacement by gravity and, therefore, poor penetration of the materials by steam.

In the operation of the sterilizer, no matter what type, the process by which sterilization is accomplished is much the same. In the stage of preparation, steam is admitted to the outer or steam jacket until the pressure of from 15 to 17 pounds is reached. In this way, the sterilizing chamber is heated and is prepared for the reception of the materials to be sterilized. After the materials have been introduced into the chamber, air is evacuated from the chamber by gravity, as explained above. The operator should keep close watch until the thermometer indicates 240° F. (115° C.); then the period of exposure, which is governed by the particular load, is timed.

At the close of the period of sterilization, the operating valve is turned to "exhaust" until chamber pressure has reduced to "zero." Jacket pressure is maintained until drying is complete. When chamber pressure has reduced to zero, the operating valve (for dry loads only) is turned to the "vacuum" or "dry" position, in which a mild degree of vacuum is created in the chamber, rarefying the vapor and hastening drying to some extent. This position is maintained for not more than 3 to 5 minutes, and the operating valve is turned to the "off" position until the chamber gauge again indicates zero pressure. Then the door is unlocked and loosened slightly but opened not more than ½ inch for about 10 minutes, depending upon the size and the density of the load. Vapor will escape into the room from the top of the door, and drying results.

For cooling down solution loads—any aqueous solution in bottles or flasks—exhaust of the chamber steam must be controlled precisely or blown stoppers and undue loss of fluid will result. This can be accomplished easily in the following way:

At the close of the period of sterilization, turn the operating valve toward the exhaust position so that the steam from the chamber will escape very slowly. Exhaust to the zero pressure should occur in not less than from 6 to 10 minutes, and the door must not be unlocked until all pressure has been exhausted completely. This will permit the fluid in the flasks or the bottles to lose its heat without violent ebullition down to the boiling point.

FACTORS GOVERNING STEAM STERILIZATION OF SURGICAL SUPPLIES*

Packaging

1. Restrict size and density of the individual pack so as to ensure uniform steam penetration.

2. Select a protective covering (wrapper) for surgical supplies—muslin, paper, parchment or cellophane.

3. Using freshly laundered fabrics to prevent superheating is important.

Loading of Sterilizer

1. Prepare all packs and arrange the load in the sterilizer so as to present the least possible resistance to

* Principles and Methods of Sterilization, American Sterilizer Co., August, 1953.

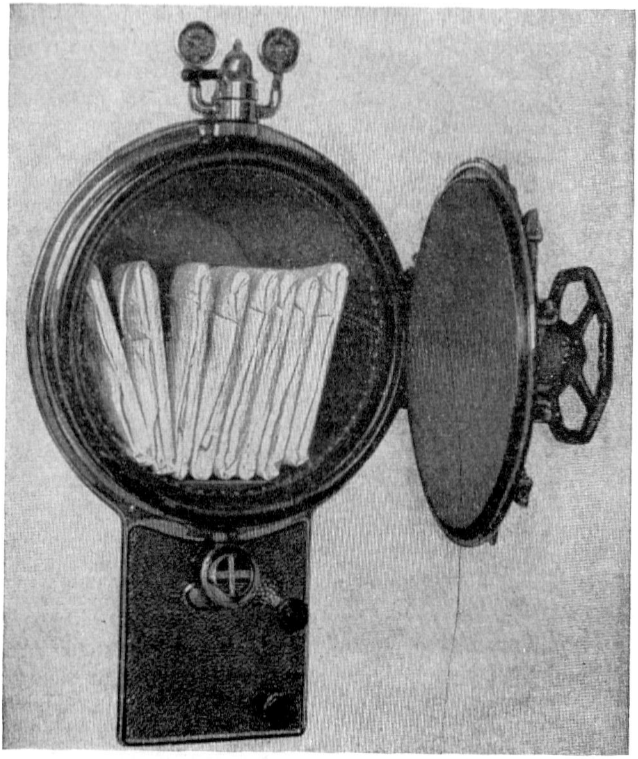

FIG. 10. Proper method of loading trays in the sterilizer—all resting on edge, with no interference from any surrounding packs. The advantage of shallow trays also is indicated: they occupy less space in the sterilizer. (*The Surgical Supervisor*, American Sterilizer Co., Erie, Pa.)

the passage of steam through the load, from the top of the chamber toward the bottom.

2. All jars, test tubes and other nonporous containers of dry material should be loaded in the sterilizer so as to provide a horizontal path for the escape of air.

Period of Exposure
(*See pp. 700, 701*)

1. Establish a period of exposure that will provide for complete penetration of the load and ensure destruction of microbial life with a liberal margin of safety.

2. Time the sterilizing period from the moment that saturated steam at 250° F. fills the chamber as indicated by the thermometer located in the chamber drain-line.

Physical Methods of Sterilization—Radiant Energy

Physical methods of sterilization are little used as yet—perhaps much less than they deserve. Those most important for mention in this connection are sunlight, the ultraviolet ray and the x-ray.

Ultraviolet Rays. These have been found to prevent the growth of bacteria in cultures, and this knowledge is being applied more and more in the treatment of wounds. Those conditions most suitable to this form of treatment are of the sluggish, sloughing type, such as one finds in a bedsore (decubitus ulcer). The rays are found in some concentration in the direct sunlight, but they are formed artificially by mercury vapor lamps, the so-called "alpine light."

Daily increasing exposure of the wound to this light frequently has a marked beneficial effect, due not only to its bactericidal function, but also to a stimulation of the reparative processes. Because of the danger of burning the patient by an overdosage, exposure should be given only under the direction of a competent physician. An alarm clock or an attendant should warn the patient when exposure is completed. Extensive burns have been known to occur when the patient fell asleep under the light.

Chemical Methods of Disinfection—Antiseptics

Since the advent of the sulfa drugs and the antibiotics, there has been less emphasis on antiseptics.

Antiseptics may either inhibit the growth of organisms or actually kill them. Therefore, being germicidal, they accomplish sterilization. Exactly what action takes place will vary with the strength of the chemical, the length of time of its application and the character of the object to be antisepticized or sterilized. For example, 70 per cent alcohol applied to the skin for one minute after soap and water will cleanse the skin effectually but will not sterilize it, whereas an instrument submerged in it for some time will be sterilized. That is to say, there is no universal antiseptic for all purposes, occasions and materials.

Today less emphasis is laid upon chemical antisepsis and more importance is attached to soap and water for cleansing in conjunction with chemotherapy.

Antiseptics are used in surgery under three main sets of conditions:

1. Application to Skin. Antiseptics are applied to the skin in a wide area about the operative field to destroy its normal and accidental bacterial inhabitants. This prevents the entrance from this source into the operative wound of infection and its development. Combined with other aseptic measures, this procedure, while not producing absolute sterility, usually is sufficient to ensure aseptic healing.

2. Application to Tissues. Antiseptics are applied to tissues that are or may be the seat of infection, in order to assist them to destroy the germs and their products rapidly and completely. When used in this way "the ideal antiseptic should effect complete sterilization within its sphere of action without causing any damage to tissue cells" (Dakin). However, the disadvantage of most antiseptics is that in killing the bacteria they tend also to destroy tissue cells. For this reason they should be used in wounds in weak solutions, and for only a short period of time. Many antiseptics have been suggested and used in tissues, and their very multiplicity would indicate that the ideal antiseptic has not been found yet. It is being recognized more and more that the body tissues have a natural resistance to infection, and that antiseptics are of value only occasionally in the treatment of certain specific types of infection, especially those on the surface of the body.

3. Sterilization of Instruments and Materials. Chemicals are used to sterilize certain instruments and materials that cannot be sterilized by heat; for example, cystoscopes, bougies and cataract knives must be immersed in a germicide. Most of the chemicals are used in the form of solutions, being dissolved in water or in alcohol. From time to time new chemical compounds appear on the market, all of them with certain advantages and disadvantages.

GROUPS OF ANTISEPTICS

The antiseptics may be divided into these groups: (1) soaps and other detergents, (2) alcohols, aldehydes and acids, (3) phenols, (4) salts of heavy metals, (5) oxidizing agents, (6) halogen compounds and (7) synthetic dyes.

Soaps and Detergents

Soaps and detergents are widely used agents for mechanical cleansing of the skin of the operative area and for removal of gross contamination from the skin surrounding traumatic wounds. They also are used in preparing the hands and the arms of the surgeon and the nurse before putting on sterile gown and gloves. The usual 10-minute scrub with soap and water may be shortened by the use of antiseptics added to the soap and by the use of detergents instead of soap.

Green Soap. This is a potassium soap which varies in color from yellowish white to greenish brown.

Tincture of Green Soap. This is an alcoholic solution of the above soap containing approximately 30 per cent alcohol.

Benzalkonium Chloride, U.S.P. (Zephiran Chloride). This is an effective surface disinfectant for skin, mucous membranes, superficial injuries and infected wounds. Solutions range in strength from 1:1,000 to 1:40,000, depending upon the purpose of treatment. All soaps should be rinsed thoroughly from areas in which it is desirous to use this detergent (cationic).

Phisoderm contains the antiseptic hexachlorophene (G-11). It has an advantage over soap in that it is close to neutrality.

Alcohols, Aldehydes and Acids

Ethyl Alcohol. This is one of the most useful antiseptics. It has a high degree of antiseptic power and has the advantage of being a fat solvent, dissolving out the fat on the surface and in the follicles of the skin, thus permitting the antiseptic to act on the more deeply situated organisms.

SPECIAL USES. In 70 per cent solution by weight (81.5 per cent by volume) it is used frequently in preoperative and postoperative disinfection of the surgeon's hands and the patient's skin and as an evaporating lotion.

Because it is a fat solvent, it is used frequently in combination with other antiseptics.

DISADVANTAGES. Alcohol causes considerable pain when applied to raw tissues; therefore, it never should be used in fresh, open wounds. It causes pronounced irritation of mucous surfaces, and for this reason it is not employed as an antiseptic for the eye, the urethra and so forth.

When used alone as a sterilizing agent for instruments, alcohol occasionally has proved to be inadequate; therefore, it must be borne in mind that sterilization by heat always is preferable whenever this is possible.

Isopropyl Alcohol. Isopropyl alcohol has shown evidence of having approximately twice the germicidal strength of ethyl alcohol. Because of this and the fact that its dilution need not be as stable as ethyl alcohol, isopropyl alcohol is more popular.

Formaldehyde is a gas with high disinfecting properties. A 40 per cent solution of the gas in water is known as formalin. Since it is too irritating for living tissue, it is mainly used as a preservative of specimens.

Boric or Boracic Acid. This is a white crystalline powder that is soluble in warm water to make about a 4 per cent solution. The drug is a feeble germicide and is used rather for restraining the growth of putrefactive organisms than for disinfection in the true sense. It is used in strengths of from 2 to 4 per cent solutions in the eye, the ear, the nose, the throat and the bladder, and as a moist dressing.

Phenols

Phenol or carbolic acid probably was the first recognized antiseptic. In its pure state it consists of pinkish-white crystals that dissolve in a small amount of water to make about a 95 per cent strength. This strength is usually known as "pure phenol" or "pure carbolic acid."

USES AS "PURE CARBOLIC ACID." To sterilize and cauterize the cut edges of intestinal mucosa; for example, the stump of the appendix is often touched with "pure carbolic" before it is inverted into the cecal wall.

Cresols are derivatives of phenol, which they have largely replaced. They are much more effective germicides and much less toxic.

Hexachlorophen, N.N.R. (Gamophen, Germa-Medica, pHisoHex). This is a preparation of cresol which is incorporated into soaps, detergent creams, etc., for application in the preoperative preparation of skin.

Salts of Heavy Metals

The germicidal activity of these salts in watery solution is great, but when the solutions are brought into contact with proteins, soaps, alkalies and so forth, this activity is reduced greatly.

Mercuric Chloride. Mercuric chloride (corrosive sublimate or bichloride of mercury) is a white crystalline substance that is extremely poisonous. It gives a clear solution in water, but its solutions for hospital use usually are dyed, generally pink, to distinguish it from other solutions.

SPECIAL USES. (1) As 1:5,000 solution in alcohol or in 1:1,000 in water as an antiseptic in the preoperative preparation of the surgeon's hands and the patient's skin.

(2) As 1:2,000 or 1:4,000 solution in water for irrigating wounds.

(3) As 1:10,000 solution in water for the irrigation of mucous surfaces, including the conjunctival sac. The solutions always should be colored with some dye and marked "Poison."

(4) As a compound tincture for the preparation of the operative field.

DISADVANTAGES. (1) It is highly poisonous. Symptoms of poisoning may arise through absorption from wounds treated with the drug. Therefore, it is never used in extensive wounds having large, exposed, absorbing surfaces. The symptoms of poisoning in the order of their appearance are metallic taste in mouth, excessive salivation, nausea and vomiting, intestinal colic, diarrhea, collapse and death.

The treatment is to stop the mercurial antiseptic and promote elimination by catharsis, forcing fluids and sweatings.

(2) It decomposes rapidly in the presence of:

(a) Soaps; therefore, it should not be used in hand preparation until after a thorough washing with sterile water. The "milky" bichloride basin seen occasionally in operating rooms is caused by a combination of the soap from the surgeon's hands with the bichloride.

(b) Albumens; therefore, it is not used in wounds having copious discharges.

(c) The gas, hydrogen sulfide (H_2S), that frequently is generated in wounds infected with *Escherichia coli*, the colon bacillus, as in anal or rectal conditions.

(3) It often causes a local dermatitis.

(4) It corrodes metal instruments.

Merthiolate is one of the newer organic mercurial antiseptics. It has been found experimentally to have high bactericidal and antiseptic properties in dilutions that are only slightly irritating to tissue and mucous surfaces. Usually, it is used in a 1:1,000 aqueous solution as a wound antiseptic. It is supplied also in the form of a tincture in alcohol-acetone colored solution for skin preparation before operation.

Metaphen is a crystalline compound of mercury with cresol, usually obtained in a yellow solution. It has been shown to have high bactericidal powers and is not irritating to the skin; nor does it corrode metal instruments. Tincture of Metaphen 1:200 is used for skin sterilization.

Silver Nitrate. This is a powerful antiseptic. It is soluble readily in water, but the water must be distilled, because ordinary tap water contains other substances that cause a deterioration of the solution. The solutions should be kept in dark bottles because they decompose when exposed to the light, forming little black specks of metallic silver. Solutions that are not clear should be discarded.

SPECIAL USES. (1) In watery solution in strengths of from ½ to 5 per cent, silver nitrate is used as an antiseptic in the eye, the urethra and the bladder. In the pure form it is called "lunar caustic" by the layman. This is prepared in stick form and often is used as a caustic. Its chief disadvantage is that, when dropped on clothing, it leaves an intense black stain.

(2) Organic compounds of silver (Protargol, Argyrol, silvol and so forth) are useful antiseptics for application on the mucous surfaces of the eye, the nose, the throat, the vagina, the urethra and so forth. They are used in watery solutions of from 0.5 to 10 per cent. These solutions must be made up fresh, as they undergo deterioration after one week's time.

Oxidizing Agents

The antiseptic properties of this group are due to their property of liberating oxygen that has a mild germicidal action.

Hydrogen Peroxide. This is a clear, watery solution that decomposes readily in the light or on heating. When applied to wound tissues, there is an immediate effervescence that marks the liberation of gaseous oxygen.

Its chief value lies probably in the mechanical effect of its effervescence, in loosening necrotic tissues and dressing and in breaking up thick adherent masses of pus that float to the surface in a sort of foam. Because of this property and its ability to give off oxygen, it is of special value in the treatment of anaerobic infections, such as those caused by the gas bacillus.

Hydrogen peroxide decomposes rapidly unless protected from light, heat and air.

Potassium Permanganate. This occurs as purple crystals, is soluble easily in water and gives a wine-colored solution.

SPECIAL USES. In solution of 1:1,000 to 1:10,000 in sloughing wounds, as an antiseptic and deodorant. It decomposes rapidly, changing from a purple to an inert brownish fluid.

DISADVANTAGES. The solutions decompose rapidly, losing their antiseptic power on contact with dead organic material, rubber or rusty metal, as in chipped enamelware. The change is accompanied by a conversion of the purple to a brown color.

Zinc Peroxide. This is a white powder or granule that must be heated to a temperature of 140° F. for 4 hours to make it active. It is prepared by mixing with distilled water to make a creamlike solution, which then has the property of giving off oxygen over a long period of time. It has been of special value in the treatment of symbiotic infections of the skin and the mouth. In such infections an anaerobic organism, usually streptococcus, is found, as well as an aerobic staphylococcus infection. The zinc peroxide cream gives off oxygen and so converts the wound into one unfavorable for anaerobic organisms. It is applied usually with petrolatum gauze over it to prevent evaporation. The dressings must be renewed daily.

Halogen Compounds

Iodine. This antiseptic ordinarily

is used as a tincture. It is one of the most useful "when conditions are such that rapid and complete sterilization may be effected by a single application."

Special Uses. (1) As a 3 to 5 per cent solution in the preparation of the skin of the patient for operation.

(2) As a 2 per cent solution for the emergency treatment of contaminated wounds.

(3) For the irrigation of infected wounds in solutions of from 1:100 to 1:500.

Disadvantages. (1) Iodine solutions often irritate the skin.

(2) On wet skin, iodine loses much of its effectiveness as a skin disinfectant and frequently causes blisters or vesicles. For this reason it is used only on dry surfaces, never on the palms of the hands, the soles of the feet, the armpits and the perineum. During the summer months, when profuse sweating occurs, iodine should not be used on the face, the scrotum and any other tender parts of the skin.

(3) The strength of iodine solutions increases on standing. This is due to evaporation of the alcoholic solvent. Therefore, they should be kept tightly corked and renewed frequently.

Iodoform. Its chief use is in the form of "iodoform gauze"—gauze impregnated with a 10 to 20 per cent emulsion of iodoform. It is used especially for packing in foul discharging wounds.

Synthetic Dyes

Acriflavine is a derivative of the coal-tar base acridine and is antiseptic in the presence of secretions. It may be applied to infected areas by swabbing or by inserting saturated gauze.

Methylrosalinine Chloride, N.F. (Gentian Violet). This is used in infected wounds and on mucous membranes. Dilutions of 1:500 and 1:1,000 are used in direct application.

Merbromin, N.F. (Mercurochrome). This has been used in a 2 per cent solution for minor abrasions; however, it is not a very active antiseptic.

Carbol-Fuchsin Paint, N.N.R. (Carfusin). A refined product of the original formula known as Castellani's paint, this is useful against superficial fungus infections.

Furan Derivative

Nitrofurazone, N.N.R. (Furacin). An effective agent against many gram-positive and gram-negative bacteria, Furacin is used in the form of a solution in the local treatment of infections and may be applied in the form of an ointment for surface lesions.

Compound Antiseptics

Many surgeons use antiseptics which are combinations of members of the above groups. Among the most important of these are the following:

Harrington's Solution

Bichloride of mercury	1.5	Gm.
Hydrochloric acid	100	cc.
Glycerin	100	cc.
Alcohol (95%)	1,200	cc.
Distilled water	2,000	cc.

It is used frequently for the disinfection of the skin and for glassware, china and so forth.

Whitehead's Varnish. This is an excellent antiseptic dressing for wounds. It is used frequently on small wounds about the face, the neck and the head when there is no ooze and when a dressing would be cumbersome and conspicuous. It is composed of

Iodoform	1 oz.
Tr. Benzoin comp.	4 oz.

Ether is used instead of alcohol in the benzoin comp.

A.B.C. Antiseptic Douche

Alum	1 oz.
Boric acid	4 oz.
Carbolic acid crystals (phenol)	3 dr.
Oil of peppermint	1½ dr.

One dram of this powder is added to a pint of water and used as an antiseptic vaginal douche.

Many other antiseptics are used or have been used, but those mentioned seem to be those employed most commonly at the present time.

Ointments are used in surgery when it is inadvisable to apply watery lotions and when it is desired to protect the surrounding skin from the irritating discharges of a wound. They are used also as mildly antiseptic applications in superficial wounds and ulcers, as stimulating applications to sluggish wound surfaces and as a means of administering medicines.

The bland ointments, such as petrolatum, lanolin and cold cream, are used to soften dry and scaly skin and to prevent dressings from adhering to secreting wounds. Mildly antiseptic ointments, such as the ointments of boric acid or zinc oxide, are used in much the same manner. The zinc oxide ointment is useful especially in the treatment of the irritating excoriation of the skin that surrounds a wound having secretion. Ointments containing scarlet red and balsam of Peru have a reputation for stimulating granulation tissue and epithelial growth. They are applied to wounds that seem to be slow in healing.

Few ointments are used in surgery as a means of administering drugs. However, there are some notable exceptions to this statement. Mercury is given in the form of mercurial ointment (blue ointment) in the treatment of syphilis. This ointment is useful also in the early treatment of local superficial infections, such as boils, infected sebaceous cysts and so forth. Methylsalicylate ointment is useful in the treatment of joint and muscle affections. It produces a local hyperemia, and its effectiveness may be due more to a local counterirritant than to its absorbed drug. Ichthyol ointment is a black, bland, oily mixture that has been used for years as a local application by the laity and the medical profession to "draw" an infection "to a head." It is probable that its only action is to keep the superficial layers of skin soft, thus making pointing somewhat easier.

Antibiotics and certain sulfonamides in the form of ointments also are used as local antiseptics for infected wounds, burns and so forth.

CHEMOTHERAPY

Sulfonamides

These drugs appear to be effective by reducing the rapidity of bacterial growth (bacteriostasis) and so permitting the phagocytic activity of the leukocytes to be more effective. Sulfadiazine, sulfamerazine and sulfathiazole are the drugs most widely used for systemic infections. Often these are given in combination because there is evidence that the mixture gives increased antibacterial effectiveness and at the same time less danger of crystal deposit in the kidney. For local action to reduce the bacteria of the colon in preparation for colon operations, sulfaguanidine, sulfathalidine and sulfasuxidine are used.

For a systemic effect, a large first dose of the drug (from 2 to 4 Gm.) is given, after which smaller doses (usually 1 Gm.) are used to maintain an adequate blood concentration. These drugs are eliminated through the kidneys and, if the urine is acid, crystals may be deposited in the renal tubules. For this reason, sodium bicarbonate usually is given with the sulfa drug to alkalinize the urine, and fluids are given in large amounts.

If medication cannot be given by mouth, a soluble form of the drug, usually sodium sulfadiazine, may be given intravenously.

Uses. The sulfonamides seem to be particularly effective in infections due to the staphylococcus and the streptococcus, but they have been found to be of value also in the treatment of meningococcal, gonococcal and various types of urinary infection.

Nursing Care

The nursing care is chiefly to administer the drug promptly, observe the patient, report toxicity in him, regulate fluid intake and keep accurate records.

As stated previously, the action of a sulfonamide depends upon its continuous concentration in the blood stream. To secure this concentration, the patient should receive the medication promptly, even being awakened, unless otherwise ordered. Vomiting of the drug should be reported promptly, and often the administration is repeated if vomiting occurs within 20 minutes.

Symptoms of toxicity associated with the sulfonamides, which should be reported immediately, are scanty or bloody urine, nausea and vomiting, fever, abdominal pain, skin rash, psychoses, dizziness, diarrhea or jaundice. Conjunctivitis is an additional toxic effect.

Urinary obstruction may be due to the precipitation of sulfa crystals in the tubules, the kidney pelvis or the ureter, and for this reason the regulation of fluid intake is important. The 24-hour output of the patient should be at least 1,000 cc. To keep the blood concentration fairly consistent and the irritation of the kidney down, the intake should be adequate and divided uniformly over the 24-hour period. Because of all these factors the need for complete and accurate records is obvious.

ANTIBIOTICS

There are 11 antibiotics now available for use in the treatment of infection. By far the most commonly used is the original one—penicillin—but as more experience is gained in the use of these substances it is found that bacteria either are resistant or develop a resistance to some of the antibiotics. Therefore, it is important to know as soon as possible to what antibiotics the bacteria causing infection are sensitive. These sensitivity tests are made by culture in which bacteria are grown on an agar plate on which are placed small disks containing a solution of the various antibiotics to be tested. Those which are found not to grow in the area surrounding the disk are sensitive to the antibiotic. Therefore, these antibiotics would be chosen for treatment of the infection.

Sensitivity tests are now made almost routinely in any infectious lesion where antibiotic therapy is contemplated, although before the antibiotic sensitivities are known, penicillin may be started empirically. This table indicates the relative sensitivity of various types of micro-organisms to the antibiotics. In addition to the fact that some bacteria

RELATIVE SENSITIVITY OF ANTIBIOTICS TO VARIOUS GROUPS OF MICRO-ORGANISMS
(After Edwin J. Pulaski)

<table>
<tr><th>GRAM-POSITIVE ORGANISMS</th><th colspan="2">GRAM-NEGATIVE BACILLI</th><th colspan="2">TUBERCLE BACILLI</th></tr>
<tr><td>(Staphylococci, Streptococci, etc.)</td><td colspan="2">(Colon Bacilli, etc.)</td><td colspan="2"></td></tr>
<tr><td>Tyrothricin</td><td colspan="4"></td></tr>
<tr><td>Bacitracin</td><td colspan="4"></td></tr>
<tr><td colspan="2">Penicillin</td><td colspan="3"></td></tr>
<tr><td colspan="5">Streptomycin — Neomycin</td></tr>
<tr><td colspan="4">Chlortetracycline Chloramphenicol Terramycin</td><td></td></tr>
<tr><td colspan="2">Erythromycin
Carbomycin</td><td colspan="3"></td></tr>
<tr><td></td><td colspan="2">Polymyxin</td><td colspan="2"></td></tr>
</table>

develop a resistance to the antibiotics, another factor often enters into the choice of the antibiotic agent, namely, the fact that the patient himself may become sensitive or allergic to one of these drugs. Therefore, in spite of the desire of the physician to use penicillin, for example, it may be necessary to use some other antibiotic because the patient is allergic to the penicillin.

Penicillin

Penicillin is a remarkably potent antibacterial agent. It can be given intravenously, intramuscularly or topically. Also, it may be given orally if in large doses (100,000 u.) every 3 hours.

Penicillin is excreted rapidly in the urine, so that, in order to maintain an effective blood level, the rapidly absorbed aqueous solution of penicillin must be given at 2- or 3-hour intervals. More slowly absorbed preparations of the drug, such as penicillin in oil and bees-wax, duracillin, ledercillin, wycillin, crysticillin and so forth, are eliminated less rapidly, and a single daily intramuscular injection will given an effective blood concentration. Insoluble salts such as procaine salt also aid in prolonging the action of penicillin. Hence, Potassium Penicillin G, Calcium Penicillin and Sodium Penicillin G are available.

Uses. Penicillin has been found to be most effective in the treatment of staphylococcic, gonococcic, pneumonococcic and hemolytic streptococcic infections. The dosage ranges from 100,000 to 1,000,000 Oxford units per 24 to 48 hours, and in some instances the treatment must continue for a week or 10 days. In empyema thoracis and in meningitis it may be given topically by injection into the pleural or subarachnoid space.

Caution. Toxic effects are rare. Chills and fever, headache and flushing of the face have been encountered. Urticaria is not uncommon, and thrombophlebitis at the injection site has occurred.

The local treatment of fresh wounds is undergoing a radical change and, although chemical antiseptics on the market are more numerous than ever, there is a distinct trend toward the employment of soap and copious amounts of water, particularly in the primary or first-aid treatment of traumatic open wounds.

Nursing Care

The patient receiving penicillin should be watched closely, and accurate records should be kept. Intramuscular injections should be made promptly.

Streptomycin

Streptomycin, like penicillin, is a highly antibacterial agent that can be given parenterally. It is produced by certain types of organisms found in the soil. Intramuscular and subcutaneous routes of administration are preferable, since the intravenous route has no advantages, and toxic reactions are more likely to occur. Also, it may be used topically or given orally.

Dihydrostreptomycin, a less toxic form of streptomycin, often is used either alone or in combination with streptomycin for intramuscular injection.

Uses. Streptomycin is most effective in the treatment of infections due to gram-negative bacilli and in certain types of tubercular infections.

The total daily dose is from 1 to 3 Gm. dissolved in distilled water and given in divided doses at 4-, 6- or 12-hour intervals.

Caution. Some patients may show sensitivity to the drug by headache, flushing, pain and tenderness at the site of injection and fever. When it is given over a long period of time, dizziness and deafness may occur.

Tyrothricin

Tyrothricin is an organic germicide and bacteriostatic agent extracted from cultures of certain types of soil bacteria. It consists principally of two fractions—gramicidin and tyrocidine. Gramicidin is effective against gram-positive organisms and tyrocidine against some gram-negative species. It is for external use only, but it may be put into abscess or empyema cavities. Its most frequent use is in the treatment of ulcers or infected open wounds. Although it may be used in higher concentrations for infections caused by more resistant organisms, it is administered usually in the dilution of 0.5 mg. of tyrothricin per cc.

Bacitracin

This new antibiotic is produced by an aerobic bacillus of the *B. subtilis* group of organisms. It is effective against many of the organisms for which penicillin is used, and it appears to have the additional advantage of greater penetration in the presence of pus and necrotic tissue. It has been used with good results in the treatment of furuncles, carbuncles and abscesses by injection into the center of each lesion of from 1 to 5 cc. of a solution containing 100 or more units of bacitracin per cc. It is used best as a topical application in infections that do not respond to penicillin therapy.

Chlortetracycline (Aureomycin)

Chlortetracycline is derived from a strain of *Streptomyces*. It has been shown to possess antibacterial activity against numerous bacteria. The drug is given best by mouth, but it may also be given intravenously. It has proved to be most useful in surgery in the treatment of infections that cannot be controlled by penicillin or streptomycin therapy. It frequently causes nausea and diarrhea.

Chloramphenicol (Chloromycetin)

This antibiotic is obtained by special culture methods from a type of *Streptomyces*. It is insoluble in water, but it is absorbed readily from the intestinal tract when given by mouth. It appears to be most effective surgically as an antibacterial agent against the gram-negative bacteria.

Oxytetracycline (Terramycin)

Terramycin is one of the broad-spectrum antibiotics which is effective against both gram-positive and gram-negative organisms. It is given both by mouth and intravenously. It is used most often in situations where the organisms are not sensitive to penicillin or in overwhelming infection. Frequently it is used to rid the bowel of organisms before colon surgery.

Erythromycin

Erythromycin also is one of the broad-spectrum antibiotics. It is most effective against the gram-positive cocci organisms, the streptococcus and the staphylococcus. It is used most often where the organisms are resistant to penicillin or where there is a penicillin sensitivity. This is administered by mouth.

Carbomycin

Carbomycin also is effective against gram-positive organisms. It is one of the newer antibiotics and is used less widely than the others previously mentioned. It is given by oral administration also.

Neomycin

Neomycin is a broad-spectrum antibiotic which is effective against both gram-negative and gram-positive organisms. Its use in surgery is mostly as a preoperative drug to rid the bowel of organisms before colon surgery.

Polymyxin

Polymyxin is used against the gram-negative bacilli. However, it is used less frequently than the other antibiotics.

CHAPTER FOUR

Preoperative Nursing Care

INTRODUCTION

When a patient goes to a hospital for an operation, he enters an environment that not only is strange and different but often is associated with much anxiety, many misgivings and even actual fear. This applies not only to the patient but often even more so to the members of his family who accompany him. The nurse, who is in most intimate contact with the patient during his stay in the hospital, must realize the large part she plays in the psychological, as well as the physical, care of the patient. With a knowledge of the probable experiences of a patient in the hospital, she can reassure him by her attention and aid. A word or two of explanation will answer many questions that arise, but all technical questions should be referred to the surgeon. A sympathetic understanding and an optimistic manner add both to the patient's mental and physical comfort. (Also see p. 6.)

ADMISSION OF THE SURGICAL PATIENT

When the routine admission requirements are completed, it is wise to obtain the name, the address and the telephone number of the nearest relative or friend. These particulars can be kept in a convenient place on the chart.

The assignment of a patient to his bed or to his room should be done with his condition and individual preferences in mind. If he is assigned to a ward, psychologically it is better for him to be placed near someone who is cheerful and convalescing from surgery rather than near one who is acutely ill or one who is bitter and pessimistic. Patients not only have been frightened out of the hospital, but they have been frightened to death. Such cases are on record.

After the temperature, the pulse and the respiration are taken and recorded, the patient should have a bath, unless he is too ill. This may be an opportune time to weigh him and to secure a urine specimen. Hospital apparel usually consists of a cotton short gown tied in the back. A dressing gown or a house coat and bedroom slippers are a necessity. Every patient should have a toothbrush and a washcloth. His clothing and valuables are given to his family or they are kept in the hospital, according to the policies of the institution.

The physician is notified of the admission of the patient. If he presents an emergency problem, medical attention takes precedence over the admission routine just outlined. A written permission for operation is obtained as soon as this method of treatment is decided upon. A patient may sign his own permit for operation if he is of age and in his right mind. Before he gives his permission, he has a right to know the nature of the operation and what to expect after it. This is the responsibility of the surgeon. If the patient is a minor, unconscious or irresponsible, permission must be obtained from a relative. For this reason, it is wise to retain a member of the family at the time of admission until this point is decided. Also, this person may contribute greatly to the history of the patient's illness.

PSYCHOLOGICAL PREPARATION

This phase of the care of the patient cannot be overemphasized. It is an important part of the entire program of his care. One knows that any kind of surgical procedure always is preceded by some type of emotional reaction in a patient, whether it is obvious or not. The usual causes for such a disturbance are fear and worry.

Fear of anesthesia was justified years ago, when little was known of the control and the effect of anesthetic agents. But with refined methods, tested drugs and skilled anesthetists, the hazards are minimized. The ease with which a patient accepts an anesthetic today is attributed to the adequate physical and mental preparation that he receives. The price of poor preparation is a difficult period of induction, followed by an unpleasant emergence from the anesthetic agent. The nurse in her daily association with her patient can do much to dispel false conceptions and information. In instances in which the anesthetist visits the patient the day before surgery, real confidence is established, and the patient accepts the anesthetic more gracefully.

Often the fear of the anesthetic is secondary to the *fear of pain or of death*. Shall I feel the knife? What if the anesthesia wears off? The patient needs reassurance that the anesthetist will be in constant attendance to take care of these problems. Some surgeons will not operate on a patient who is convinced that he will die. This is a real fear, and it cannot be dismissed lightly. Good rapport between patient and nurse, together with tact on the nurse's part, may bring him to a realization that his fear is magnified. It will help him greatly if those responsible for his care build up his confidence.

The significance of *spiritual therapy* must not be forgotten. Regardless of the religious affiliation of the patient, the nurse must recognize that faith in a Higher Power can be as therapeutic as medication. Every attempt must be made to help the patient achieve the fullest spiritual help that he requests. This may be accomplished by participating in prayer, by reading passages of Scripture or by calling a clergyman. Such ministration by the nurse implies that she be informed about different religious beliefs. Faith has great healing power; the beliefs of each individual patient should be respected.

The average person has many *worries* when he is well, but he has more when he is ill. He may have financial problems, family responsibilities and employment obligations; in addition to these, he may fear a poor prognosis or the probability of a handicap in the future. These problems can be investigated by the nurse. If the difficulty is of such a nature that a medical social worker can give assistance, the aid of such a person should be enlisted. If the worry stems from fear of what the prognosis is likely to be, the physician should be informed.

Often the interval of time preparatory to surgery may drag. *Recreational and diversional activities,* such as reading, listening to the radio, handcrafts, games and so forth, are useful. The nurse can arrange for individuals with similar interests to meet. Many times patients can help one another.

The *fear of the unknown* is the worst of all. Therefore, the more understanding one has of the probabilities for the future, the better is the adjustment. The nurse can do much to allay the anxieties of her patient and induce a certain peace of mind. A patient frequently will express fears and misgivings to the nurse but hide them from the surgeon. In such circumstances the nurse should communicate these evidences of anxiety privately to the surgeon.

In her association with her patient, the nurse must be cautious and tactful. A detailed discussion of the medical problems of her patients does not come within her sphere. It is the physician's place to discuss surgical procedures, prognosis and future treatment. By doing so, much trouble can be avoided if the nurse knows her limitations, as well as her strong points, in her relationship to her patient.

Perhaps the most valuable facility at the disposal of the nurse is her ability to *listen* to the patient. By engaging in conversation and using the principles of tactful interviewing, the nurse can acquire invaluable bits of information. An unhurried, understanding and kind nurse invites confidence on the part of her patient.

Lastly, every patient should be treated as an individual who has fears and hopes quite apart from the fears and hopes of the next person. To understand and help one patient may require a completely different approach from that used on another.

EARLY PHYSICAL PREPARATION

Before treatment is initiated, the patient will be given a physical examination. The physician and the nurse must respect his feelings and his sense of modesty. In bathing her patient, the nurse may make significant physical findings, such as a rash, decubitus ulcer and so forth, that may be contributory.

There may be many diagnostic tests, such as blood specimens, roentgenographic studies, gastric analyses, tissue biopsies and stool and urine specimens. In all these tests the nurse plays an important part. She is in a position to help her patient to understand the need for diagnostic studies. She is aware that it is important to collect specimens and to describe them accurately in her charting. She must arrange for their safe transportation to the laboratory. The nurse knows that blood pressure, temperature, pulse and respiration are important indices of the condition of the patient and, therefore, must be charted correctly.

Preoperative Condition. Common conditions that affect a surgical risk may be dehydration and malnutrition. Perhaps the patient has been vomiting a considerable amount and, as a result, there is a disturbed fluid and electrolyte balance. To remedy this condition, the physician may order parenteral fluids, plasma and amino acids. In such a situation it is important to keep a good record of total intake and output. Malnutrition may be alleviated by high caloric diets with adequate vitamins and proteins. This is important, because vitamin C and protein are significant in tissue repair. Dental caries and poor mouth hygiene should be taken care of by the frequent use of a toothbrush and a mouthwash. The nurse has an opportunity to serve food attractively so that it will tempt the appetite of her patient. Hot foods should be served hot, nothing should be spilled, and the tray should be placed within comfortable reach of the patient.

Patients with associated cardiac, diabetic or respiratory complications may require appropriate treatment before operation. Obesity increases the seriousness of these complications to a great extent. For example, they shock easily, do not stand dehydration and often have crippled hearts and kidneys, the result being cyanosis, dyspnea and edema. Their fatty tissues are not highly resistant to infection; therefore, dehiscence and infected wounds are more common. They are difficult to nurse because of their weight, they breathe poorly when lying on their side and so are subject to hypoventilation and postoperative pulmonary complications, distention and phlebitis.

It is important for the nurse to remember the effect of old age or senescence. Reactions to injury are less pronounced and slower in appearing. Muscle rigidity often is almost nil, as in the case of acute appendicitis. The aged do not stand dehydration at all well. Their old chronic conditions of diabetes, anemia, obesity, hypoproteinemia and so forth must be considered. Certain drugs are dangerous because they are poorly tolerated. Scopolamine, morphia and the barbiturates are likely to cause confusion and disorientation, even excitement and apprehension. Some drugs have a cumulative effect. Sleeping and eating habits and the use of alcohol and laxatives, as well as the nightly "sleeping" medicine, must not be dismissed as unimportant.

To summarize, the preparation and the care of the patient before operation are guided by an understanding of him as an individual. *Our objective is known; that is, to get the patient into the best possible condition for surgery. The means of achieving that goal are determined by the needs of the individual patient.*

General Preoperative Nursing Care

Surgeons and hospitals differ greatly in the detail of preparation for operation, but the general principle remains the same: to make the patient as clean as possible, externally and internally, and to cause the least possible amount of physical and mental exhaustion in doing so. The reasons for preoperative procedures are obvious. All sources of infection must be eliminated, hence the scrupulous cleanliness of the operative site. The intestines and the bladder must be empty to prevent their contents from being discharged involuntarily while the patient is under the influence of the anesthetic and to preclude an accidental incision in them, as sometimes occurs in an abdominal operation when these organs are distended. This is true particularly of the bladder and is the chief reason why it must be empty before a patient is sent to the operating room for a laparotomy.

Any preparation of the patient before operation should be carried out in the most efficient and capable way. Never approach a patient with an air of indecision: to do so causes him to lose confidence at once, and lost confidence is not regained easily. Determine exactly what procedures or orders are to be performed and proceed with them in a systematic manner. If the treatment seems to be at all alarming to the patient, explain to him what you are about to do. Always work quietly and as quickly as possible, with thoroughness and neatness: bustle, confusion and noise harass the patient.

During this period of preparation, from the time of admission to the actual operation, one of the most important duties of the nurse is very close observation of the patient. Any sneezing, snuffling and coughing must be reported to the attending surgeon at once. Failure to do so may lead to postoperative pulmonary complications.

It should be the aim of every nurse to send her patient to the operating room in the best condition possible, so that convalescence will not be impaired. To this end she must remember that there is a great difference in the complaints of patients, and that any technic may have to be altered to suit individual needs. She must use her judgment and, when in doubt as to the advisability of a certain procedure, ask for instructions.

Bath. The patient should have a warm bath the night before operation.

Hair. A shampoo several days before operation is advisable, unless the condition of the patient does not warrant it.

Mouth and Teeth. The teeth should be brushed thoroughly twice a day and the mouth rinsed with a mild antiseptic solution at least three times a day.

Diet. When the operation is scheduled for the morning, the meal the evening before may be an ordinary light diet. Water may, and should be, given freely up to 4 hours before operation. In dehydrated patients, and especially in older ones, fluids often are encouraged by mouth before operation. In addition, and especially in cases in which fluids cannot be given by mouth, they are administered by venoclysis. If the operation is scheduled to take place after noon and is not to be upon any part of the gastro-intestinal tract, the patient may be given a soft diet for breakfast when nourishment is very necessary.

Starvation, exhaustion, prolonged loss of fluids from fistulous tracts or vomiting results in loss of calories, vitamins and proteins (hypoproteinemia). The preparation of such patients for operation demands the use of transfusions of blood, plasma or amino acid preparations. The particular vitamins needed may be added as indicated.

Enema. A warm soapsuds enema is given the evening before operation, and may be repeated if ineffectual. Unless the condition of the patient presents some contraindication, the commode, and not the bedpan, should be used in evacuating the enema.

Local (Skin) Preparation by Nurse

"The purpose of skin care preoperatively is to render the skin as clean and free of bacteria as possible without causing irritation or damage to the skin, without impairing its natural protective function, and without interfering with subsequent wound healing" (Knocke and Knocke). The patient should be prepared the evening prior to the day of operation. After the bath, the area in the region of the operative field is cleansed particularly by the use of warm water and soap. Any adhesive or grease may be removed readily with a sponge moistened in benzene or ether, if the odor is not objectionable to the patient. All hair must be shaved from the part to be operated upon. Be very sure to have a sharp razor and to shave thoroughly a sufficiently wide area. (It is embarrassing to have a surgeon call for a razor after the patient is placed on the operating table.) Scratches should be avoided, and any skin eruptions must be reported because they are potential sites of infection.

Instructions as to special preparation will be found under the various operations.

Some surgeons require nothing further in the way of local preparation than thorough shaving and cleansing of the part until the patient reaches the operating room. Others prefer to have the operative area washed further with an antiseptic solution, such as 1:1,000 Zephiran Chloride, and the area covered with a dry, sterile dressing. This procedure is carried out the evening before operation and is followed in the morning by applications of a germicide and another sterile dressing. Aseptic technic, sterile covers and sterile cotton swabs must be used in the method mentioned. An abdominal bandage usually is the most satisfactory to hold the sterile gauze dressings in place. This may be made of light-weight muslin and need not in itself be sterile. Extremities receiving sterile preparation should have sterile covers tied securely in place in such a way that they are not cramped. Before applying iodine, the skin must be perfectly dry. Washing and shaving should be done at least 6 hours before iodine is to be applied, as moisture interferes with the action of the drug. For this reason, shaving must be done without soap, and water must be omitted entirely when iodine is to be used in preparation for an emergency operation. Also, because of the danger of blistering, great care must be taken

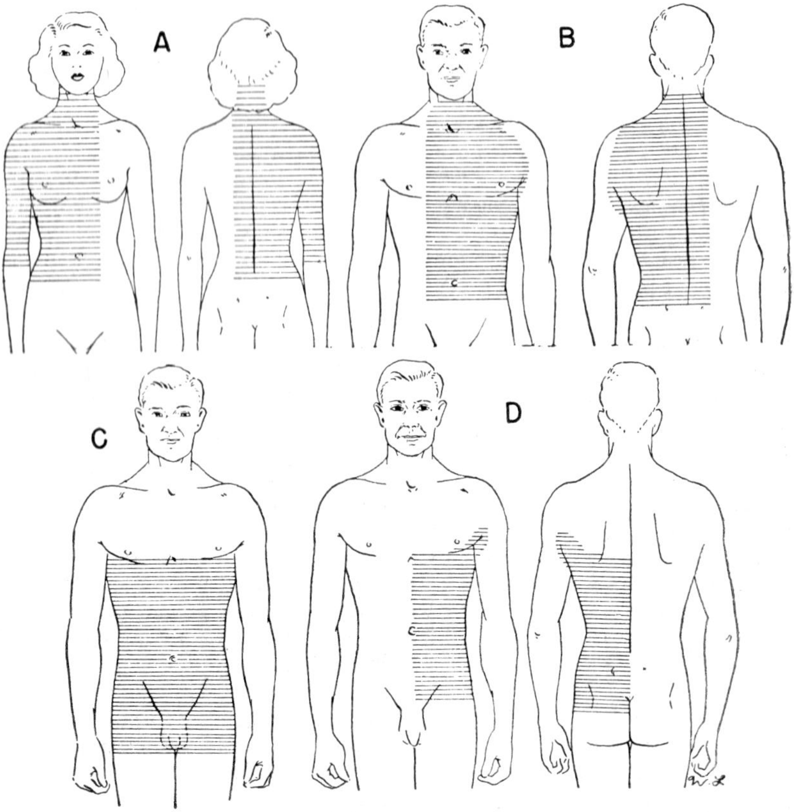

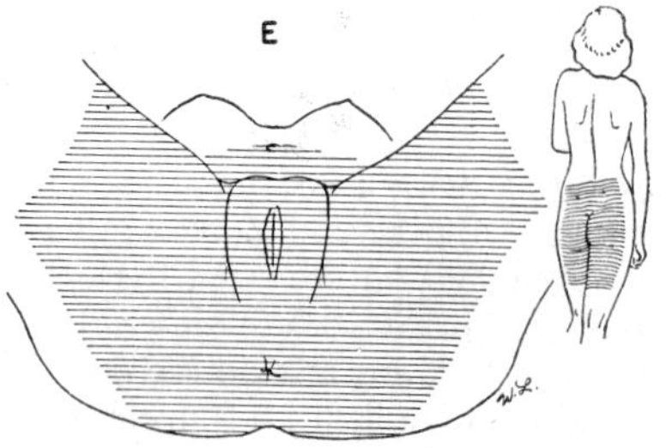

FIG. 11. Areas to be prepared for operation. The shaded areas are those to be shaved. (A) Preparation for amputation of breast. Note that the area to be prepared includes the front and the back of the trunk and extends from the neck to the umbilicus. The axilla and the upper portion of the arm also are included. (B) Area of preparation for operation on the thorax. (C) Area of preparation for operation upon the abdomen (laparotomy) and for hernia. The preparation should extend from the nipple line to well below the crest of the ilium. For herniorrhaphy the upper limit of preparation may be the area of the umbilicus. (D) Area to be prepared for nephrectomy. Note that the preparation should be on both the anterior and the posterior sides of the trunk. (E) Area to be prepared for operations on the perineum. These areas should be shaved completely for all gynecologic operations, operations around the anus and for such combined operations as an abdominoperineal resection of the rectum.

not to apply too much iodine. The skin never should be more than a very light brown in color. More than this is an excess and should be removed with alcohol. Iodine should not be used on the scalp, the face, the axilla, the perineum or the scrotum. In summer, iodine may, and often does, blister the sweaty skin.

When using solutions on the abdomen, be careful to prevent any excess from trickling down into the groins, as this may cause severe burns of the scrotum or the labia.

Nursing Preparation of Operative Field

Cranial Operations. Obtain specific instructions from the surgeon as to the extent of shaving that is necessary.

Thyroid and Neck Operations. Shave the anterior neck from under the chin to the nipple line. The area should be shaved back to the hair line and to meet the bed line when the patient is lying in the supine position.

Operations upon the Chest. Shave the affected side from the spine posteriorly to beyond the mid-line anteriorly, and from the clavicle to the umbilicus.

Breast Amputation. Shave the axilla on the affected side. Skin preparation should extend from above the clavicle to the umbilicus, from beyond the mid-line anteriorly to beyond the mid-line posteriorly. Particular care should be taken in cleansing the folds underneath the breast.

Operations upon the Abdomen. Shave from the nipple line in males and from below the breast in females to, and including, the pubic area. Laterally, shaving should extend to the anterior axillary line. Particular care should be taken in cleansing the umbilicus and the inguinal creases.

Inguinal Hernia. Shave the lower abdomen from the umbilicus downward, including the suprapubic area and about 6 inches of the upper thigh on the affected side. Particular attention should be paid to cleansing the groin.

Operations on the Lower Bowel and the Rectum. Shave the entire abdomen, as for any abdominal operation and, in addition, prepare the perineum as for any anal operation.

Anal Operations. Shave the area for a distance of about 10 inches from the anus. A suprapubic preparation is not necessary in male patients, but a partial perineal shave should be carried out in female patients.

Amputations. The area should be shaved and the skin cleansed for a distance of about 12 inches above and below the proposed site of amputation. It is important for the nurse to know where the amputation is to be performed. Thus, in gangrene of the foot, the amputation often is through the thigh, and it is necessary, therefore, to prepare the thigh.

Skin Grafts. Shave both anterior thighs or the area from which a graft is to be taken. Request instructions.

Operations upon the Spine. Shave and prepare the skin for an area of 12 inches above and below the site of operation. Ask the surgeon for instructions.

When the nurse is not sure about the area to be prepared, she always should ask for instructions.

Final Preparation of Patient by Nurse

The patient is called for by the nurse in the operating room about 20 minutes before the anesthesia is to be started. Previous to this the ward nurse clothes the patient in the regulation short gown, open in the back. Occasionally, long flannel stockings are added. Further, for a woman, long hair is plaited in two braids, all hairpins are removed, and the head and the hair are covered entirely with a lawn or thin muslin cap. The mouth must be inspected and all false teeth or plates, chewing gum and so forth removed. Jewelry should not be worn to the operating room; even wedding rings should be taken off. All articles of value, including false teeth, should be labeled clearly with the patient's name and left in charge of the head nurse. If a patient has any real objection to the removal of a ring, a narrow tape may be tied to the ring and then fastened securely around the patient's wrist.

All patients (except urologic cases) should void immediately before being sent to the operating room. Unless the patient is in a weakened condition, the use of the commode or bathroom rather than the bedpan should be urged. The bladder must be empty but, since catheterization is associated with 40 per cent of all cases of postoperative cystitis, this method of emptying it should not be resorted to except in an emergency. The amount of urine voided should be measured and recorded on a special slip or the anesthesia chart.

PREOPERATIVE MEDICATION

The administration of any anesthetic (general, spinal, regional or local) is facilitated greatly by use of preoperative medication. Such medication is ordered to meet the needs of the particular patient. The drugs used most commonly are (1) the opiates—morphine, Demerol, Pantopon, Dilaudid, (2) the belladonna derivatives—atropine, scopolamine, and (3) the barbiturates—phenobarbital, pentobarbital.

Opiates and barbiturates tend to allay the anxiety and the apprehension of the patient. They reduce also the metabolic rate and, by so doing, permit the induction of surgical anesthesia with smaller quantities of anesthetic agent. The belladonna derivatives reduce the amount of secretions in the mouth and the respiratory tract and help thereby to maintain a clear airway. They tend also to obtund certain harmful reflexes that may occur during operation on the chest and the abdomen.

These drugs should be given from 45 to 75 minutes before anesthesia is begun. Therefore, it is most important that the nurse give this medication precisely at the time it is ordered, otherwise it will have worn off or—what happens more often—it will not have begun to act when anesthesia is started.

Very frequently operations are delayed or schedules changed, and it becomes impossible to order medication for a given time. In these situations the preoperative medication is ordered "on call from operating room." Although this is far from ideal and should be avoided

GRACE-NEW HAVEN COMMUNITY HOSPITAL

DIVISION OR CLINIC: TOMP 3
NAME: Taylor, Roberta — 11333 UNIT NO.
ADDRESS: 247 Oak St. NH — 764170
BIRTH DATE: 8/5/17 NH BSM — Ward ACCOMMODATION

Check List for Pre-Operative Preparation

Check each item as it has been completed in the Pre-Operative preparation of the patient.

Operative permit (F.89): Signed by patient ✓ husband .... parent .... guardian ....

Dated 12-13-49 Witnessed ✓ Joanna Foster

Skin preparation: Done by Joanna Foster Checked by Miss Eachwell

Surgical bed prepared: ✓ Patient voided 600 cc. 10:10 P.M.

Medication given Demerol 0.075 gm. Atrop. Sulf. 0.0004 gm. Time given 10:10 P.M. Charting complete ✓

Anesthesia record (F.677) on chart ✓ Doctor's orders (F. 677-B) on chart ✓

Patient's Charge Card (F. 1141) (3 copies) on chart ✓

Artificial denture removed Removed Eyes —

Jewelry removed ✓ Wedding ring tied ✓ Hairpins, etc. removed ✓

Remarks:

Signature Joanna Foster
Nurse

F. 1165 — 62

FIG. 12. Preoperative check list which is attached to the patient's chart and is checked immediately before the patient is taken to the operating room.

whenever possible, the nurse can help by having the medication ready to give and by administering it as soon as the patient is called for. It usually takes from 15 to 20 minutes to get a patient ready for the operating room. If the nurse gives the medication before she attends to the other details of preparing the patient, she will have allowed the patient at least partial benefit of the preoperative medication and will have contributed thereby to a smoother and more pleasant anesthetic and operative course. A last-minute check concludes the preparation. (Fig. 12.)

TRANSPORTATION TO THE OPERATING ROOM

The patient then is transferred to the operating room in bed or on a previously prepared stretcher. This should be made as comfortable as possible and must be made up with a sufficient number of blankets to ensure against chilling from draughty corridors. A small pillow at the head usually is acceptable. There should be no question about the length of the top covers of the stretcher. They should be long enough to tuck in at both the patient's feet and shoulders. A shoulder blanket adds extra protection for the chest. The nurse always should remain with the patient until excused by one of the anesthetists. Often she is expected to aid in the transfer of the patient from the bed or stretcher to the operating table and to reassure the patient during the preliminary draping. The chart should be given to the anesthetist or a nurse; it never should be left with the patient.

Extremely ill patients, patients with fractures of the lower extremities, and all upper abdominal cases always should be sent to the operating room in bed.

CARE OF EMERGENCY CASES

Patients admitted as emergency cases may be classified conveniently as follows:

Acute inflammations—for example, acute appendicitis, ruptured duodenal or gastric ulcer and acute osteomyelitis.

Acute intestinal obstruction, due to strangulated hernia, peritoneal adhesions and carcinoma.

Acute traumatic conditions—for example, serious fractures, gunshot or stab wounds, severe burns and severe injuries of thorax, head or abdomen.

All such cases demand immediate attention. Therefore, every effort must be made to expedite the details of admission. The patient should be transferred at once from the receiving to the surgical ward, in order that no time may be lost in starting treatment. Even a short delay may be fatal.

The patient should be removed from the stretcher as soon as possible and placed in bed. To avoid delay, an emergency bed should be in readiness at all times. This should be made like a postoperative bed, with the addition of extra plastic sheet protection of the mattress so that the patient may be placed between blankets immediately. Any lifting or moving of the patient must be done with extreme caution, not only for the sake of comfort but for the prevention of further injury. Any bumping or jarring of the bed or stretcher is inexcusable.

Shock. After the patient has been placed in bed, he should be covered at once with warm blankets. Emergency cases are more or less shocked and must be protected thoroughly from draughts and exposure. In the presence of severe shock—rapid, thready pulse; subnormal temperature; irregular, shallow respirations; cold, moist skin, and marked general apathy—usually it is wiser to postpone removal of clothing until orders for stimulation and the treatment of shock have been carried out. The patient should be placed in the head low dorsal (Trendelenburg) position

(p. 108). If hypodermic injection or other medication is ordered, prepare and administer it immediately. Tetanus antitoxin is given in case of gunshot wounds and also in those which may have been contaminated with dirt. The efficient nurse prepares and is ready to give the antitoxin as soon as the resident physician arrives to prescribe it.

Hemorrhage. If hemorrhage has occurred and bleeding still persists, determine its nature and origin and make every attempt to arrest it. Arterial bleeding is characterized by spurts of bright red blood and is controlled best by the application of a tourniquet above the bleeding, or, when this is not possible, by direct pressure on the artery involved. In case of severe arterial hemorrhage, make pressure with anything, regardless of sterility, as unchecked arterial bleeding causes death in a very short time. Firm pressure with the thumb or the finger may be sufficient to save a life. Venous bleeding is darker in color than arterial bleeding and occurs as a steady flow. Oozing of blood is capillary in origin. Both of these may be checked by firm pressure with gauze pads and bandage (see p. 140).

Any temporary dressings or splints that have been applied before admission should be left intact until the doctor arrives. To disturb them may cause fresh hemorrhage or further trauma to the parts.

Undressing. Severely injured patients usually are given a hypodermic injection of morphine (by the doctor's orders, of course) before disturbing them for removal of clothes. Garments should be removed always from the uninjured or the least injured part first and then, with all gentleness, from the injured part. Cut the clothing when necessary but do not use the scissors thoughtlessly. Avoid as much as possible moving and turning the patient. Never expose the patient unnecessarily and provide ample protection from draughts. Work quickly and very carefully, as new injuries may be discovered in the process of undressing. Always be on the alert for these and report to the surgeon any unusual tenderness, bruises and contusions.

When removing clothing from severely burned patients, proceed with extra care and caution because of the added danger of hemorrhage. Often baths of saline will relieve the patient's pain and make removal of clothing easier.

Temperature, pulse and respiration should be taken and recorded as soon as possible after admission and hourly thereafter for 3 hours, after which every third hour is sufficient unless otherwise ordered.

Nothing should be given by mouth to an "emergency" patient until ordered by the physician. This precaution is taken in case an immediate operation has to be performed.

The first urine voided should be sent to the laboratory with a request for a "stat" report. If this specimen is not saved, much valuable information, as well as time, may be lost.

The preparation of emergency patients for operation usually is confined to the operative field and is essentially the same as the routine preparation. The area of operation is shaved and cleansed with green soap and an antiseptic, as already mentioned (p. 57). Do not try to remove temporary dressings in preparation for operation in cases of fracture or hemorrhage. Such dressings are left in place until after the patient has been anesthetized.

If at all feasible, the emergency patient more than any other should be sent to the operating room in bed rather than on a stretcher.

CHAPTER FIVE

The Patient in the Operating Room

GENERAL CONSIDERATIONS

The surgical patient usually is interested in and even concerned about the type of anesthesia that he is to receive. He has heard friends or relatives discuss the subject on the basis of personal experience or hearsay, and not infrequently he has formed definite opinions as to the merits or the demerits of the various methods in vogue. Therefore, it is helpful for the anesthetist to visit the patient in his own room before operation, introduce himself and point out that he has come for the purpose of allaying the fears that he knows exist in the minds of so many people. This preoperative contact builds up confidence and enables the patient to recognize a familiar face as he is being wheeled onto the operating floor. Uncertainty and anxiety are relieved, in part at least, and a much smoother course can be anticipated.

Today, with the increasing technical demands placed on the surgeon through bolder abdominal surgery, chest surgery, brain surgery and so forth, it is of the utmost importance that he be freed of the responsibility of watching the patient's anesthetic progress while he is operating. Consequently, the physician-anesthetist, especially trained in the art and the science of anesthesiology, has come into existence. To him, after consultation with the surgeon, can be delegated the choice of anesthesia, the technical problems relating to the administration of the anesthetic agent and the supervision of the patient's condition during the operation. This enables the surgeon to devote his entire energy to the operation proper. Such a "sharing" of responsibility obviously benefits the patient.

In the event that physicians so qualified are not available, the skill of nurses trained especially in anesthesia, preferably by a physician, must be called upon.

THE ANESTHETIZING ROOM

Upon arrival on the surgical floor, the patient should be met by the anesthetist and accompanied to the anesthetizing room. This room should adjoin the operating room: it should

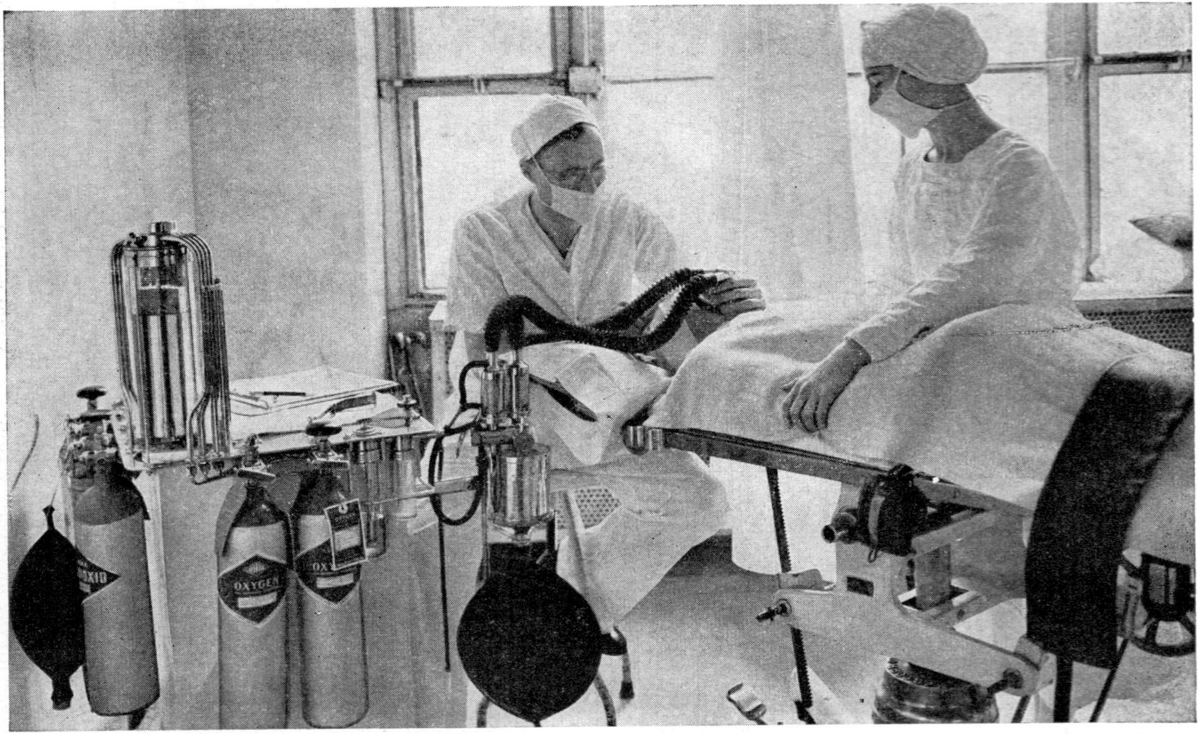

Fig. 13. Anesthesia, using nitrous oxide and oxygen. Note presence of nurse. Restraints are at hand, but they are not applied until the patient is under the influence of the anesthetic. The ether screen is placed in position just before the patient is draped.

be quiet, well lighted and commodious, and the personnel should reflect an air of cheerful and efficient activity, without rush and hurry. In this room the patient is transferred to the operating table, and a last-minute check of his condition is made, blood pressure, pulse and respiratory rates in particular being noted. Then the anesthetic previously selected is administered. When all is in readiness for the beginning of the operation, the patient is wheeled into the operating room.

TYPES OF ANESTHESIA

Anesthetics have been divided into two classes according to whether they suspend the sensations (1) of the whole body (general anesthetics) or (2) of parts of the body (local, regional or spinal anesthetics). General anesthesia can be obtained by inhalation, intravenous or rectal technic.

Inhalation Anesthesia

The inhalation anesthetics in common usage are:

Ether, chloroform, ethyl chloride and Vinethene—liquids producing anesthesia by inhalation of their vapor.

Nitrous oxide, ethylene and cyclopropane—gases also administered by inhalation, usually in combination with oxygen.

These substances, when inhaled, enter the blood through the pulmonary capillaries and, when in sufficient concentration, act on the cerebral centers in such a manner as to produce loss of consciousness and of sensation. When the administration of the anesthetic has been discontinued, the vapor or gas is eliminated via the lungs in respiration.

STAGES OF ANESTHESIA

Anesthesia generally is described as having four stages, each of which presents a rather definite group of symptoms.

Stage of Beginning Anesthesia

As the patient breathes in the anesthetic vapor, a feeling of warmth steals over his body, dizziness is experienced, and he seems to be detached from the world. He experiences a ringing, roaring or buzzing in his ears and then, though still conscious, he is aware that he is unable to move his limbs voluntarily. During this stage noises are greatly exaggerated; even low voices or minor sounds appear distressingly loud and unreal. For this reason, unnecessary noise or motion must be prevented at all costs while anesthesia is being started.

Stage of Excitement

This stage—characterized variously by struggling, shouting, talking, singing, laughing or even crying—frequently may be avoided by judicious suggestion before anesthesia is begun and by its even and slow administration. The pupils of the eyes are dilated, but contract if exposed to light, the pulse rate is rapid, and respiration is irregular.

Because of the uncontrolled movements of the patient during this stage, the anesthetist always should be attended by a nurse and an orderly, who should be ready to apply restraining straps if occasion demands. The patient should not be touched except for purposes of restraint, and in no circumstances should there be any palpation of the operative site.

Stage of Surgical Anesthesia

The stage of surgical anesthesia is reached by continued administration of the vapor or gas. The patient is then entirely unconscious, lying quietly on the table with muscles relaxed and with most reflex actions abolished. The pupils are small, but they retain their contractile power on exposure to light. Respiration is regular and slightly more shallow than normal, the pulse rate is about normal and of good volume, and the skin is pink or slightly flushed. By proper administration of the anesthetic this stage may be maintained for hours.

Stage of Danger

This stage is reached when too much anesthesia has been given and when the patient has not been observed carefully. The respiration becomes shallow, the pulse weak and thready; the pupils become widely dilated and no longer contract when exposed to light. Cyanosis develops gradually and, unless prompt action is taken, death follows rapidly. If this stage should develop, the anesthetic is discontinued immediately, and artificial respiration is given. Stimulants may be administered.

During the administration of an anesthetic, there is, of course, no sharp division between the various stages. The patient passes gradually from one stage to another, and it is only by close observation of the signs exhibited by the patient that an anesthetist can have complete control of the situation. The condition of the pupils and the respiratory and the cardiac rates are probably the most reliable guides to the patient's condition. The anesthetist should focus his attention entirely on the patient and not be diverted by an interest in the details of the operation or by other activities of the room.

The administration of an anesthetic is attended by other physiologic activities that have not been mentioned. Some anesthetics, especially ether, produce a hypersecretion of mucus and saliva. This may be eliminated largely by the preoperative administration of atropine. Vomiting occurs not infrequently, especially when the patient comes to the operating room with a full stomach. The head should be turned sharply to the side, if gagging occurs, and a basin provided to collect the vomitus. The head of the table should be lowered to permit material to flow out of the mouth by gravity. Suction apparatus always should be available.

During the anesthesia, the temperature may fall. Because of this, every precaution should be taken against chilling him. A warm bed and blankets always should be provided. Sugar metabolism is much reduced, with the result that acidosis may develop.

In addition to the dangers of the anesthetic itself, the anesthetist must guard against asphyxia. If the operation is in the mouth or the nose, this may be due to foreign bodies in the mouth or falling back of the tongue or aspiration of vomitus, saliva or blood.

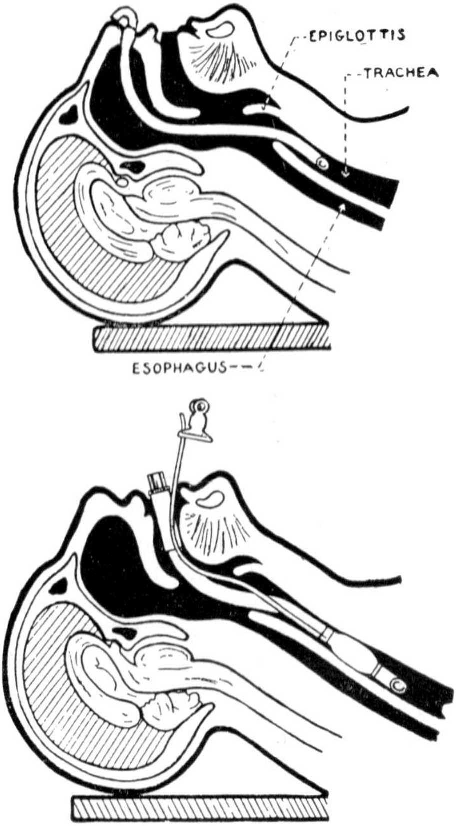

FIG. 14. Endotracheal anesthesia. (*Top*) Magill tube in proper position, intranasal intubation being used. Note metal elbow at proximal end of tube. This adaptor is used to keep the tube from entering the nose beyond reach of extubation. It can be used also to attach to anesthetic equipment. (*Bottom*) Oral intubation. The tube in position with the cuff inflated. (Surgical Equipment, September, 1949)

METHODS OF ADMINISTRATION

Open-Drop Method

This method is used for the anesthetics that are liquid. The fluid is dropped slowly on several (eight) layers of gauze held over the patient's nose and mouth. The patient inhales the vapor that evaporates from the gauze. Care must be taken to prevent a drop of the anesthetic from entering the eye. If this occurs, the eye should be irrigated immediately with saline solution and followed by a drop of sterile liquid petrolatum.

Vapor or Gas Administration with Mask

Liquid anesthetics may be given by causing the patient to breathe air or oxygen containing the vapor arising from the fluid. Ether, especially, is used in this manner, frequently in combination with the gas anesthetics. The vapor is conducted to the patient by a tube and a mask.

The gases (nitrous oxide, ethylene, cyclopropane and oxygen) are contained in tanks under pressure and are allowed to escape at the proper rate through valves opening into a mixing chamber, usually a large rubber bag. The bag is connected by a flexible tube to a mask, which is put over the patient's face. A reservoir containing ether often is attached to the mechanism so that, by turning a valve, a regulated amount of ether vapor may be given with the gas if this is desired.

Intrapharyngeal Anesthesia

Many operations upon the mouth and the lower part of the face will not permit the use of the ordinary inhaler. After anesthesia has been induced in these cases, it is possible to continue its administration by the introduction of ether by the vapor method, through small rubber tubes that lead into the pharynx by way of the nostrils.

Endotracheal Anesthesia

The endotracheal technic consists of introducing a soft rubber or other variety of tube directly into the trachea, either by exposing the larynx with a laryngoscope or by passing it "blindly." It may be inserted either through the nose or the mouth.

This technic has many advantages, but the most important is the most obvious—the patient has an almost perfect airway. There is no danger of respiratory obstruction, either from the falling back of the tongue against the posterior pharyngeal wall (swallowing the tongue) or from spasm of the vocal cords. The endotracheal method has its greatest use in chest surgery, in which the thorax is open and the patient must depend upon the anesthetist to assist him in breathing or take over breathing for him completely by rhythmic compression of the breathing bag. But many other types of operation have been made possible or made safer by this technic: for example, neurosurgical, dental, plastic and nose and throat procedures, in which the anesthetist does not have immediate access to the patient's face, or any procedure on a patient in whom, because of obesity or anatomic abnormality, the airway may become compromised under anesthesia.

Another important advantage of endotracheal intubation is that it provides a convenient method of aspirating secretions, blood or other foreign material from the trachea and the bronchi. This is not only important in anesthesia, but it is invaluable in the nursing care of very ill patients.

INHALATION ANESTHETIC AGENTS

Ether

Ether generally is considered the best and the safest of the general anesthetics. It is a clear, volatile, inflammable fluid. It may be given by any of the methods mentioned.

Advantages. It produces anesthesia with relaxation admirably suited for surgical operations.

It is not highly toxic and it has a wide margin of safety between the dosage required for anesthesia and the toxic dose. The signs of a toxic dosage usually appear in sufficient time to allow for resuscitation of the patient and avoid a fatal outcome.

No accurate statistics are available, but various authors give mortality figures at from one death in 16,000 to one in 30,000.

In emergencies, ether may be given by unskilled persons under the guidance of the surgeon.

Disadvantages. Ether vapor, especially in high concentration, irritates the respiratory mucous membrane only when it has been administered improperly or when the patient has not received adequate care in the immediate postoperative period. Nonetheless, in the presence of respiratory diseases it is advisable to avoid ether whenever possible.

The period of induction and of "coming out" is longer than for most of the other anesthetics.

There are certain complications that not infrequently follow ether administration. Pulmonary complications are supposed to occur more frequently after ether due to irritation of the respiratory mucosa. The commonest forms of complication are acute bronchitis, bronchopneumonia and atelectasis. Ether causes some irritation of the renal epithelium and, for this reason, it should be used sparingly in cases of nephritis, especially of the acute type associated with septic diseases. Diminution or suppression of urine may result.

Vinethene

Vinethene is a clear, colorless volatile liquid. When given by the slow-drop method on gauze over the nostrils, it produces a rapid and a not unpleasant anesthesia from which the patient recovers rapidly with little or no nausea or vomiting. It is useful for short anesthesia. Kidney damage and liver damage may follow its use, particularly if it is given for operations of long duration.

Chloroform

Chloroform is a colorless, sweet-smelling liquid. It is noninflammable and less volatile than ether. Its anesthetic strength is about seven times greater than that of ether; therefore, its administration requires more skill and more careful observation than ether.

It is given commonly by the most open method possible. The drug is dropped very slowly upon the gauze or inhaler at a rate of about one drop for each inhalation. Chloroform produces rapid anesthesia with little struggling on the part of the patient.

Advantages. The patients go under and emerge from the influence of the anesthetic rapidly. For this reason it is used at times for short operations on children and in obstetric cases.

It produces practically no respiratory irritation; therefore, it may be useful at times when operation is necessary in the case of a patient suffering from a respiratory disease.

Disadvantages. It is such a powerful anesthetic that it is too dangerous for ordinary use. "The danger of chloroform is that it is possible for a healthy person to inhale a poisonous dose in a single breath." The margin of safety, therefore, is very small. It is contraindicated when there is an associated disease of the heart.

The administration of chloroform for any length of time may cause degenerative changes in the liver (acute yellow atrophy) and the adrenals that may prove fatal several days after operation.

Chloroform is considered to be a rather dangerous anesthetic by most

American surgeons, and for this reason it is used little in this country.

Ethyl Chloride

Ethyl chloride at ordinary room temperature is a gas, but it is dispensed usually under compression and put up in glass tubes with a tiny hole in one end through which the fluid is allowed to escape as desired.

As an anesthetic it is rapid in its action and is administered by inhalation. It is used occasionally for short anesthesia and as a preliminary to ether. The rapid action of the drug makes it very dangerous for general use.

Nitrous Oxide

Nitrous oxide ("laughing gas," "sweet air," N_2O) is a colorless gas with a sweetish odor. It is administered from compression tanks through tubes that connect with a tight-fitting mask. It may be given in the pure state for a few minutes, in which case it produces narcosis, but it has the disadvantage of giving rise to a deep cyanosis due to its exclusion of oxygen from the lungs. For this reason it is given generally so that 8 parts of oxygen are mixed with 92 parts of nitrous oxide. This mixture may be varied by easily adjustable valves (according to the needs of the patient). If cyanosis develops (which is looked upon as the surest danger signal for this anesthesia) more oxygen may be given until the normal color returns. Nitrous oxide frequently is administered in combination with ether vapor.

Advantages. It produces rapid anesthesia from which the patient recovers quickly; therefore, it is useful for short procedures on patients who are to remain ambulatory.

For long, shocking operations, especially abdominal sections, it is, in combination with the slightest possible amount of ether, one of the best of the general anesthetics.

Its after-effects (nausea and vomiting) are slight.

It produces little respiratory irritation; therefore, it may be used when patients have a respiratory disease.

Disadvantages. Nitrous oxide can be administered only by a skilled anesthetist who has had special experience in its use.

Such large amounts of nitrous oxide are required for the production of anesthesia that often the concentrations of oxygen available are not adequate. For this reason it must be used with caution in those individuals whose reserves are low and who cannot withstand even short periods without oxygen. Such individuals include those suffering from arteriosclerosis, high blood pressure, heart disease, anemia, brain damage and so forth.

It does not act well in prolonged operations upon alcoholics.

It is difficult to use in the dark-skinned races, because of the fact that the color of the skin, the index of cyanosis, cannot be of much service.

Ethylene

Ethylene is a colorless, highly inflammable gas possessing a characteristic sweetish odor that reminds one somewhat of burnt matches. It is dispensed in pressure tanks that are used with an inhalation apparatus such as that used for nitrous oxide. The concentration employed for surgical anesthesia is generally 90 per cent ethylene and 10 per cent oxygen, though after a prolonged period of anesthesia a deep anesthetic state may be maintained on 80 per cent ethylene.

Advantages. Rapid induction of anesthesia and rapid recovery.

No irritation of the respiratory mucous membrane.

Satisfactory relaxation without cyanosis.

Disadvantages. It has an odor that is offensive to some.

Oozing from wounds seems to be increased, and the clotting time is prolonged.

Cyclopropane

Cyclopropane is one of the more recent anesthetic gases. It is much more potent than nitrous oxide or ethylene and can produce anesthesia in concentrations of from 15 to 20 per cent. The remainder of the anesthetic mixture can consist of oxygen; therefore, the patient has a more than adequate supply at all times. Cyclopropane is particularly nonirritating and is of value for surgical patients who have respiratory diseases as a complicating factor. It is a powerful depressant to breathing, and for this reason should be administered only by an expert. Occasionally, marked disorders of the heart rate and rhythm occur during cyclopropane anesthesia.

Explosibility

All the inhalation anesthetics discussed, with the exception of nitrous oxide and chloroform, form explosive mixtures with air or oxygen. Therefore, they should be avoided if possible when the electric cautery, the electric desiccator and so forth are to be used. In addition, the spark of static electricity may set off an explosion. For this reason woolen blankets should not be used to cover the patient on the operating table. Nor should sharkskin or silk uniforms be permitted near the gas machine or the anesthetized patient. Finally, no one should touch the patient in the vicinity of the breathing mask lest a spark be generated and cause an explosion. The hazard of explosion is present always, but such unfortunate accidents will be extremely rare if common sense is exercised.

D-Tubocurarine Chloride

D-tubocurarine, a synthetic drug with the peculiar property of preventing nerve impulses from reaching striated muscles, is being used now as an adjunct in anesthesia. It is in no sense an anesthetic agent, but it is given in conjunction with the various general anesthetic agents to provide muscular relaxation without deep anesthesia. Serious depression of respiration may occur if the dose given is too great, and careful observation of the volume of breathing is of particular importance.

Other similar acting drugs are succinylcholine, Syncurine and Metubine.

Intravenous Anesthesia

General anesthesia also can be produced by the intravenous injection of various substances. Two extremely short-acting barbiturates—Pentothal and Surital—are the anesthetics in most common use today for this purpose. These substances lead to unconsciousness within 30 seconds. The onset of anesthesia is extremely pleasant; there is none of the buzzing, the roaring or the dizziness known to follow the administra-

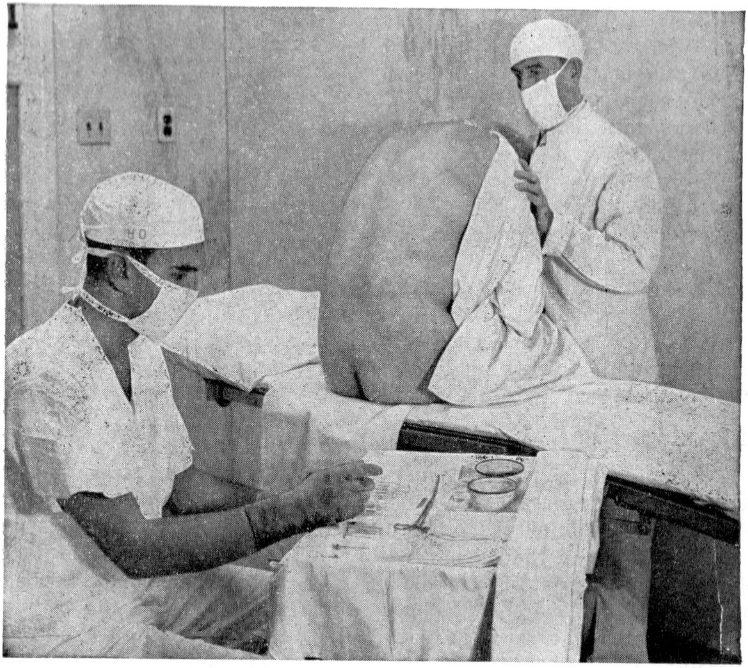

FIG. 15. Sitting position for spinal puncture.

tion of an inhalation anesthetic. For this reason intravenous anesthesia is the favorite of patients who have experienced various methods. The duration of action is brief, and the patient awakens with little nausea or vomiting. Pentothal frequently is given in addition to other anesthetic agents. It is especially useful to relieve the anxiety of the patient with spinal anesthesia.

Pentothal and Surital are powerful depressants of breathing, and their chief danger lies in this characteristic. They should be administered only by skilled anesthetists and only when some method of giving oxygen is available immediately should trouble arise. Sneezing, coughing and choking are noted occasionally.

Intravenous anesthesia has the advantage of being nonexplosive, of requiring little equipment and of being so easy to take. The low incidence of postoperative nausea and vomiting makes the method useful in eye surgery, in which retching endangers vision in the operated eye. It is useful in short procedures, but is used less often for abdominal surgery. It is not indicated for children, who have small veins and who are more susceptible to respiratory obstruction. The reasons in both instances are apparent.

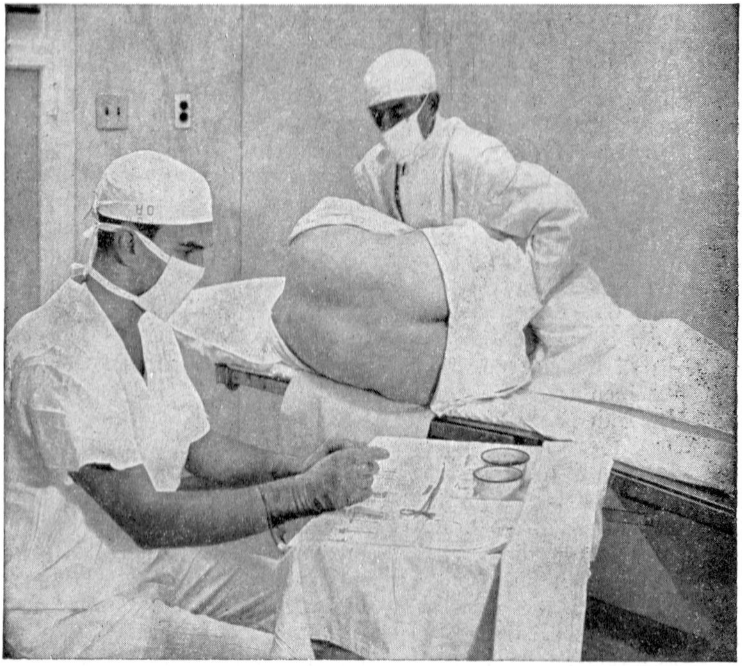

Fig. 16. Spinal anesthesia being given in lateral position. Note position of assistant, one arm behind the patient's knees and the other behind patient's neck in order to arch the back.

Rectal Anesthesia

This term really is incorrect. It is not safe to produce total anesthesia by placing anesthetics in the rectum. A more proper use of the method is the production of *basal narcosis*. This means a partial anesthesia, the rectal anesthetic being supplemented by some other form of anesthesia, either inhalation or local as a rule.

Avertin fluid (tribromethyl alcohol) is used most frequently for this purpose. It is dissolved in water to make from 2.5 to 3 per cent solution. Dosage is based on body weight and, in the average case, varies from 60 to 100 mg. per Kg. The solution should be tested for acidity before being injected, since the drug may decompose into acids that will irritate the rectum. Injection of the solution is made slowly, with the patient lying on his side. After from 5 to 15 minutes, the patient falls into an apparently natural sleep. He must be watched carefully lest there be any obstruction to breathing. The duration of the narcotic effect is prolonged, and careful attention must be paid in the postoperative period, since occasionally depression is profound.

Spinal Anesthesia

It must never be forgotten that the patient under spinal, regional or local anesthesia is awake and aware of his surroundings. Careless conversation, unnecessary noise, unpleasant odors—all are noticed by the patient on the operating table and reflect discredit on the operating room staff. Quiet must be insisted upon. The diagnosis must not be made aloud if the patient is not to be made aware of it at once.

Anesthesia of the lower extremities, the abdomen and even of the chest may be induced by the introduction of anesthetic drugs into the subarachnoid space (Figs. 15 and 16). A spinal puncture is made with sterile precautions, and the drug is injected in solution through the needle. As soon as the injection has been made, the patient is placed on his back and shoulder braces are adjusted. As a rule, the head and the shoulders are lowered, depending on the height of anesthesia desired. In a few minutes anesthesia and paralysis appear, first of the toes and the perineum and then gradually of the legs and the abdomen. The drugs generally used are procaine, Pontocaine and Nupercaine.

Advantages. It is administered easily, it is inexpensive and it requires a minimum of equipment. The anesthesia produced usually is rapid in onset, and there is excellent muscular relaxation. The patient may remain awake, if that is desirable. It is a relatively safe anesthesia in experienced hands. Mortality figures compare favorably with those of the safer general anesthetics.

Disadvantages. Soon after the administration of the drug there may be a marked fall in blood pressure, caused by a paralysis of the vasomotor nerves. This phenomenon is noted most often when the anesthesia ascends to the upper abdomen and the chest. It has been shown that the preoperative administration of drugs such as ephedrine or methoxamine may be used to prevent the marked decrease in blood pressure. If the pressure becomes low, the patient's head usually is lowered to maintain an adequate cerebral circulation. The inhalation of oxygen, the intravenous administration of blood, plasma or saline and the injection of stimulant drugs such as ephedrine, Neosynephrin and methoxamine, or phenylephrine, are measures of value once the blood pressure has fallen. Nausea, vomiting and pain not infrequently occur during surgery under spinal anesthesia. As a rule, this is due to traction on various structures, particularly those within the abdominal cavity. These reactions may be avoided by the simultaneous intravenous administration of a weak solution of Pentothal.

When the anesthetic drug reaches the upper thoracic and cervical cord in high concentration, a temporary, partial or complete respiratory paralysis may occur. This complication is treated by maintaining artificial respiration until the effects of the drug on the respiratory nerves have worn off. The Drinker respirator has been used occasionally for this purpose.

Such postoperative complications as headaches, paralysis or meningitis may occur. Research continues to be done in an effort to establish the cause of lumbar puncture headache.

Evidence seems to indicate that several factors are involved: the size of the spinal needle used, the leakage of fluid from the subarachnoid space, the activity of the patient and the degree of the patient's hydration. Any measure which can increase the cerebrospinal pressure is helpful in relieving headache. These include keeping the patient flat and quiet, applying a tight abdominal binder and injecting fluid into the subarachnoid space.

In addition to taking the blood pressure, the nurse should observe these patients closely and make notes as to the time of return of motion and sensation in the legs and the toes. When there is complete return of sensation in the toes, the patient may be considered to have recovered from the effects of the spinal drug.

SERIAL SPINAL

Two real objections to spinal anesthesia are (1) that the surgeon has to work to time—he must finish his work before the anesthesia wears off and (2) that the entire dose must be given at once, and harm may result if one's calculations are incorrect: the patient may not have enough anesthesia or he may have too much.

To overcome these objections a method of prolonging spinal anesthesia was devised—so-called continuous or serial spinal. A malleable needle made of German silver is used for the lumbar puncture. This is left in place, and to accommodate it when the patient is turned on his back a special mattress is employed. This is 5 inches thick and has a large hole cut in it. The needle protrudes into this hole. From the needle a small-bore rubber tube is connected to a syringe containing the anesthetic solution. In some hospitals a fine ureteral (Touhy) catheter may be introduced into the dural sac through a needle. The needle is removed, leaving the catheter in place. With this technic a special mattress is not necessary. Repeated injections of the spinal anesthetic are possible. Anesthesia can be prolonged indefinitely, and for poor-risk patients small doses can be used at first. If these are sufficient, well and good; if not, more can be added. The hazard of guessing at the dose thus is minimized.

Regional Anesthesia

Regional anesthesia is that branch of local anesthesia in which, by an injection into or round the nerves, the area supplied by these nerve trunks is anesthetized. There are many types of this anesthesia, depending upon the various nerve groups that are injected.

Brachial Plexus Block. This produces anesthesia of the arm.

Paravertebral Anesthesia. This produces anesthesia of the spinal nerves supplying the abdominal wall and the viscera.

Transsacral Caudal Block. This produces anesthesia of the perineum and, occasionally, the lower abdomen.

The most recent addition to obstetric anesthesia has been an adaptation of caudal block analogous to the change from a single-injection spinal to serial spinal. This adaptation is called *continuous or serial caudal.* A malleable needle or a nylon ureteral catheter is inserted into the caudal canal just above the tip of the coccyx. This is allowed to remain in place and is attached by a rubber tube to a reservoir of anesthetic solution. When the woman in labor complains of pain, an injection is made, and subsequent injections are given as indicated. These may be continued for from 20 to 30 hours. The patient is conscious during the entire labor, and the fetus is spared the depression caused by drugs given to relieve maternal distress. The mechanism of labor is changed somewhat by this method. The second stage is longer, and operative deliveries are more frequent.

The method is not entirely without harm. Infections have occurred at the site of the injection. The level of anesthesia may become too high, and respiratory and circulatory difficulties may follow. With a drop in blood pressure the fetus may be endangered. Convulsions can occur, and the nurse should report at once any marked restlessness, anxiety, tremor or twitching.

Local Infiltration Anesthesia

Infiltration anesthesia is the injection of a solution containing the local anesthesia into the tissues through which the incision is to pass. Often it is combined with a local regional block by injection of the nerves immediately supplying that area.

In operations upon the abdominal viscera, complete anesthesia is not obtained by infiltration or local block of the anterior abdominal wall, because the viscera are supplied by nerves that have not been affected by the anesthetic. For this reason, a separate injection must be made into the region of the splanchnic nerves, which supply the abdominal organs, except those of the pelvis. This injection may be made from the back (posterior-splanchnic anesthesia), or anteriorly, after opening the abdomen.

COCAINE

Cocaine is a white crystalline powder that is soluble readily in water.

Uses. In from 1 to 4 per cent for anesthesia of the eye or of the mucous surface of the nose, the mouth, the urethra and so forth.

In from 0.1 to 1 per cent solutions for anesthetizing the skin.

In crystalline form for application to mucous surfaces.

Disadvantages. It is highly poisonous, 1 gr. being regarded as the maximum dose for subcutaneous injections. Even this dose may produce acute toxic symptoms if rapidly absorbed or injected into a vein. The cause of the poisoning is the action of the drug on the centers of the medulla, causing respiratory failure and cardiac depression. The first symptom is a feeling of faintness. Nausea and vomiting occur, the pulse rate increases, and respiratory failure follows. In the event of cocaine poisoning with respiratory paralysis, life may be saved if artificial respiration is practiced until the effect of the drug wears off.

Prolonged sterilization by heat decomposes the drug.

PROCAINE

Procaine is the least toxic of the local anesthetics. It is used in ½ and 1 per cent solutions, and as much as 2 Gm. may be injected without toxic effects. It has supplanted cocaine for general use. Although its effects as an anesthetic are not quite as marked as those of cocaine, its lack of toxicity recommends its use.

Advantages. It may be sterilized by heat.

It is very slightly toxic.

Its anesthetic effects are sufficiently potent for all ordinary requirements.

NUPERCAINE (PERCAINE)

This drug is a much more powerful anesthetic agent than procaine. It is used in concentrations of 1:1,000 physiologic saline for injection anesthesia and in concentrations of 1:50 physiologic saline for application to the surface in nose and throat surgery. The appearance of anesthesia is less rapid than with the other anesthetic agents, but its duration is much longer, lasting often for from 2 to 3 hours. It is the most toxic of the local anesthetics.

EPINEPHRINE (ADRENALIN)

Local anesthesia is administered often in combination with epinephrine (5 to 10 minims to the ounce). Epinephrine has the property of causing a local constriction of the blood vessels, which in turn prevents rapid absorption of the anesthetic drug and so prolongs its local action.

CONTRAINDICATIONS FOR LOCAL ANESTHESIA

Local anesthesia is the anesthesia of choice in every operation in which it can be used. However, it is contraindicated in surgical operations upon highly nervous, apprehensive patients. The trauma, both mental and nervous, experienced by these individuals under a local anesthesia may be more harmful than that following a general anesthetic. A patient who begs to be put to sleep rarely does well under local anesthesia.

TECHNIC OF LOCAL ANESTHESIA

The technic for the introduction of local infiltration requires few extraordinary materials. For the ordinary case the following are all that are needed:

1. Flask of sterile ½ per cent procaine solution.
2. Sterile beaker or medicine glass.
3. Sterile syringes and needles to fit. If the syringe and the needles are kept in alcohol, they should be rinsed thoroughly in sterile water before being used.
4. Sterile sponges.

The skin is prepared as for an operation and, with a small-gauge needle, a little of the anesthetic is injected into the skin layers. This produces a blanching or wheal. The anesthetic then is carried ahead of the needle in the skin until an area as long as the proposed incision is anesthetized. A larger, longer needle then is used to infiltrate the deeper tissues with the anesthetic. The action of the drug is almost immediate, so that the operation may begin as soon as the injection is finished. The anesthesia lasts from ½ hour to 1 hour.

Refrigeration Anesthesia

This means the chilling of tissues in an extremity. It is not freezing and does not damage tissues, which freezing does. It has many advantages in certain conditions of trauma, infection and gangrene in the extremities, particularly in face of the factors of age and the necessity for delayed surgery.

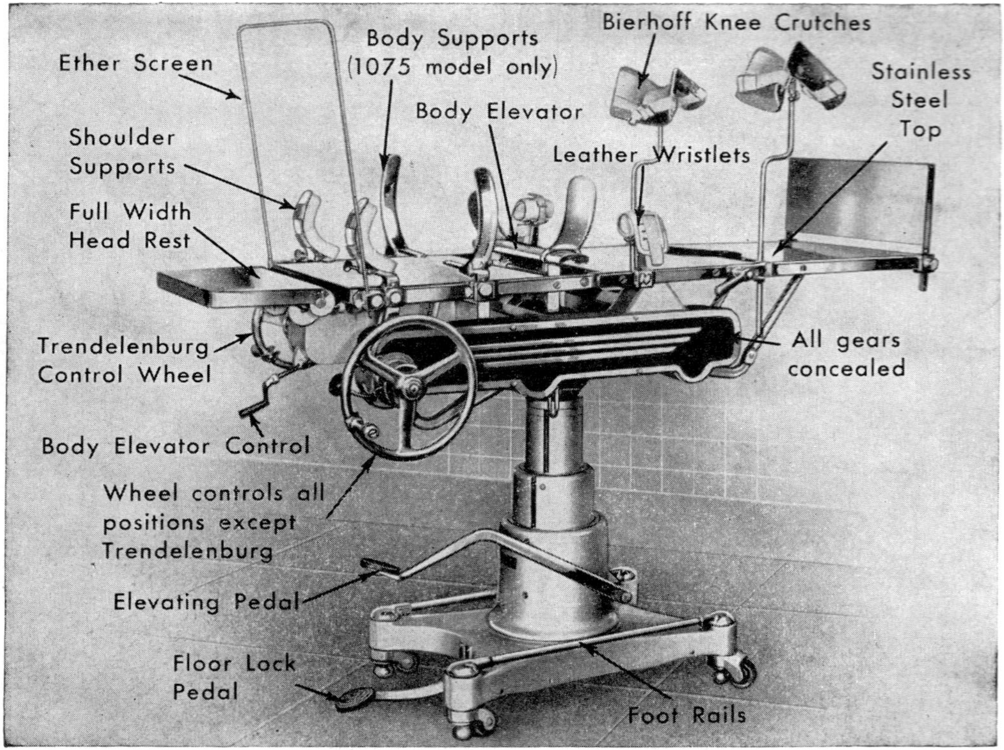

FIG. 17. Operating table. (American Sterilizer Co., Erie, Pa.)

Technic of Administration. Refrigeration anesthesia is done on the ward. The patient is told about the procedure and receives his preoperative medication. His leg is elevated for about 5 minutes, and ice bags are placed around the area where the tourniquet is to be applied to reduce discomfort due to pressure. Any method may be used to enclose the ice as it comes in contact with the extremity. However, several precautions must be observed. The patient must be protected from chilling by applying an extra blanket around his uninvolved leg, protecting his genitalia with additional covering and providing a shoulder blanket. Pro-

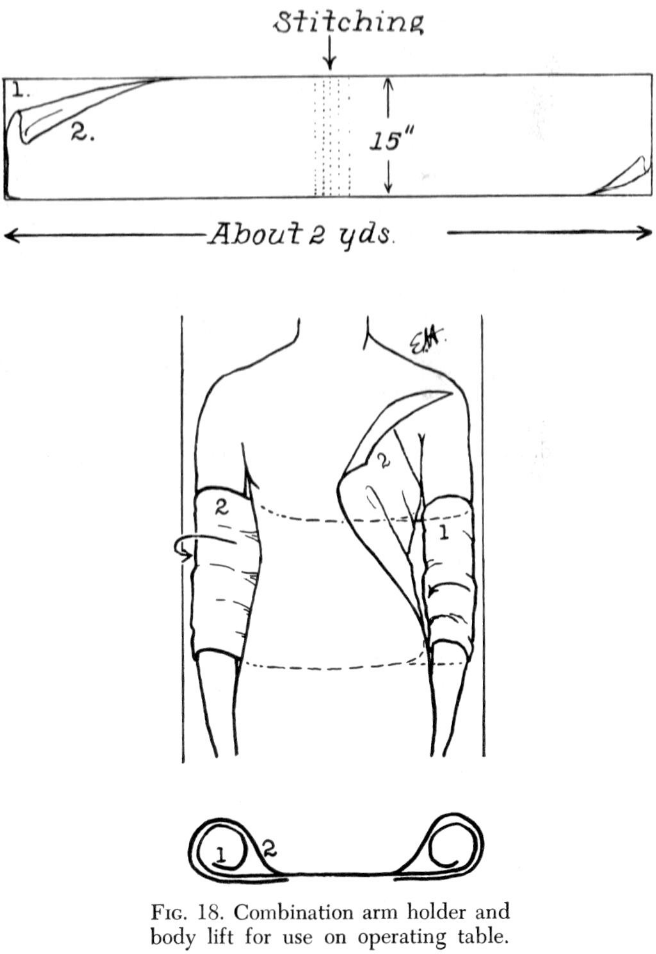

FIG. 18. Combination arm holder and body lift for use on operating table.

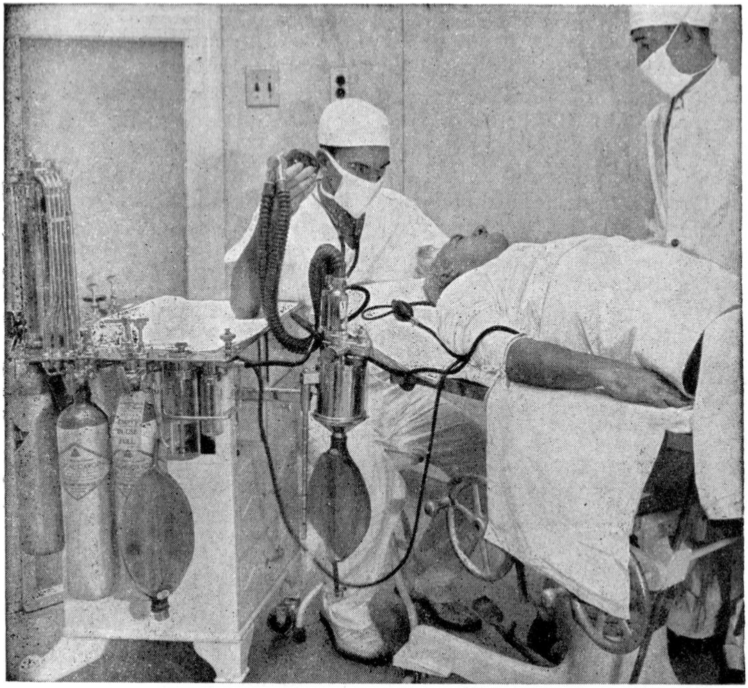

FIG. 19. Patient on operating table ready for anesthesia, with blood pressure cuff applied. Note presence of orderly. Arm holder-lift ready for use.

vision should be made to allow for drainage of the melted ice by forming a trough which slopes downward into a bucket at the foot of the bed. As was mentioned before, it is disastrous to freeze the limb. The temperature should not fall below 2° C. This requires from 1½ hours in the lower leg to from 2½ to 3 hours in the thigh. The refrigeration is not interrupted until the operation is about to start. The anesthesia will last from 1 to 1½ hours.

Postoperative Nursing Care

The stump usually is surrounded with icebags for from 48 to 72 hours, the number being reduced gradually during the 4 days after operation. Pneumonia, in older patients in particular, is a threat. The usual precautionary measures of deep breathing, change of position, restricted sedation, exercises and shortening of the convalescent period in bed are indicated.

ARTIFICIAL HIBERNATION

A new technic, *artificial hibernation,* has been used successfully in the field of cardiac surgery. By this method, the body temperature of the patient is reduced to about 80° F. in order to decrease the rate of me-

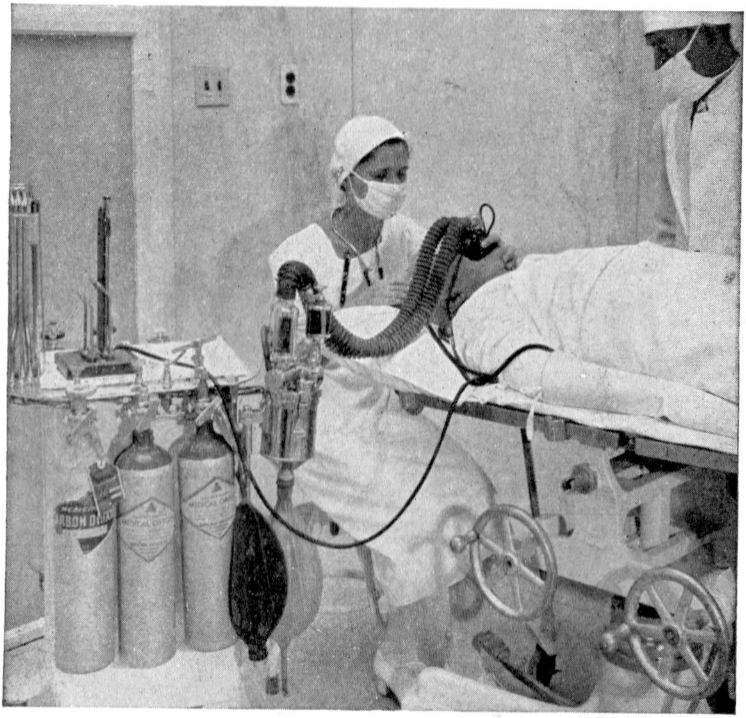

FIG. 20. Lower portion of the arm holder is wrapped over the arm. Top portion then is turned down, over and under the arm. This encloses the arm and the hand and holds the entire extremity on the table. This type of holder is an improvement over the old type of cuff in that the arm cannot drop over the edge of the table.

tabolism. A complication is that of ventricular fibrillation.

ARTIFICIAL HYPOTENSION DURING OPERATION

Another new development is that of producing *deliberate hypotension.* This is accomplished by spinal or intravenous injection of drugs which affect the sympathetic ganglia. The resultant hypotension reduces bleeding at the operative site, thereby allowing for more rapid surgery. Such a technic has been successful in brain surgery, radical neck dissection and radical pelvic surgery.

POSITION ON OPERATING TABLE

The position in which the patient is placed on the operating table depends upon the operation to be performed as well as the physical condition of the patient. The excessively obese person may require a pillow under head and shoulders, or may find it impossible to stand the lithotomy or the overextended back or

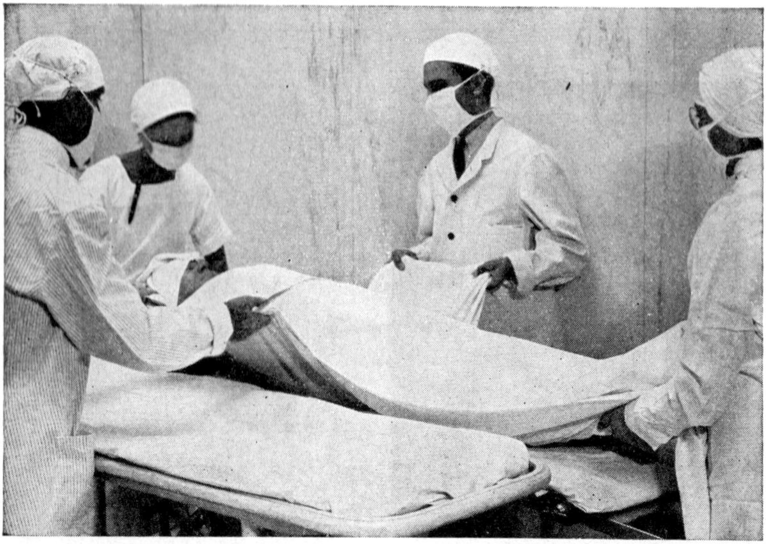

FIG. 21. At completion of the operation, the arms are unwrapped, and the arm holder may be used as a body lift to transfer the patient from the operating table to the litter or the bed.

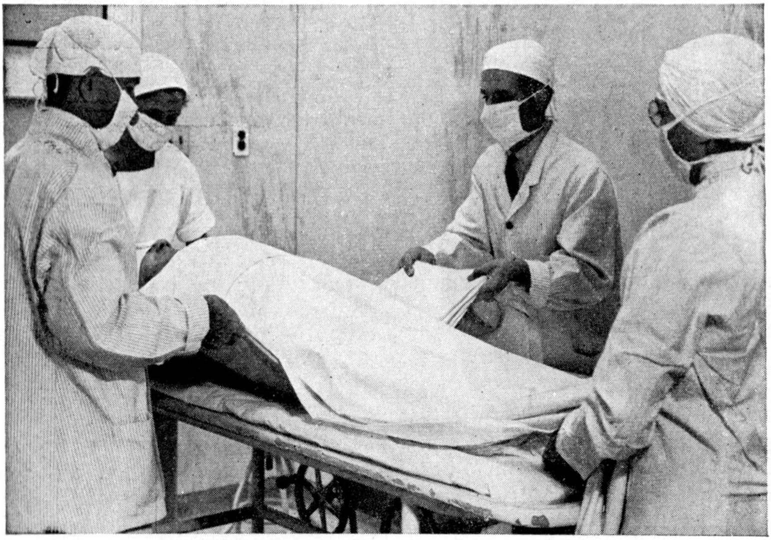

FIG. 22. The patient has been lifted onto the litter with the muslin arm holder. This is left in place and used again in the ward or the room to transfer the patient from the litter to the bed.

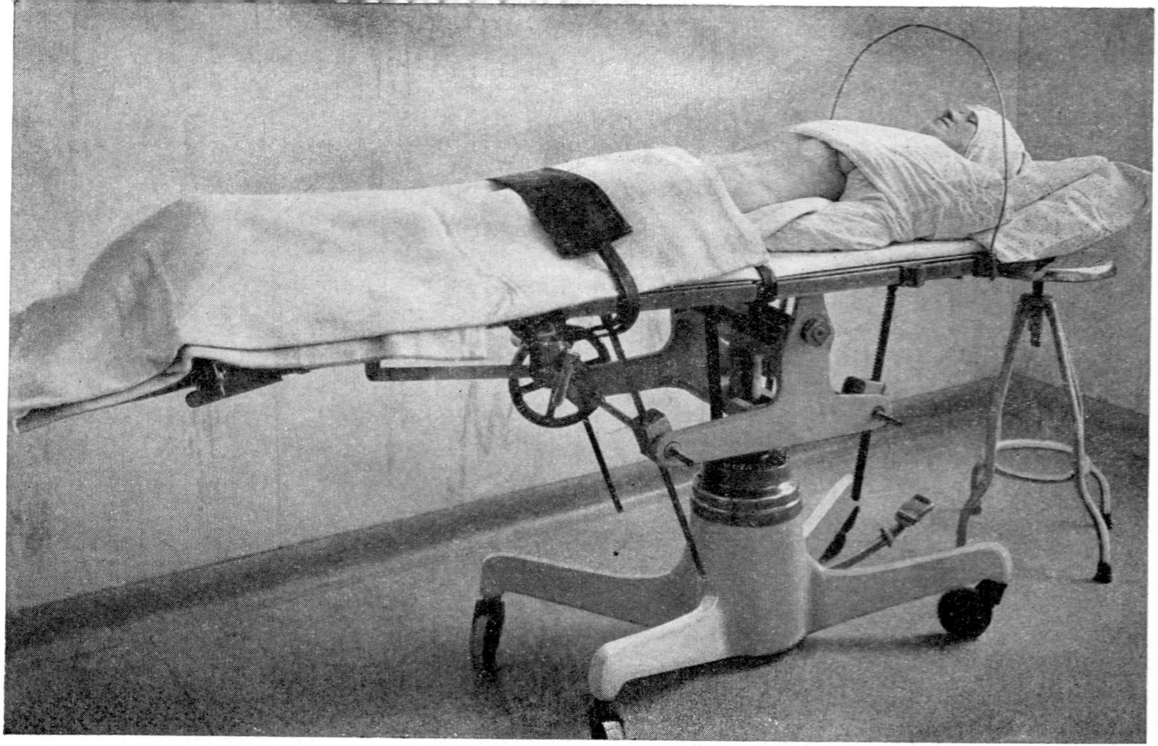

FIG. 23. Position on the operating table. Patient prepared for laparotomy. Note the strap above the knees and the wrist straps with the hands under the patient's hips.

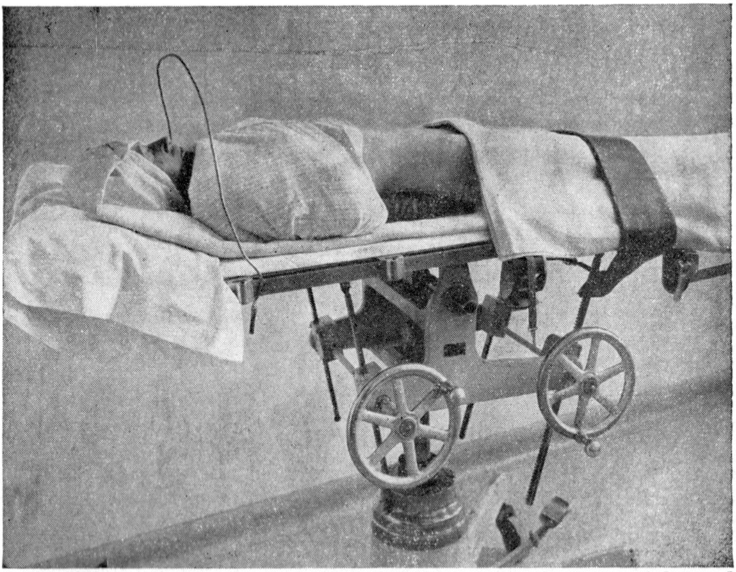

Fig. 24. Position on the operating table. Preparation for lower abdominal operation. Note the arms held by the gown; also the pillow in the small of the back.

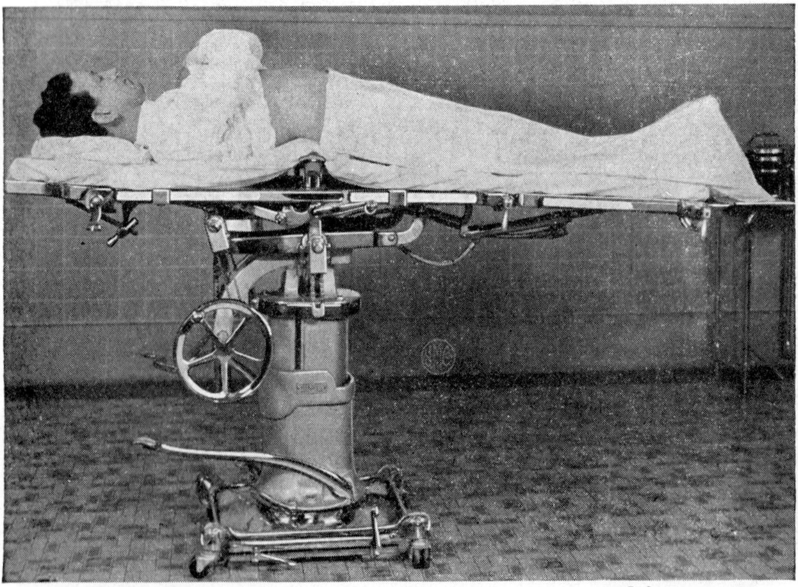

Fig. 25. Position on the operating table. Patient is prepared for operation on the gallbladder. A mechanical lift instead of the air pillow is used under the lower chest.

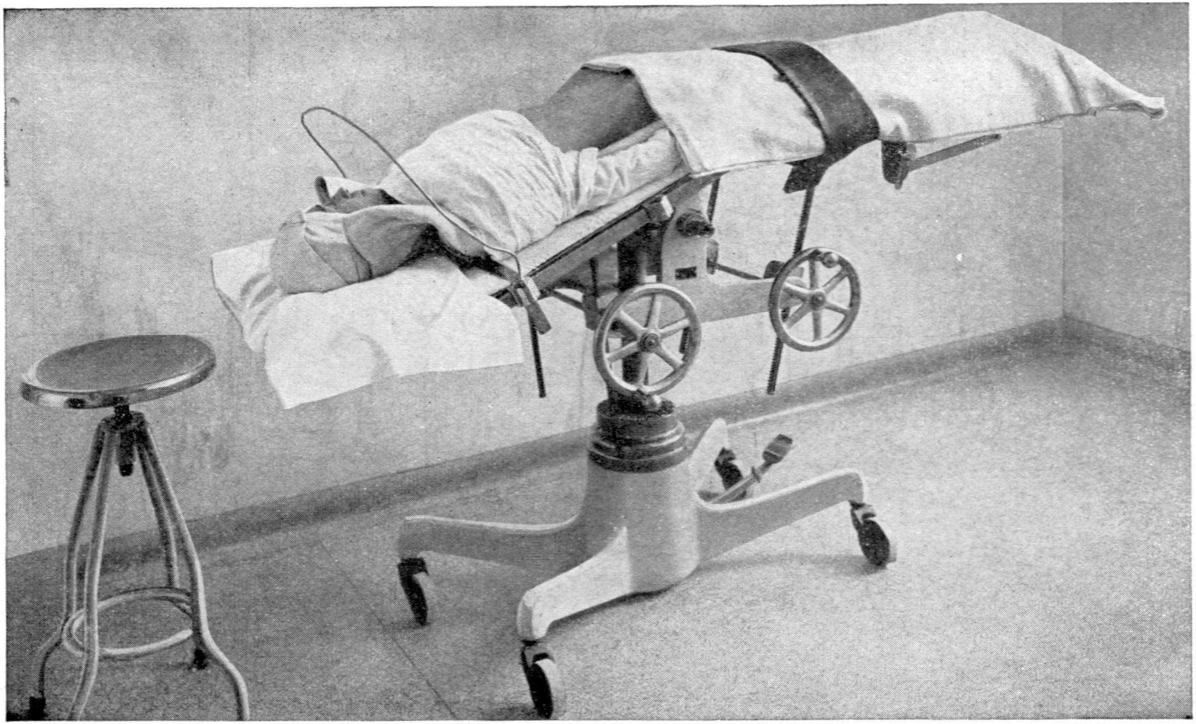

FIG. 26. Trendelenburg position on operating table. Note padded shoulder braces in place.

neck because it "shuts off" his breathing. Pressure points must be cushioned adequately to prevent irreparable nerve damage (Figs. 24 to 32).

The usual position is flat upon the back, with the arms at the side on the table, palms down. The wrists should be secured in this position with straps or a bandage to prevent wristdrop, which may occur from pressure on the nerves if the arms are allowed to fall over the edge of the table. A small pillow in the small of the back often will prevent backache. This position is used for most abdominal operations, except for those upon the gallbladder and the

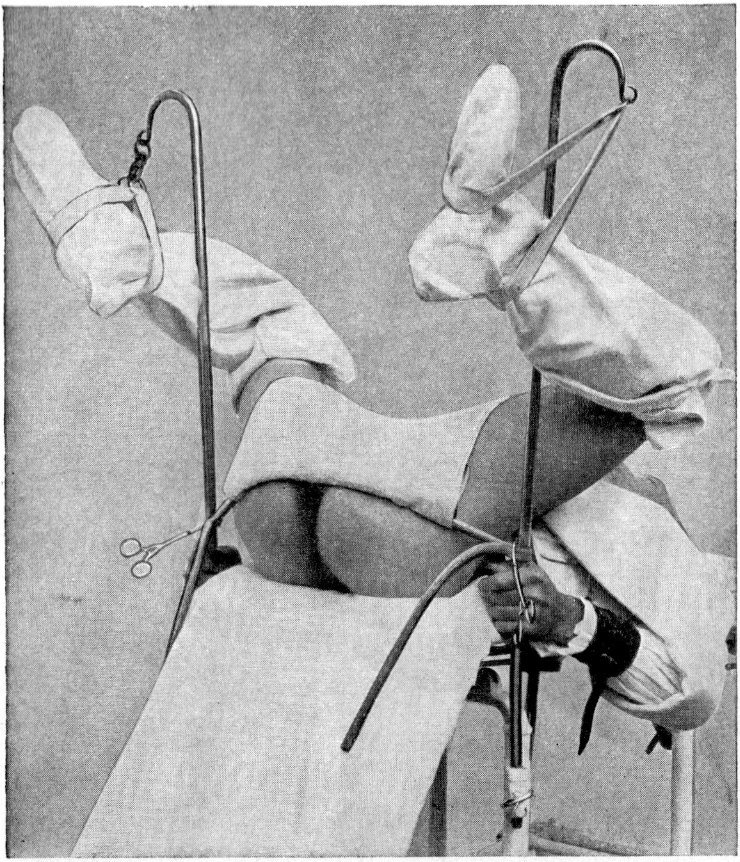

FIG. 27. Lithotomy position. Note that the hips extend over the edge of the table. Towel and tube method of covering patient.

pelvis, and for other operations as described below.

Trendelenburg Position. This position usually is employed for operations on the lower abdomen and the pelvis to obtain good exposure by displacing the intestines into the upper abdomen. In this position the head and the body are lowered, so that the plane of the body meets the horizontal at an angle. The knees are flexed by "breaking" the table, and the patient is held in position by padded shoulder braces (Fig. 26).

Lithotomy Position. This is the position in which, with the patient on his back and under the influence of an anesthetic, the legs and the thighs are flexed to right angles. The position is maintained by placing the

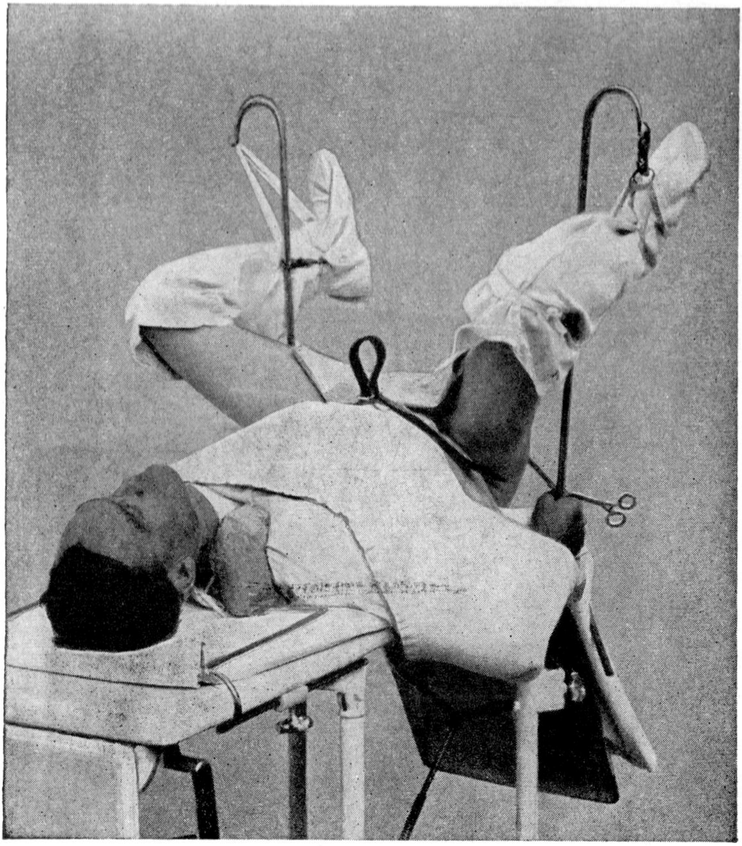

FIG. 28. Lithotomy position. Note the shoulder braces and the strap over the pelvis.

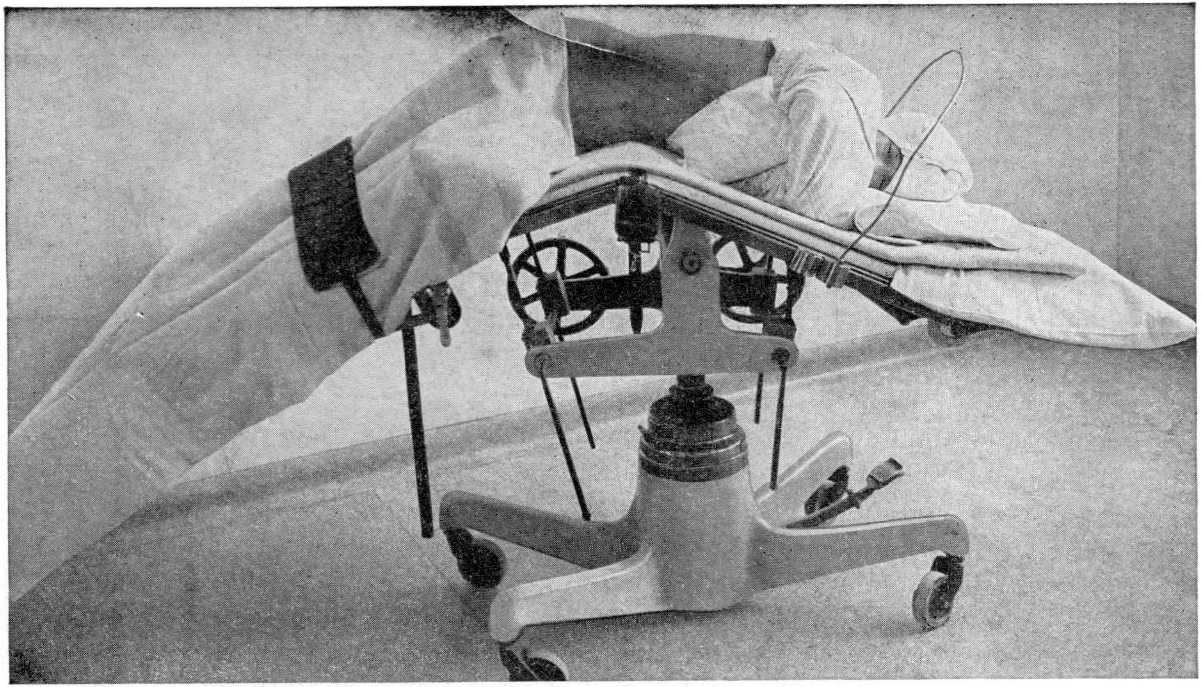

FIG. 29. Patient on operating table for kidney operation, lying on his well side. Table is broken to spread apart space between the lower ribs and the pelvis. The upper leg is extended; the lower leg is flexed at the knee and the hip joints; a pillow is placed between the legs. Note the sandbag, which helps to support patient's chest.

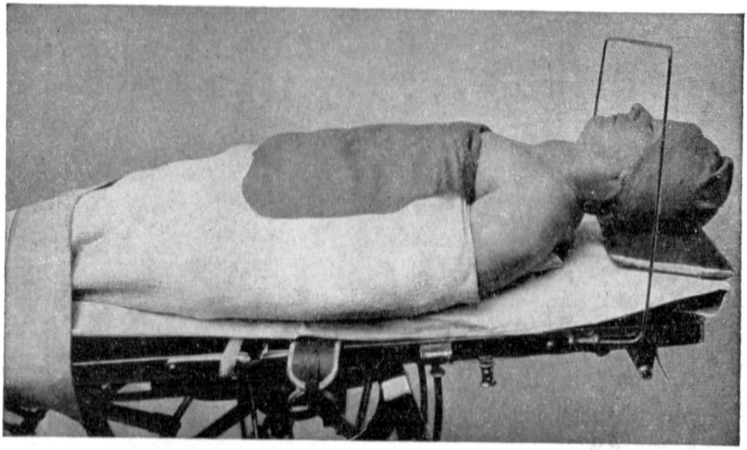

FIG. 30. Patient prepared for thyroid operation. Note air pillow under the shoulders.

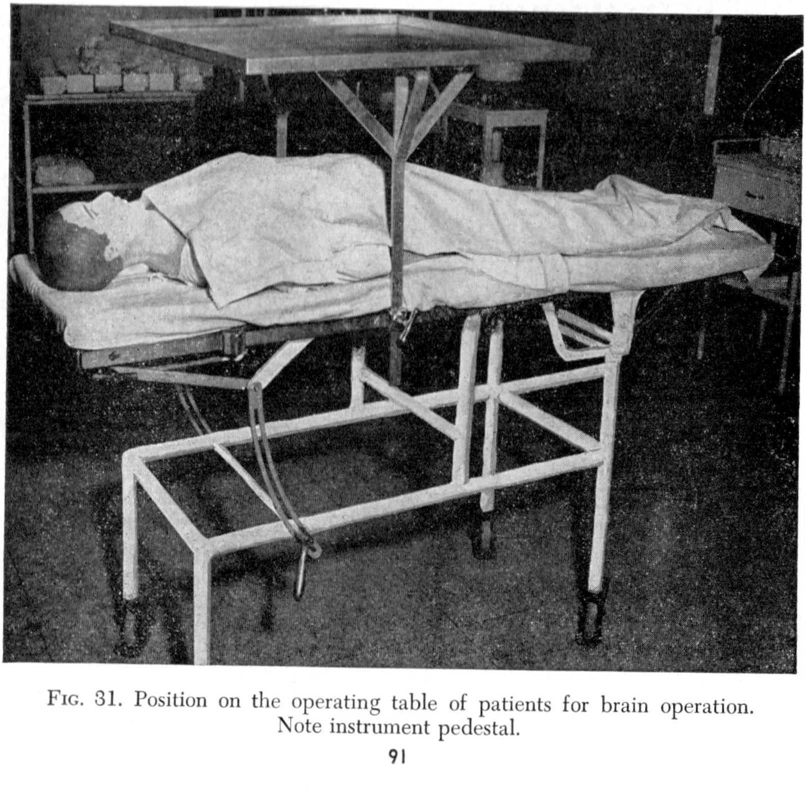

FIG. 31. Position on the operating table of patients for brain operation. Note instrument pedestal.

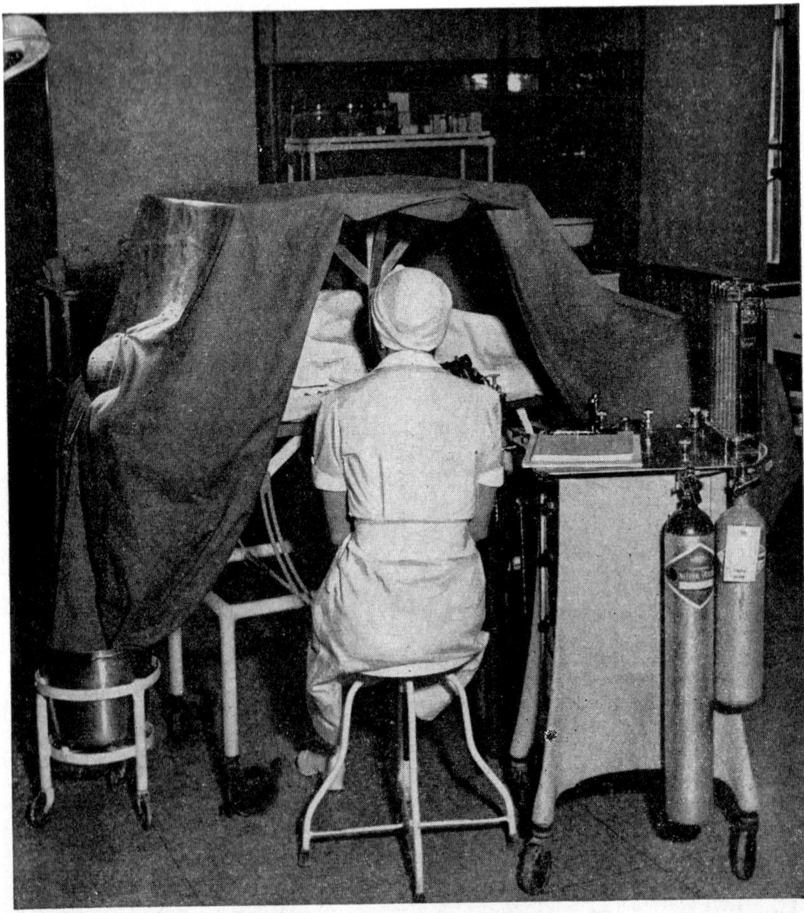

FIG. 31 (*Continued*). Position on the operating table of patients for brain operation. Drapes applied, showing the position of the anesthetist under the drapes, which should cover the instrument pedestal.

feet in stirrups. Nearly all perineal, rectal and vaginal operations require this posture (Figs. 27 and 28).

For kidney operations, the patient is placed on his well side in Sims's position with an air pillow 5 or 6 inches thick under the loin, or he is placed on a table with a kidney or back lift (Fig. 29).

Operations for empyema thoracis frequently are performed with the patient in the sitting position, the affected side projecting slightly over the edge of the table and the hand of that side placed on the opposite shoulder.

Operations on the neck for goiter and so forth are performed with the patient on his back, the neck extended somewhat by a pillow beneath the shoulders (Fig. 30).

Operations on the skull and the brain demand special positions and apparatus, and these usually are adjusted by the surgeon in charge (Fig. 31). Restraining straps are applied after the anesthetic is begun.

RESPONSIBILITY OF THE ANESTHESIA SERVICE

The ever-increasing extent and magnitude of surgical procedures are making more and more demands on the anesthetist. These demands are being met admirably by the employment of physicians to give or to supervise the giving of the anesthesias. Furthermore, the combining of two or more methods for the same operation increases the efficiency and the safety of the procedure. The early use of transfusions is demanded more frequently. To accomplish all this and to meet the immediate postoperative needs, many hospitals now are having postoperative patients sent to a recovery or postanesthesia ward or room next to the operating room.

Even though there are many people in an operating room directing their attention to the care of one patient, accidents have happened, and the patient has been the victim. The nurse must assume her share of the responsibility.

Preoperatively, the patient who is under sedation must be watched constantly. Usually, he has fasted all night and has had no breakfast; the possibility of his fainting is always present. While he is on a stretcher or an operating table, two well-placed straps are usually in position; in addition, someone must be in constant attendance so that the patient does not fall or injure himself.

Proper identification of each patient is also essential. In the hurry and bustle of many active clinics, it is possible for an individual to have the "wrong" operation.

CHAPTER SIX

Postoperative Nursing Care

The nursing care of the patient after operation is second in importance only to the operation itself. The knowledge, the skill and the ability required by the surgical nurse make this type of nursing one of the most satisfying. She is a most valuable person to the patient, to his family and to the surgeon. (Also see p. 7.)

POSTOPERATIVE RECEPTION OF THE PATIENT

Postoperative Bed

As soon as the patient is taken into the operating room the attending nurse should prepare his bed and room for his reception after the operation. The bed should have a firm mattress. As it is necessary to raise the head and the knees of the patient, a Gatch or Deckert bed is desirable. Provision should be made to raise the foot end of the bed if necessary. This can be accomplished by the use of bed pins or wooden blocks. The ordinary hospital bed usually fulfills these requirements. The bed may be made so that it will be open and ready to receive the patient. A cotton blanket may be placed over the bottom bedding. This will aid in absorbing perspiration. Later it can be removed easily, and the bottom bedding will still be fresh. A rubber sheet or a 24-inch square of plastic material can serve as a protection under the sheet at the head of the bed. An extra patient gown should be available so that the gown on the patient can be changed if it is wet from perspiration. Also, an emesis basin and a box of paper wipes can be placed near the head of the bed or stretcher.

The Recovery Room

Usually this unit is on the same floor as and near the operating rooms. The room should be quiet, neat and clean. Unnecessary equipment should be removed. The temperature of the room should be kept uniform, about 68° to 70° F. during the day and about 60° F. at night.

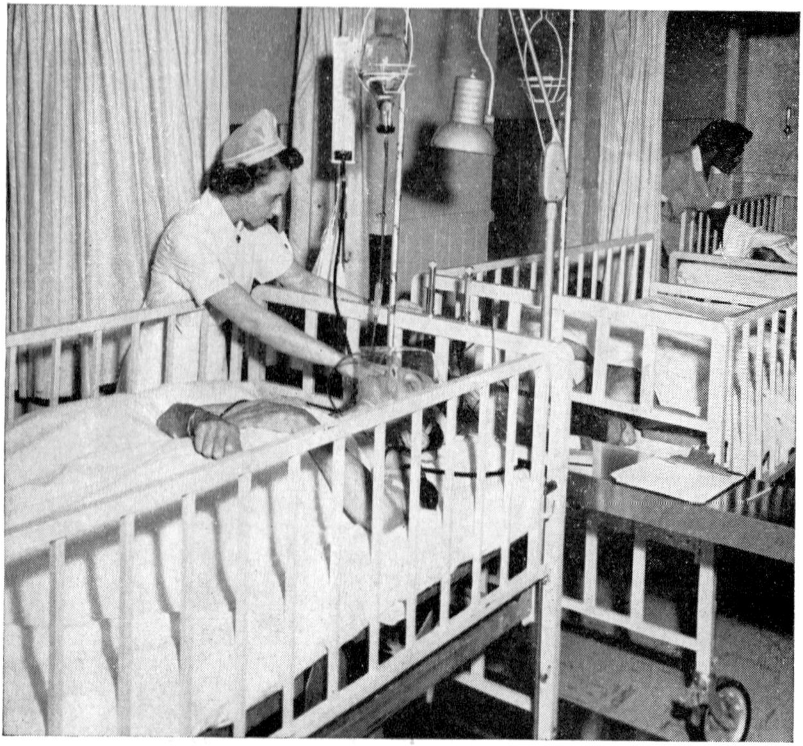

FIG. 32. Recovery room.

There should be an abundance of fresh air, but no draughts.

This room is under the control of the anesthesia department and is furnished with their equipment for immediate use. Their personnel is set up for the employment of artificial respiration—if necessary, intubation, suction and so forth. The chief immediate postoperative hazards are those of shock and anoxemia due to respiratory difficulties. Shock can be avoided largely by the timely administration of intravenous fluids and blood, and by appropriate drugs. The respiratory difficulties may be treated as they arise or, better, the patient can be treated so that they do not arise. Airways or endotracheal tubes may be left in place until respiratory reflexes return. Mucus obstructing the pharynx or the trachea should be aspirated. Oxygen may be given by mask or tent, if necessary. Such service has reduced greatly the hazards incident to prolonged shock and anoxia with the possible associated postoperative psychoses.

The careful and frequent observation of vital signs (blood pressure, pulse, respiration, temperature) is the responsibility of the specially prepared recovery-room nurse. She is not to be distracted by other routine nursing care, nor should her equipment be taken to other parts of the hospital, except in the case of emergency. The recovery-room nurse is a great help to the entire hospital because she not only gives the patient expert and necessary care during the period of recovery from anesthesia, but she also frees the remaining nursing personnel from the exacting burden of watching the patient during this time.

A patient remains in this unit until he has reacted from the anesthetic agent. In some hospitals, it is the policy to keep the patient overnight and return him to his unit the next morning after he has had morning care.

Immediate Postoperative Nursing Care

Removing Patient from Operating Table

The removal of the patient from the operating table to the bed or the stretcher should be done with the least possible delay and exposure. Exposure of the perspiring patient predisposes to pulmonary complications and postoperative shock. The site of the operation should be kept in mind every time a newly operated patient is moved. Many wounds are closed under considerable tension, and every effort should be made not

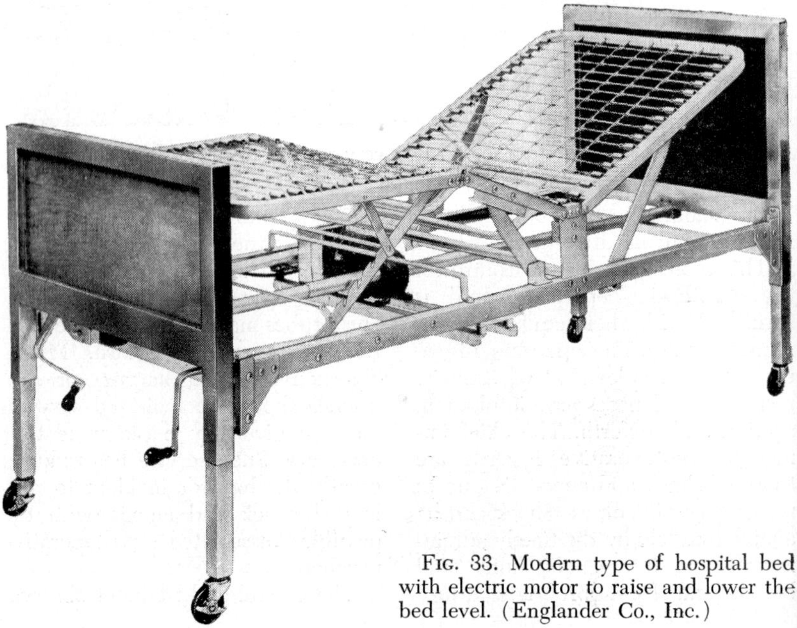

Fig. 33. Modern type of hospital bed with electric motor to raise and lower the bed level. (Englander Co., Inc.)

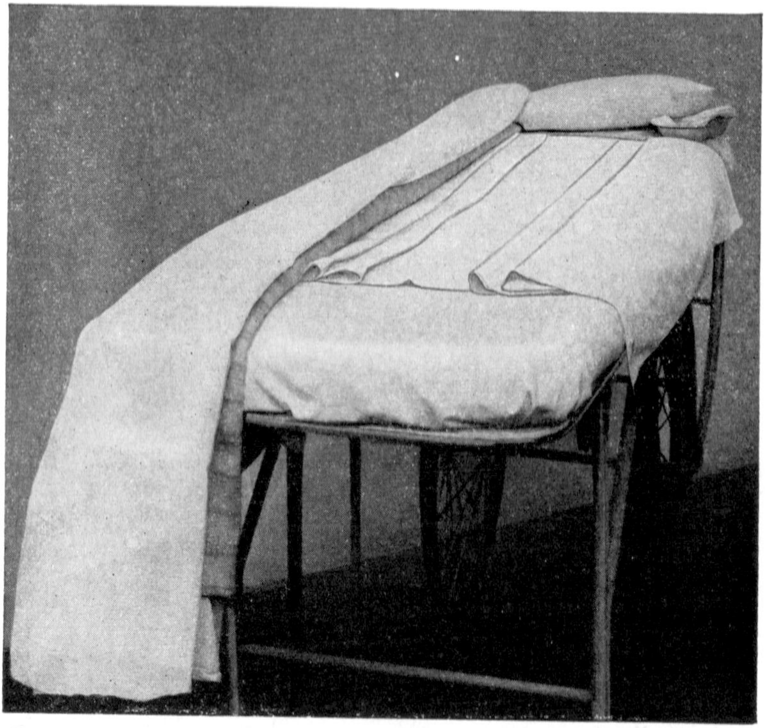

FIG. 34 A. Preparation of stretcher for lifting patient with sheet, which is used when the patient is not transferred directly to his bed.

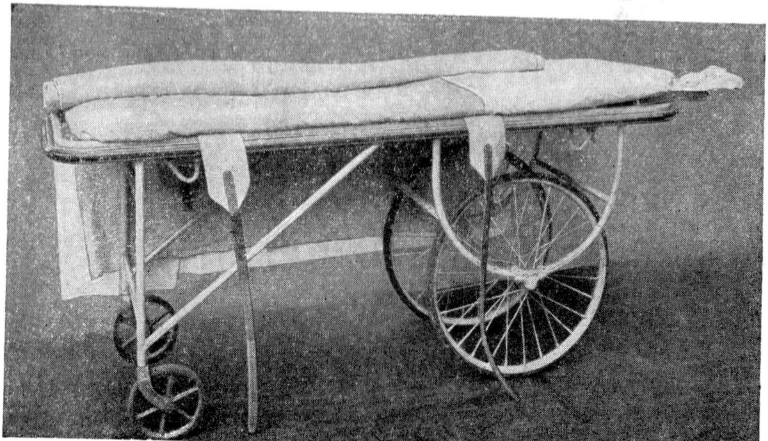

FIG. 34 B. Stretcher prepared for reception of a patient. Note the blankets folded at the side of the stretcher, the nurse's basin and gauze under a corner of the mattress, and restraining straps in place.

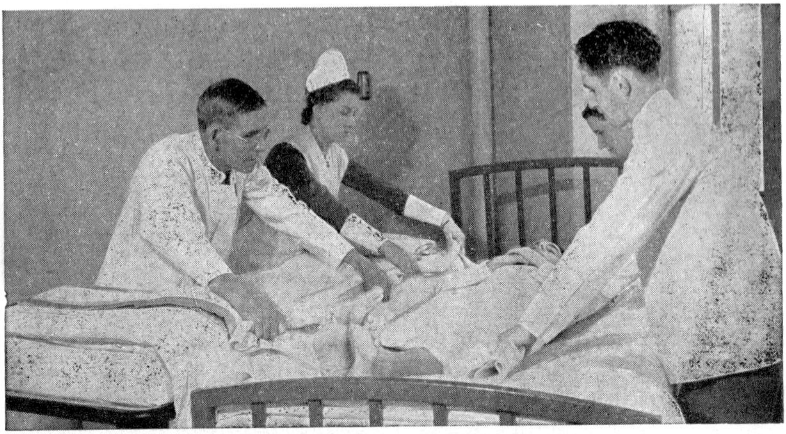

FIG. 35 A. Lifting the patient on a blanket from bed to stretcher. Feet should be covered.

to place any further strain on the sutures. Thus, in cases in which a thyroidectomy has been performed, the head should not be allowed to fall backward; in breast amputations the arm of the operated side should be held close to the body; in nephrectomy, the patient should not be allowed to lie on the affected side; and so on.

As soon as the patient is placed on the stretcher or bed, he is covered with warm blankets that have been arranged previously on the

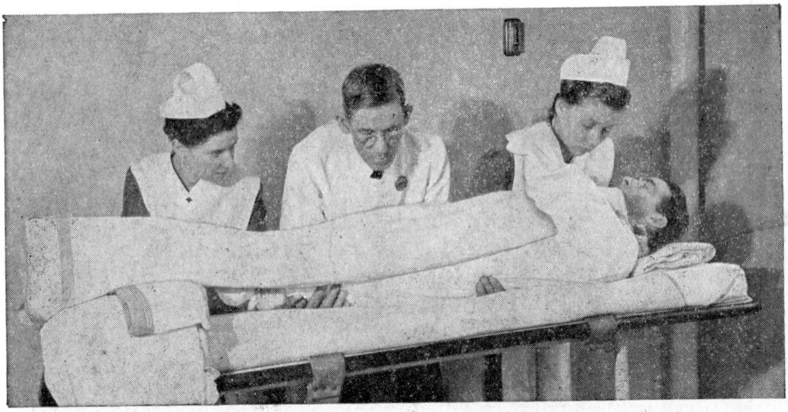

FIG. 35 B. Arm carry for lifting patients from stretcher or operating table. Attendants place their arms under the patient. If conscious and strong enough, the patient holds onto the attendant at his head; if not, their arm is held at his side.

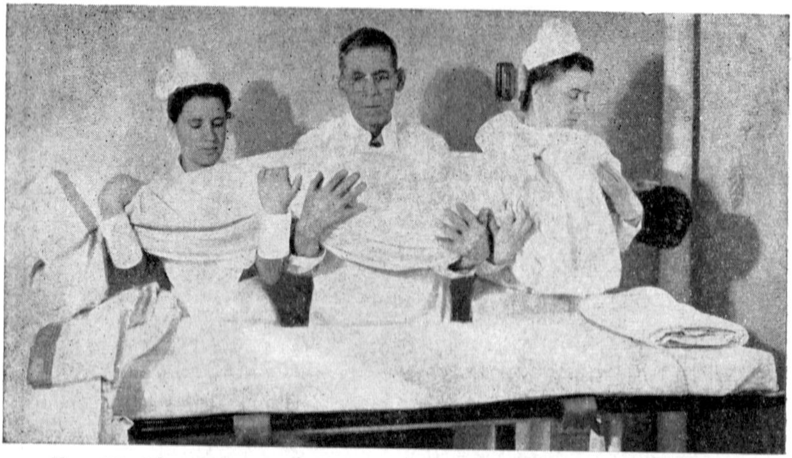

FIG. 36. The patient is rolled onto the chests of the attendants. The attendant at the head of the patient must support the elbow and the arm of unconscious or weak patients.

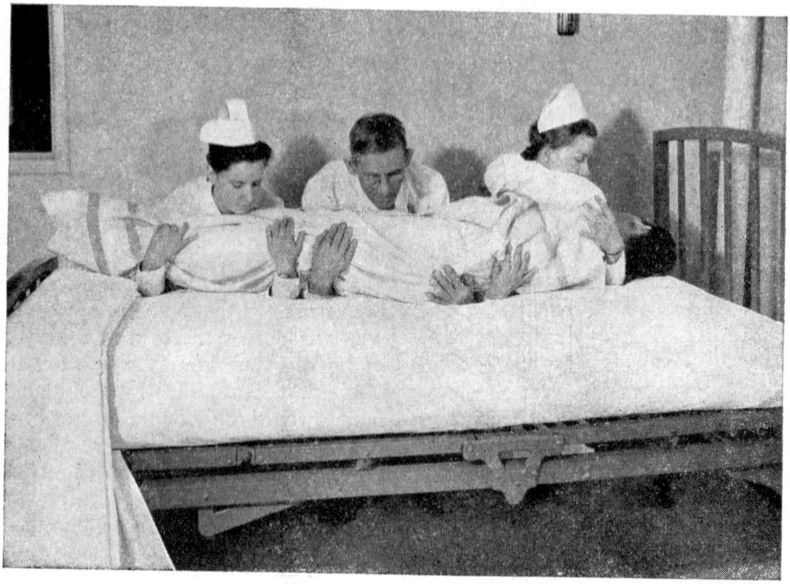

FIG. 37. Arm carry, placing the patient in bed. Attendants lean forward, placing their elbows on the bed and letting the patient roll backward slowly onto his back.

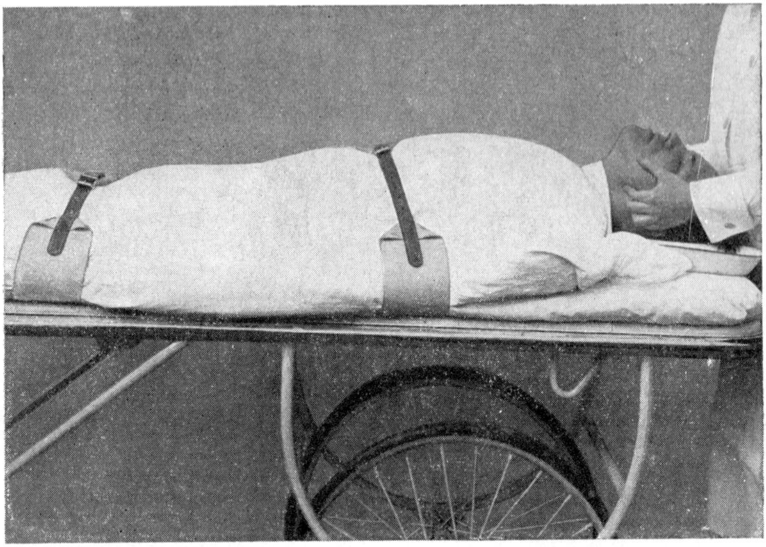

FIG. 38. Patient prepared for return to the ward from the operating room. Note restraining straps; the nurse holds the jaw forward to prevent respiratory difficulty.

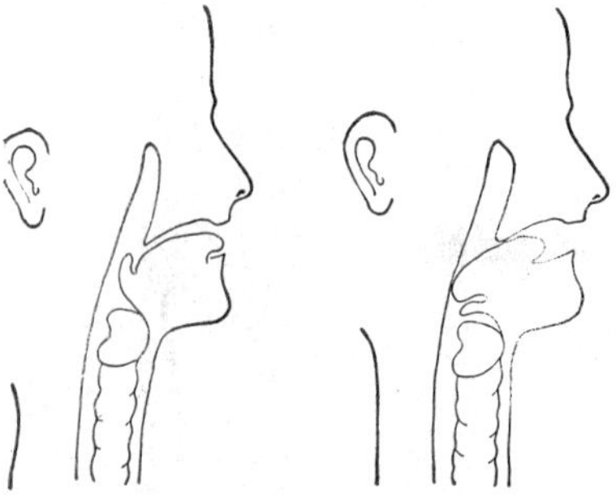

FIG. 39. Respiratory obstruction. (*Left*) With the tone of muscles normal, the tongue is in its usual position. (*Right*) With the muscles relaxed, the chin drops back, and the tongue comes in contact with the posterior wall of the pharynx, thereby shutting off the respiratory passages. (Greisheimer, Esther: The Physiological effects of anesthesia, Am. J. Nursing **49**: 338)

stretcher. The wet and soiled gown and socks should be removed, a warm and dry gown applied, and the bedding tucked in along the sides as well as at the bottom. On the stretcher the patient is held with straps above the knees and the elbows. The straps serve the double purpose of securing the blankets and of restraining the patient should he pass through a stage of excitement as he recovers from the anesthetic. Without the aid of straps a single nurse would be unable to restrain many patients, and there have been times when the patient in his struggles has fallen from the stretcher and done himself considerable injury.

THE FIRST HOUR AFTER OPERATION

If at all possible, it is recommended that the nurse be in the operating room during the operation. Only in this way can she know exactly the kind of surgical procedure carried out on her patient. If she has not witnessed the operation, she should ascertain as soon as possible:

1. The condition of the patient.
2. The nature of the operation performed.
3. The anesthetic agent used.
4. Any unusual experiences that the patient had in the operating room which would influence his immediate postoperative care, such as undue hemorrhage, respiratory difficulties, drug therapy, etc.
5. The presence of drainage tubes and how they are to be connected.

In the first hour after operation, and especially in the first few minutes after the patient leaves the operating room, during the return to his room, the attending nurse should be on guard for the first serious postoperative complication. i.e., disturbances of respiration. These disturbances are confined almost entirely to those patients who have had a general anesthetic, especially ether. Patients given local anesthesia, nitrous oxide or ethylene usually are "awake" a few minutes after leaving the operating room. However, those patients having ether usually are completely unconscious, with all muscles relaxed. This relaxation extends to the muscles of the pharynx; therefore, when the patient lies on his back the lower jaw and the tongue fall backward, and the air passages close more or less completely (Fig. 39). The patient gives evidence of this difficulty in breathing by choking and irregular respirations, and in a short time a

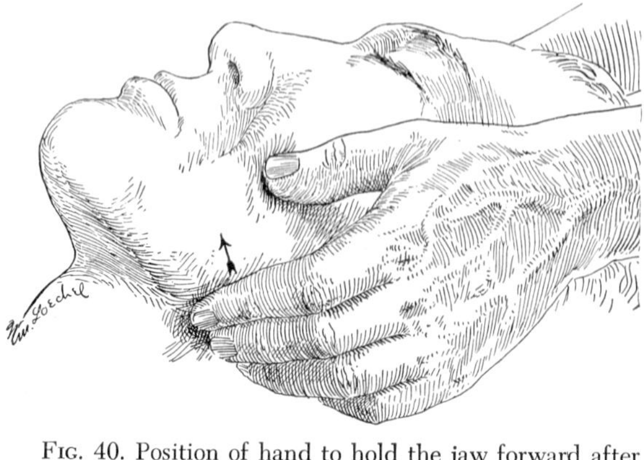

FIG. 40. Position of hand to hold the jaw forward after inhalation anesthesia. Note that the fingers are placed behind the angle of the jaw, and the direction of the arrow shows the direction of pressure being exerted on the jaw. As the jaw is pushed forward the tongue is brought forward so as to keep an open airway. This is important, especially after operation under general anesthesia in children, for instance, in tonsillectomy.

blue duskiness (cyanosis) of the skin appears. The treatment of this complication is to push forward on the angle of the lower jaw as if to push the lower teeth in front of the upper. This maneuver pulls the tongue forward and opens the air passages. At times it may be necessary to grasp the tongue between gauze and pull it forward for a time. This prevents

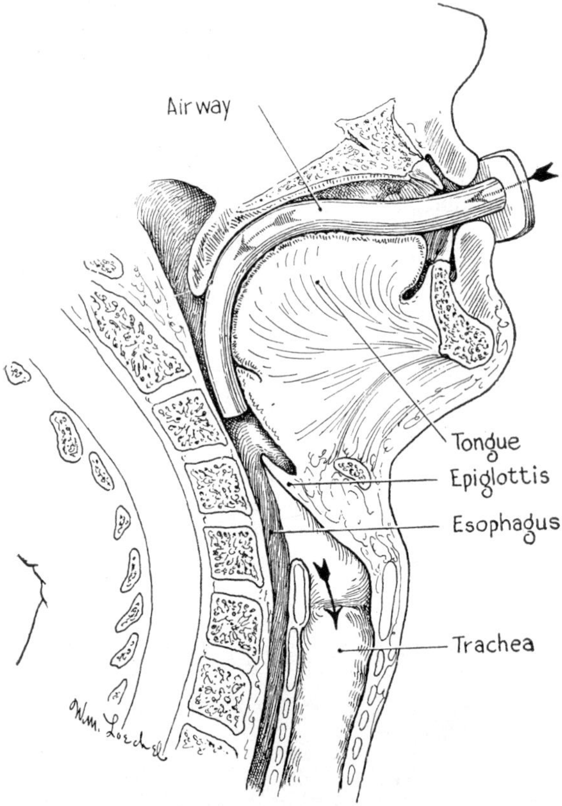

FIG. 41. Diagrammatic view to show methods by which an airway prevents respiratory difficulty after anesthesia. The airway passes over the base of the tongue and delivers air into the pharynx in the region of the epiglottis. Patients are often brought from the operating room with an airway in place. This should remain in place until the patient recovers sufficiently to breathe normally. Usually, as patients regain consciousness, the airway causes irritation; then it should be removed.

the respiratory obstruction, and the maneuver should be continued when necessary until the patient has regained reflex functions sufficiently to carry on normal respiration.

Often the anesthetist leaves a hard rubber or plastic "airway" in the mouth or a rubber nasal catheter in the nose. By both devices a patent airway is maintained. Such a device should not be removed until the patient expresses a desire to emit it. As this equipment is the property of the operating room, it should be cleaned thoroughly and returned. (See Figs. 41 and 42.)

Not infrequently the respiratory difficulty is produced by an excessive secretion of mucus. Turning the head to the side will allow the collected fluid to escape from the side of the mouth. If vomiting occurs, the head should be turned sharply to the side, and the vomitus collected in the basin previously provided. The face should be wiped with gauze or paper wipes carried for that purpose.

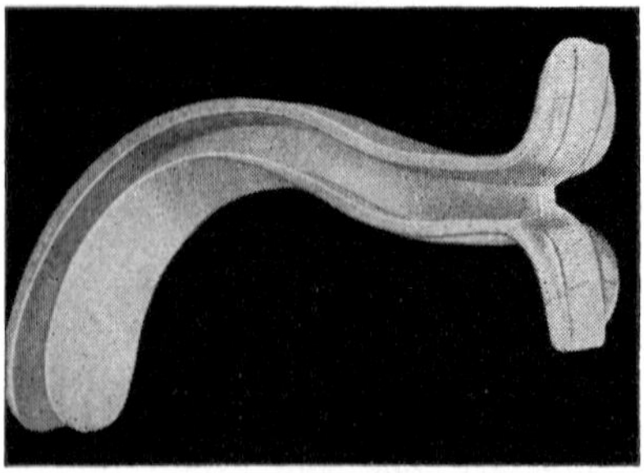

FIG. 42. The Berman Disposable Oral Airway is made of polyethylene and features a central partition which leaves either side free for easy insertion of catheters and easy cleaning. It is inexpensive enough to permit the use of a fresh, uncontaminated airway for each patient.

Nursing During Recovery from Anesthesia

A nurse should be in constant attendance while the patient is recovering from anesthesia. *Never leave a patient alone, even for an instant.* Until the patient regains consciousness, the bed is kept flat to guard against postoperative shock. When and how much the bed may be raised will be taken up later. As soon as the patient is settled in bed, the temperature, pulse, respiration and blood pressure should be taken and recorded. External heat (hot-water bottles or electric pads) may be ordered when the temperature is below 97° F. Always remember that burns occur very readily after anesthesia, due to the general depression of the nervous and the circulatory systems. There should be at least one fold of blanket between the patient and the hot-water bottle or electric pad, the object being to place the heat near, rather than against, the patient. In the case of a change of nurses, the one going off duty should inspect the skin of the patient and report to the relieving nurse the condition of the skin, the number of hot-water bottles or pads and their location. It is not safe to use electric pads near wet dressings because of the danger of a short circuit in the heating unit of the pad. Warm blankets to keep the patient's clothing dry and prevent exposure generally are sufficient to combat a subnormal temperature and shock.

In hot weather, it is important that the patient should not lose large amounts of fluid by unnecessary perspiration. Therefore, it is usual during the summer not to cover the patient with blankets, and the recovery bed is prepared without them.

The following are the chief responsibilities of the nurse attending the patient during recovery from anesthesia:

1. **Carry out any "stat" orders immediately.** This usually refers to drug or oxygen therapy.

2. **Turn the patient's head to the side** when he vomits. Wipe the lips and the mouth with paper wipes or gauze. Note the amount and the nature of the vomitus and record them. Allow the patient to rinse his mouth with mouthwash if he is able to do so. Moisten the lips to relieve thirst.

3. **Observe the patient for signs** of respiratory obstruction, shock and hemorrhage. The chief guides are the appearance of the patient, the pulse, the respiration and the temperature. The pulse and the respiration should be counted every 15 minutes for the first 2 hours, and every half hour for the next 2 hours. Thereafter they may be taken less frequently if they remain stable. The blood pressure is taken as often as ordered. A temperature of over 100° or under 97° F., respirations of over 30 or under 16 and a systolic blood pressure of under 90 are usually considered reportable at once. Make notes on the general condition of the patient—for example, his color, good or cyanotic; skin, cold and clammy, warm and moist; excessive mucus in the throat and in the nostrils.

4. **Keep the patient as quiet and as comfortable** as possible. When he is coming out of the anesthesia he may be restless. If it is at all possible, he should not be restrained, but he must be protected from injuring himself. Usually an infusion is running. If the arm is splinted, the needle will not be dislodged. However, the patient can pull the needle out with his free hand. Patients who have had hyoscine (scopolamine) or Amytal before operation should be watched closely for several hours after they have recovered from the effects of the anesthesia. Not infrequently, these drugs cause a type of delirium. Patients have been known to get out of bed and do other injurious things while under their influence. When the patient is fully conscious, deep breathing and turning every hour are necessary to prevent atelectasis or other pulmonary complications.

5. **Attach any drainage apparatus** when drainage is to be collected in a bottle—for example, cholecystostomy or choledochostomy tubes, catheters or enterostomy drains.

6. **Begin postoperative treatment** as ordered—for example, attach gastric or Miller-Abbott tube to Wangensteen suction-drainage apparatus.

7. **Inspect dressings** from time to time to detect signs of undue hemorrhage or abnormal drainage. Reinforce dressings, if necessary, making note of them, with time, on nurse's record.

8. **Report any alarming or peculiar symptoms** to the surgeon at once. This includes any mental phenomena or uneasiness on the part of the patient. A patient's statements concerning his condition never should be disregarded entirely.

9. **Keep an intelligent and accurate nurse's record.** (See page 126.)

Often this is the only way the physician can follow the condition of his patient. A good record gives immeasurable help to the evening and night nurses.

Important and Unimportant Symptoms

Often the inexperienced nurse will be at a loss to differentiate between important and unimportant symptoms; and, in fact, the experienced nurse sometimes may be puzzled as to whether or not to notify the surgeon of a certain change in condition. The safest plan always is to call for advice when in doubt. However, in order to be able to decide intelligently, there are a few general rules that may be of some assistance. Of course, any severe symptom always is important. Any apparently slight symptom that tends to recur repeatedly or to increase in severity should be regarded as significant—for example, hiccough may or may not be of importance, depending on the duration. A symptom seemingly may be of no consequence in itself, but when associated with other definite changes may foretell danger—for example, a repeated sigh means nothing but, when accompanied by great restlessness, increasing pallor, rising pulse rate and so forth, it becomes one of the clinical signs of dangerous hemorrhage. Any progressive and steady change for the worse in the general condition, even with no outstanding symptoms evident, is of the gravest importance. And, as has been mentioned already, the patient's complaints and statements never should be passed over without investigation.

If the doctor in charge of the patient is to be notified for any reason, be sure to have all necessary information literally at your fingertips before going to the telephone. Know the latest temperature, the pulse and the respiration figures, and always take the patient's chart and the nurse's record with you to the telephone, in order to refer to them should occasion arise. Learn to state the patient's condition concisely and accurately, and be prepared to answer all questions intelligently.

RETURN TO COMPLETE CONSCIOUSNESS

With the return of complete consciousness come increasing pain and discomfort. Hypodermic injections of morphine, Dilaudid, Demerol or Methadon often are ordered for pain and restlessness. Such an order usually is written "p.r.n." (Latin for "pro re nata"—as required by circumstances) for a certain number of doses. The time of administration frequently is left to the judgment of the nurse, but she should first exercise her resourcefulness in making the patient comfortable without them. There is seldom any method of relieving pain in the operative region, but the following suggestions may be useful in assuaging general discomfort temporarily and rendering the hypodermic more effectual when finally it is given:

1. **Change Position.** Give added support with pillows. A small pillow in the hollow of the back is comforting, as is a pillow under the knees.

2. **Encourage Deep Breathing.** A most important point in the care of the patient after the anesthesia is to prevent pulmonary complications. This is another significant reason

why the *radical alteration in the position* of the patient is important. He is able to expand his lungs better when this is done. Patients are *encouraged to cough* in an effort to clear the respiratory passages of secretions. A third method of causing gas exchange in the lung is to encourage the patient to *take deep breaths.* This may be done by the use of a blow bottle. This is merely a gallon bottle half filled with water. A length of rubber tubing with a mouthpiece is attached to the bottle and the patient is asked to "blow bubbles" for five minutes in every hour. Unless the patient is told why it is important for him to do this simple procedure, the nurse may not get his co-operation. Another method of stimulating deep respirations is by the use of carbon dioxide inhalations. This may be carried out by using a face mask attached to a gas tank or simply by instructing the patient to blow in and out of a paper bag. In a fourth method the patient should be shown how to take a deep breath, hold it a second and then give a hard cough as he starts to expel the air. On the second or the third exercise of this kind, he will expectorate suddenly a viscid mass of mucus and clear his lung.

3. **Wash the Face and the Hands.** Cold cloths applied to the forehead often are soothing.

4. **Give a Mouthwash Freely.** At the same time wipe the lips with a cool gauze sponge when water by mouth is not permitted.

5. **Rub the Back with Alcohol.** The limbs may be stroked very lightly with alcohol. *They never should be rubbed vigorously.* To do so may dislodge a thrombus and result in embolus and death.

6. **Give water if permissible in small quantities when nausea ceases.** If small amounts are retained by the patient, the quantity given at one time may be increased gradually. Water is best either hot or cold, otherwise it is likely to cause nausea. There are times when a large glass of water will do a patient no harm, even when he is nauseated, but this never should be given without the proper authority. Patients usually ask for cracked ice, and frequently it does no harm in small amounts. If orders are that the patient is to have nothing by mouth, cracked ice wrapped in a piece of gauze is refreshing and soothing to the lips.

7. **Remove blankets.** If the patient has been put between blankets, they should be removed upon complete recovery from the anesthesia —when the temperature, the pulse and the respirations are within normal limits; or they may be removed promptly but carefully when they are the cause of excessive perspiration. Recovery beds should be made in such a manner that the patient is left between sheets when these extra blankets are withdrawn. Cool sheets usually are a most gratifying change and often very soothing. However, care must be taken that the change is not too abrupt: if the patient complains of excessive heat, remove the under blanket first and the upper blanket a little later. In warm weather too many blankets will cause marked perspiration and the consequent loss of a large amount of fluid. Therefore, it is advisable as a rule not to use blankets on the recovery bed during warm periods in the summer months. Remember that patients who have been anes-

thetized are susceptible to chills and draughts. Remember, also, that the obese patient perspires profusely and so loses fluid and salt much more rapidly than the patient who is of normal weight; therefore, shock due to fluid loss will occur earlier.

8. **Elimination.** URINATION. The length of time a patient may be permitted to go without voiding after operation varies considerably with the type of operation performed. In gynecologic and abdominal patients catheterization may be required at the end of 8 or 10 hours (sometimes sooner), and in others it may be put off for from 16 to 18 hours. Generally speaking, every effort must be made to avoid the use of the catheter. Exhaust all known methods to aid the patient in voiding—let water run, apply heat and so forth. Never give a patient a cold bedpan. When a patient complains of not being able to use the bedpan, some surgeons permit the use of the commode rather than resort to catheterization. Of course, this applies only to suitable cases. Male patients sometimes are permitted to stand beside the bed, but this should not be allowed unless an orderly is in attendance to prevent any accidents from falling or fainting. All urine, whether voided or catheterized, must be measured and the amount noted on the nurse's record. A separate intake and output chart (p. 126) should be kept on all aged and all very ill patients. (See also p. 149, Urinary Retention.)

DEFECATION. Each defecation should be recorded. If the bowels do not move spontaneously every day or every other day, a cleansing enema usually is given. As a rule, cathartics are not given to postoperative patients, especially if the operation has beer on the abdomen.

BODY ALIGNMENT AND GOOD BODY MECHANICS

Regardless of whether the patient is lying, sitting, standing or walking, the nurse must be able to recognize at a glance whether he is maintaining proper physiologic position. If not, it is her responsibility to correct it. Poor posture for the surgical patient can result only in the development of complications with subsequent delay in convalescence. Such untoward effects include pulmonary complications which result from inadequate chest expansion, improper drainage from body cavities, contractures, decubiti, circulatory impairment and urinary and gastro-intestinal difficulties.

The principles of proper body alignment and good body mechanics are an essential part of good surgical nursing. These apply to the nurse as well as to her patient.

DORSAL POSITION

The patient lies on his back without elevation of the head. In most cases this is the position in which the patient is placed immediately after operation. The head usually is turned to one side to facilitate easy evacuation of vomitus and to prevent its aspiration into the lungs. Bed covers should not restrict the movement of the toes and the feet of the patient.

This position is maintained until the patient has recovered from the effects of the anesthetic and has regained sufficient reflex activity to swallow, cough and so forth. This position may be employed to advan-

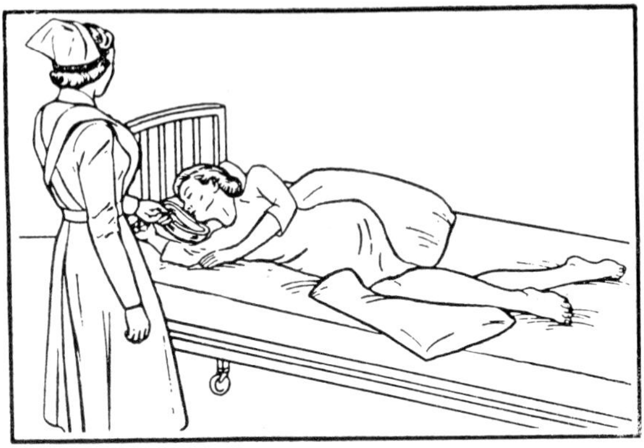

FIG. 43. Position for immediate postoperative patient which permits drainage of mucus from the mouth and general relaxation. (Winters, M. C.: Protective Body Mechanics in Daily Life and in Nursing, Philadelphia, Saunders)

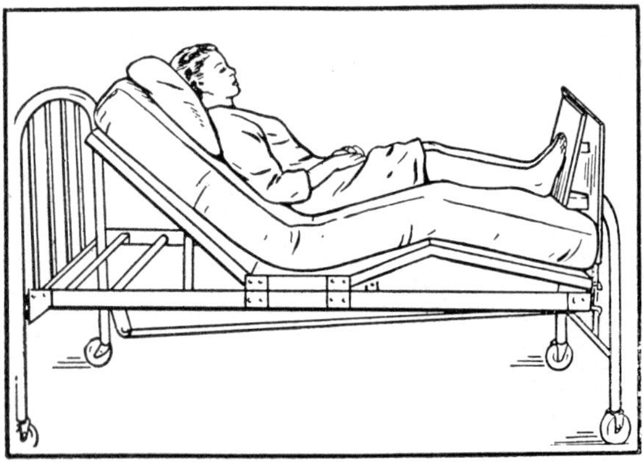

FIG. 44. In Fowler's position the patient's position is arranged so that flexion of hips and knees corresponds to the bend in the mattress provided by the gatch. The trunk is in good alignment. Foot support adds to comfort and helps prevent patient from sliding down in bed. (Winters, M. C.: Protective Body Mechanics in Daily Life and in Nursing, Philadelphia, Saunders)

tage many times when the necessity for drainage does not demand the Fowler position. It is believed that when the patient is flat in bed, respiration often is more free and turning is easier, advantages that are important in the prevention of respiratory complications.

Head Low Dorsal (Trendelenburg) Position

The patient lies on his back with or without a pillow under his head, and the foot of the bed is raised from 1 foot to 3 feet. This position increases the blood flow to the cerebral centers. It is indicated in the treatment of shock and hemorrhage, both before and after operation. It is used often after spinal anesthesia.

Sims' or Lateral Position

The patient lies on either side with the upper arm forward. The under leg lies slightly flexed, the upper leg is flexed at the thigh and the knee. The head is supported on a pillow, and a second pillow is

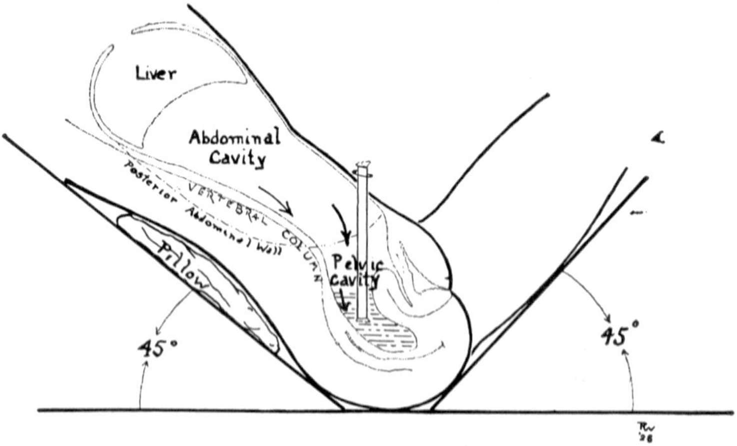

FIG. 45. Illustrating effect of Fowler position in a case of peritonitis with pelvic drainage.

placed longitudinally under the flexed knee. This position is used when it is desirable to have the patient change position frequently to aid in the drainage of cavities, as of the chest, the abdomen and so forth, and to prevent postoperative pulmonary, respiratory and circulatory complications. (See Fig. 43.)

FOWLER POSITION

Of all the positions ordered for a patient, perhaps the most common, as well as the most difficult to maintain, is the Fowler. The difficulty in most instances lies in trying to make the patient fit the bed rather than having the bed conform to the needs of the patient. The patient's trunk is raised to form an angle of form 60° to 70° F. with the horizontal. (Fig. 44.) This is a comfortable sitting position. Operative cases usually are put in Fowler position as soon as they have recovered consciousness, but great caution must be observed in raising the bed. It is not an unusual occurrence for a patient to feel faint following the raising of the head of the bed, and for this reason a close watch must be kept on the pulse rate and the color. If the patient complains of any dizziness, the bed must be lowered at once. However, if the condition of the patient is good, the head of the bed may be raised within an hour or two. It will be found that there is less slipping of the patient when the knee area is elevated before the head is raised.

The nurse must determine whether or not the patient is in correct position and comfortable. Often very short people are most uncomfortable in the ordinary hospital bed and must be supported by pillows. Sometimes it is more satisfactory to place a pillow under the knees rather than to raise the spring. If this is more comfortable, it is advisable to place a support against the feet to prevent slipping down in bed, to prevent footdrop and to make the patient feel more secure.

When the Fowler position is ordered for a patient, it is the nurse's responsibility to see that this position is maintained at all times. It is not sufficient to arrange the patient in a faultless manner: he must remain so. No matter how correctly placed or how well supported by pillows the patient is, he will slip down in the course of time and frequent lifting up in bed and readjustment of the pillows will be necessary. A particularly strict Fowler position is important in all abdominal drainage cases. (Figs. 45 and 46.) The reason for this should be obvious—a sitting posture permits free drainage to the pelvis, where nature provides more resistance to infection. Another significant reason for maintaining good body posture is that it affords better functioning of all organs, including those of respiration.

Jackknife or Semi-Fowler Position

This position is one used to relieve tension following the repair of inguinal or abdominal hernia. It is produced by raising the head of the patient from 10 to 12 inches and flexing the knees. In the Gatch bed, the elevation of the head and the knees one notch will give the proper position.

The Patient's Comfort and Changes of Position

Hampered by dressings, splints or drainage apparatus, the patient very frequently is quite unable to shift his position. Lying constantly in the same position may be the cause of pressure sores or hypostatic pneumonia, to mention only two of the more serious resulting complications. Turning a pillow from one side to another presents a cooler side as it touches the patient. Proper support for the arms and the hands offers a measure of comfort. A foot support encourages the patient to stretch his foot muscles and spread his toes, which is a relaxing maneuver. The helpless patient must be turned from side to side at least every two hours, and he should have his position changed as soon as he becomes uncomfortable.

When a patient is unable to turn himself, it may be necessary for the nurse to have one or two assistants. The number of persons needed de-

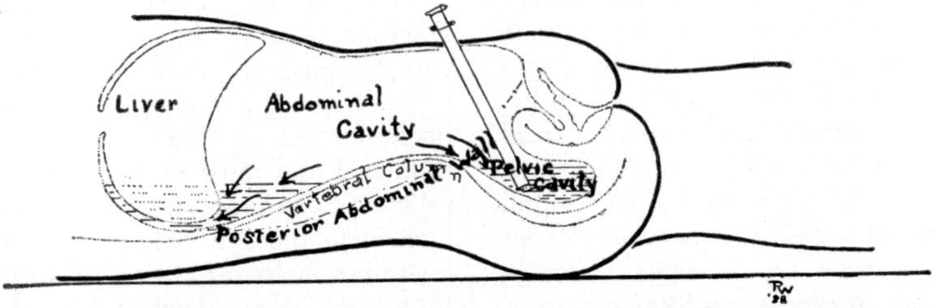

Fig. 46. Illustrating puddling of pus beneath diaphragm in a case of peritonitis treated in horizontal position.

pends upon whether the patient must be moved in one unit or not and upon his height and weight. At all times, the nurse should practice good body mechanics herself. Often back strain can be prevented if, instead of bending at the waist, the nurse can lift her patient with her back erect, bending at the knees and the hips.

EARLY POSTOPERATIVE AMBULATION

Almost all types of surgical patients are allowed and encouraged to be out of bed within 24 to 48 hours after operation. The advantages of early ambulation are seen in a reduction of postoperative complications. Atelectasis and hypostatic pneumonia are relatively infrequent when the patient is ambulatory. Ambulation increases respiratory exchange and aids in preventing stasis of bronchial secretions within the lung. Postoperative distention is almost absent, due to the increased tone of the gastro-intestinal tract and the abdominal wall. Frequent enemata, therefore, are unnecessary. Thrombophlebitis or phlebothrombosis are less frequent because ambulation increases the rate of circulation in the extremities, thereby preventing stasis of venous blood. There is clinical as well as experimental evidence to show that the rate of healing in abdominal wounds is more rapid by early ambulation, and the occurrence of postoperative evisceration has been no greater than formerly: in some series of cases actually it has been less when the patient was allowed to be out of bed soon after operation. Statistics indicate that pain is decreased, as shown by the number of hypodermics required. Comparative records also indicate that the pulse rate and the temperature return to normal sooner when the patient attempts to regain his normal preoperative activity as quickly as possible. Reestablishing a normal physiology includes a resumption of a full diet. Normal intestinal function occurs only on an adequate diet. Unless definitely contraindicated, such a diet should be given within the first 48 hours. Finally, there are the further advantages to the patient of a shorter stay in the hospital, with the consequent lower expense. And the shorter stay means an increased turnover of patients. It is almost certain that with the constantly improving surgical technic, patients will become ambulatory much sooner than in the past, unless some complication supervenes that calls for absolute rest in bed. Such complications would include acute infections with drainage, those with Wangensteen or Miller-Abbott suction or those requiring constant intravenous therapy.

Early ambulation should not be overdone. The condition of the patient must be the deciding factor. The very ill and feeble aged patient must be given every consideration. First of all, he must be placed almost upright in bed until all suggestion of dizziness has passed. This position can be obtained by raising the head of the bed. Then, he may be placed completely upright and turned so that his legs hang over the edge of the bed. After this preparation, he may be helped to stand beside his bed. When he has become accommodated to the upright position he may take a few steps to a chair or around the bed. The nurse should be at his side to give support, both physical and moral. Care must be taken not to tire the patient, and the extent of the first few periods of ambulation should vary with the type of operation and the physical condition and the age of the patient.

CONVALESCENT BED EXERCISES

When early ambulation is not feasible due to circumstances already mentioned, convalescent bed exercises may accomplish to some extent the same desirable results. These should begin as soon after operation as possible—preferably within the first 24 hours—and they should be done under supervision to ensure their adequacy.

All movements are repeated a prescribed number of times, usually from three to five. They are performed slowly, and the patient should be conscious of effort and concentration upon each part. Exercises include three phases: (1) strong contracture or tensing of muscles, (2) conscious relaxation and (3) complete rest. Leg exercises consist of flexion and extension of the foot and the toes, and internal and external rotation of the foot. If the patient can move the leg and the thigh, the thighs are abducted and adducted. In addition, flexion and extension of the leg on the thigh and the thigh on the pelvis may be carried out. Exercises with the arms and the shoulders are almost identical with the usual setting-up exercises. They consist of thrusting the arms and the forearms forward and backward, up and out, flexing and extending the fingers and rotation of the hand on the wrist. If the patient will co-operate, neck exercises may be employed in the same manner. Deep breathing exercises are a requisite and consist of deep inhalations with strong, forceful exhaling followed by coughing. Additional exercises for those who may be turned upon the abdomen include extension of the trunk upon the pelvis and the lower extremities upon the pelvis. Finally, an attempt is made to exercise all muscle groups at regular intervals as frequently as toleration will permit.

POSTOPERATIVE DIET

Patients have nutritional and fluid needs even more after operation than before it. Although these requirements may be supplied fairly well by the intravenous administration of amino acids, glucose, saline and blood (see pp. 161-178), this method of feeding a patient is much less efficient than by giving food by mouth. However, in some cases food or fluid cannot be given immediately after operation. Oral feeding usually is withheld for a time after operations on the stomach or the duodenum, or after operations that require the packing away of intestinal coils from the operative field, such as the removal of the gallbladder, the colon or the rectum. In other patients, nausea and vomiting may occur due to the anesthetic or other causes, even though the operation has not required the opening of the abdomen. In such cases intravenous feeding must be relied upon until food and fluids can be taken by mouth.

In many instances, even though a major operation has been performed, there is no reason why a normal diet cannot be given. Thus, after a thyroidectomy, a breast amputation, a lung resection or a herniorrhaphy, the patient may receive a full diet if he desires it. The patient should be encouraged to eat normally, because many patients are afraid to eat. By eating a normal diet, many of the unpleasant "gas pains" and enemas can be avoided. However, food should not be forced on the unwilling patient. The desire of the patient for food is one of the best indications of a normal recovery.

Liquid Diet

Usually liquids are desired first by the patient after operation. They also are tolerated by him. Water, fruit juices and tea with lemon and sugar may be given in increasing amounts if vomiting does not occur. The fluids supply relatively few calories. If fluids are tolerated well, gelatin, junket, custard and cornstarch pudding may be added gradually; even buttered toast, milk and creamed soups.

As soon as the patient tolerates liquids well, solid food may be given. In some cases—for instance, after operations upon the upper intestinal tract—some special precautions as to diet are taken, but in many cases—especially those patients operated upon under local or spinal anesthesia—a full diet may be given during the first 24 hours after operation.

Patients having dry mouths—especially those who are extremely ill—should have chewing gum or fruit lozenges to stimulate salivary secretion in prophylaxis against parotitis.

Soft Diet

Except in special cases (stomach, rectum and so forth) a simple soapsuds enema is given in from 48 to 72 hours after operation and, if effective, the patient may have soft diet (1,700 calories), which consists of all of liquid diet plus toast or zwieback, milk toast, well-cooked cereals, eggs (soft-cooked or poached), butter, rice, potatoes (baked or mashed), stewed fruits, simple desserts (ice creams, sherbets, ices, fruit whips, custards, plain gelatin and cornstarch), creamed chicken, creamed fish, milk, coffee, cocoa, tea. This diet may include a small portion of white meat of chicken and a baked potato. It then may be increased to an easily assimilated *light diet,* including meat, vegetables, salads and more substantial desserts.

High Caloric Diet

A high caloric diet is indicated for those patients suffering from diseases of long standing, hyperthyroidism, and especially after operation in cases of empyema, osteomyelitis and so forth, when the period of convalescence usually is one of months rather than of days or weeks. By building up body weight and strength the patient is able more easily to overcome the disease from which he is suffering.

Since fat produces more than twice as many calories as do carbohydrates and protein, this portion of the diet is made as large as possible by an abundance of such foods as butter, cream, fat meats (bacon), and olive oil. The remainder of the diet is composed of protein, and the higher carbohydrate foods. A sample diet of about 3,000 calories follows:

Breakfast:

Egg	1
Bacon	3 slices
Toast	2 slices
Butter	2 squares
Cooked cereal	1 cup
Cream	¾ cup
Sugar	2 teaspoonfuls
Fruit	1 serving

Luncheon:

Egg	1
Potato	1 (medium size)
Lettuce	4–5 leaves
Mayonnaise or French dressing	1 tablespoonful
Bread	2 slices
Butter	2 squares
Milk	½ glass
Cream	½ glass
Green vegetable	1 serving
Fruit	1 serving

Dinner:

Creamed soup	1 cup
Meat, fish or chicken	¼ lb.
Bread	2 slices
Butter	2 squares
Potato	1 (medium size)
Vegetable, such as peas, beets, carrots, Lima beans and so forth	1 serving
Vegetable, such as celery, asparagus, tomato	1 serving
Milk	½ glass
Cream	½ glass
Pudding	1 serving

The doctor must be consulted for instructions in rectal cases. The diet for stomach and duodenal cases is given on p. 314.

CARE OF THE WOUND

Rigid Asepsis. The most important requisite for the successful care of wounds is rigid asepsis. Bacteria are excluded from wounds during the period of operation to the full extent of the facilities for sterility of the operating room. Those that enter the wound usually are destroyed by the natural powers of resistance of the body. Accidental wounds are potentially infected wounds. Therefore, the surgeon is concerned with the removal of as much of the infection as possible and with the protection of the wound from further invasion by bacteria.

Wound Classification

Wounds are classified as (1) incised, (2) contused, (3) lacerated or (4) puncture, according to the manner in which they were made.

Incised wounds are those made by a clean cut with a sharp instrument. They are made by the surgeon in every operation.

Contused wounds are made by blunt force and are characterized by considerable injury of the soft parts, hemorrhage and swelling.

Lacerated wounds are those with jagged, irregular edges, such as would be made by glass, barbed wire and so forth.

Puncture wounds have small openings in the skin, such as those made by a bullet, a knifestab and the like.

Clean wounds (those made aseptically) usually are closed by sutures after all bleeding points have been ligated carefully. All other wounds are potentially infected and cannot be closed until every effort has been made to remove all devitalized tissue and infection. Therefore, a formal operation is performed for the purpose of cutting out the infected and devitalized tissue. This operation is called *débridement*. Often it is well to insert a small drain before suturing the wound to prevent the collection of blood and lymph, which would retard healing if it were allowed to remain.

A New Trend in Dressings*

There is an increasing trend toward the elimination of dressings, either shortly after surgery or within the immediate postoperative period, wherever possible or feasible. On clean, dry incisions, it is noted that when the initial dressing (applied in the operating room) is removed, usually it is not replaced. Generally, initial dressings on clean, dry incisions are left in place until the sutures are removed, and if a dressing is replaced at all, its purpose is more an esthetic than a necessary one. Substitute materials, such as sprayed plastic dressings, are being tested, and the few observed seem to be providing satisfactory service for clean and dry incisions. Then, on clean, dry wounds it seems superfluous to be concerned with the ability of the dressing to absorb secretions, since there are practically no secretions to be absorbed. Texture and comfort and perhaps screening ability against microorganisms (although this latter is a doubtful prerequisite) can be given more emphasis than powers of absorption in such dressings.

* Adapted from Postoperative Wound Care Study Report, Department of Nursing, University of Chicago Clinics.

Criteria of a Good Dressing

Certain criteria apply to all kinds of dressings. In general, these include:

1. The assurance of positive sterility of both materials and the technics of their application.
2. Economy in the use of materials and the unit cost per dressing.
3. Durability of materials, so that dressings will hold up even under the stress of motion, including early ambulation.
4. Simplicity of packaging of sterile goods to allow ease in application while assuring good aseptic technic.
5. Comfort to the patient in both the texture of the materials used and the total bulk of the dressing.
6. Availability on the wards in sufficient quantity at all times, but supplied so that overstocking and its inherent risk of loss of sterility be prevented.
7. Adequate means for safe disposal of used and contaminated dressings.
8. Adequate facilities for handwashing for protection of both the patient and the practitioner.

While a dressing placed over a clean, nondraining incision should afford protection and maintenance of a clean area, the problems of a dressing used where drainage is present must meet certain other qualifications. In addition to those listed above, these would include the following:

1. Adequate absorption to preclude soiling of bed linen and potential contamination.
2. Durable materials which retain shape and form even when soiled and can withstand motion by the patient without matting or disintegrating.
3. Comfortable fit and minimum bulk to the draining area and so applied as to serve the purpose of absorbing the maximum amount of drainage (i.e.,

SPONGES: SURGICAL AND POSTOPERATIVE TYPES

Type	Description	Use	Capacity	Approx. Cost
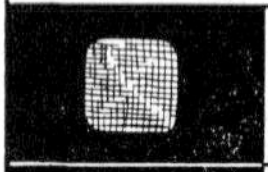	2"x 2" Gauze – 12ply	Small dressings	6cc.	35¢ per 100
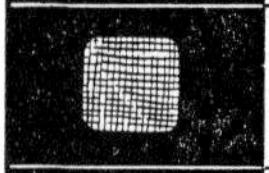	2"x 2" Gauze – cotton filmated	Skin prep	9cc.	35¢ per 100
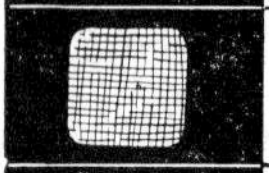	3"x 3" Gauze – 12 ply	Minor or major surgery	12cc.	89¢ per 100
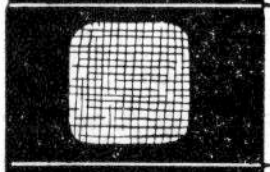	3"x 3" Gauze – cotton filmated	Postoperative and surface dressings	14cc.	63¢ per 100
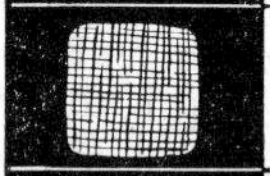	4"x 4" Gauze – 8ply	Minor surgery	11 cc.	½¢ each
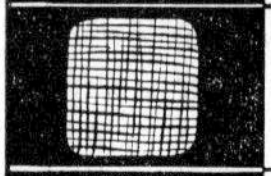	4"x 4" Gauze – 16ply	Minor or major surgery	17cc.	1½¢ each
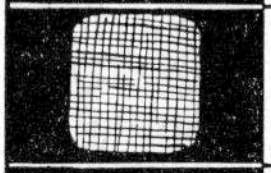	4"x 4" Gauze – cotton filmated	Postoperative dressings	22cc.	1½¢ each
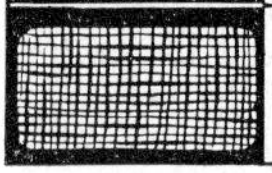	8"x 4" Gauze – 12ply	Major surgery large dressings	22cc.	2½¢ each

Fig. 47. A description of a large assortment of surgical sponges. Each sponge is described, with columns listing the sizes and the absorbent capacities, other nomenclature, the general uses and applications and the value of individual dressings.

applied with consideration of the direction of maximum flow of drainage).

4. Secure placing, so that position is retained when the patient moves.

The Economies of Surgical Dressings

In discussing the cost of dressings, one must be aware constantly that in addition to the obvious unit cost of the materials themselves, the cost of processing and sterilizing in the hospital must be included. The largest percentage of such additional cost is that which may be attributed to labor, although other considerations such as the costs of autoclaving, packaging of materials and equipment necessary to do the job, also must be estimated. (Figs. 47 and 48.)

The ideal processing of dressings materials should be done by an efficient central supply unit, and ward personnel should not be utilized for any step in the processing when a central supply is available.

Materials should be supplied to

COTTON BALLS

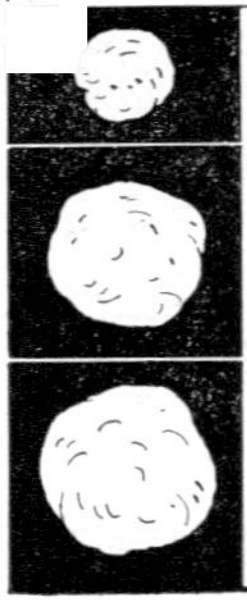

Type	Description	Uses	Capacity	Approx. Cost
	Medium	Skin preps	9cc.	$.91 per M
	Large	Perineal	31cc.	$2.23 per M
	Perineal	Applicator for Medications	40cc.	$3.27 per M

OBSTETRIC PADS

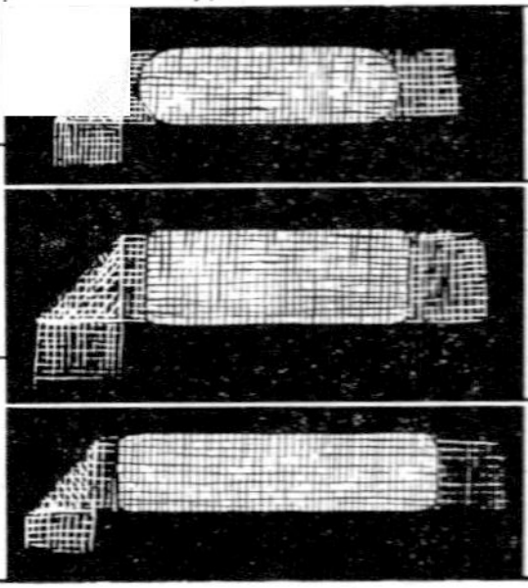

Type	Description	Capacity	Approx. Cost
	$8\frac{3}{4}$" Cellulose filler	142 cc.	$1\frac{1}{2}$¢ each
	9" cotton filler	192cc	2¢ each
	12" cotton filler	234cc	$2\frac{1}{2}$¢ each

COMBINE PADS

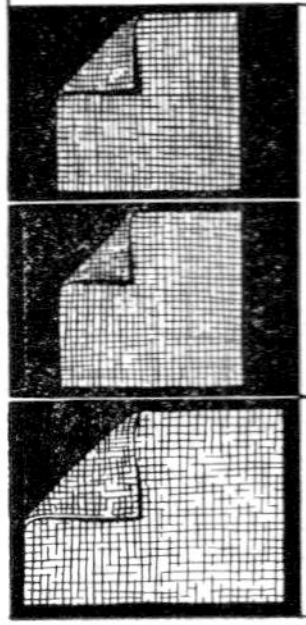

Type	Description	Uses	Capacity	Approx. Cost
	Absorbent cotton with nonabsorbent backing 8"x $7\frac{1}{2}$"	Postoperative secondary dressing; Drainage pads; Compress dressing	177cc.	$2\frac{1}{2}$¢ each
	All-absorbent cotton 8"x $7\frac{1}{2}$"	Postoperative secondary dressing; Drainage pads; Compress dressing	197cc	$2\frac{1}{2}$¢ each
	Absorbent cotton with nonabsorbent backing 10"x 12"	Postoperative secondary dressing; Drainage pads; Incontinent pad	290cc	$4\frac{1}{2}$¢ each

FIG. 48. An illustration of obstetric pads, combine pads, cotton balls, underpads and disposal diapers. Descriptive information includes the general uses and applications, the sizes and the absorbent capacities, other nomenclature and the value of individual items.

each ward in accordance with an established standard of use, so that the clerical task of filling out necessary requisition forms is left to ward clerical help. It is particularly expensive to use a professional nurse for this task.

A continuing plan for education of personnel in the proper use of dressing materials is also essential to good economy. In addition to the obvious conservation of materials and restriction of use to proper tasks, this must include a standardized method for the application of all kinds of surgical dressings (e.g., to stop the futile use of nonabsorbent combine pads on top of nonabsorbent combine pads).

Absorption by Dressings

Absorption is a decided problem in the application of dressings to draining wounds, particularly such types of draining wounds as colostomies, ileostomies, cystostomies, bile duct drainage, etc. While no dressing can be substituted for good nursing care, including change of dressings as often as necessary, a dressing designed to provide absorption without excessive bulk is certainly desirable. It is widespread practice in many hospitals to provide a fluffed gauze dressing of some kind for this purpose. The practice of fluffing washed gauze is impractical from an economic viewpoint unless (as is done sometimes) it is manufactured by patient labor—certainly an undesirable situation. The practice of fluffing the regular 4x4 or 4x8 gauze pad at the bedside is also ridiculously wasteful of labor; at the same time, using such pads as they are provided, stacked one on another, provides a dressing which repeatedly becomes matted, heavy and soggy and lacks adequate absorption. This is particularly true of very fluid drainage. Heavy drainage packs have performed satisfactorily in many cases. These heavy drainage packs are a combination of the following dressings:

4 CHIX cleaners which are used to cleanse the incision and the wound area.

2 strips of Zobec cotton filmated gauze, each 15 in. long, to be used as a fluff or a wrap around the wound area, i.e., for stoma, drains, etc. (functions as a wick).

2 all-absorbent cotton combine pads 8x10 in. to be placed over the gauze (functions as a well).

1 combine pad 12x16 in. with nonabsorbent backing to cover the complete assembly of dressing (functions as a cap).

Surgical Dressing Technic

The prerequisite to flawless surgical dressing technic is for surgeons and nurses to agree on a standard. Thereafter, it becomes a matter of repeated teaching and supervision to ensure that such handling of dressings actually is carried out.

Surgical Dressing Cart. A surgical dressing cart is essential on a surgical floor. It should be easily movable, with well-oiled wheels to prevent noise. It is easier to keep clean if it has a metal surface rather than a painted one. A tray on an extended arm, which can be set up as a sterile field near the patient, is desirable. The cart also should have a covered receptacle for soiled dressings.

The dressing carriage should contain sufficient supplies for routine dressings. Those materials which are used infrequently ought to be stored in the nearby treatment room.

SURGICAL DRESSING CART EQUIPMENT

Transfer forceps in a container with an antiseptic.

Unsterile forceps in a container with an antiseptic, to handle soiled dressings.

Sterile Supplies
- Trays, each containing
  - Scissors
  - Dressing forceps
  - Hemostat
  - Grooved director or probe
- Surgical sponges, large and small
- Combine pads
- Cotton balls
- Towels or covers
- Applicator sticks and tongue depressors
- Culture tubes and plain tubes
- Petrolatum gauze
- Safety pins

Medications and Solutions
- Alcohol, 70 per cent
- Zephiran 1:1,000
- Benzene or carbon tetrachloride
- Tr. benzoin compound or Whitehead's varnish

Ointments
- Sterile petrolatum

Unsterile Supplies
- Adhesive tape, various widths
- Montgomery straps
- Bandage, gauze, 1-6 in.
- Bandage scissors
- Paper bags for soiled dressings

Nursing Responsibility. The surgical nurse should be available to assist the physician in the changing of dressings for several reasons:

1. The "team" working together assures the patient of expert care.
2. The nurse, as a witness to the dressing, is better informed concerning her patient and therefore can give him more intelligent care.
3. The use of a nurse in the handling of equipment (such as the dressing cart) eliminates the risk of contamination of equipment which serves many patients.
4. The use of the doctor's time in changing dressings which a trained, professional nurse is entirely capable of doing is uneconomical. While all initial postoperative dressings are done properly only by the surgeon, subsequent applications should be done by the nurse, in whom the surgeon must have sufficient confidence to trust that unfavorable changes in the incision will be reported promptly.

Surgical dressings should be noted on the patient's chart as carefully as any other medication or treatment, and pertinent observations should be recorded by the nurse.

Dressing Technic. PREPARATION OF THE PATIENT. The patient should be told that the surgeon is going to change his dressing, and that it is a simple procedure associated with little discomfort. *Dressings should not be done at mealtime.* If the patient is in an open ward, the curtains should be drawn to ensure his privacy. When the dressing has a foul odor or the patient is unusually squeamish, it is better to wheel his bed to the ward treatment room, away from other patients. He should not be exposed unduly; his sense of modesty should be respected.

USE OF TRANSFER FORCEPS. To carry out aseptic technic, the nurse must know how to handle the transfer forceps correctly. This is an essential instrument which has the unique quality of possessing a sterile and an unsterile section. Naturally, the unsterile handle is grasped by the unsterile hand of the user. The sterile end usually is kept submerged

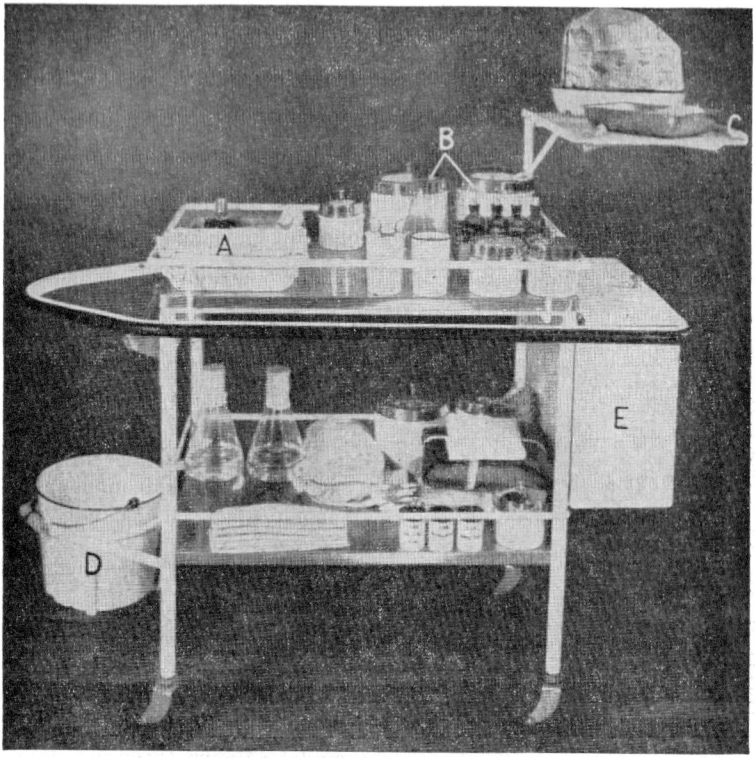

FIG. 49. Dressing carriage for use in bedside dressing in surgical wards. (A) Trays enclosed in muslin envelope. These contain instruments for dressing one patient. (B) Jars for sterile dressings. (C) Dressing tray which may be rotated over bed and on which is placed sterile tray with dressing instruments and basin with paper lining for soiled dressings. (D) Receptacle for soiled dressings enclosed in paper. (E) Compartment for soiled covers, gloves and so forth.

in a germicide. It is necessary to observe the following precautions in order to maintain sterility:

1. Always keep the tips of the forceps pointing downward. If this is not done, solution will run down to the unsterile handle and consequently will contaminate the tips. In the newer commercially made transfer forceps (Fig. 306), this problem is eliminated by the use of a rubber guard.

2. These forceps should not touch anything on a sterile field which is being used currently for a particular patient.

3. In grasping petrolatum gauze, it is better to use another sterile instrument rather than the transfer forceps. It is obvious that petrolatum on the tips of the transfer forceps would be an annoying handicap.

A ROUTINE DRESSING. The dressing carriage is equipped with a small tray in one corner that can be turned so as to be convenient for the surgeon (Fig. 49). On this tray are the materials for the dressing. For the routine dressing the equipment usually consists of scissors, forceps, hemostat and grooved director placed in a small enamel tray that has been sterilized in an envelope cover of muslin. An individual tray is used for each patient.

If there is any doubt concerning the sterility of an instrument or a dressing, it should be considered to be unsterile. In no circumstance should the nurse touch soiled dressings with her hands.

Dressing Procedure

Stitches or clips used to approximate the skin edges are of no value after the fifth, the sixth or the seventh day. The nurse should be prepared for the first dressing at that time. The adhesive then should be removed by pulling it parallel with the skin surface and not at right angles. The nurse removes the old dressing by means of an unsterile forceps and places this dressing in a paper bag for easy disposal. She then hands the surgeon a sterile cover which becomes the sterile field. A sterile set of simple instruments are provided. Then the nurse drops 2 or 3 sterile cotton balls on the sterile field. Using a forceps, the surgeon grasps a cotton ball and holds it over the emesis basin as the nurse pours a small quantity of the desired antiseptic. After cleansing the wound and surrounding skin with alcohol, the stitches are removed, and the nurse provides sterile gauze compresses and adhesive strips for the new dressing. Tension sutures are allowed to remain in place for a longer period of time in some instances.

THE DRESSING OF DRAINING WOUNDS. It may be necessary to dress draining wounds as soon as

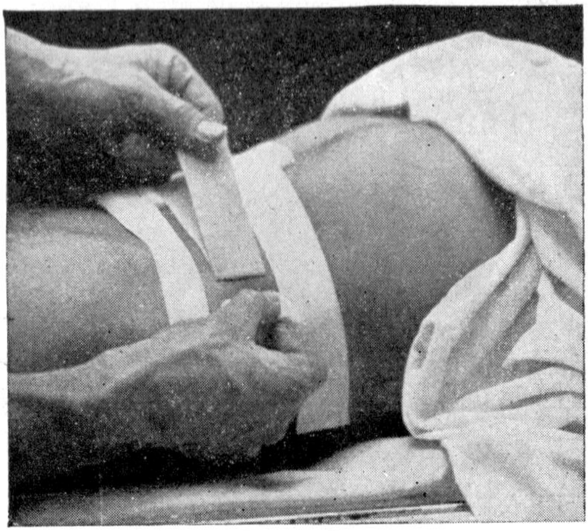

FIG. 50. Removing adhesive strips.

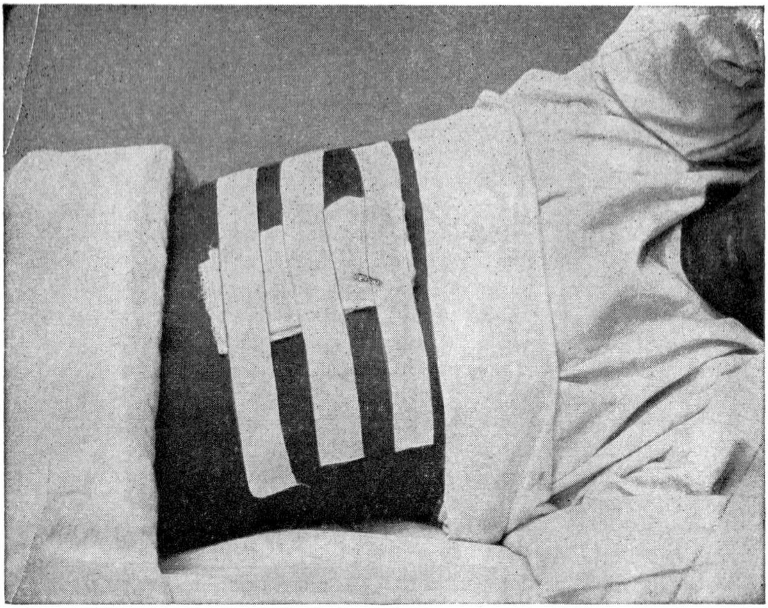

FIG. 51. Adhesive strips applied to abdominal wound. Note that sufficient gauze is exposed between adhesive to allow for inspection and ventilation.

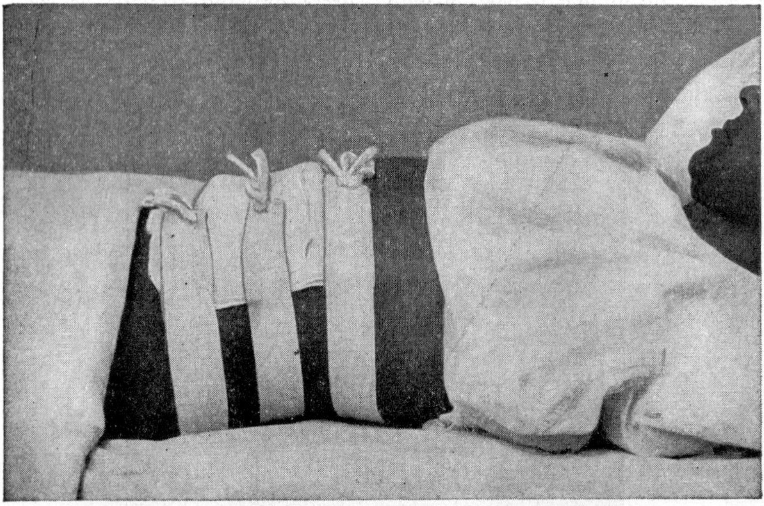

FIG. 52. Montgomery tape dressing, for use when dressings have to be changed frequently.

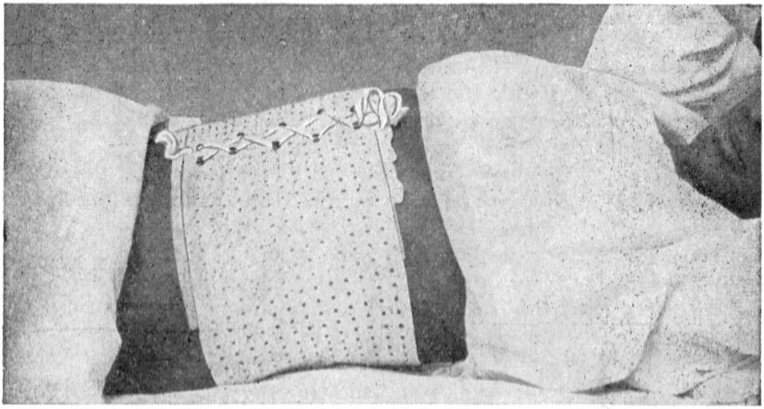

Fig. 53. (*Top*) Laced dressing. (*Bottom*) Adhesive matchstick dressing with rubber bands. For use when dressings have to be changed frequently.

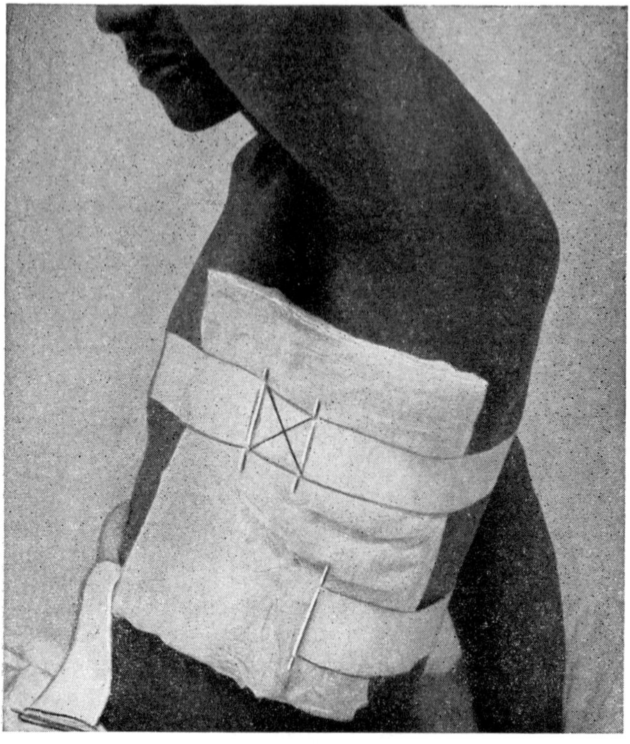

24 hours after operation. Nothing causes a patient more unnecessary discomfort than a dressing saturated with drainage fluids. It dries on the edges and becomes stiff and scratchy, and the odor frequently is very offensive, if not actually nauseating. The nurse may relieve such a situation by changing the outer layers of the dressing at frequent intervals between dressings.

When it is necessary to dress the wound daily, either adhesive with tapes or a laced dressing is more convenient than simple adhesive strips. (Figs. 51 to 53.) These should not be applied so tightly that the dressings underneath are unable to retain drainage. A scultetus binder also makes an effective, convenient dressing. (Fig. 54.)

When the edges of the wound gape and the gauze has become adherent to the tissues, the patient may be spared considerable pain by moistening the dressings with peroxide of hydrogen. For this purpose a syringe and a basin containing the solution must be provided. As the surgeon applies the peroxide, the

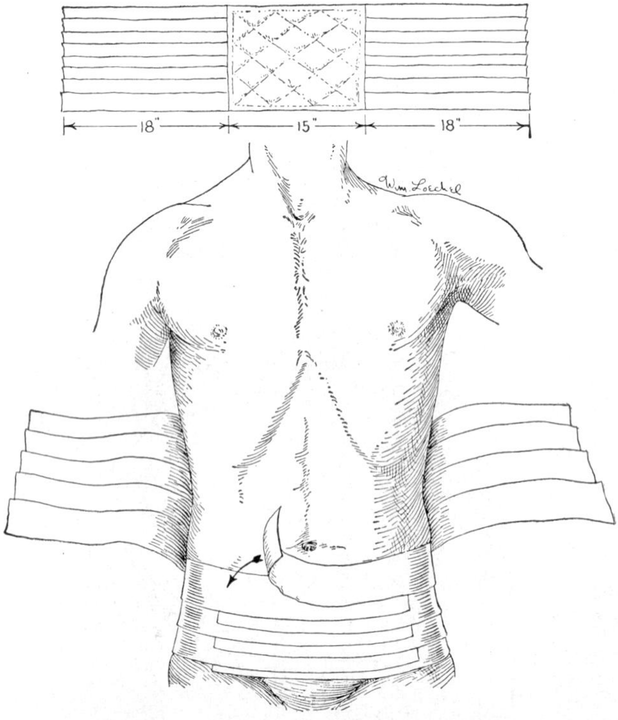

FIG. 54. Scultetus binder. Dimensions of binder and method of sewing are shown, also the method of application of binder. The tails should overlap from below upward, and the binder should fit snugly.

nurse should hold a waste pan to prevent the solution from soiling the bed.

When drainage tubes are being shortened, the nurse should have a sterile safety pin ready to insert in the new tube end. If the tubes are removed, the surgeon frequently inserts a piece of rubber tissue or packing to prevent too early a closing of the drainage tract. These materials should be at hand and ready for use.

The drainage from an infected wound frequently proves to be irritating to the surrounding skin. Often this situation may be avoided by the use of a protecting ointment or dressing. Petrolatum gauze and zinc oxide ointments are favorite preparations. When the discharge from the wound contains the digestive enzymes, as in pancreatic or intestinal fistulae, ileostomy and cecostomy wounds, more active measures to protect the skin must be taken. In some cases, the enzyme-containing secretion may be aspirated by constant suction. In others, the skin surrounding the wound may be protected by such adhering ointments as zinc oxide ointment containing aluminum filings or better by a creamy paste mixture of aluminum hydroxide gel and kaolin (Protogel, Wyeth) which is both soothing to the skin and a neutralizer of the enzymes in the secretions. These must be applied to an absolutely dry skin surface.

The nurse who assists with dressings has a most important part in the care of the surgical patient in that, by her interest, alertness and readiness, dressings can be changed efficiently with economical use of the surgeon's time and a minimum of discomfort for the patient. By knowing beforehand the nature of the surgery performed on her patient, the nurse will be able to anticipate the surgeon's needs. The surgeon will not expect her to have on hand materials that are unusual or out of the ordinary, but on request she should have them ready for use at the time of the next dressing.

The Completion of a Dressing. When the dressing is completed, the soiled dressings are wrapped in the bag and placed in a large covered bucket on the side of the cart. One end of the lower shelf of the cart is reserved for used or contaminated materials: instruments, trays, covers, gloves and so forth. When all the ward dressings are completed, the bucket is emptied into a covered dressing can. Eventually, these dressings go to the incinerator; the cart is cleaned and restocked for subsequent use. Each night the dressing carriage is cleaned thoroughly: the containers are refilled and autoclaved, and the supplies are replaced. Thus, the cart is made ready for dressing each morning.

Special Dressings

For dressings on special surgical services some variation in supplies is necessary. For dressing patients on the urologic service the cart is equipped with various types and sizes of sterile catheters and connecting tubes. Frequently, special types of bandages and dressings are employed. These are supplied according to the needs of the surgeon.

For the dressing of patients in private rooms a tray containing the following articles should be available:

Sterile simple tray containing
- Plain forceps
- Scissors
- Hemostat
- Probe or grooved director

Sterile packages of
- Assorted sponges
- Combine pads
- Assorted packing
- Plain and culture tubes
- Draping covers
- Applicator sticks
- Safety pins
- Gloves

Container with sterile drainage tubes and rubber dam
Container with dry sterile cotton balls
Alcohol, 70 per cent
Peroxide of hydrogen
Flask of sterile saline
Collodion
Adhesive, ½ in., 1 in., 2 in.
Bandage, 1 in., 2 in., 3 in.
Paper envelope for waste

CHARTS AND NURSES' RECORDS

To keep a record of all observations and treatments bearing on patient care is an essential function of the nurse (Fig. 55). Accuracy and neatness in the matter of charts and records usually bespeak thorough nursing with keen observation and attention to detail. For this reason, the record should be kept up to date. Such a nurse's report is worth more than one in which the whole record for the day is written in 5 minutes before the nurse reports to her successor.

In general, printing rather than script is preferable since usually it is more legible. Statements should be concise, pertinent and brief. The recording of the reactions of a patient to a treatment may be more important for his future therapy than the treatment itself. Hence, significant conversation, facial expressions, and general behavior of an individual ought to be charted when such activities seem to be worthy of attention. Cultural practices of the patient which reflect past experiences and indicate future tendencies may affect future treatment; therefore, these should be recorded by the nurse. This will be of value not only to the physician but also to the next nurse coming to care for this patient.

The nurse prepares the very important temperature chart that shows fluctuations in the vital signs of the patient. Of course, all medications and treatments should be recorded with the time of administration. The effects produced and/or the results noted must be recorded. For example, in recording an enema, the kind, the amount of solution given and the effectiveness are desired. Merely to chart "Eff." or "Not eff." is not sufficient. By effectiveness is meant, What type of return (color and consistency as well as amount)? Was there much flatus? How did the patient feel during and after the enema?

At the end of each 8- or 12-hour period, a brief summary is charted, depending on the desires of the surgeon. This may be merely fluid intake and output or it may be more extensive. A 24-hour résumé is more nearly complete and should include the condition of the patient, the medications and the treatments given during that time, the intake and the output and so forth.

Complete fluid intake and output charts are essential on some patients. The nurse must remember that the

NURSES' RECORD

Tomp. 3 — Taylor, Roberta — 247 Oak St. N.H. — (3)

DATE AND HOURS	INTAKE		OUTPUT		STOOL	B P	MEDICATION AND TREATMENT	REMARKS
Dec. 14								
	1st. P.O. Day beginning 8 A.M. Dec. 14,							
8:30 A.M.						128/86		Morning bath. Back
								care. Moves about
								in bed and turns
10:00								without difficulty.
	Cracked ice						Demerol 0.075 Gm.	Thirsty. Complains
								of some discomfort
								at incision site.
								Has not voided yet.
								No distention or
								discomfort.
								Infusion, N. Saline
10:30 - 11:30								started by Dr. Kerin.
								Resting comfortably.
			Urine	600				Voided. Amber color.
11:30								Sitting upright and
								"dangling" over edge
								of bed for 5 min.
								Pulse regular.
12:15 P.M.	Water	100				130/88		M. S. Jackson
	N. Saline (I.V.)	1000					Vitamin C 200 mgm.	Infusion continued
								with 5% glucose in
:30								H_2O. Vitamin added.
								Sat on edge of
								bed, for a few min.
								Up in chair. After
								being in chair for
								5 min. pulse became
								elevated from 72-88
								Said she was feel-
								ing weak and dizzy.
								Back to bed.
	5% gluc. (I.V.)	1000						Infusion discontin-
								ued.
	Hot tea							Tea and 2 pieces
	with lemon	120						of unbuttered toast.

© 2239 REMINGTON RAND INC.-22

FIGUR

NURSES' RECORD

Pomp. 3. — Taylor, Roberta — 247 Oak St., N.H. — (4.)

DATE AND HOURS	INTAKE		OUTPUT		STOOL	B P	MEDICATION AND TREATMENT	REMARKS
Dec. 14								
3 P.M.	Water	200	Urine	300				Visited by husband.
								Drs. Lindsay and
								Kerin in.
								Afternoon care.
								Moves and turns
								when reminded. Uses
								blow bottle hourly.
4:00						128/88	Penicillin 200,000 U.	Lt. Thigh (I.M.)
5:00	Grapefruit						Acetyl Salicylic	
	Juice	200					Acid 0.065 Gm.	For headache and
	Tea	120						discomfort.
6:00								"Dangled" Up and
								out of bed. Walking
								with nurse to window
								and then to door.
								In chair for 30 min.
								Enjoyed being up.
								"Surprised that I
								could do it."
7:00			Urine	700				Resting in bed.
	Fluid Summary for 12 Hrs. Ending 8 P.M. Dec. 14, 1953							1st P.O. Day
	Per Mouth	740	Urine ∴	1600				Out of Bed 30 min.
	Per Infusion	2000						Good Day
	Intake	2740	Output	1600				Jane James.

fluid intake includes all fluids given to the patient by any method during the 24-hour period. This includes liquid foods as well as water taken by mouth and all fluids given parenterally. Fluids used for irrigating gastro-intestinal suction tubes likewise should be included. Fluid output consists of all measurable fluids given off by the patient in 24 hours. This includes urine voided, vomitus and drainage. These fluids are recorded in cubic centimeters and are totaled at 12- and 24-hour periods.

In many hospitals it is required that each nurse sign or initial that portion of the nurse's record which represents the time she was responsible for the patient's care. When the patient is discharged, the nurse is responsible for seeing that the complete chart is in order and is sent to the record room. This completes her responsibility.

CHAPTER SEVEN

Postoperative Discomforts and Complaints

By knowing that her patient may experience some discomforts postoperatively, the nurse will be alerted to recognize their early manifestations and then to proceed to alleviate them as best she can. This chapter should help the nurse to achieve these objectives.

PAIN

Pain is among the earliest postoperative symptoms. It can be expected as soon as the patient returns to consciousness. During the first 24 hours the pain is considered to be due to the cutting, the retracting and the suturing incidental to the operation, and for this discomfort morphine or a similar narcotic should be given as ordered. If the patient still complains, the surgeon should be notified.

The pain in abdominal operations is aggravated continually by vomiting, coughing and respiratory movements, and often in these cases it is wise to administer the morphine before the patient has recovered entirely from the anesthetic, so that he will pass several additional hours in quiet sleep and thus be spared a large part of the immediate postoperative nausea and vomiting. When hyoscine has been given before operation or when a basal anesthetic (pp. 74, 75) such as Avertin or Pentothal Sodium has been used, often recovery from anesthesia is long. In such cases, morphine may be withheld until the necessity for its use arises.

Although pain in the first 24 hours usually is due to the operative procedures, the nurse never should omit a thorough inspection of the wound and the dressings for causes of discomfort. Pins from dressings or drainage tubes may be sticking into the patient, or the bandage may be too tight. Pain occuring after operations upon bones or joints in which splints or a cast has been applied demands immediate attention. Pressure points occur very frequently because of insufficient padding or because the bandages have been applied too firmly. These difficulties may be overcome easily if they are found early but, if the danger sign, pain, is disregarded, the patient may go without treatment until pressure causes necrosis of skin or tendons or paralysis of nerves. The pain in these patients may be very short-lived, but it never should be neglected for a single moment.

Pain is a symptom that differs markedly in acuity in various patients. A neurotic patient with a small wound may complain much more than a phlegmatic individual after an extensive operation. Not only does the mental state of the patient affect the amount of pain he experiences but there seems to be an actual difference in the amount of pain experienced by individuals of the same type. Some races—the Negro, the Chinese and the Germanic types—seem to bear pain well, while the Jewish, the Italian and other Latin races do not. Pain seems to be experienced less keenly in old age than in youth and middle age. "Pain is the resultant then of two factors, the lesion and the patient, and in order to arrive at an intelligent appreciation of its true significance, both must be thoroughly understood." When the patient complains of pain, the nurse should find its location, whether it is intermittent or constant, and whether it is dull, sharp or colicky in character. She should ascertain whether there is any constant radiation of the pain—whether it is down the legs; whether it is in the back; whether it occurs on taking a breath; or whether it is worse at night than during the day. These facts should be noted on the nurse's record and communicated to the surgeon, because with this information he may be able to diagnose the cause more accurately and prescribe for its relief.

Headache after spinal anesthesia may be severe for a few days. By keeping the patient flat and quiet and administering aspirin, the headache may be controlled. (See p. 76.)

Treatment. The treatment of postoperative pain depends upon its cause. After making sure that there is no removable cause for discomfort in the wound or the dressings, other reasons for discomfort should be investigated, and proper specific treatment instituted. As a general rule, pain that occurs after 24 hours usually is due to causes other than the operation.

Abdominal distention is a common cause, and often relief may be given by the insertion of a rectal tube or, better, by the use of a small enema. The sharp pains of a postoperative pleurisy may be relieved almost completely by tight adhesive strapping.

Drugs should be used in conjunction with other forms of treatment rather than instead of them. Morphine, above all others, is the most effective, and it should not be withheld if the indications for its use arise. The morphine habit rarely develops in a patient to whom it is given for actual pain. However, as soon as possible it may be replaced by codeine and the coal-tar group, such as aspirin, sodium salicylate and Phenacetin. In patients who exhibit an idiosyncrasy to morphine, Demerol, Pantopon or Dilaudid often is substituted with good results.

Certain patients come to depend upon their "hypodermic," especially at night, and complain of pain and discomfort that obviously are not as severe as they represent them to be. In such cases a hypodermic of sterile saline solution may act as a placebo. This trick never should be resorted to without the knowledge and the consent of the surgeon.

VOMITING

Vomiting is perhaps the most frequent postoperative symptom, and the nurse should know this. She should have a basin at hand to catch any vomitus and she should turn the patient's head to one side. Also, she should keep the patient and the bed clean. In case of an abdominal operation, the patient will appreciate it if she will support the wound with her hand during the retching. The nurse should provide a mouth wash after the patient has vomited.

There are three types of postoperative vomiting, according to its duration: (1) vomiting when coming out of the anesthetic, (2) vomiting that is continuous through the first day and night, and (3) vomiting that is excessive or prolonged.

When Coming Out of the Anesthetic

The vomiting that occurs as the patient is coming out of the anesthetic relieves the stomach merely of mucus and saliva swallowed during the anesthetic period. This type of vomiting also may occur occasionally after operations done under local anesthesia. Its duration is short (from 2 to 8 hours at most), and it requires no special treatment beyond the washing out of the mouth and the withholding of fluids for a few hours.

When Continuous Through the First Day and Night

Vomiting that continues for the first day and night may be due to one of several causes:

Effects of the Anesthesia. These may persist so that some patients may be nauseated and vomit long after they have regained consciousness. This idiosyncrasy occurs especially in patients who have had ether. If such patients are given a large glass of warm water with a half teaspoonful of sodium bicarbonate dissolved in it, they usually will vomit immediately, bringing up with the fluid considerable amounts of ether-laden mucus. After one or two such spontaneous gastric lavages, the patient usually will be relieved, and, after an hour or two, fluids may be given by mouth. Very frequently a hypodermic of morphine may give the patient several hours' rest, at the end of which time the nausea and the vomiting will have ceased.

Paralysis of Intestinal Activity. Frequently, there is considerable injury to the abdominal organs during an operation, with resultant paralysis of intestinal activity for a period longer than usual. Such patients have what in effect is a sterile peritonitis: fluids from the upper intestinal canal do not move onward; they dam back and are vomited. Nasal catheter drainage of the stomach for a time is the most effective treatment.

Idiosyncrasy. The patient may be affected in an unusual way by morphine. Usually he vomits soon after the administration of the drug. An experienced nurse will recognize this idiosyncrasy and will report her suspicions to the surgeon and ask for instructions.

When Excessive and Prolonged

The causes of vomiting that continues without much remission for from 3 to 7 days, retarding the patient's recovery or even threatening his life, usually are serious and will be discussed separately. Such conditions may be enumerated as follows:

1. Intestinal obstruction
2. Acute dilatation of stomach
3. Uremia or kidney insufficiency
4. Hemorrhage in operations upon stomach
5. Peritonitis

At times, even without any apparent marked organic cause, vomiting will continue longer than usual. Such patients usually are highly nervous, apprehensive individuals, and it frequently taxes the ingenuity of both doctor and nurse to the utmost to keep anything in their stomachs. In these cases, charged water, gingerale or champagne may be tried after evacuation of the stomach through a nasal catheter.

RESTLESSNESS

Discomfort. Restlessness is a postoperative symptom that should not be passed over lightly. The most common cause probably is the general discomfort following an operation, especially pain in the back, headache and thirst. This discomfort may be relieved largely by a gentle massage with alcohol, followed by a dose of aspirin (which may be repeated if necessary).

Tight Drainage-soaked Bandages. Often these cause enough discomfort to make a patient restless and ill at ease. Fresh dressings usually improve the patient's spirits and make him more comfortable. Severe pain should not be permitted to be the cause of restlessness. Morphine or other narcotics should be given until relief is obtained. They should not be given for restlessness or sleeplessness. Milder somnifacients should be used.

Retention of urine, which occurs not infrequently after operation, may be the sole cause for restlessness.

Severe Toxemia. This condition frequently produces a very restless patient. For such a patient little can be done until the toxins have been eliminated from the blood. He is quieted best by adequate doses of morphine.

Flatulence and Hiccough. Flatulence and hiccough may be causes of restlessness. Their recognition and their treatment will be discussed later (pp. 133 and 147).

Hemorrhage. Probably the most serious cause of restlessness is hemorrhage. This is discussed in the next chapter.

SLEEPLESSNESS

Frequently, sleeplessness is associated with restlessness in patients after operation. However, there are many patients who simply cannot sleep. When this situation continues for 2 or 3 days, it is the cause of considerable anxiety to the surgeon. It is in such a situation that a competent nurse is most valuable. She must recognize that a patient taken suddenly from an active life and put to bed in strange surroundings may have cause for inability to sleep. The prolonged rest and periods of sleep secured during the daytime leave him wide awake at a time when in ordinary circumstances he would be asleep.

Treatment. The nurse, anticipating such a result, will provide diversion for her patient and cut the daytime naps short, so that at night he is ready to welcome a "good sound sleep." At bedtime she may give a gentle massage, particularly of the back and the neck, ventilate the room thoroughly and dim the lights. If these ordinary measures do not promote sleep, further causes of insomnia must be looked for. Many patients are used to some form of food before going to bed. These patients frequently will go to sleep after they have been given a cup of warm milk or cocoa and crackers or other food that is easily assimilated.

Worry and anxiety keep many patients awake. If it is possible to ascertain the cause of their worry, attempts can be made to relieve it. Perhaps it concerns their surgery, length of convalescence, readjustment to a new way of life—whatever it may be and however deep the worry, there is always a bright side of the picture. An understanding nurse can help such an individual. Spiritual comfort can provide an inner peace.

Medications. To this type of patient, bromides or barbiturates may be given with benefit. They should be given cautiously and in doses just sufficient to produce the desired effect.

Demerol and Dilaudid are useful as analgesics. Alcohol in 5 per cent solution frequently is used intravenously to reduce pain, restlessness and sleeplessness. The alcohol may be introduced into the usual intravenous solutions. Commercially prepared solutions also are available. The solution is given by the drip method.

THIRST

Thirst is a troublesome symptom after many general anesthetics, and even after some cases of local anesthesia. It is due in large measure to the dryness of the mouth and the pharynx, caused by the inhibition of mucous secretion by the usual preoperative injection of atropine. Many patients operated upon under local anesthesia will complain of thirst during the operation. In addition, there is a considerable loss of body fluids due to perspiration, increased mucous secretion in the lungs and more or less loss of blood, so that the factor of dehydration also enters into the cause. To combat the loss of fluids, solutions are given into the vein for the first few hours after operation. Even though an adequate amount of fluid is taken by these methods, often it does not relieve the thirst.

The sticky, dry mouth demands fluids, and fluids may be given to most patients as soon as the postoperative nausea and vomiting have passed. Sips of hot water or hot tea with lemon juice serve to dissolve the mucus better than cold water. Iced water never should be used, although small pieces of ice given to the patient may be very much enjoyed, and the amount of fluid given by this method is so small relatively that it is permitted even in cases in which fluids are withheld by mouth. As soon as the patient can take water by mouth in sufficient quantities, the parenteral administration should be discontinued.

When operations have been performed upon the mouth, the esophagus and the stomach, and about the duodenum, water usually is withheld for about 24 hours—often longer. To relieve the thirst of these patients often taxes the ingenuity of the most experienced nurse. Mouthwashes containing some weak alkali to dissolve the mucus are the best—for example, liquor antisepticus alkalinus diluted 1 to 4 with water. A solution of equal parts of boric acid 4 per cent and glycerin also may be used. It seems to leave the mouth "wet" and allays thirst somewhat. A damp cloth laid over the mouth will tend to moisten the air breathed and will be gratifying to many patients. Hard candies, chewing gum, even paraffin wax, may be chewed. This stimulates the flow of saliva and tends to keep the mouth moist.

ABDOMINAL DISTENTION

Distention of the abdomen after operation is very common. The trauma to the abdominal contents by operation produces a loss of normal peristalsis for 24 to 48 hours, depending on the type and the extent of the operation. Even though nothing is given by mouth, swallowed air and gastro-intestinal secretions enter the stomach and the intestines and if not propelled by peristaltic activity, they collect in the intestinal coils to produce distention. Most often the gas collects in the colon; hence, a rectal tube or a small enema may be expected to give relief. Following major abdominal operations, distention may be avoided by the prophylactic use of a gastric or an intestinal tube. By this means the air which is swallowed (swallowed air provides most of the gas that produces distention) may be aspirated from the stomach and the upper intestine.

Certain patients swallow air as a part of anxiety reaction. If these characteristics can be recognized, the gastric suction tube may be used for a longer time than usual, until full peristalsis activity (passage of flatus) is resumed.

Distended Bladder. A distended bladder frequently is the cause of a distention of the lower abdomen. This is discussed below (see p. 149).

CONSTIPATION AND DIARRHEA

The care of the bowels after operation is a responsibility shared alike by surgeon and nurse. The nurse, who is with the patient constantly, must be prepared to give accurate reports as to the number and the character of the stools, the effectiveness of enemas and so forth.

Constipation

The causes of constipation after operation may be innocent or serious. The irritation and the trauma to the bowel at the time of the operation may inhibit intestinal movements for several days, but usually peristaltic function returns after the third day, following a simple enema and an increase in diet. Local inflammation, peritonitis or abscess may cause constipation, but the treatment of the causal condition is indicated. Constipation has been mentioned as being a constant symptom of intestinal obstruction.

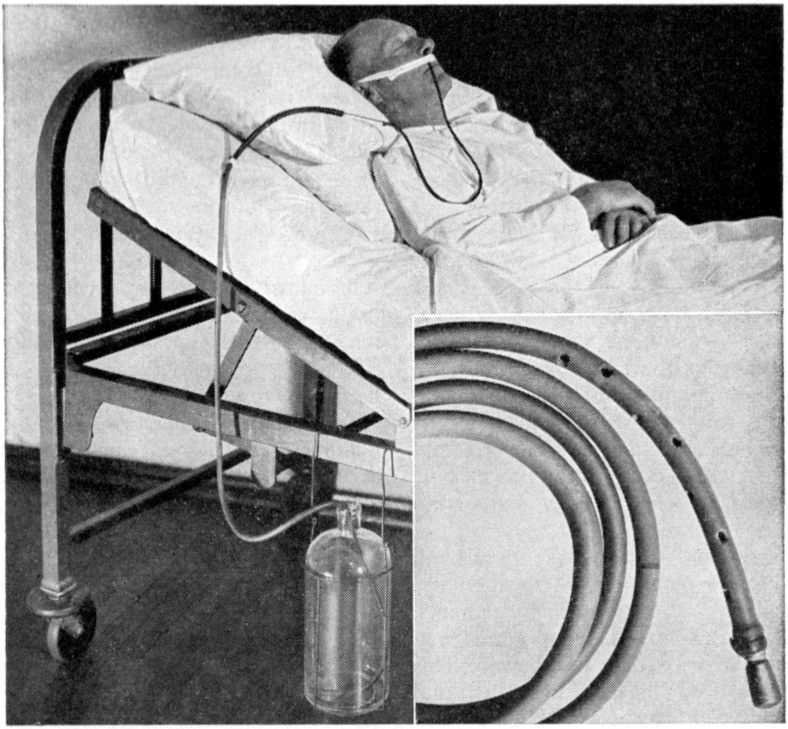

FIG. 56. Jutte tube used for continuous siphon drainage of the stomach, shown both in detail (*inset*) and in position when in use.

Fecal Impaction. An avoidable cause of postoperative constipation is fecal impaction. This complication is a result of neglect and never should be permitted to occur. The patients usually are individuals past middle age, weakened somewhat by operation, whose bowel movements have been small in amount for several days. Enemas appear to be fairly effective, but distention usually will continue and the patient will have both general abdominal and local discomfort. He often states that he feels that the bowel wants to move but that movement gives no relief. Diarrhea may occur and persist, due to irritation of the upper rectum and the sigmoid by dammed-up fecal material. The diagnosis is made easily by inserting the gloved finger into the rectum. A hard fecal mass that fills the rectum will be palpated.

Treatment. The treatment of the condition is to remove the impaction. Enemas of 6 ounces of liquid petrolatum (oil enema) often are effective in softening the mass and helping its discharge. The harder masses may not be moved by this treatment. In these cases, the impaction may be broken up with the gloved finger, or by injecting from 1 to 2 ounces of hydrogen peroxide into the rectum. The foaming action of the drug tends to break up the fecal masses, which then may be evacuated.

It must be borne in mind also, in this connection, that many people, especially thin females and older people, are constipated habitually, and often give a history of having taken some form of laxative drug every day for years. These patients should be allowed to return to their former bowel habits as soon as possible after operation—at least until they have recovered from their operation. As a general rule it is best not to give cathartic drugs for at least a week after abdominal operations, and for a much longer time when drains have been inserted. Enemas usually are effective in evacuating the lower bowel, and cathartic drugs never should be given except on the physician's orders. An exception to this rule may be made in the case of liquid petrolatum (paraffin oil). This substance causes no irritation to the bowel and may be used without danger in doses of 1 ounce once or twice daily.

Diarrhea

After operations diarrhea is not rare. The patient may have from 5 to 10 liquid stools of small amount a day. This should be reported at once. Fecal impaction has been mentioned as the most frequent cause of this complication in the aged.

Intoxication, especially that of intestinal origin, often results in diarrhea. Often a thorough purge may relieve this symptom entirely, but this treatment should not be attempted until other causes have been excluded.

Local irritation, such as a pelvic abscess, is the most frequent cause of diarrhea after operations in which a peritonitis was found. The gloved finger will find a tender mass bulging into the rectum. Surgical drainage usually is required, although at times these abscesses will rupture spontaneously and drain into the rectum. Diarrhea due to a pelvic abscess is usually "spurious" in type—that is, not a true diarrhea but simply the expulsion of small amounts of liquid from the rectum. It is associated often with *tenesmus* (straining). The patient also may have painful urination.

CHAPTER EIGHT

Postoperative Complications

INTRODUCTION

The danger from surgical disease is not only the risk of the operative procedure; there is also the very definite hazard of postoperative complications that may prolong the convalescence or even be an important contributing cause in an unsuccessful operative result. The nurse plays an important part in the prevention of these complications and in their early treatment should they arise. The signs and symptoms of the more common postoperative complications are discussed in this chapter. In each instance the most improved methods of prevention and the usual treatment are emphasized.

It should be borne in mind constantly that attention must be paid to the patient as an individual as well as to his particular surgical condition.

SHOCK

Postoperative Shock. One of the most serious postoperative complications is shock. It was, for a time, the cause of many operative fatalities. However, adequate attention in recent years to preoperative fluid balance and surgical preparation, together with the intelligent use of whole blood and blood substitutes during and after operation, has prevented this complication to a large extent.

Shock, for practical purposes, may be defined as "a disproportion between the circulating blood volume and cardiovascular tree." It may be due either to an inadequate amount of blood in the circulation or, if a normal amount of blood is present, to a relative insufficiency due to dilatation of the vascular tree.

There are many causes of shock, and in almost all instances it is due to a combination of two or more factors. These factors may be grouped under three types. The first is *neurogenic,* sometimes called *primary* shock. It may result from anesthetics, especially spinal anesthesia, or neurogenic factors such as fear of operation, the sight of blood or the hustle and bustle in the strange atmosphere of the operating room. The second type is that due to blood loss or *hematogenic* shock. Often there is more blood loss at operation than the surgeon realizes. The handling of body tissues may cause local trauma and loss of blood and plasma from the circulation, thereby creating a decrease in the circulating blood volume. The third type is *toxic* shock. This is rather ill-defined and is not well understood. It is characterized by a change in the capillary endothelium that permits loss of blood and plasma through the capillary walls into the surrounding tissues. This is thought to be caused by a toxic factor that enters the blood stream from traumatized or infected tissue.

Symptoms of Shock. No matter what the cause, the symptoms of shock are due to a depression of the vascular system, and the circulation becomes insufficient to carry on its normal functions. The result then is an apathetic patient in whom all sensations are markedly dulled. The skin is cold and moist, the lips are somewhat cyanotic, the pulse is rapid and thready, the respiration is rapid and shallow, and the temperature is subnormal. The blood pressure is low, 90 or less, systolic.

Effects of Shock. Continued shock and its associated low blood pressure with decreased rate of circulating blood result in undesirable body changes. One of these is anoxia. *Anoxia,* a lack of oxygen in the body tissues, may be the result of *anoxemia,* decreased oxygen content in the blood. Oxygen, which combines with the blood for transportation throughout the body may be insufficient to provide the tissues with their normal requirements. This may result from a depressed circulation of an inadequate quantity of blood. Some of the more specialized tissues, the brain, the spinal cord and the kidneys, undergo degenerative changes rapidly when they are not supplied with adequate oxygen. These changes in the brain may be manifested by a permanent lack of nervous control to the vascular system and vascular collapse, paralysis of one or more parts of the body, or by *hyperpyrexia.* The last is an excessive fever, sometimes as high as 108° or 109° F., that presages usually a fatal outcome and is the result of changes in the hypothalamic area. Later symptoms may include loss of memory and psychogenic alterations. When the kidney is deprived of oxygen for a sufficient period of time, kidney depression or failure may occur. Kidney depression, *oliguria,* is manifested by a decreased kidney secretion and urinary output. Kidney failure or *anuria* is evidenced by a lack of urinary secretion. Thrombosis with subsequent emboli also may occur throughout the body due to stasis of blood resulting from decreased circulation (see p. 144).

Principles of Treatment. The best treatment for shock is prophylaxis. This consists of adequate preparation of the patient, mental as well as physical, and anticipation of any complication that may arise during or after operation. The proper type of anesthesia should be chosen after careful consideration of the patient and his disease. Blood transfusion and plasma should be available if indicated. Operative trauma should be kept at a minimum. After operation, factors that may promote shock are to be prevented. Pain is controlled by making the patient as comfortable as possible and by using narcotics judiciously. Exposure should be avoided. In some hospitals a "postoperative station" is available. There the patient can be watched and cared for by nurses trained especially in the recovery of patients from anesthesia. In addition, a quiet room is advantageous in the immediate postoperative period in reducing mental trauma.

Treatment. (1) BODY HEAT. Present opinion is that body heat should be maintained by warm, dry blankets at only slightly higher than normal body temperature. If temperatures above body heat are employed, further dilation of blood vessels throughout the body may occur. This creates an even greater disproportion between the circulating blood volume and the cardiovascular tree. Warm drinks, such as hot tea or coffee, may be given by mouth unless they are contraindicated.

(2) RELIEF OF PAIN. Pain should be relieved as far as possible by the intelligent use of narcotics. However, when the circulation is depressed, as it is in shock, the effect of morphine or other narcotics will be delayed. Therefore, one must avoid overloading the patient with drugs that may accumulate during shock and become overwhelming when the circulation has been restored to normal. Other measures are used sometimes to alleviate pain. One of the most useful is procaine block of the peripheral nerves. This is satisfactory especially after operations upon the chest, where relief can be obtained by intercostal nerve blocks.

(3) RESTORATION OF BLOOD VOLUME. This, of course, is the most important goal to be achieved in the treatment of shock. However, if the depressed circulation cannot be restored immediately, one must protect the vital centers of the brain. Irreversible changes may take place in a short period of time if the volume of the circulating blood is inadequate. The foot of the bed should be elevated and the head lowered, so that the heart can maintain the circulation more easily to these vital centers. In addition, some surgeons apply tight bandages to the extremities, bandaging toward the trunk. By this procedure the available blood may be kept in a smaller circulating area, the affected blood pressure being raised thereby.

The quickest method of supplying an adequate amount of circulating blood is by transfusion. When blood is not available, a blood substitute, such as plasma or plasma volume expanders (Dextran), should be employed. Solutions of the electrolytes, glucose and saline solutions, should be used only when blood or plasma is not available, and then only until one or the other can be obtained.

(4) OXYGEN. As patients in shock have some anoxemia, to increase the available oxygen to the blood may

be beneficial. This can be done most easily by mask or intranasal catheter. An oxygen tent is bulky and cumbersome, and it takes too long to assemble it. However, if one is immediately available, it will achieve the same purpose.

(5) DRUGS. Certain drugs may cause a temporary rise in blood pressure. These act by constricting the vessels in the peripheral circulation or by stimulating the brain centers, but they have a transient effect, and sometimes the effects are more harmful than beneficial. They should be used with caution, and only on the surgeon's orders. These drugs include epinephrine or an extract of the adrenal cortex known as desoxycorticosterone, Pituitrin, ephedrine and caffeine-sodium benzoate.

The Nurse's Responsibility. From a glance at the above outline, the nurse's responsibility should shock develop is (1) to keep the patient on his back and elevate the foot of the bed, (2) to apply dry, warm blankets, (3) to call the surgeon, (4) to obtain a tank of oxygen and a mask or an intranasal catheter with tubing and attachments and (5) to have the following articles ready for immediate use: a sphygmomanometer and a stethoscope; an intravenous tray, preferably with plasma or glucose and salt solution; a hypodermic syringe in case the surgeon decides to use some drug mentioned above.

HEMORRHAGE

Classification. Hemorrhage is classified as (1) *primary,* when it occurs at the time of the operation; (2) *intermediary,* when it occurs within the first few hours after an operation, due to a return of blood pressure to its normal level and a consequent washing out of the insecure clots from untied vessels; and (3) *secondary,* when it occurs some time after the operation, due to the slipping of a ligature because of infection, insecure tying or erosion of a vessel by a drainage tube.

A further classification frequently is made according to the kind of vessel that is bleeding. *Capillary* hemorrhage is characterized by a slow general ooze; *venous* hemorrhage bubbles out quickly and is dark in color; *arterial* hemorrhage is bright in color and appears in spurts with each heartbeat.

When the hemorrhage is on the surface and can be seen, it is spoken of as *evident;* when it cannot be seen, as in the peritoneal cavity, it is spoken of as *concealed.*

Symptoms. Hemorrhage presents a more or less well-defined syndrome, depending on the amount of blood lost and the rapidity of its escape. The patient is apprehensive, restless and moves continually; he is thirsty; and the skin is cold, moist and pale. The pulse rate increases, the temperature falls, respirations are rapid and deep, often of the gasping type spoken of as "air hunger." As the hemorrhage progresses, the blood pressure and the hemoglobin of the blood fall rapidly, the lips and the conjunctiva become pallid, spots appear before the eyes, a ringing is heard in the ears, and the patient grows weaker but remains conscious until near death. The nurse must notify the surgeon immediately and carry out emergency measures until he arrives.

Treatment. Often the effects of hemorrhage after an operation are masked by those due to the anesthetic and to shock; therefore, the treatment of the patient is in a general way almost identical to that described for shock, viz., (1) keep the head low, (2) administer morphine to keep the patient quiet and (3) apply heat. The wound always should be inspected to find out, if possible, the site of the bleeding. A sterile gauze pad and a snug bandage with elevation of the part, arm or leg, are indicated.

A transfusion of blood is the most logical therapeutic measure, and in the case of serious operation, the blood of the patient is typed and blood is secured beforehand. If blood is not available when needed, saline solution, plasma or a plasma volume expander (Dextran) may be given intravenously to tide the patient over temporarily until the blood can be secured (see pp. 169 to 173).

In giving fluids by vein in cases of hemorrhage it must be remembered that too large a quantity may raise the blood pressure enough to start the bleeding again, unless the hemorrhage has been well controlled.

PULMONARY COMPLICATIONS

Respiratory complications are among the most frequent and serious with which the surgeon has to deal. Experience has shown that they may be avoided in large measure by careful preoperative observation and by taking every precaution during and after the operation. It is well known that those patients who have some respiratory disease before operation are more prone to develop serious complications after operation. Therefore, the careful surgeon will perform only emergency operations when acute disease of the respiratory tract exists. The nurse may aid by reporting any symptom, such as cough, sneezing, injected conjunctiva and nasal discharge, to the surgeon before the operation.

During and immediately after the operation, every effort should be made to prevent chilling and to keep the patient warm.

After the operation the nurse should provide a warm bed and warm dry garments; frequently a small blanket folded and pinned over the shoulders may be used in the prophylactic treatment of respiratory disorders.

The predisposing and exciting causes of pulmonary complications may be any of the following:

1. Infections in the mouth, the nose and the throat.
2. The irritating effect of the anesthetic, especially ether, on the respiratory mucous membranes, with a resultant increase in mucous secretion.
3. The aspiration of vomitus.
4. Shallow respiration after operations, especially those on the upper abdomen, because of the pain in the wound that deep respiration will cause.

It seems probable then that in many cases the cause is largely a lack of complete aeration of the lungs. The mucus formed is not coughed up, bacterial action comes into play and, when the affection is limited to the larger air passages, a *bronchitis* results. If the process involves the pulmonary alveoli, a *bronchopneumonia* occurs. Penicillin and the sulfa drugs frequently are used both in the prophylactic and the active treatment of respiratory complications.

The increased metabolism and the general improvement of all body functions incidental to getting the patient up out of bed have led many surgeons to regard getting him up as one of the best prophylactic measures against pulmonary complications. When the patient's wound or condition otherwise permits, it is not unusual to allow him to get up on the second or the third day after operation, and even on the first day. This practice is especially valuable in preventing pulmonary complications in older patients.

Atelectasis

When the mucous plug closes one of the bronchi entirely, there is a collapse of the pulmonary tissue beyond, and a massive *atelectasis* is said to result (Fig. 57). The prophylactic treatment of these conditions then would seem to include measures to promote full aeration of the lungs. The nurse should instruct her patient to take at least 10 deep inhalations every hour. Frequently, some surgeons recommend some apparatus (a spirometer, blow-bottles or common paper bags) into which the patient blows in an effort to expand the lungs fully. Turning the patient from side to side results occasionally in coughing, with expulsion of the mucous plug, and recovery. At times the mucous plug may be removed by aspiration through a bronchoscope.

Bronchitis

This pulmonary complication may appear at any time after operation, usually within the first 5 or 6 days. The symptoms vary accord-

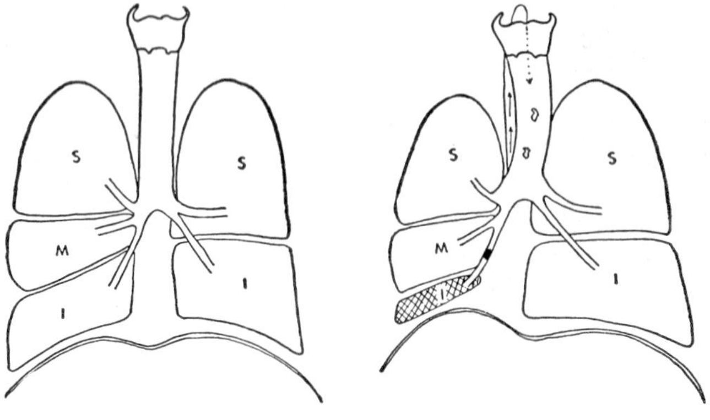

Fig. 57. Atelectasis. (*Left*) Normal expansion of all lobes of lungs. (*Right*) Plug of mucus or vomitus in bronchus leading to inferior lobe of right lung, with atelectasis of lobe. Arrows indicate the path followed by vomitus from the esophagus into the trachea before protective reflexes have returned following anesthesia. (Greisheimer, E. M.: The physiological effects of anesthesia, Am. J. Nursing **49**:339)

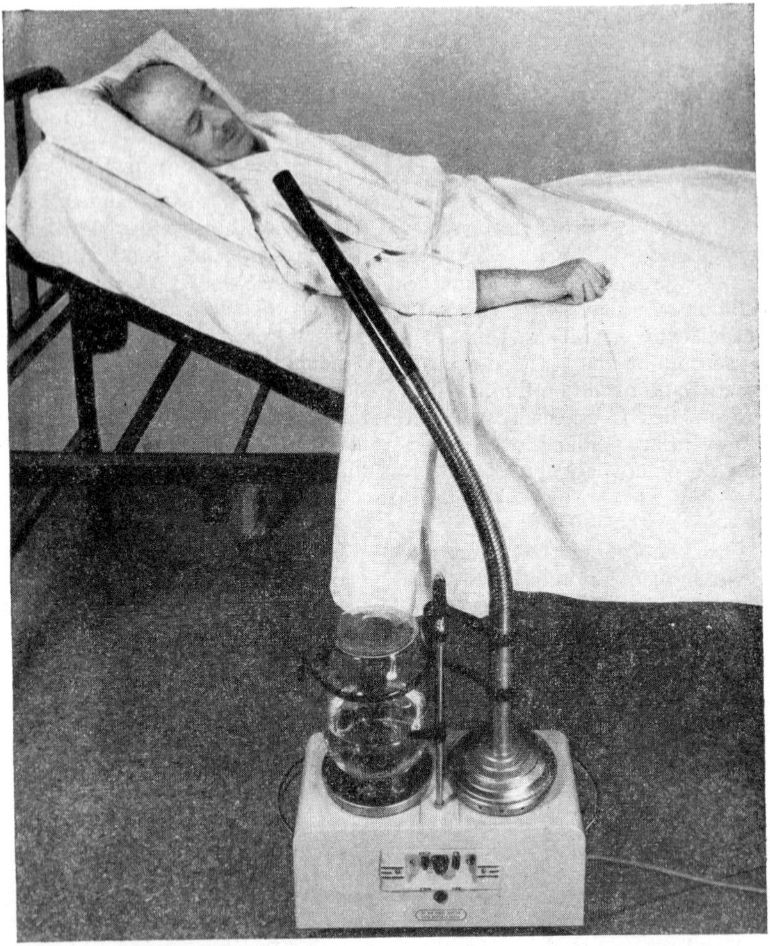

FIG. 58. Patient receiving inhalation from Colson vaporizer. The tube also may be inserted under a croup tent to supply steam and medication.

ing to the disease. A simple bronchitis is characterized by cough productive of considerable mucopus, but without marked temperature or pulse elevation.

Treatment. A most effective method of treatment of bronchitis is the inhalation of steam. Often various medications are added. The old-fashioned croup tent is used less frequently than formerly, its place now being taken by the newer types of electric vaporizers. In using these the nurse must be careful to see that they are kept filled with water and are so placed that burning of the patient would be impossible. Figure 58 shows a vaporizer than stands on the floor. Smaller types for table use are more apt to be spilled.

Bronchopneumonia

Bronchopneumonia is perhaps the second most frequent pulmonary complication. Besides a productive cough, there is considerable temperature elevation, with an increase in the pulse and the respiratory rates.

Treatment. The patient is encouraged to take fluids, and expectorant and supportive drugs are given him. Distention should be watched for and prevented, if possible, so as to avoid added respiratory or cardiac embarrassment.

Pleurisy

Pleurisy is not an uncommon occurrence after operation. Its chief symptom is an acute, knifelike pain in the chest on the affected side that is particularly excruciating when the patient takes a deep breath. Also, there usually is some slight temperature and pulse rise, and respirations are rapid and more shallow than normal.

Treatment. A tight adhesive strapping, applied during full expiration, will relieve the pain almost at once. Aspirin, 0.6 Gm. (gr. x), may be added if it is needed.

Pleurisy with effusion may result secondary to a primary pleurisy. In these cases aspiration of the chest frequently becomes necessary.

Lobar Pneumonia

Lobar pneumonia is a less frequent complication after operation. Usually it begins with a chill, followed by high temperature, pulse and respiration. There may be little or no cough, but the respiratory embarrassment, the flushed cheeks and the evident illness of the patient make a combination of clinical signs that are distinctive. The disease runs its usual course with the added complication of the operative wound.

Treatment. The treatment is as for bronchopneumonia, with liberal use of the antibiotics and the sulfonamides.

Hypostatic Pulmonary Congestion

Hypostatic pulmonary congestion is a condition that develops too often in old or in very weak patients. Its cause is a weakened heart and vascular system that permit a stagnation of blood at the bases of both lungs. It occurs most frequently, perhaps, in old people who have sustained a fractured femur, a condition that necessitates a long stay in bed in one position. The symptoms frequently are not marked for a time—perhaps a slight elevation of temperature and pulse and respiratory rate, also a slight cough. But physical examination will reveal dullness and rales at the bases of the lungs. If the condition goes untreated, the outcome may be fatal.

Treatment. Prophylaxis is the important thing. When the surgical condition permits, such a patient should be turned from side to side frequently and given cardiac stimulants. Also, he should be allowed out of bed as soon as possible to sit in a chair or a wheelchair. Many times this pulmonary complication becomes more serious than the original surgical condition, in which case the surgical condition may be disregarded in measure to permit proper treatment of the hypostatic pneumonia.

Because of reduced aeration in many of the pulmonary complications, which means that less oxygen reaches the blood, many clinics are employing an oxygen tent in treatment. This apparatus, which consists of a large hood that encloses the patient's head and shoulders, delivers oxygen in high concentration combined with a small amount of carbon dioxide. By this means the patient receives more oxygen with each respiration, cyanosis is lessened, and the general condition is improved. The nurse is required to see that the tent fits closely about the shoulders of the patient. (See p. 178).

Pulmonary Embolism

An *embolus* is defined as a foreign body in the blood stream. In most cases it is formed by a blood clot that becomes dislodged from its original site and is carried along in the blood. When the clot is carried to the heart, it is forced by the blood into the pulmonary artery, where it plugs the main artery or one of its branches. The symptoms produced are among the most sudden and startling in surgical practice. A patient passing an apparently normal convalescence suddenly cries out with sharp, stabbing pains in the chest and becomes breathless, cyanotic and anxious. The pupils dilate, cold sweat pours out, the pulse becomes rapid and irregular, then imperceptible, and death usually results. If death does not occur within 30 minutes, there is a chance of recovery.

This complication may arise at any time after operation, but it occurs most frequently during the second week when the patient is beginning to become more active. It is probable that the movements of the patient dislodge the clot, because pulmonary embolism seems to occur most frequently immediately after the patient has been taken out of bed or put to bed again for the first time after operation.

Treatment. If death does not occur at once, oxygen or fresh air should be given in abundance, with the patient in the sitting position to help respiration. Attempts should be made to quiet and reassure the patient, and drugs (morphine) should be given to prevent the panic that rapidly will wear out the overworked, dilating heart.

FEMORAL PHLEBITIS OR THROMBOSIS

This complication occurs most frequently after operations upon the lower abdomen or in the course of severe septic diseases, such as peritonitis, ruptured ulcer and so forth. An inflammation of the vein occurs associated with a clotting of blood; this may be mild or severe. The cause of the complication may be injury to the vein by tight straps or leg-holders at the time of operation, concentration of blood by loss of fluid or dehydration, or, more commonly, probably the slowing of the blood flow in the extremity due to a lowered metabolism and depression of the circulation after operation. It is probable that several of these factors may act together to produce the thrombosis commonly

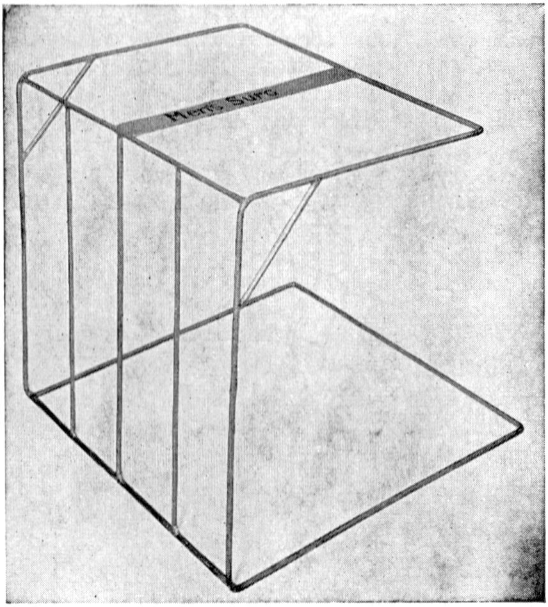

FIG. 59. (A, *Top*) Eliason cradle, built to slip under mattress at side, head or foot of bed. (B, *Bottom*) Eliason cradle, with bedclothes in place. An electric light may be fastened to top to provide heat in cases of inflammation of the feet and the legs.

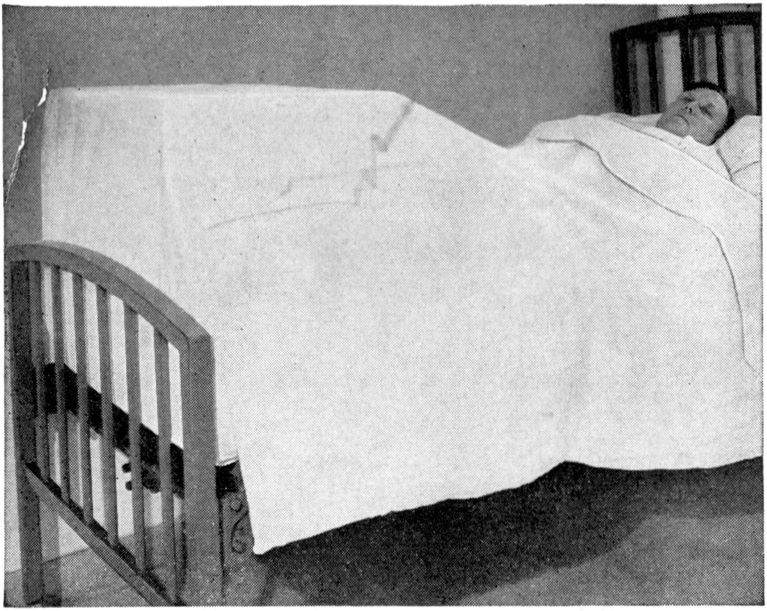

seen. The left leg is affected more frequently. The first symptom may be a pain or a cramp in the calf. Pressure here gives pain, and a day or so later a painful swelling of the entire leg occurs, often associated with a slight fever and sometimes with chills and sweats. The swelling is due to a soft edema that pits easily on pressure. There is marked tenderness over the anteromesial surface of the thigh, and frequently the vein itself may be palpated as a firm pencil-like mass that may be rolled under the fingers.

A milder form of the same disease is termed *phlebothrombosis,* to indicate intravascular clotting without marked inflammation of the vein. The clotting occurs usually in the veins of the calf, often with few symptoms except slight soreness of the calf. The danger from this type of thrombosis is that the clot may be dislodged and produce an embolus. It is believed that most pulmonary emboli (p. 144) arise from this source.

Treatment

The treatment of thrombophlebitis or phlebothrombosis may be considered as (1) prophylactic and (2) active.

Prophylactic Treatment. Efforts are directed toward preventing the formation of a thrombus and include such measures as adequate administration of fluids after operation to prevent blood concentration, leg exercises, bandaging of the legs and getting the patient out of bed early to prevent stagnation of the blood in the veins of the lower extremity.

Active Treatment. It has been shown that the pain and the edema of phlebitis are due in large measure to a stimulation of the sympathetic nerves. The thrombophlebitis produces this stimulation, which results in a spasm of the smaller veins and arteries. The swelling appears to arise from an increased permeability of the capillaries that is brought about by this phenomenon. A block of the sympathetic ganglia with procaine will relieve the vascular spasm quickly, with resultant relief of pain and disappearance of the edema. The sympathetic block may be produced "chemically" by the use of drugs. Etamon and Priscoline are drugs of this class. A more direct effect may be produced by procaine solution injected into the epidural space (caudal block). A plastic tubing may be inserted through which repeated injections may be made. The block also may be performed by injecting an anesthetic solution around the lumbar sympathetic ganglia. This injection may have to be repeated.

In addition to the foregoing methods, some surgeons believe that ligation of the femoral veins is an important therapeutic method. The idea behind this method of therapy is to prevent pulmonary embolism from the breaking off of thrombi.

Anticoagulant therapy has taken a prominent place in the prophylaxis and the treatment of phlebitis and phlebothrombosis. Heparin, given intravenously by the drip method or intramuscularly in an oily menstruum, reduces the coagulability of the blood rapidly and is used most often when an immediate effect is desired. Repeated checks of the coagulation time of the blood are necessary to control its administration. Dicumarol is a second drug that is used for a similar purpose. It is given by mouth and does not become effective for about 24 hours. Its daily dosage is controlled by daily estimations of the prothrombin time of the blood.

Both as a prophylactic and an active treatment of phlebitis and thrombosis, wrapping the legs from toes to groin with snug elastic adhesive bandages has much virtue. These bandages prevent swelling and stagnation of venous blood in the legs and do much to relieve pain in the phlebitic extremity.

HICCOUGH (SINGULTUS)

Hiccough occurs not infrequently after abdominal operations. Often it occurs in mild transitory attacks that cease spontaneously or with very simple treatment. When hiccoughs persist they may produce considerable distress and serious effects such as vomiting, acid-base and fluid imbalance, malnutrition, exhaustion and possibly wound dehiscence.

Hiccough is produced by intermittent spasms of the diaphragm. It is associated with a coarse sound, a result of the vibration of the closed vocal cords as the air rushes suddenly into the lungs. The cause of the diaphragmatic spasm may be any irritation of the phrenic nerve from its center in the spinal cord to its terminal ramifications on the undersurface of the diaphragm. This irritation may be direct—such as a stimulation of the nerve itself by a distended stomach, peritonitis or subdiaphragmatic abscess, abdominal distention, pleurisy or tumors in the chest pressing on the nerves; or indirect—such as toxemia, uremia and so forth that stimulate the center; or reflex—such as irritations from a drainage tube, exposure to cold, drinking very hot or very cold fluids or obstruction of the intestines.

Treatment. The multitude of remedies suggested for the relief of this condition is proof that no one treatment is effective in every case. The best remedy, of course, is removal of the cause, which in some cases is easy—for example, gastric lavage for gastric distention, shortening or removal of drainage tubes causing irritation, or adhesive strapping in pleurisy. At other times the removal of the cause is almost impossible; then attention must be directed toward the treatment of the hiccough itself. Many simple remedies—such as drinking a half glass of water in which a teaspoonful of sodium bicarbonate has been dissolved, swallowing ice, stopping the patient from talking, sucking a lemon, taking a little vinegar, salt or sugar—have been used and often with success. Probably the most efficient of the older and simpler remedies is to hold the breath while taking large swallows of cold water.

After studying the problem recently, a group of anesthesiologists recommend treatment ranging from the simplest to the most drastic until relief is obtained. Their suggestions, in order, are:

1. Finger pressure on the eyeballs through closed lids for several minutes.
2. Induced vomiting.
3. Gastric lavage.
4. Intravenous injection of atropine.
5. Inhalation of carbon dioxide (breathing in and out of a paper bag or more technical administration).

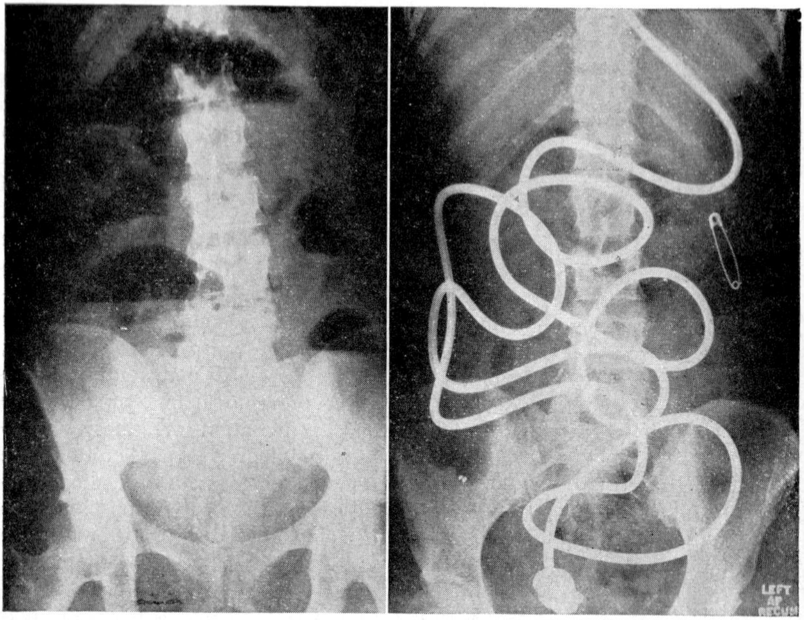

FIG. 60. (*Left*) Marked intestinal distention 4 days after exploratory operation. (*Right*) Twenty-four hours later, after Miller-Abbott tube had decompressed the intestines by constant suction. The tube may be seen following the coils of the intestines.

6. Should these fail, a phrenic nerve block.
7. As a final resort, a phrenic nerve crush.

INTESTINAL OBSTRUCTION

Intestinal obstruction is a complication that may follow abdominal operations. It occurs most often after operations on the lower abdomen and the pelvis, and especially after those in which drainage has been necessary. The symptoms usually appear between the third and the fifth days. The cause is some obstruction of the intestinal current—frequently a loop of intestine that has become kinked from inflammatory adhesions or that has become involved in the drainage tract. A typical situation is that of a patient with a ruptured appendix, having pelvic drainage. He had his enema on the third day, and it was reported to be effective. He was fed a soft diet and, after a day or two, he complained of sharp, colicky, abdominal pains with a pain-free interval between. Usually there is no temperature or pulse elevation. At first the pains are localized, and this point should be noted by the nurse, because the localization of the early pains represents in a general way the loop of intestine that is just above the obstruction.

Usually, the patient will continue to have abdominal pains, with shorter and shorter intervals between. If the ear or a stethoscope is placed on the abdomen, sounds may be heard that give evidence of extremely active intestinal movements, especially during an attack of pain. The intestinal contents, being unable to move forward, distend the intestinal coils, are carried backward to the stomach and are vomited. Thus, vomiting and increasing distention gradually become more prominent symptoms. Hiccough often precedes the vomiting in many cases. The bowels do not move, and enemas return nearly clear, showing that very little of the intestinal contents has reached the large bowel since the enema on the third day. Unless the obstruction is relieved the patient continues to vomit, distention becomes more pronounced, the pulse becomes rapid, and the end is a toxic death.

Treatment. Sometimes the distention of the intestine above the obstruction can be prevented by the use of the constant-suction drainage of the Wangensteen apparatus with the Miller-Abbott, Harris or Cantor tubes, in which case the inflammatory reaction of the bowel at the site of the obstruction may subside and the obstruction is relieved. (See Fig. 60). However, at times it is necessary to relieve the obstructed intestine by operation. In addition, intravenous infusions of saline usually are given. (See the section on intestinal obstruction for a more complete discussion of the treatment and the postoperative care, pp. 315 to 326.)

URINARY RETENTION

Urinary retention may follow any operation, but it occurs most frequently after operations on the rectum, the anus and the vagina, and after herniorrhaphies and operations on the lower abdomen. The cause is thought to be a spasm of the bladder sphincter.

Not infrequently patients are unable to void in bed but, when allowed to sit or stand up, do so without difficulty. When standing does not interfere with the operative result, male patients may be allowed to stand by the side of the bed or female patients to sit on the edge of the bed with their feet on a chair or a stool. However, many patients cannot be permitted this liberty and other means of encouraging urination must be tried. Some people have what has been called a "stammering" bladder and cannot void with another person in the room. These patients should be left alone for a time after being provided with a warm bedpan or urinal.

Frequently the sound or the sight of running water may relax reflexly the spasm of the bladder sphincter. A bedpan containing warm water or an irrigation of the perineum with warm water frequently will initiate urination for female patients. A small warm enema often is of value in such a situation. If the retention of urine continues for some hours, the patient will complain of considerable pain in the lower abdomen, and the bladder frequently can be palpated and seen in outline distending the lower anterior abdominal wall.

When all conservative measures have failed, catheterization must be practiced. If the patient has voided just before operation, this procedure may be delayed in most cases for 12 to 18 hours. There are two reasons for wishing to avoid catheterization: (1) there is the possibility of infecting the bladder and producing a cystitis; and, (2) experience has shown that once a patient has been catheterized, frequently he needs subsequent catheterizations.

Many patients may exhibit a palpable bladder, with lower abdominal discomfort, and still void small amounts of urine at frequent intervals. The keen nurse will not mistake this for normal functioning of the bladder. This voiding of from 1 to 2 ounces of urine at intervals of from 15 to 30 minutes is, rather, a sign of an overdistended bladder, the very distention being sufficient to allow the escape of small amounts of urine at intervals. The condition usually is spoken of as the "overflow of retention." A catheter usually will relieve the patient by draining from 20 to 30 ounces of urine from the bladder. "Incontinence of retention" may be evidenced by a constant dribble of urine, yet the bladder remains overdistended. Overdistention injures the bladder; catheterization is indicated. There often is a definite psychic element in urinary retention.

After fractures of the spine, there frequently is a paralysis of the part of the body supplied by nerves that arise below the site of the fracture. Among other nerves that are paralyzed are those that supply the bladder. Such patients nearly always are very much shocked and, if they recover, they are unable to control either bowels or bladder. Catheterization in these patients is dangerous because of the certainty of infection that develops sooner or later. It has been found that these individuals may escape this danger by the development of what is know as an "automatic bladder." By this term is meant the ability of the patient to empty his bladder by suprapubic pressure. By this simple procedure the life of these patients may be prolonged many months. (See also Tidal Drainage, p. 521.)

URINARY INCONTINENCE

Incontinence of urine is a frequent complication in the aged, either after operation or after shocking injuries. It is due probably to weakness with loss of tone of the bladder sphincter. This symptom frequently disappears as the patient gains in strength and normal muscular tone is regained.

Treatment. Treatment of urinary incontinence is difficult. In many cases, an indwelling catheter may be inserted. In some cases the giving of a bedpan hourly may keep the bed dry. It is well to place a large pad under the patient to absorb the urine. A pad placed against the vulva also may be used. The incontinent patient must be watched carefully to prevent the development of bedsores.

DELIRIUM

Postoperative delirium occurs occasionally in several groups of patients. The most common types are:

Toxic

Toxic delirium occurs in conjunction with the signs and the symptoms of a general toxemia. These patients are very ill, usually with a high temperature and pulse rate. The face is flushed, and the eyes are bright and roving. These patients move incessantly, often attempting to get out of bed and disarranging the bedclothes continually. They present a marked degree of mental confusion. These states are seen in surgical conditions, most often in cases of general peritonitis or other septic conditions.

In such cases elimination is promoted by encouraging the intake of fluids, and the causative condition is treated by other methods. Usually, however, the outcome is fatal.

Traumatic

Traumatic delirium is a mental state resulting from sudden trauma of any sort, especially in highly nervous people. The malady may take the form of wild maniacal excitement, of simple confusion with hallucinations and delusions or of melancholic depression. Sedative drugs—chloral, paraldehyde and morphine—are used in treatment. Usually the state begins and ends suddenly.

Delirium Tremens

Individuals who have used alcohol habitually over a long period of time are very poor surgical risks. The alcohol has damaged practically every organ and in the event of accidents or serious surgical procedures their resistance is much below that of the average person. These patients always take anesthesia poorly.

After operation the patient may do well for a few days, but the prolonged abstinence from alcohol causes him to become restless, nervous and irritated easily by little things. The facial expression changes entirely. Also, he sleeps poorly and often is disturbed by unreal dreams. When approached by the doctor or the nurse he appears to awake suddenly, asks "Who are you?" and, when he is told where he is, he will appear to be fairly normal for a short time. These symptoms should be watched for in patients who have been alcoholics, because by active treatment at this stage the more violent delirium may be avoided.

Active delirium tremens may come on suddenly or gradually. After a period of restless, nervous, semidelirium, the patient finally loses entire control of his mental functions and "horrors reign supreme." "His mind is a chaos of ever-changing ideas." He talks incessantly, tries to get out of bed to get away from the hallucinations of fear and persecution that torment him continually. If attempts are made to restrain him, he may fight maniacally and often will injure himself and others. "In this stage the patient is obviously sick." He is sleepless, he perspires freely and the limbs display a marked tremor. Finally, after many hours of torture, the patient becomes stuporous.

Treatment. When possible, the treatment of these patients should begin 2 or 3 days before operation by most thorough elimination from the kidneys, the bowels and the skin. These measures should be continued after operation, especially if any of the early signs of the condition develop. Sedative drugs—chloral, bromides, paraldehyde and morphine—should be given in quantities to keep the patient quiet. Stimulation often is required, espe-

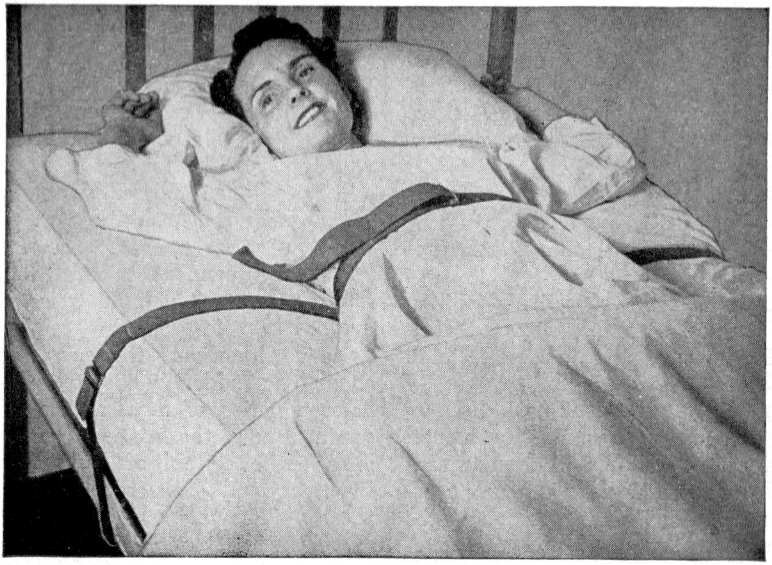

FIG. 61. The Posey safety belt. This restraint allows the patient to turn over or sit up in bed.

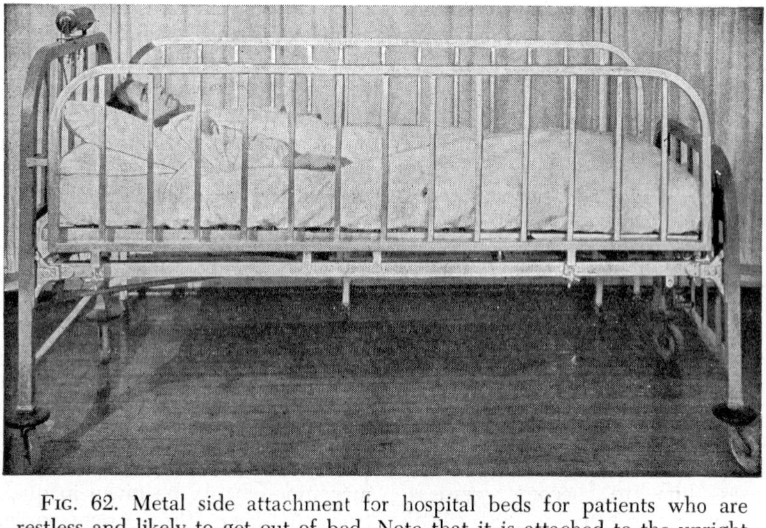

FIG. 62. Metal side attachment for hospital beds for patients who are restless and likely to get out of bed. Note that it is attached to the upright headpiece and is held to the side of the bed by screws.

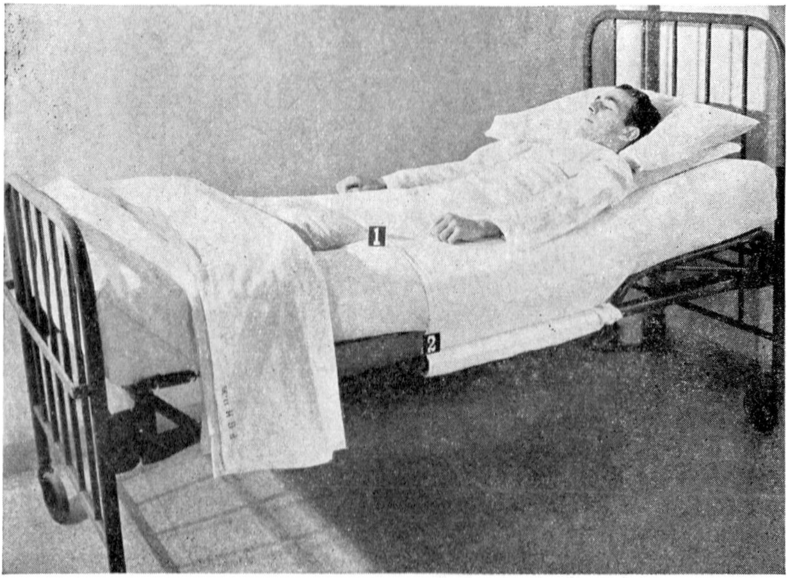

FIG. 63. Restraining sheet. Folded sheet (1) passes over patient's body and (2) is held fast by being wrapped round the side of the bed.

cially in the older alcoholics, in the form of whisky, strychnine, caffeine and so forth. The chief cause of the symptoms in chronic alcoholics has been shown to be a depletion of the carbohydrate stores of the body and an inadequate ingestion of vitamins. Therefore, glucose is given intravenously, and vitamins are administered in concentrated form by mouth and by injection.

RESTRAINT

In the postoperative care of patients, it is wise for the nurse to explain the necessity for the patient's remaining in bed until the surgeon permits him to get up. Often patients prefer to get out of bed to void or get a drink of water rather than bother the nurse. This may lead to serious complications that a word or two of explanation can prevent. However, in some cases it may be impossible for the patient to grasp this. This is true of patients who are disoriented, and especially of older individuals. In such cases, the simplest form of restraint is the use of a bed with sideboards or side protection. This permits the patient to move about in bed at will but prevents him from getting out of bed easily and injuring himself. Most hospital beds are provided with such sideboards for use as necessary.

To protect both patient and nurse, often it becomes necessary to apply some form of restraint in cases of delirium. In the milder forms, a restraining sheet may be used: an ordinary sheet folded lengthwise to

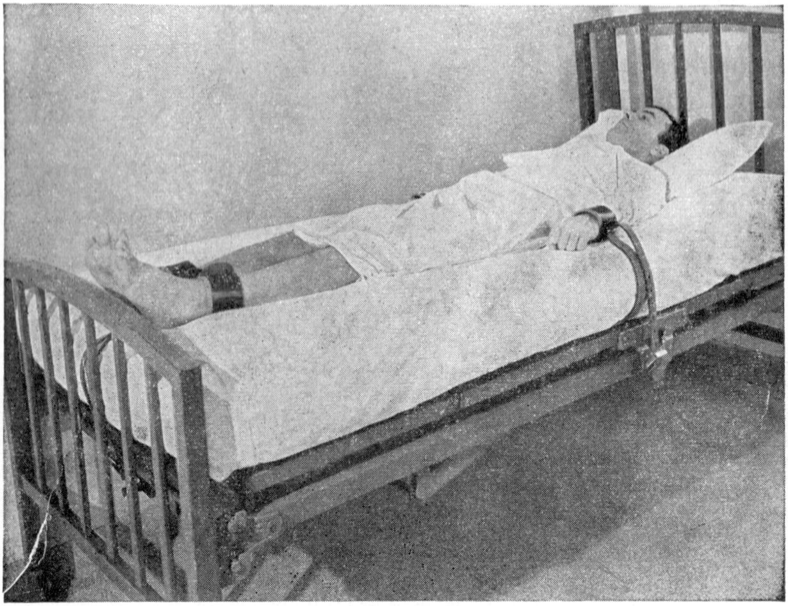

FIG. 64. Restraint by use of straps and cuffs. The cuffs are covered by cotton and bandage (omitted here for illustrative purposes).

be from about 12 to 15 inches wide, applied firmly over the thighs and held by wrapping each end round the bed frame (Fig. 63).

Restraint of the upper extremities may be obtained by applying straight splints to hold the elbow joint in extension or by bandaging the fingers over a roller bandage held in the palm.

Nursing Care

The psychological effect of being restrained can be severe; therefore, any form of restraint should be applied only as a last resort. All other means of making the patient quiet should be tried first. If possible, he should be isolated from other patients. Any article in his vicinity which could be used harmfully should be removed.

When restraints are used, the patient should be in a comfortable and natural position. Restraint to the chest should be avoided, if possible. When restraints are applied, care should be taken that the part is not so constricted as to interfere with the circulation. The appearance of cyanosis in hand or foot indicates that the appliance is too tight. The appliances should be padded carefully and so used as to prevent chafing or pressure sores. The skin underneath them should be inspected frequently, bathed carefully and rubbed with alcohol at least every 2 or 3 hours. The key to locked restraining straps should be kept in a definite place, and all nurses caring for the patient should know its location. Even though restraints are applied, the patient never should be left unwatched. Any patient needing restraint should have constant and careful nursing attention.

WOUND COMPLICATIONS

Infection

In spite of all aseptic precautions, supposedly clean wounds become infected at times. The inflammatory process usually begins to show symptoms in from 36 to 48 hours. The patient's pulse rate and temperature increase, and the wound usually becomes somewhat tender, swollen and warm. At times, when the infection is deep, there may be no local signs. When the surgeon makes a diagnosis of wound infection, usually he removes one stitch or more and, under aseptic precautions, separates the wound edges with a pair of blunt scissors or a hemostat. The infection opened, he will call for a drain of rubber or gauze, which an alert nurse will have ready for him. In addition, many surgeons will require some form of warm antiseptic solution with which to flush the wound.

Hematoma (Hemorrhage)

The nurse should know the location of the patient's incision so that she may inspect the dressings for hemorrhage at intervals during the first 24 hours after operation. Any undue amount of bleeding should be reported to the surgeon. At times concealed bleeding occurs in the wound but beneath the skin. This hemorrhage usually stops spontaneously but results in clot formation within the wound. If the clot is small, it will be absorbed and need not be treated. When the clot is large, the wound usually bulges somewhat, and healing will be delayed unless it is removed. After the removal of several stitches, the clot is evacuated, after which the wound is packed lightly with gauze. Healing occurs usually by granulation, or a secondary closure may be performed.

Rupture (Disruption, Evisceration or Dehiscence)

This complication is especially serious in the case of abdominal wounds. It results from the giving way of sutures and from infection; also, more frequently, after marked distention or cough. The rupture of the wound may occur suddenly, with the escape of coils of intestine onto the abdominal wall. Such a catastrophe causes considerable pain and often is associated with vomiting. Frequently the patient says that something gave way. When the wound edges part slowly, the intestines may escape gradually or not at all, and the presenting symptom may be the sudden drainage of a large amount of peritoneal fluid into the dressings.

When rupture of a wound occurs, the attending surgeon should be notified at once. The protruding coils of intestine should be covered with sterile gauze.

A scultetus binder, properly applied, is an excellent prophylactic measure against an accident of this kind, and often it is used in the primary dressing, especially for operations on individuals with weak or

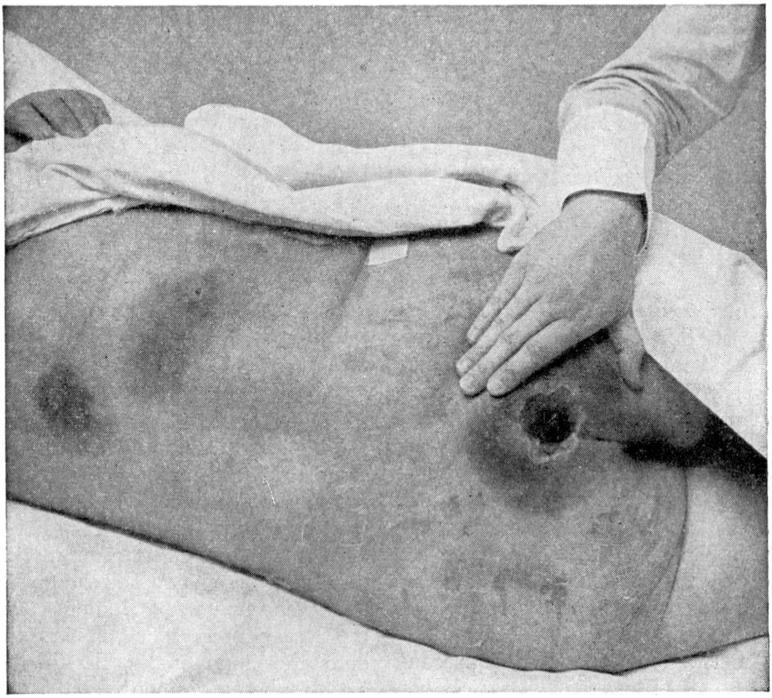

Fig. 65. Decubitus ulcer or bedsore over sacrum.

pendulous abdominal walls (Fig. 54). It is used often also as a firm binder when rupture of a wound has occurred. Vitamin deficiency or serum protein or chloride may require correction.

Keloid

Not infrequently in an otherwise normal wound the scar develops a tendency to excessive growth. Sometimes the entire scar is affected; at other times the condition is segmented. This keloid tendency is unexplainable, unpredictable and unavoidable in some individuals. (See p. 409 and Fig. 175.)

A great deal of investigation has been done along the lines of prevention and cure. Careful closure of the wound, complete hemostasis, pressure support without undue tension on the suture lines—all are reputed to combat this distressing wound complication.

DECUBITI

The development of bedsores is a reflection on the care given the patient by the nurse attending him. Bedsores are due to a local anemia caused by prolonged pressure at one point. They are most prone to occur over bony prominences, such as the sacrum and the coccyx, the shoulders, the elbows and the heels. They occur most frequently in emaciated and otherwise weakened individuals, although they may occur in any patient if there is prolonged local pressure on the tissues. Patients with diabetes are especially prone to develop this complication.

The exciting cause of bedsores is pressure, but the predisposing causes may be a wrinkled sheet, crumbs and other articles in the bed, incontinence of urine and feces, excessive perspiration and so forth: in other words, patients who are kept clean and dry usually escape this misfortune.

The lesion begins with a reddening of the skin, usually but not always with a short-lived burning pain. After this a bluish discoloration appears at the point of pressure. This is somewhat mottled at first, but it turns to a solid brown or black later. At times there are tiny blisters filled with a brown fluid that break and leave ulcerating surfaces. Soon or late the dead tissue separates and leaves a crater that must heal by granulation. At times it may be possible to excise the entire ulcer and close the resulting defect by a plastic operation.

Nursing Care

Prophylaxis. The most important part of the treatment of bedsores is prophylaxis. A bath followed by an alcohol rub (50 per cent) twice daily keeps the skin clean and tends to harden it somewhat. In addition, the rub is a form of massage that should stimulate the circulation in the areas in which pressure is the most constant. The bed should be kept scrupulously clean, free from crumbs and foreign particles, with the sheet tightly stretched to prevent wrinkles. The skin should be kept dry at all times. Occasionally the rubber sheet generally used on the hospital bed causes patients to perspire freely. In such event it may be well to replace the rubber sheet with an extra draw sheet. Dusting powders of zinc stearate or even talcum powder, should be used freely and as frequently as is necessary to keep the skin dry.

If the patient is incontinent of urine or feces, or both, a very strict watch should be kept over him. As soon as the bed is soiled, the patient should be washed with soap and warm water and then given a brisk alcohol rub. The bed should be changed immediately, and pads made of cotton and gauze should be placed so as to catch the excretions in the event of a recurrence.

If any redness of the skin appears, rub with zinc oxide ointment. The patient should be examined twice daily for evidence of beginning pressure sores, and an effort should be made to distribute the pressure points by changing the position of the patient at frequent intervals. Rubber air-rings half inflated with air may be used to advantage to relieve pressure over the sacrum and the coccyx. Cotton "doughnuts" are contraindicated since they tend to decrease circulation to the area, which needs a good blood supply. Bear in mind that measures that tend to build up the patient serve to increase his resistance and lessen the chance of development of a bedsore. An abundance of fresh air and sunlight, good food and stimulating drinks may be included under this category. A low-serum protein often contributes to tardy healing.

If bedsores develop (and they do, occasionally, in spite of every precaution taken against them), steps should be taken immediately to relieve all pressure and tension from the affected area. Often air cushions, water or air mattresses are used, but the best treatment is to place the patient in a position in which no weight is borne by the sore or the surrounding area. Thus, if the sore develops over the sacrum, the patient should be first on one side, then on the other, care being taken that other sores do not develop over the hips.

The lesion itself should be kept clean and protected with a sterile gauze dressing.

When the ulcer involves deeper structures, the sloughs should be removed as soon as they separate. Frequent massage of the tissues about the ulcer tends to increase the circulation and to hasten healing.

For deep decubiti which refuse to heal by conservative means, excision of the ulcer, and often of the underlying bony prominence, with plastic closure by skin flaps may be necessary. Before any such operative intervention can be carried out, active correction of the hypoproteinemia and the infection must be undertaken by the use of a high-protein diet, blood transfusions and antibiotics.

CHAPTER NINE

Special Therapies: Fluid Balance and Gas Therapy

THE NURSE AND FLUID THERAPY

The nurse is a key member of the team whose responsibility it is to meet the fluid and the nutritional needs of the surgical patient. An increasing knowledge of the chemical composition of body fluids in recent years has brought with it a greater awareness of the importance of restoring normal water and electrolyte balance in the bodies of patients subjected to surgery. To attain this end, parenteral fluid therapy, whether for nutrition, maintenance or replacement, now is planned and adapted to meet the particular need. The only way a surgeon can meet adequately the fluid needs of a patient is by knowing his intake and fluid losses. In surgical nursing, it is as imperative to keep accurate intake and output records as it is to administer medications, oxygen and so forth.

In this chapter, an attempt will be made to clarify some of the physiologic, the chemical and the nutritional changes which take place in the normal adult and in individuals who have a surgical problem. Although the whole subject of fluid balance is a complex one, the nurse ought to have an understanding of the problem. As a result, she will be of greater assistance to the surgeon and be better able to administer more intelligent nursing care to her patient.

PHYSIOLOGY

The total body water is divided into two main divisions: extracellular and intracellular fluid. Extracellular fluid includes plasma (about 5% of body weight) and interstitial fluid (about 15% of body weight). Intracellular fluid is equal to about 50 per cent of body weight. Hence, 70 per cent of body weight is water (Fig. 66).

Fluid exchange occurs in a definite way. For instance, the skin can lose fluid only, the gastro-intestinal tract can absorb or lose fluid, the lungs lose fluid by evaporation, and the kidneys lose fluid and many other substances. Ordinarily, fluid is taken through the gastro-intestinal tract and is excreted in the urine, the feces and the perspiration and through losses from the lungs (Fig. 68 A). Abnormally, fluid is lost by vomiting, diarrhea, fistula, perspiration, hemorrhage and exudation. It is estimated that water loss by evaporation is approximately 2,000 cc.; water loss in the urine averages

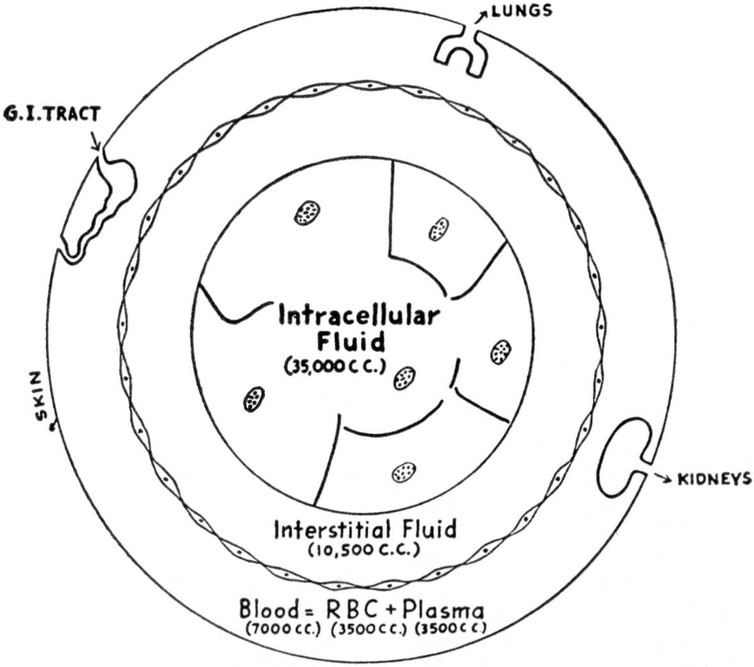

FIG. 66. A diagram illustrating the 3 main compartments of the body separated from each other by definite anatomic barriers, i.e., the capillary and the cell walls. The inner sphere is the intracellular space containing the fluid inside the cells of muscles, liver, etc., separated from the rest of the body by cell membrane. The outer space represents circulating blood. In the space between is the interstitial (or intercellular) fluid. The barrier between the blood and the interstitial fluid is the wall of the blood capillary membrane. (Elman, Robert: Fluid balance from the nurse's point of view, Am. J. Nursing **49**:222)

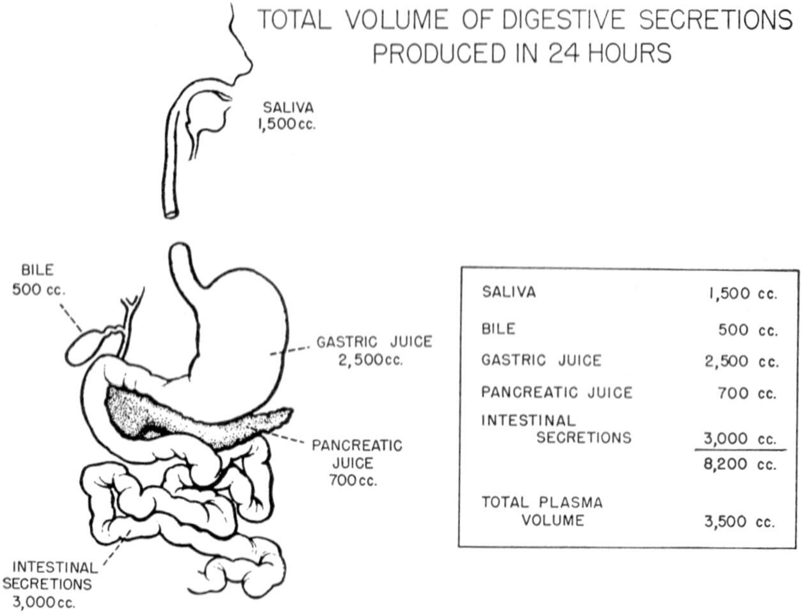

SALIVA	1,500 cc.
BILE	500 cc.
GASTRIC JUICE	2,500 cc.
PANCREATIC JUICE	700 cc.
INTESTINAL SECRETIONS	3,000 cc.
	8,200 cc.
TOTAL PLASMA VOLUME	3,500 cc.

FIG. 67. Total volume of digestive secretions produced in 24 hours. (Bowen, Arthur: Intravenous Alimentation in surgical patients, Mod. Med.)

about 1,500 cc. To this total daily loss of 3,500 cc. must be added the approximate amount of fluid loss in vomiting, drainage, diarrhea or any other abnormal or unusual loss. These losses are corrected by oral intake of food and fluid and/or parenteral injection.

SPECIFIC NEEDS OF THE SURGICAL PATIENT

WATER

Water is second only to oxygen as a vital physiologic necessity. Man can be starved, can lose almost all of his glycogen and fat, half of his body protein, 40 per cent of his body weight and still live. However, a loss of 10 per cent of his water content is serious, and a loss of 20 per cent is fatal.

According to Bowen (Fig. 67), the amount of fluid secreted by the gastro-intestinal tract in 24 hours is close to 8,000 cc., an amount equal to the total blood volume. Consequently, vomiting, diarrhea and draining fistulae can and do result in the loss of considerable amounts of water and electrolytes.

The water loss sustained during surgical procedures by evaporation and perspiration is about 1,000 to 1,500 cc. In addition, fluid losses due to hemorrhage may vary from 1,000 to 3,000 cc. Furthermore, due to anesthesia and the operative procedure, it is usually impossible to give

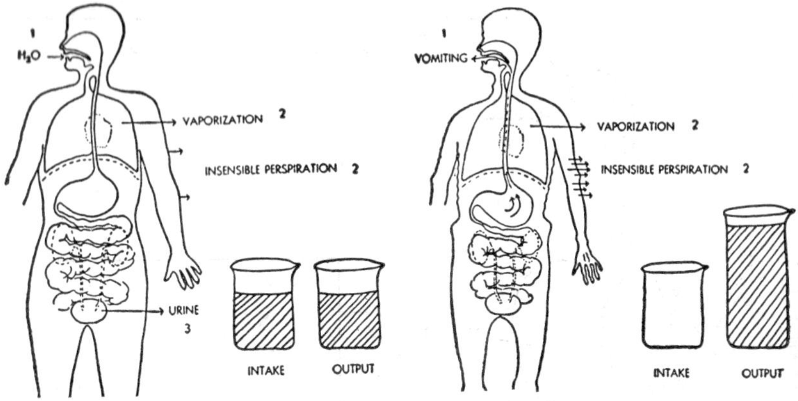

FIG. 68. Fluid balance and imbalance in a surgical patient. (*Left*) Normal fluid balance. (1) Water taken in as such. (2) Water lost by vaporization from the lungs and the skin (insensible loss). (3) Water lost in urine. The small amount normally lost in the feces is not indicated. The amount lost as sensible perspiration is highly variable and is not indicated. Daily intake and output are equal. (*Right*) Output exceeds intake. (1) Water lost by vomiting. None is taken in either as such or in food. The only source is the water of oxidation produced in the cells as the body tissues are consumed. (2) Water lost by vaporization. The insensible loss from the skin is increased, due to the elevation of the body temperature or to hot weather. Little or no urine is formed. The variable loss by sensible perspiration is not shown.

fluids by mouth for one or two days and even longer. Therefore, in order to maintain a fluid balance (fluid intake equal to fluid loss) fluid must be given parenterally. In addition to the loss of fluid at operation, many patients may lose fluid by vomiting or from drainage due to intestinal, biliary, pancreatic or other fistulae. In these patients also, the fluid balance is disturbed. In some cases, especially those in which there has been an inability to take fluids as in carcinoma of the esophagus, or in those in which there has been prolonged fluid loss by vomiting, as in pyloric or intestinal obstruction, the fluid deficit may be present even before operation. Cases in which there is a marked and prolonged fluid deficit are said to be *dehydrated* (Fig. 68). Accompanying symptoms are hot, dry skin, thirst, dry tongue, sunken eyes, temperature elevation and scanty urine. Fluid replacement is given preferably by mouth, but in those situations where fluids cannot be given orally they must be administered parenterally, usually intravenously. When fluids are given intravenously, they usually are given at the rate of 60 drops per minute. However, this speed may be varied, depending upon the fluid needs of the patient and the condition of the cardiovascular system. Thus, in patients who are markedly dehydrated, fluids may be given very rapidly. In older patients, where the heart muscle is not of the best, replacement is done more cautiously and slowly.

A fairly accurate clinical estimate of the fluid balance may be obtained by the amount of the urinary output; hence, it is extremely important to measure the urine. In most cases an output varying between 1,000 and 1,500 cc. is considered to be adequate.

Electrolytes

The electrolytes are the various salts of sodium, potassium, calcium and magnesium which are found in solution in the body fluids. These salts are normal and necessary in the body metabolism. When fluids are lost from the body, there is likewise a loss of the body electrolytes; thus, in vomiting, diarrhea or intestinal or biliary fistulae, electrolytes as well as fluids are lost. Because of the fact that these fluids vary in their electrolyte composition, there is a difference in the electrolyte loss by these various means. Thus, in vomiting, the loss is mostly the hydrochloric acid of the stomach, and the ion loss is chloride; the basic ion, sodium, is retained. On the other hand, the loss from intestinal fistulae contains more of the basic ions—calcium, sodium and potassium. Under normal conditions, the acid-base balance is maintained by urinary excretion, but under certain conditions, such as immediately after operation, sodium excretion may be less than normal, and potassium excretion may be increased. These variations also produce disturbances in acid-base balance and must be taken into account in administering postoperative electrolyte solutions.

It is possible to follow the electrolytes in the blood by chemical examination and thus to administer fluids to make up for the deficits which appear. The most commonly used electrolyte solution is that of physiologic sodium chloride. This means that the sodium chloride is in an aqueous solution in the same concentration as that found in the blood. In 1,000 cc. of this solution there are 9 Gm. of sodium chloride. Because of the fact that the kidneys do not excrete sodium well immediately after operation, the administration of more than 1,000 cc. of physiologic saline may result in sodium retention and various systemic disturbances. Therefore, it is usual to make up the fluid needs of the patient by giving glucose in distilled water in addition to the 1,000 cc. of saline solution.

Often potassium is added to intravenous solutions in the immediate postoperative period because excessive potassium is lost in the urine during this time. It also is used to make up for the loss of this ion in cases of gastric and intestinal fistulae.

The other basic ions, calcium, magnesium and so forth, are less important in acid-base equilibrium, but occasionally, specific disturbances of these ions also may be met. For example, in parathyroid deficiency or in tumors, disturbances of the calcium ion are found.

In some cases of electrolyte disturbance, fluids containing more than one of the basic ions are employed. These are such solutions as

Ringer's solution, Hartmann's solution, etc.

Carbohydrates

The body stores carbohydrates as glycogen in the liver, the muscles and other tissues, but the storage supply is relatively small and is used rapidly when food cannot be taken to replenish it. The carbohydrates are found in solution in the blood stream in the form of glucose. This is readily available commercially and may be administered in aqueous solution to make up for at least a part of the deficit produced by the inability to take food by mouth. It is used in a 5 and sometimes 10 per cent solution. In addition, invert sugar has been found useful in supplying carbohydrate needs of the body. Finally, alcohol in 3 to 5 per cent solution may be used as an easily available source of energy.

Protein

Since all cells require protein in their formation and metabolism, the inability to take protein foods by mouth or the loss of protein containing fluids from the body produces a condition which we term *hypoproteinemia.* This most often occurs when food cannot be eaten, such as in diseases of the esophagus and the stomach. The most striking example is the patient with an obstructing carcinoma of the esophagus. The hypoproteinemia due to the loss of protein containing fluids is seen in various ways—in ulcerating tumors of the gastro-intestinal tract, in inflammatory ulcerations of the colon and the intestine (colitis, ileitis) and in exudates from large denuded surfaces such as burns or extensive wounds.

The maintenance of a normal protein content of the blood is extremely important if the surgical patient is to recover rapidly. The clinical manifestations of hypoproteinemia are peripheral and visceral edema, inhibition of gastro-intestinal motility and interference with wound healing.

The protein and nutritional balance is maintained best by oral feeding, but there are many instances in which food cannot be given by mouth in attempts to overcome the protein deficit. In such instances, protein-containing fluids must be given by vein, and of these there are available blood, plasma and amino acids in solution. Each of these fluids has its own indications and uses.

Vitamins

Vitamins are recognized as being important in maintaining nutrition and general health. Under normal conditions and with a normal food intake, vitamins are taken in adequate amounts. However, in situations in which food cannot be given by mouth, as in esophageal, pyloric and intestinal obstruction and in the postoperative state, vitamin deficiencies of more or less degree may occur. Furthermore, abnormal losses of vitamins may be present following vomiting or diarrhea. In some instances where fat ingestion is restricted or absorption does not take place, such as jaundice, a deficiency of the fat-soluble vitamins may occur.

The water-soluble vitamins may be administered parenterally with intravenous solutions to make up for

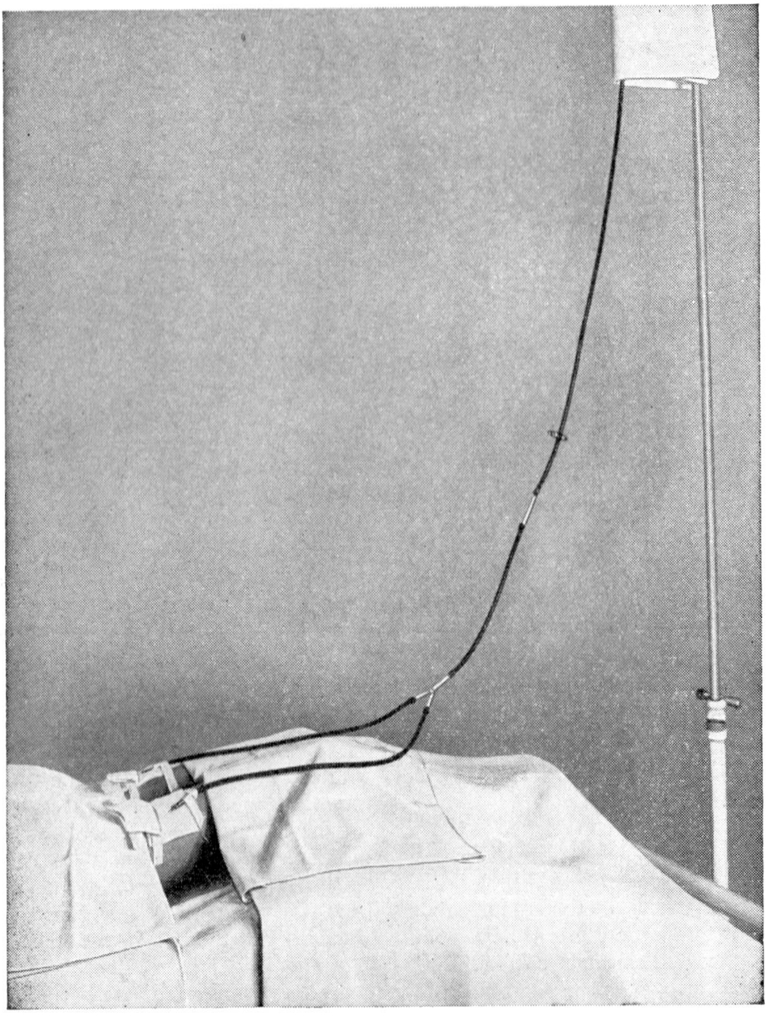

FIG. 69 A. Hypodermoclysis—continuous-drip method. Note needles anchored in place with adhesive and sterile gauze covers to be placed over needles.

the deficit and occasionally they may be given intramuscularly in cases where specific vitamin needs appear, e.g., vitamin K in jaundice.

It is important to supply adequate amounts of vitamins to permit the normal metabolic processes to function and to avoid the consequences of deficiency which may result in poor nutritional state of the patient

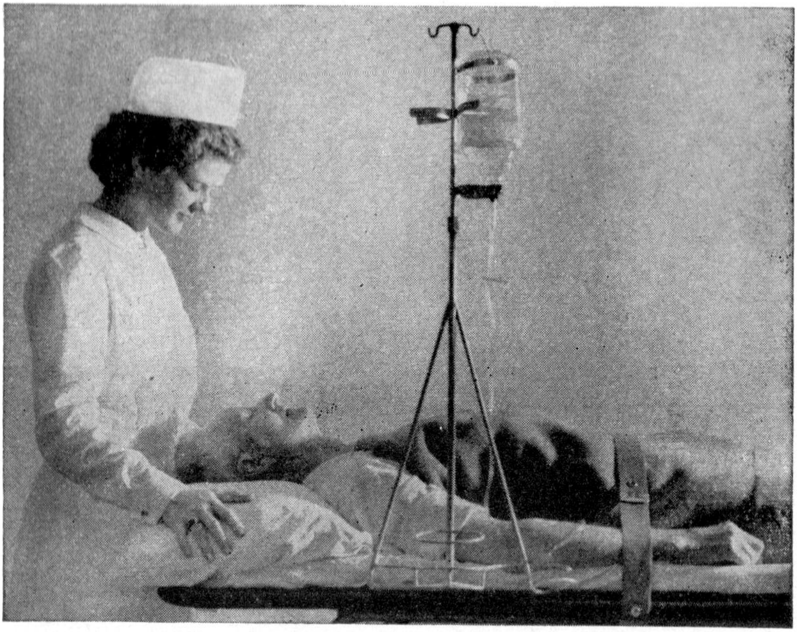

FIG. 69 B. Patient returning from the operating room. Note the stretcher standard for holding the intravenous fluid container during transport. The fluid is in a commercial container with plastic disposable tubing.

and inhibit normal reparative processes.

METHODS OF ADMINISTRATION

The usual methods for giving fluids to a patient are (1) by mouth, (2) by hypodermoclysis, (3) by intravenous infusion, and (4) by peritoneum. In selected patients with inaccessible veins, fluids have been given through a needle inserted into the sternum.

MOUTH

Fluids are given by mouth in large quantities in the preoperative preparation of anemic and dehydrated patients and in the postoperative period after the cessation of the nausea that often follows the administration of an anesthetic. This is the natural and the easiest method, and the fluids that may be given include water (not ice water), hot tea and fruit juices, often combined with egg albumen. (See Liquid Diet, p. 113.)

Fluids must not be given by mouth (except by order) after operation on any part of the gastro-intestinal tract, except the region of the anus and except in cases of simple appendectomy. Often post-anesthetic nausea and vomiting make fluid administration by mouth impossible. In such event, one or more of the following methods may be employed.

Hypodermoclysis

Hypodermoclysis is the subcutaneous injection of fluids for absorption by the lymphatics of the connective tissue. It may be used when the administration of fluids is indicated, irrespective of the site of operation. Often it is used in conjunction with the other methods when it is desired to administer large amounts of fluid fairly rapidly. When a failing circulation makes absorption slow, the method is of little value.

All apparatus, fluids and instruments must be sterile, and the technic must be carried out with full aseptic precautions. (Fig. 69.) The solution should be checked carefully before being used to prevent error and serious complications.

Rapid Method

Fluid is allowed to flow from a reservoir through a rubber tube and a needle into the connective tissues beneath the breasts or into the outer portion of the thighs. As the fluid runs into the tissues, the needle is moved in different directions and the tissues are massaged gently to increase the rate of absorption. This method is used in pediatric surgery for administration of fluid to small infants. Usually, a syringe and a needle are used.

Continuous Method

After thorough preparation of the skin on the anterior and the lateral surfaces of the thighs with an antiseptic (the area previously having been shaved when necessary), the nurse washes her hands with soap and water and puts on sterile gloves. Then she drapes the patient with sterile covers and exposes the prepared areas. Taking up the sterile apparatus, the sterile nurse holds the reservoir (usually glass), into which is poured some of the sterile solution to be given. If a closed flask is used, such as the Fenwal, it is attached. The clamp on the main delivery tube is released until the solution fills all tubes below the glass dropper. In this manner, all the air is excluded from the tubes. (If this precaution is not taken, air frequently will collect in one of the small tubes, and its presence will prevent the flow of fluid on that side.) The tube is clamped below the dropper to prevent the escape of the fluid, and the needles are inserted into the prepared areas, covered with sterile gauze and held in position with a strip of adhesive. The tip of the needle should lie in the loose subcutaneous fatty tissue just beneath the skin surface.

The temperature of the solution may be that of the room. Since the flow is drop by drop, it is not believed that the difference between room and body temperatures makes any difference in the absorption of the fluid in the subcutaneous tissue or has any deleterious effect on the patient.

The reservoir is elevated until the height of the pressure column (the glass dropper) is about 2 feet above the bed, and the fluid is allowed to drop slowly from the dropping tube.

This method of fluid administration is used occasionally when lack of available veins makes intravenous administration difficult or impossible.

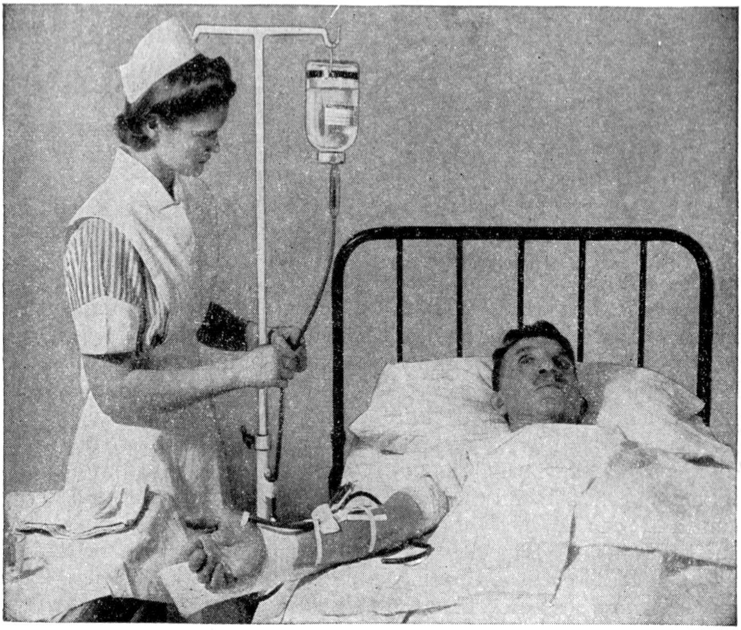

FIG. 70. Commercial apparatus for continuous intravenous infusion. The sterile solutions may be obtained in special containers, ready for immediate use. Illustration shows the nurse adjusting the flow of intravenous fluid after the introduction of the needle by the surgeon.

Solutions

The solutions generally used for hypodermoclysis are:

1. **Physiologic sodium chloride** (saline) solution, which is about 0.85 per cent solution of sodium chloride in distilled water.

2. **Glucose** (from 3 to 5 per cent solutions) in normal salt is employed sometimes as an extreme measure. The authors do not recommend it because of the danger of sloughing of tissue.

3. **Hyaluronidase.** The addition of hyaluronidase, an enzyme that decreases surface tension, to the infusion solutions appears to speed absorption by hypodermoclysis to a degree almost approximating that of intravenous infusion. It is most effective when it is added to the first few cubic centimeters of the infusion fluid.

Dangers

1. The needles may puncture a large blood vessel. If this happens, as shown by back flow of blood into the glass tube, the needle should be withdrawn slightly before the flow of solution is allowed to start. For this reason, injections always are made at sites at which there are no important vessels—for example, at

the lateral aspects of the thighs, under the breasts and, less often, the lateral aspects of the abdominal wall.

2. The needles may puncture a cavity—for example, abdominal or pleural cavity—especially in thin people.

3. Abscess may develop, due to infections at the site of injection, unless all aseptic precautions are taken.

4. Sloughing may occur if the fluid is permitted to run in too fast. The pressure of the solution compresses the blood vessels, prevents absorption and causes death of the tissues due to a local loss of blood supply. Such a condition often is associated with infection. This danger can be forestalled easily by frequent observance of the areas receiving the fluid. If the area is blanched, firm to the touch and painful, the rate of flow should be decreased and the tube leading to that area clamped temporarily until pain ceases and color returns.

Intravenous Infusion

Fluid introduced by vein enters directly into the circulation. It is the surest and the most rapid method available; therefore, it is used almost entirely in present-day surgery.

If the circulation is good, the fluid is lost rapidly through the kidneys and other excretory organs or by absorption into the tissues, so that the procedure must be repeated frequently. For this reason, intravenous infusion should be considered as having only a temporary effect in increasing the volume of circulating fluids. More lasting effects are obtained by a transfusion of blood or plasma. (For equipment, see p. 172.)

Methods

Sterile solutions are introduced into a vein, usually near the bend of the elbow, through a needle or cannula. The same precautions as to asepsis are taken as for hypodermoclysis. The solution in the reservoir should be at room temperature. The solution is given at a rate of about 40 to 60 drops a minute or as ordered by the physician, and the amount and the type of solution are indicated in the surgeon's written orders. Drugs may be introduced into the tube by a hypodermic syringe and needle. Adrenalin and caffeine often are used in this way.

VENOCLYSIS

Often better results are obtained, when the administration of fluids is not an emergency measure, by giving the intravenous infusion by the drip method over a long period of time. The needle, polyethylene tubing or cannula is inserted into a convenient vein and fixed by tapes to the arm. Often the arm is held in a pillow splint. In very restless patients, wooden or plaster splints must be used. A slight flexion of 10° at the elbow gives most comfort to the patient.

The solution is given at a rate of about 150 cc. an hour. The nurse must keep a strict watch over the patient during the procedure to prevent him from dislodging the needle. The temperature of the solution need not be above that of the room in this slow method of venoclysis. The administration of intravenous solutions is the responsibility of the surgeon, but once the infusion is started the nurse is called upon to watch it and to report to the physician should the fluid stop running or should it appear to be entering the tissues instead of the vein.

Solutions for intravenous administration must be not only sterile but also chemically free from the products of bacterial or fungous growth that occur before sterilization. All containers for solutions to be used for intravenous administration should be cleaned chemically and washed with freshly distilled water just before sterilization (within 3 hours). Tubing through which such solutions are to be given must be cleaned similarly just before sterilization. Commercially prepared intravenous solutions have disposable bottles, disposable connections and tubing. All solutions for intravenous use, including the citrate and ether solutions used in collecting blood from donors, should be prepared in freshly cleaned containers with freshly distilled water immediately before sterilization (within 3 hours). There must be no interval during which bacteria or molds can grow in material to be injected intravenously before it is sterilized: the sterilized products of bacterial or mold growth may be highly toxic. The reactions from intravenous infusions appear to arise from (1) improper cleansing of the apparatus, (2) improper preparation of the solutions and finally (3) too rapid administration of the solution. Reactions are characterized by elevation of temperature, at times accompanied by a chill. As a rule, these reactions are not serious but, when the infusion is administered properly, they should not occur.

Polyethylene tubing is used in intravenous therapy as an indwelling catheter. Eight-inch lengths with beveled ends are used as disposable cannulas and may be left in veins up to 4 weeks. Following the taking of a blood specimen or the giving of an infusion, the tube is sealed off with heat and reopened the next day.

Polyethylene tubing is sterilized with Zephiran Chloride 1:1,000. The solution must be drawn into the tubing to expel all air bubbles, and the tubing immersed in the solution for at least 18 hours. Before using, the tubing should be rinsed with sterile saline both outside and inside. Sterilization methods which are destructive to polyethylene are boiling, autoclaving and immersion in alcohol or formalin.

Dangers

Infection, unless full asepsis is practiced.

Embolus. The introduction of a foreign body into the blood stream may cause symptoms immediate and grave. The foreign body or embolus may be air, blood clot, foreign bodies in the fluid and so forth. Care must be taken that the solution introduced is absolutely clear, and that air is removed entirely from the tubing system.

Dilatation of Heart. This danger is encountered only when the solution is introduced too rapidly. Its signs are (1) dyspnea (difficult respiration), (2) pain in the chest, (3) engorged veins of face and neck, cyanosis, especially of the lips and the eyelids, and (4) cardiac embarrassment (often followed by death). Report any of these signs immediately or stop the flow and obtain instructions.

Solutions

The fluids used for intravenous injection are:

1. **Physiologic sodium chloride solutions,** 0.85 per cent solution.
2. **Glucose solutions,** from 5 to 50 per cent strengths, according to the purpose for which it is used.
3. **Physiologic saline and 5 or 10 per cent glucose.**
4. **Hartmann's Solution.** This is a solution of sodium, potassium and calcium chlorides and sodium lactate. It may be obtained prepared sterile in hermetically sealed ampules. As it is in concentrated form, it is diluted according to instructions on the label before being employed intravenously and also subcutaneously or intraperitoneally in the treatment of dehydration. It is of special value in the treatment of acidosis and alkalosis because it is a buffer solution. In acidosis it is of value because it supplies the needed salts and fluid, and the lactate is converted slowly but effectively into a sodium bicarbonate. In alkalosis its action is almost equally effective. Because of its chloride and water content it enables the kidney to excrete the alkali bicarbonate more rapidly.
5. **Ringer's Solution.** This is a solution of the chlorides of sodium, potassium and calcium in the proper proportions. Its special value is in the treatment of dehydration, when, because of its more complete salt content, it may be more effective than ordinary physiologic saline.
6. **Protein Hydrolysates and Amino Acids.** The restoration of blood elements with substitutes derived from human blood is an expensive form of therapy. As a result, much work has been done in the search for other materials of a less costly source. By the hydrolysis of such cheap forms of protein as casein or lactalbumin to polypeptides or amino acids, a substance is formed, which, when placed in 5 per cent solution (50 Gm. per 1,000 cc.), can easily be administered intravenously, and it supplies the building stones for the formation of new body tissues. This is valuable especially in preparing the malnourished patient for surgery or for use during the postoperative period when oral alimentation is interfered with for long periods of time. These protein hydrolysate and amino acid preparations are supplied by commercial manufacturers under various trade names, and they are available in most hospitals. Reactions are not uncommon; therefore, a careful watch should be kept during the administration of these preparations. They must be given slowly (from 40 to 50 drops a minute). If they are given more rapidly, the patient may complain of a feeling of warmth. From 4 to 6 hours is required to give a liter of the solution. Once a flask of the solution is opened, it should be given at that time or discarded, as it is an excellent culture medium for bacteria, and storage is unwise. A cloudy solution never should be given. Depending upon the needs of the patient, from 1 to 3 liters of the solution may be administered daily. This would supply the nitrogen

equivalent of from 50 to 150 Gm. of protein. As the conversion of amino acids or protein hydrolysates into body proteins proceeds at a rather inefficient rate, 3 liters often is necessary to meet the daily minimal body requirements of protein.

7. **Lactate Solutions.** These usually are used in the correction of acidosis.

8. **Plasma.** Although fresh whole blood is the best substitute for blood in most instances, it became apparent during World War II that plasma had a permanent place in surgical therapy. Plasma is made by siphoning the supernatant fluid from blood after the red cells have settled to the bottom of a container with the aid of a centrifuge. It can be preserved for three years at least when frozen (maintained below–15° C.) or indefinitely when its water content is removed and it is kept in a dry state in sealed containers. To prepare for use, thawing is all that is necessary when it is preserved in the frozen state, or adding distilled water when it is in the dry form. Plasma has almost all the properties of blood, except the ability to carry oxygen; and it can be used in most instances in which red blood cells are not needed. It is relatively free of reactions and allergic manifestations; it can be used for shock and burns and for supplying antibodies in treating infections and correcting hypoproteinemic states.

As it can be stored easily on the ward or in the accident room for emergency use, and can be administered without time-consuming typing and cross-matching, it does have two advantages at least over whole blood. These advantages alone made it invaluable in the forward combat areas during the war. In civil life it is used chiefly for emergencies, for the replacement of blood proteins in states of malnutrition and for burns when there is a concentration of red blood cells in the circulation due to loss of plasma through damaged capillaries.

After being prepared for administration, it is passed through a fine mesh filter to remove undissolved particles and given intravenously. Even though rare, reactions in the form of chills, dyspnea and a feeling of warmth must be watched for.

Equipment

The trays for a venoclysis or intravenous infusion are obtained from the central supply room in many hospitals. Occasionally, it may be necessary to expose the vein before a needle or a cannula can be inserted into it, in which case a tray for phlebotomy (venesection) also should be procured. The nurse also should obtain from the central supply room the solutions requested by the surgeon. In addition, the following scrub-up tray should be prepared on the ward:

Alcohol sponges
Tincture of iodine
Curved basin
Curved hemostat
Rubber-tube tourniquet
Forceps in 70 per cent alcohol
Dressing mackintosh and muslin cover
Small gauze dressings
½-inch adhesive
2-inch bandage

An adjustable irrigating pole likewise will be necessary.

Procedure for an Intravenous Infusion

The nurse should assemble all the necessary equipment and see that the irrigating standard is placed properly at the side of the bed. She should count and record the patient's pulse. The sterile tray and the solution flask should be placed on a table at the side of the patient's bed within easy reach of the surgeon.

After washing her hands, the nurse prepares the site of puncture in the arm. The gown is removed from the arm on the side to be used, the chest meanwhile being protected with a blanket to prevent exposure and chilling. A pillow or splint, protected with a mackintosh and a cover, is placed underneath the elbow. The rubber-tube tourniquet is placed underneath the upper part of the arm but not tied. Then the site of injection, as selected by the surgeon—usually the anterior portion of the elbow region—is prepared with an antiseptic designated by the surgeon. This is done with a cotton ball, saturated with the antiseptic, held in forceps. The tourniquet is tightened. The sterile cap from the flask of solution is removed by the nurse, and the plastic tubing of the infusion set is attached to the bottle by introducing the sterile needles through the rubber stopper. After inverting the bottle, air is expelled from the tubing by allowing a small amount of fluid to run through it. When the needle has been inserted into the vein, the tourniquet is removed, and the nurse provides sterile gauze pads and half-inch adhesive to hold the needle in place.

After the intravenous infusion has been started, the nurse must make frequent observations of the patient's pulse, respiration and color. It is her responsibility to see that the bottle does not become empty and so cause air to be introduced into the blood stream. When commercially prepared solutions are used, the bottles must be changed as they become empty. Sterile precautions must be observed throughout. She must also observe the rate of flow of the fluid as ordered by the surgeon. In restless patients it may be necessary for the arm to be held to the side of the bed with a bandage. The nurse should inspect the tissues around the needle frequently to see if infiltration of the tissues is taking place. If it is, it means that the needle has been displaced. The flow should be stopped and the physician should be notified.

Charting. The nurse's record should contain a note concerning the time of the starting of the intravenous infusion, the kind and the quantity of the solution used and any unusual symptoms that may occur. As each additional flask of solution is added, it must be recorded on the nurse's record so that the surgeon may know by looking at the nurse's chart exactly how much fluid has been administered.

BLOOD TRANSFUSION

Blood transfusion is the transfer of blood from the veins of one person to the veins of another. It is used in the treatment of the acute anemia following hemorrhage. It is also of value in any kind of anemia, shock, infections and blood diseases—for example, purpura and leukemia. Frequently blood transfusions are used in the prophylaxis against shock during and after operation.

The person who gives the blood is termed the *donor*, and the one who receives it, the *recipient*. Before a transfusion is attempted, the bloods of the donor and the recipient must be typed and cross-matched. The donor usually selected is one whose blood is the same type as that of the recipient. (There are 4 main types of blood, and the blood of one type may not mix well with that of another.) When a donor has been selected, specimens of his blood and that of the recipient are mixed and examined to make sure that they are compatible. This is called *cross-agglutination*.

Rh Factor

In 1940 it was discovered that there was an additional substance present in the blood of most individuals that should be considered in giving transfusions. The substance, about the exact nature of which little is known, was given the name *Rh factor* because it appeared to be identical with a substance found in the blood of all Rhesus monkeys. Approximately 85 per cent of the general population has the factor, in which case the designation is *Rh positive*, and the remaining 15 per cent does not have the factor, in which case the designation is *Rh negative*. This factor, like the 4 blood groups, follows a Mendelian dominant pattern of inheritance.

Little concern is experienced when blood is given to an Rh-positive individual, as his blood already contains the factor, and no reaction occurs when additional substance is given. However, when an Rh-negative recipient receives blood from an Rh-positive donor, the recipient's body forms antibodies against the factor (becomes sensitized). At a later date, when he is given an additional transfusion of Rh-positive blood, he may experience a violent reaction, characterized in many cases by jaundice and anemia.

An Rh-negative mother may develop antibodies (become sensitized) during a pregnancy with an Rh-positive fetus and be the subject of a serious reaction, even at a much later date, when given Rh-positive blood. In such a case the father of the child would be an Rh-positive individual.

Most cases of erythroblastosis fetalis (a disease of the newborn similar in many respects to a transfusion reaction) result from agglutination of the infant's red cells by antibodies transmitted from an Rh-negative mother who had been sensitized previously by either a pregnancy with an Rh-positive fetus or a transfusion of Rh-positive blood containing none of the harmful antibodies.

Even though only the 15 per cent Rh-negative population is subject to a possible reaction due to the Rh factor, it should be considered in every case, and the compatibility ascertained prior to transfusion.

Methods

Many methods of transfusion have been used and discarded, largely because of the difficulty of their technic. There are two main groups:

Direct Transfusion. The blood vessels of the donor and the recip-

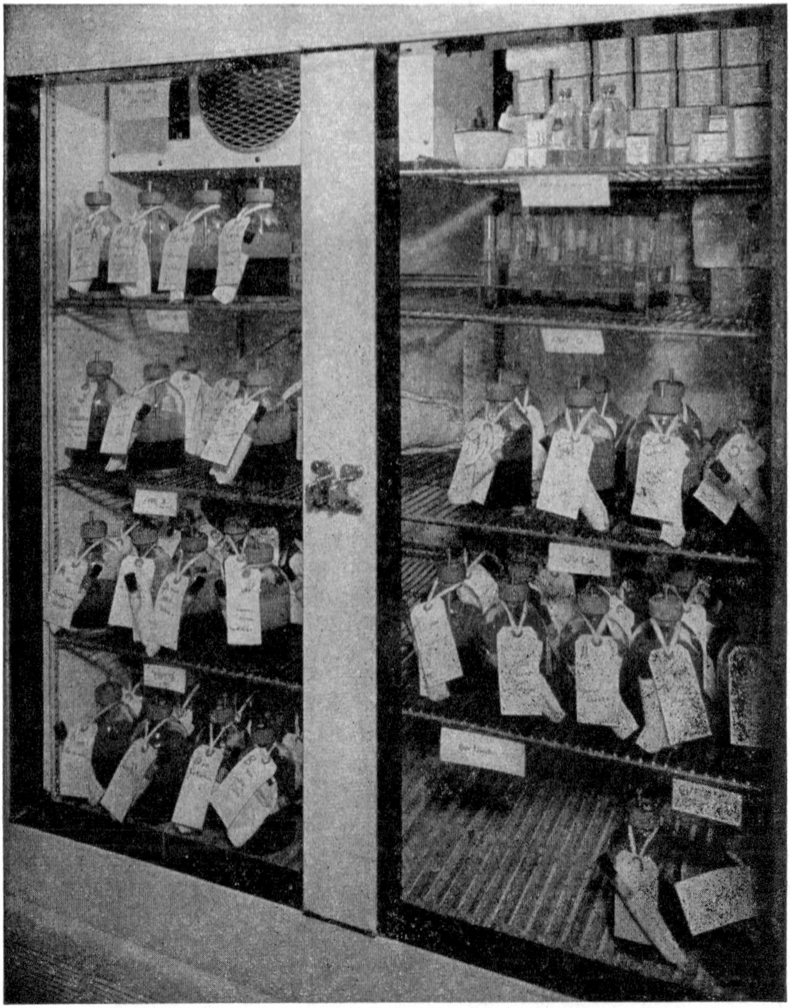

Fig. 71. Refrigerator in use as a depository for the blood bank. Note flasks of blood properly capped and tagged. On each flask is a small tube of citrated blood that may be used for cross agglutination, which avoids the necessity of opening the flask.

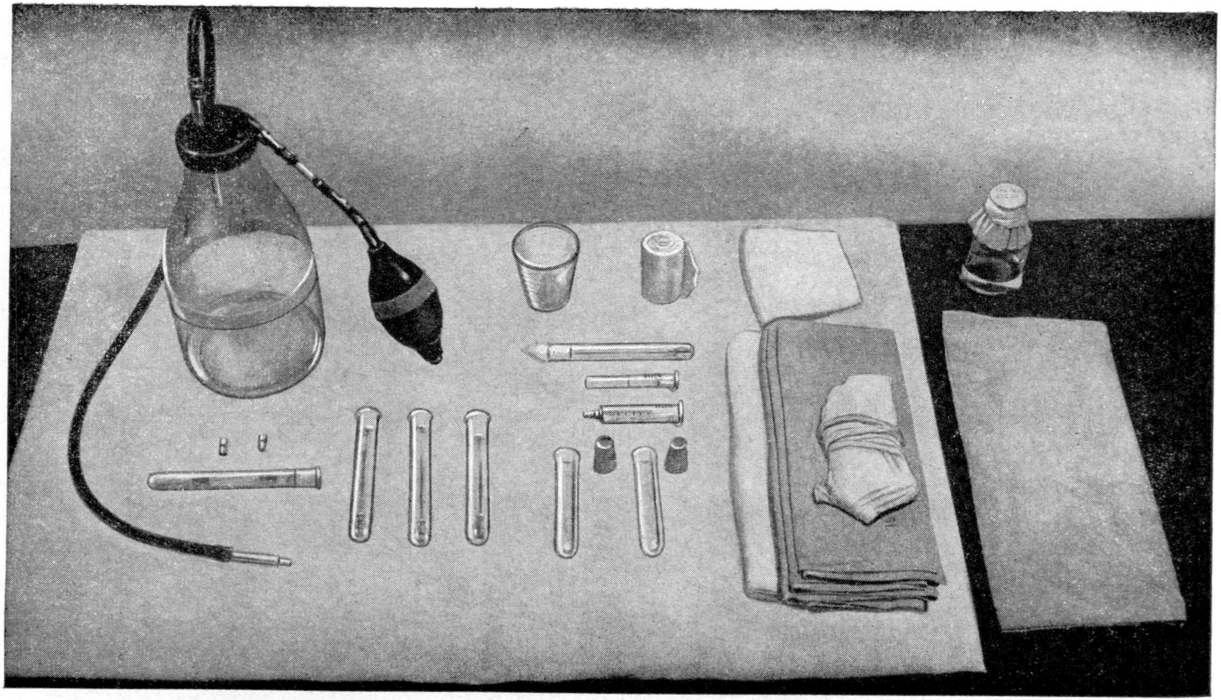

Fig. 72. Donor's tray, with blood flask containing citrate, suction bulb, sterile gloves and small flask of procaine. Note rubber stopper on blood flask that covers the lips of the bottle completely. In front of the flask are the BD adapters No. 425, which were removed to attach the tubing and the filter. In the sterile tube are a second set of adapters to be used when the blood has been taken.

ient are joined. It is rarely that this method is used now.

Indirect Transfusion. Blood flows from the veins of the donor into a receptacle before it enters the veins of the recipient.

Unmodified Blood

Many methods have been devised. Those used most commonly consist of a U tube connected to a syringe, whereby blood is drawn from the vein of the donor, a valve is turned, and the blood is injected immediately into the veins of the recipient.

Modified Blood

Blood is drawn from the donor into a vessel containing some anticoagulant, and then is allowed to flow into the veins of the recipient. Modified or citrated blood can be kept in a stoppered flask in the refrigerator at 4° C. (39° F.) for as long as 5 days. If glucose has been added to give a final concentration of from 1 to 3 per cent, the blood may be kept 30 days in the refrigerator. The discovery of this fact has led to the formation of blood repositories or banks in numerous hospitals. Citrated blood of the various types is kept on hand and is available for transfusion as soon as a cross-agglutination is obtained.

When citrated blood is given to the patient, the technic is essentially the same as that used in giving fluid by intravenous infusion, the only difference being that after the fluid is started by the administration of a small amount of physiologic saline, the blood instead of saline is added. When blood is administered from the bottle in which it was collected, a filter must be introduced into the connecting tubing to remove small clots before the blood enters the vein. The same precautions as for the giving of fluid by intravenous infusion must be observed. The nurse should observe and record the time at which the blood is given and the amount, any rise in temperature, rise in pulse, difficulty in respiration, nausea and vomiting (see dangers on p. 178).

After the giving of a transfusion or the withdrawing of blood from a donor, the nurse must wash carefully in cold water all the apparatus that has been used. Using one of the syringes on the tray, cold water should be forced through the needles, and water should be run generously through the rubber tubing in order to wash away as well as possible all the blood particles that may be adhering to it. The apparatus then must be assembled carefully on the tray and returned to the central supply room for further cleaning and resterilization.

In many hospitals use is made of disposable donor sets composed of plastic tubing fitted with a filter. They are fitted readily into special containers into which the blood is drawn. Sterile needles, of course, must be available. In using these sets, which usually are sterilized and dispensed in cellophane, the nurse must take sterile precautions, being careful not to contaminate the end that goes into the blood bottle or the end to which the needle is attached. These sets prepared commercially have the advantage of being standardized. They are not used again and so reactions due to retained impurities in the flask and the tubing are avoided. In addition, they save much valuable time for the busy nurse, in that there is no after-care of tubing and flask; the needles only must be cleaned.

Transfusion in Infants

Transfusion of blood in infants is more difficult because of the small size of the veins. Usually only relatively small amounts of blood are given (from 10 to 20 cc. per kilo of body weight) so that often the blood may be given by a needle and a syringe. The large veins of the neck, and even the longitudinal sinus, may be used. Occasionally in older children, when there are no available veins, the blood may be introduced into the large blood sinuses of the bone marrow. The sternum and the tibia are the bones used most often in these "marrow transfusions."

Dangers

The dangers associated with transfusion of blood are essentially those described for an intravenous infusion plus another danger that is encountered sometimes due to the character of the blood itself. If the blood of both donor and recipient has not been matched carefully, the patient may complain of pain in the back and the chest, and cyanosis and dyspnea may develop, followed by death.

Often, even when all details of technic have been observed carefully, a post-transfusion reaction may occur. This usually is characterized by a chill, occurring from 10 to 15 minutes to an hour after the transfusion. Following the chill there is a rise in temperature to 101° or 102° F. and a commensurate rise in pulse rate. In most cases the temperature and the pulse return rapidly to the level present before the transfusion. This type of reaction usually can be avoided if the blood is given slowly enough. When any sign suggestive of a transfusion reaction occurs, the nurse should stop the transfusion and call the doctor.

Peritoneum

Fluids may be given into the peritoneal cavity for absorption. This method may be used in infants by injecting fluid through a needle into the peritoneal cavity.

GAS THERAPY

Oxygen has been administered as therapy for many years, but it has assumed greater importance as methods of administration have improved. Oxygen is supplied in concentrations above that found in normal air, thus raising the oxygen tension in the inspired air. As a result, a more complete respiratory exchange in the lungs becomes possible, the hemoglobin leaving the lungs with a higher percentage of oxygen than is possible when ordinary air is inspired and the deficiency of oxygen in the tissues is overcome. Normal air contains 20.93 per cent oxygen, 79.04 per cent nitrogen and 0.03 per cent carbon dioxide. A concentration of 45 per cent oxygen usually is required to relieve cyanosis.

Indications for Use

The medical conditions in which the administration of oxygen has been especially helpful are pneumonia, pulmonary edema, coronary occlusion, congestive heart failure and asphyxia from various causes. In

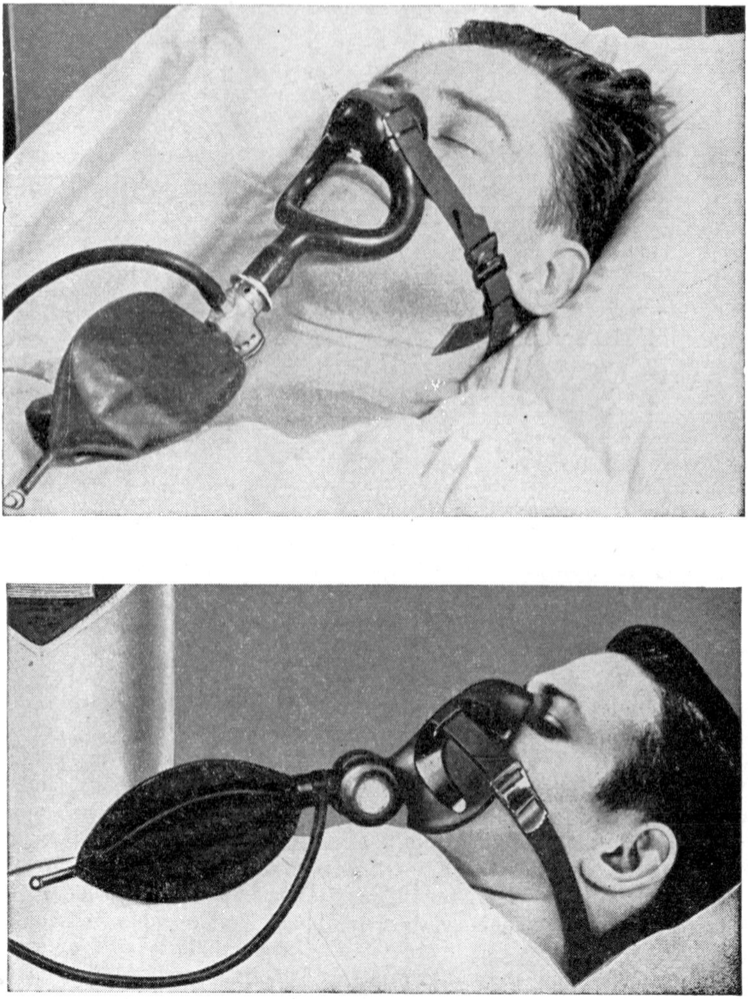

FIG. 73. Method of administration of oxygen by (*top*) the Boothby, Lovelace and Bulbulian (B-L-B) mask, and (*bottom*) the oronasal mask.

surgery it is used as a prophylactic measure both during and after operation.

During Operation. At this time the factors that may contribute to a reduction of the oxygen in the tissues are the preanesthetic medication, the anesthetic drugs and the condition of the patient's circulatory system. To combat this deficiency,

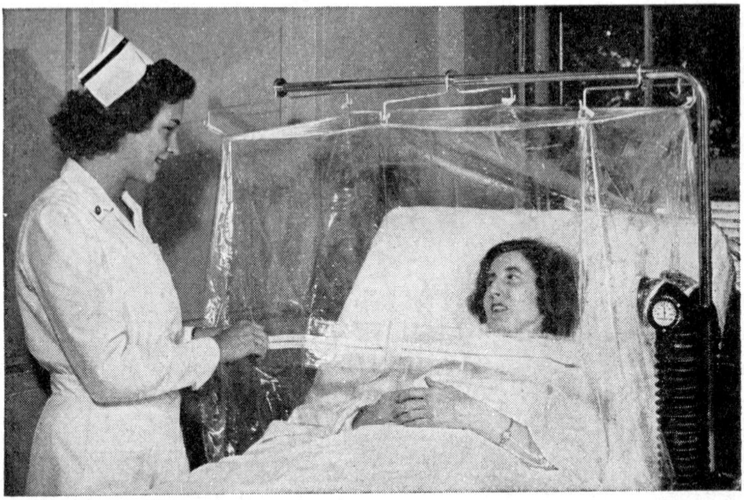

FIG. 74. Plastic type of oxygen tent with zipper front. Note the flow regulator at the intake pipe. In this type of transparent tent the patient does not feel as enclosed as in the old type, in which small windows gave the only view of the outside. In addition, the nurse is able to instruct the patient within the tent without opening it or disturbing its oxygen contents. (National Cylinder Gas Company)

oxygen usually is given in high concentration during the period of anesthesia in any operation of long duration or of a serious nature.

After Operation. At this time, the sedative drugs, the pain incidental to the operative wound and the nature of the operation *per se* may all contribute in reducing the oxygen-carbon dioxide exchange and, therefore, the oxygen supply to the blood and especially to the brain. Pulmonary complications (especially atelectasis, pneumonia and pulmonary embolism) result in a deficient oxygen-carbon dioxide exchange in the lungs, with the resulting reduction of circulating oxygen and even cyanosis. Oxygen therapy also is indicated in the treatment of patients who have some temporary partial obstruction in the air passages (as after thyroidectomy), in patients with disease of the lungs, and in those who have a deficient respiration due to pain in an upper abdominal wound. Inhalations of oxygen have been found to aid in the treatment of ileus when it is of the reflex or paralytic type. Cyanosis is a danger sign, and it should be combated promptly by correcting its cause.

After operations on the thyroid gland, after operations for empyema and pulmonary diseases, and frequently after extensive gastric and bile-duct operations, gas therapy may be used as a prophylactic measure.

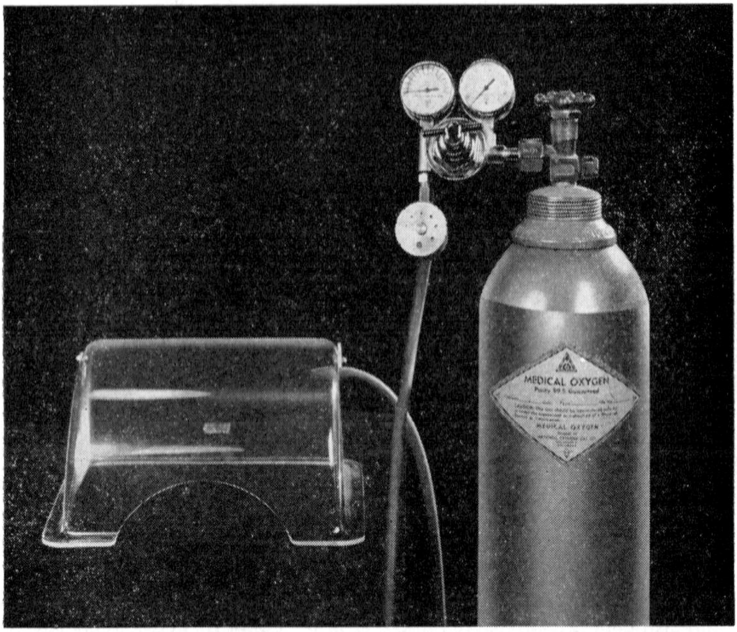

FIG. 75. Plastic head tent which is used instead of oxygen tent for application of oxygen in high concentration. The plastic box is placed over the patient's head and oxygen is administered as it would be through a mask. The head tent is removed easily and is used and transported more easily than is the large-size tent. (Natural Cylinder Gas Company)

METHODS OF ADMINISTRATION

Oxygen may be administered by nasal catheter; by nasal inhalator, funnel or face mask; by B-L-B (Boothby, Lovelace and Bulbulian) inhalation apparatus; by oxygen tent; or by an oxygen chamber. When a tent is used, it may be operated with or without a motor. The Burgess-Collins or open-top type, which runs without a motor, necessitates keeping the patient flat.

In all but the B-L-B inhalation apparatus, oxygen seldom reaches a greater concentration than from 40 to 60 per cent. Some authorities claim that concentrations higher than 70 per cent will be injurious because of the irritating effect on the mucous membrane of the lungs and the change in the oxygen tension of the tissues. Dr. Boothby and his associates report that "100 per cent" oxygen has been administered continuously for 48 hours without pulmonary irritation. This high oxygen concentration may be given for pulmonary embolism, coronary thrombosis, surgical and traumatic shock, reduction of acute gaseous

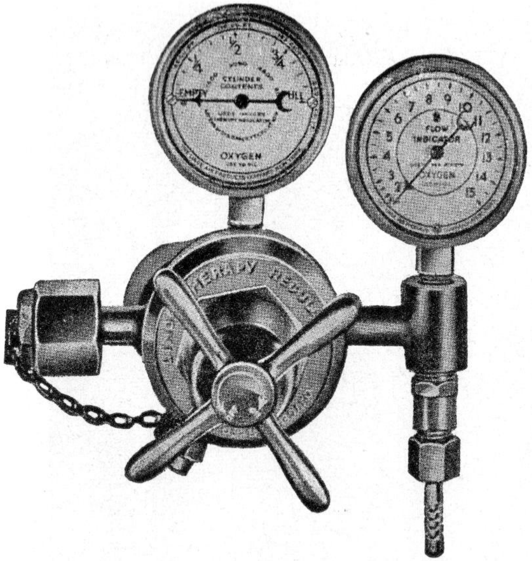

FIG. 76. Oxygen regulator to be attached to the oxygen tank. See above for a description of its use. (Barach, A. L.: Physiologic Therapy in Respiratory Diseases, ed. 2, Philadelphia, Lippincott)

abdominal distention, massive atelectasis and prevention of headaches after encephalography, also in the treatment of infections with anaerobic or partially anaerobic bacteria, particularly those caused by the organisms of gas gangrene and tetanus.

Nursing Care

The nurse must be familiar with the type of apparatus to be used in administering oxygen, and she should follow all directions carefully. The nurse's responsibilities may be enumerated as follows:

1. **Prepare the Patient Psychologically as Well as Physically.** Many individuals associate oxygen therapy with a critically ill patient who is at death's door. A reassuring explanation should be given to the patient beforehand so that these fears are minimized. Present-day uses of oxygen therapy include supportive and comfort measures as well as therapeutic. Patients may object to the confinement and the limitations of a tent. The use of transparent plastic tents can reduce this feeling of claustrophobia.

2. **Attach the Regulator to the Oxygen Tank.** This is the nurse's responsibility if an oxygen technician is not available. It must be done before any form of oxygen therapy can be given. The purpose of the oxygen regulator is twofold: (1) to indicate the amount of oxygen in the tank; and (2) to "step-down" the force of the oxygen that is under pressure to a usable and regulated level. Consequently, a regulator has two gauges that indicate both.

A. Before a regulator can be attached to an oxygen tank, the cylinder valve must be loosened slightly ("cracked") to allow the gas to blow dust particles from the outlet.

B. Attach the regulator by screwing the metal band of the regulator over the projecting tip of the cylinder.

C. Turn regulator valve "Off."

D. Open the cylinder valve *gradually* and the indicator on one gauge will show the amount of oxygen in the tank.

E. Turn regulator valve "On," and the flow indicator gauge will show the number of liters of oxygen flowing per minute. Turn the valve to number desired by the physician.

3. **Provide an Oxygen Concentration as Ordered by the Physician.** The oxygen content of the tent atmosphere can be analyzed by withdrawing a measured sample and forcing it through a liquid that absorbs the oxygen. The decrease in the volume of the liquid gives the percentage of oxygen present. The device is attached to certain models, or it may be secured separately.

To prevent the escape of oxygen from an oxygen tent, a rubber mackintosh is placed over the mattress, the sides of the tent are tucked in securely under the mattress and a draw sheet is placed over the free front edge. In giving nursing care through the openings, the nurse should see to it that the tent is kept close round her arm. Morning care can be given with the tent in place.

To administer "100 per cent" concentration of oxygen or oxygen helium in the B-L-B apparatus, the holes should be closed and enough gas allowed to flow into the inhalation apparatus so that the reservoir rebreathing bag is almost, but not quite, emptied with each inspiration. Such administrations of high concentrations seldom are given longer than from 36 to 40 hours. For lower concentrations with this apparatus, two or three holes are opened, and the bag should collapse with each inhalation.

The accurate administration of oxygen is as important as the accurate measurement of any medication.

4. **Prevent Fire and Explosions.** This may be done by keeping all open flames and electric devices away from the apparatus. Before using an alcohol lamp, the tank should be closed and the room aired. Patients in oxygen tents should be given a hand bell and not the electric signaling cord. Avoid the use of oil on any oxygen regulator. Do not rub the patient's back with alcohol but bathe thoroughly and powder.

5. **Maintain the Relative Humidity at about 50 Per Cent.** When administering oxygen by nasal catheter, the gas should bubble through a jar of water. To supply adequate moisture the jar should be kept from one-half to two-thirds full. The ice compartment attached to the oxygen tent cools the air and condenses excess humidity. For adequate surface exposure of the ice the pieces should be about the size of a man's fist. The B-L-B apparatus retains sufficient moisture from the exhaled air in the rebreathing bag to humidify the air for inhalation. The metal nasal inhalator condenses moisture on its surfaces, and in this way sufficient humidity is supplied.

6. **Regulate the Temperature in the Oxygen Tent** to about 68° F. A shoulder blanket may be used to cover the shoulders, and the incoming air should be directed away from the patient.

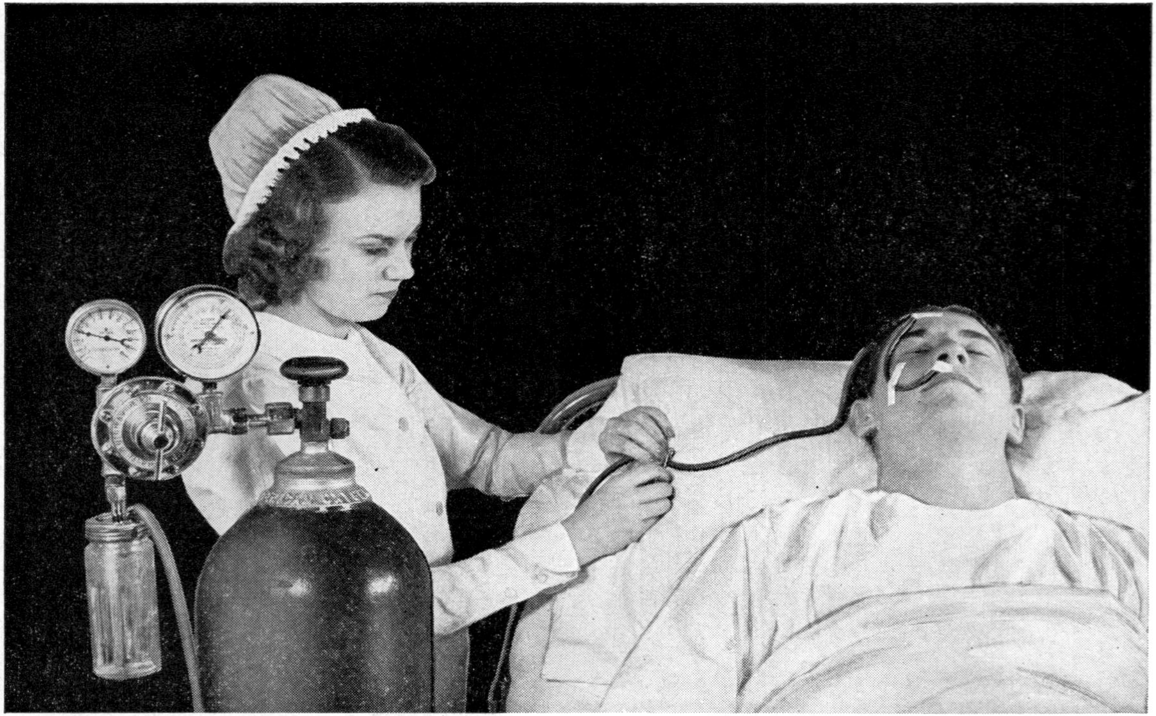

Fig. 77. Oxygen administration through a nasal catheter. Note that the line from the tank is through a pressure gauge, and that the gas passes through a water reservoir before entering the nose. Note also the method of attaching the catheter to the patient's face with adhesive.

7. **Prevent tanks from being upset** by placing them on special standards or by strapping them to the bed.

Nasal Oxygen

Oxygen by nasal catheter is one of the simplest and most convenient methods of administration. The chief disadvantage is that it may be irritating to mucous membrane. A No. 12 catheter with many pinhead holes for a distance of about 2 to 3 cm. from the tip is ideal. The distance a catheter is to be passed is determined by measuring the distance from the tip of the patient's nose to the tip of his ear. This length is marked on the catheter, a piece of adhesive tape being used for the purpose. Then, with the oxygen flowing through the catheter, moisten the catheter with water and pass it through the nostril up to the adhesive marking. Such a catheter should be removed by the nurse every 8 hours. A clean catheter should be available to reinsert immediately. Such technic will prevent undue crusting of secretions on the catheter and possible blocking of the oxygen outlet. Changing from one nostril to the other may be more comfortable for the patient. Catheters should not be forced into the nostril. Oxygen flow usually is ordered at from 6 to 8 liters per minute.

CHAPTER TEN

Nursing Care of the Geriatric Surgical Patient

The society which fosters research to save human life cannot escape responsibility for the life thus extended. It is for science not only to add years to life, but more important, to add life to the years.

(Piersol, G. M., and Bortz, E. L.: Ann. Int. Med. **12**:964, 1939)

Much attention is being focused on how to age gracefully and on how to be healthier, happier and more active in later years. The reason for increasing emphasis on this age group is that the number of persons 65 years old or more has almost quadrupled in the past half century. With the many advances in surgical technic and anesthesiology and the introduction of chemotherapy as well as the antibiotics, it is not surprising to note that many of our surgical patients are in this older age group. An attempt will be made in this chapter to emphasize the needs of the older patient who faces, experiences and recovers from surgery.

THE NURSE AND THE ELDERLY SURGICAL PATIENT

Is the nursing care which the older person should receive any different from that given to those of a younger age group? Essentially, it is not different but it has more depth; more is required of the surgical nurse.

The nurse who cares for the elderly must possess and display an emotional maturity. On greeting the newly admitted patient the nurse should make him feel welcome and at home. If his condition permits, he should be introduced to nearby patients. At this early meeting, the nurse can observe any incapacities such as difficulty in hearing, tremor of an extremity, a stiff joint and so forth. If he can be placed near another patient with whom he can talk it will help him to adjust to the hospital environment.

By listening to her patient, a nurse may not only enhance his self-esteem but also may gain an over-all

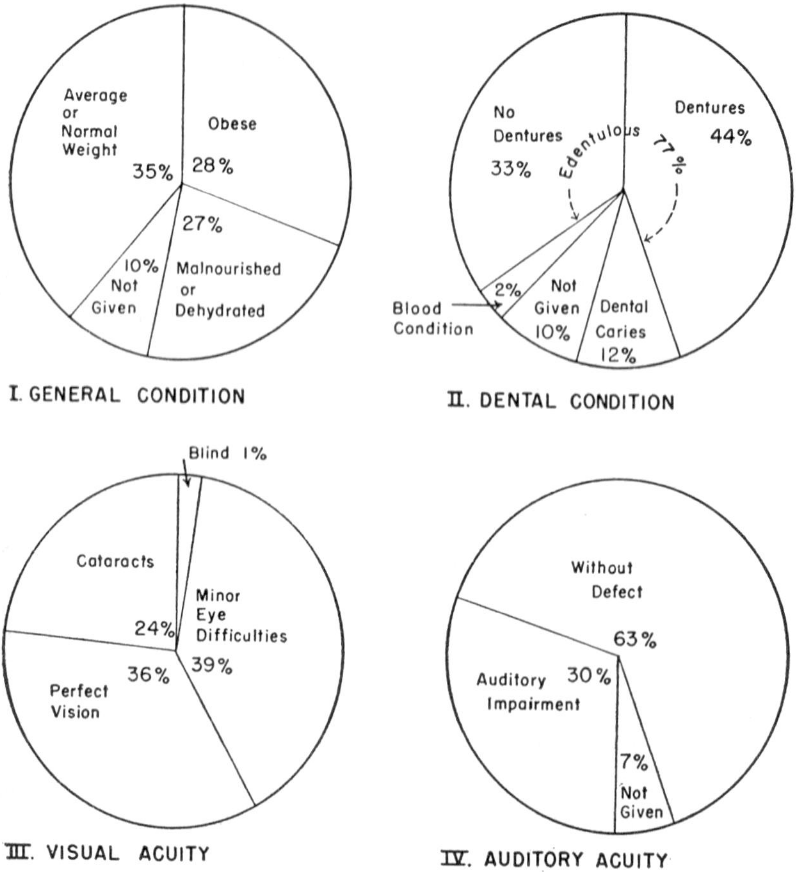

FIG. 78. This chart shows the general physical conditions of an unselected group of surgical geriatric patients. (Sholtis, L. A.: Nursing the elderly surgical patient, Am. J. Nursing **51**:727)

picture of his interests, beliefs and reactions. These can be helpful in diagnosis, prognosis and in planning for his total care. An illustration of this is a patient who harbored false concepts about medicine which were accepted as sound medical practice in his youth. Until these ideas were expressed and corrected, they served as a hurdle to effective therapy.

The successful nurse early recognizes differences in older people. Some may be old and decrepit physically but are alert mentally and fresh in spirit. Very readily one may detect an inherent sense of humor, a philosophical frame of mind or a thwarted and depressed personality. Often the patient's temperament will direct his course of progress. Keen observation of these manifestations will present a challenge to the nurse as she develops a plan of care for her geriatric patient.

A fixed routine may provide a sense of security for some elderly persons. To know that a certain activity will take place at a certain time provides a schedule which allows him to anticipate and to do a certain amount of his own planning. The nurse can strengthen his further belief that he matters when she remembers his desires and idiosyncrasies even when they seem trivial. Having very little ice in the water pitcher may account for an adequate or an inadequate intake of fluids. These little things are significant aspects of individualized patient care.

During the period of preoperative build-up, diversional aids such as visits, radio, television, newspapers, letters and gifts are significant. The older person has less tendency to live in the past if his present is filled with interesting activities.

Before procedures or examinations are done they should be described to the older patient in order to eliminate fears and tensions. Most of these individuals object to being hurried; therefore, sufficient time should be planned in preparation for a treatment. Every effort should be made to establish the confidence of the older patient in those individuals responsible for his care. If it is possible to learn of the socio-economic background of the patient, a more tolerant understanding of his present condition and problems will result.

SIGNIFICANT CHARACTERISTICS OF THE OLDER PATIENT

One of the most disturbing *environmental factors* to the geriatric person is noise. Therefore, every attempt should be made to control unpleasant sounds such as dropping metal objects on a hard floor, handling dishes carelessly in the kitchen, banging elevator doors and so forth.

In general, the older patient does not like very much fresh air; therefore, indirect means of ventilation must be utilized. It is difficult to alter the sleeping habits of an individual; hence, any adjustments which can be made in the patient's behalf is desirable. Frequently, one has a patient who takes naps during the day and then complains of inability to sleep at night. In most instances, day napping should be discouraged in favor of a good night's sleep.

The aging process and the inelasticity of the *skin* predispose to decubiti. The older patient is often content to lie in bed without moving. He must be encouraged to move and get out of bed as frequently as is permissible. Mineral oil, lanolin creams or baby oil can be used on dry skin; alcohol should not be used, since it causes drying of the cutaneous tissues. Some authorities say that bathing once or twice a week is sufficient, since frequent bathing removes the natural oil from the skin. The feet especially become dry. It is well to remember that before cutting nails, the feet should be soaked in warm water. Shower or bathtub bathing using water of moderate temperature is preferred to the bed bath. The nurse should anticipate that the geriatric patient needs help to prevent accidents. Safety measures should be utilized. The patient often experiences stiffness and pain when he begins to move or change his position. Because neuromuscular control as well as sensory function may be impaired, the aged bone structures are injured easily.

Further, *visual impairment* may predispose the patient to accidents (Fig. 78). Side rails in the bathroom should be available, and all rooms should be well lighted. At the bedside there should be a footstool with a broad base and nonskid tips. The older patient's bed is equipped with side rails to remind him to remain in bed at night. They are useful to hold onto when raising oneself to the sitting position and when turning over in bed.

The nurse who takes care of the older patient should know of any *hearing impairment.* Perhaps only one ear is involved, or he may not hear certain ranges of sound; whatever the difficulty, often by the nurse's practicing a simple procedure the patient may understand clearly. Most patients who have diminished hearing are reluctant to call attention to it; therefore, it is up to the nurse to take the initiative in discovering this or any other handicap.

Many of our older patients have lost a number of their own *teeth* or possess remnants of them. Those who have dentures occasionally present difficulties with poorly fitting sets. This can be serious, inasmuch as constant irritation from a jagged tooth or an ill-fitting denture can lead to cancer of the mouth. Dentures should be cleaned at least twice daily; when they are not being worn a receptacle should be available for them. Frequently, the mouth is the most neglected part of the body. The nurse should encourage and help the patient in carrying out good mouth hygiene. By a careful evaluation of the condition of the mouth, the nurse is able to meet the patient's nutritional needs better, to request dental attention if necessary and to prevent postoperative pulmonary and systemic infections.

Nutritional Needs. A diet that is well planned and served attractively is of no consequence if the elderly individual is unable to eat it because of poor or absent teeth. If this is not the reason, the nurse should investigate further. Poor eating practices often are caused by habit, isolation, prejudice, lack of money, improperly fitting dentures, a reduced amount of salivary and gastric secretion or an impression that food is unimportant.

With a decrease in physical activity, fewer calories and less carbohydrate and fat are necessary. Protein and mineral requirements remain the same. Because of the decrease in absorption of calcium, more is needed in the diet. It is well to remember that a diet low in protein contributes to poor wound healing.

Food tastes vary in individuals. For one whose sense of taste is keen, it may be extremely difficult to make a radical change in his food habits when his physical condition requires it. The nurse must be aware of the emotional and the social values of food, particularly in the obese. One usually eats to obtain fuel for energy, for building and repairing tissues; however, one may eat for pleasure as well as for comfort when sad and lonely.

Often a patient's progress will depend upon whether he has had too little fluid with resultant dehydration or too much fluid which may result in cardiac failure and edema. Some patients are reluctant to take fluids when urinary difficulties are present such as frequent voiding, pain on urination or the inconvenience of using the bedpan. These conditions should be reported or corrected as the case may be. Fluids given intravenously must be given very slowly to avoid circulatory overloading. Hyaluronidase often is added to subcutaneous fluids to hasten their absorption.

PREOPERATIVE CARE

Preparation for surgery demands a careful evaluation of the cardiovascular and the urinary systems as well as the nutritional status in the older patient. Although he may be admitted for a specific problem, it is usual for him to have several other difficulties. Ideally, all deficiencies should be eliminated before he goes to the operating room; practically, some compromises are necessary.

Psychological Aspects. Confidence will be strengthened if the geriatric patient fully realizes that the contemplated operation is less hazardous than the disease it is expected to remedy. Years of living have a tendency to broaden his ability to adjust to crises. He accepts adjustments more easily; this is particularly advantageous when he is given an anesthetic, for usually he has a smooth induction, maintenance and recovery. On the other hand, one must not assume that he is unconcerned. His attachment to life may be as real as the younger individual's, because in old age one is more conscious of the shortness of the remaining years.

Preoperative Medication. Drug sensitivity usually is increased in elderly individuals, so that dosages are generally smaller. Preoperative medication is given earlier in the aged because of delayed absorption. In those individuals who have cerebral arteriosclerosis, barbiturates and scopolamine may cause excitement; therefore, paraldehyde, chloral hydrate or tincture of opium may be preferable. Some physicians do not prescribe morphine for the older person. When it is given, the respiratory rate must be observed carefully. If sedatives are given, often one third to one half the usual adult amount is prescribed.

Enemas may be ordered the evening before rather than the morning of surgery because of the inclination of the rectum to retain fluid for several hours.

Position on Operating Table. In the operating room the older patient should be handled thoughtfully with no unnecessary exposure. One must have utmost patience in positioning him, since he cannot relax and allow others to move him as desired. Often his joints and muscles are painful when moved. His final position should be relaxed and as comfortable as possible. Extremes in positioning are to be avoided since they hinder circulation.

Anesthesia. Practically all the anesthetic agents used in the younger patient can be used in those past 65. Intravenous Pentothal Sodium has been used as a very satisfactory induction anesthetic. Complicated gas machines may be frightening; consequently, the prick of a needle may be more tolerable than a rubber face mask. Frequently it is used preliminary to a general inhalation anesthetic. Most experienced anesthesiologists prefer to give a mixture of cyclopropane and oxygen by the intratracheal method. This, combined with the curare drugs as needed for relaxation, has the advantage that there is complete control of the anesthesia at all times. The gas concentration can be varied as needed, and adequate oxygenation can be maintained at all times.

Spinal anesthesia also may be used for geriatric patients. It must be remembered that even though their blood vessels may be quite inelastic, they may have a profound drop in pressure. If the blood pressure drop is sudden and prolonged it may lead to circulatory insufficiency. This in turn may cause thrombosis, followed by embolism, infarction and anoxemia. To maintain blood pressure at a normal level is of utmost importance in these individuals.

Going to the other extreme, it is well to remember that sudden increases in blood pressure from excessive or over-rapid infusions may cause pulmonary edema.

POSTOPERATIVE CARE

The immediate postoperative care is the same as that for any patient. However, the older person can chill more easily, and the possibility of shock is greater. Keeping him warm and turning him from side to side after he regains consciousness are essential. His position should be changed frequently not only for his comfort, since he often complains of aches when lying in one position, but also to avoid pulmonary and circulatory complications.

Since lung expansion is decreased, the geriatric patient is more prone to develop pneumonia. Secretions in the upper respiratory tract usually are removed by the anesthetist with an endotracheal aspiration tube. Thereafter, in the recovery room the nurse should encourage the patient to cough and take deep breaths. If secretions continue to accumulate, it may be necessary to do a temporary tracheotomy to facilitate breathing.

Fluids should be encouraged for many known reasons. Occasionally, the older patient will not take liquids because the nurse has used too much ice, and he may not be used to that. One older man did not drink fluids because the nurse always filled his glass full; the prospect of drinking a glass full of water overwhelmed him. When another nurse poured a quarter of a glassful at a time, he drank it willingly.

The above incident illustrates the fact that each individual is a person in his own right. Many of the older folks have set ways which may seem unusual to the nurse, but the sooner such a quirk is recognized, the more successful will the nurse be in her total care of that patient.

Usually the oldster needs to be coaxed to drink enough fluids. An output of one liter or more indicates that his intake is sufficient for his needs. The recording of intake and output is important, obviously.

In giving postoperative intravenous fluids, some surgeons prefer to give them slowly over a 24-hour period rather than more rapidly at 2 or 3 separate times. If this regimen is followed, it is wise to splint the patient's arm (unless a plastic cannula is used). The nurse should be on the watch for any swelling or discomfort at the intravenous site. When fluids are given by hypodermoclysis, hyaluronidase usually is given to facilitate absorption.

Disorientation and Confusion. The older patient even in normal life may show evidences of disorientation and confusion as to time and space. Operation or injury may precipitate such a state in patients who heretofore have been mentally clear. The nurse must recognize the dangers of these mental changes and guard against injury or accident by the use of side rails and by careful observation. In particular, these patients must be watched to see that they do not remove dressings, infusion needles, suction tubes and catheters.

Postoperative Distention. Most often this is due to retention of swallowed air in the intestinal tract. This can be avoided by aspiration of the air from the stomach through a suction tube introduced through the nose and the esophagus into the gastric lumen. Suction may be provided in many ways, Wangensteen, Steadman pump and so forth, and in many cases is maintained until peristalsis is recovered, usually on the second or third day.

In older people, the sluggish peristalsis in the colon frequently results in incomplete evacuation and therefore retention of fecal material in the sigmoid colon and the rectum. The absorption of fluid produces a hard fecal mass which is irritating to the gut and often produces frequent small stools, a sort of pseudodiarrhea. Digital examination reveals a hard mass of fecal material in the rectum. When this mass is broken up by the finger and by enemas, the symptoms are relieved.

Incontinence. In the older person, there is a loss, temporary or even permanent, of control over the bladder and the bowel, resulting in incontinence. Often these symptoms are most apparent when the patient is below par, either following operation or after a debilitating illness or trauma. They often disappear as the patient recovers and returns toward his normal strength and vigor. Then the problem is one of keeping the patient clean and avoiding complications which arise secondary to the moisture and the uncleanliness. Thorough washing with soap and water followed by drying and a change of bed linen will go a long way toward the prevention of decubiti.

Pain. Enough drug to relieve pain but not enough to make it difficult for the patient to perform his exercises may be given. Gone are the days when oversedation was the rule because it was thought that the repair process could continue only when the body and the mind were completely at rest.

Exercise. Activity in bed as well as out of bed is essential to recovery. Bed exercises include turning from side to side, flexing and extending the legs and the arms, deep breathing and deliberate coughing. In getting out of bed, the patient should turn to his operated side and bend his knees up. As he swings his feet over the side of the bed, the nurse can assist him to a sitting position. A stool should be available for him to stand on for a few moments before he steps down. Ambulation means that he walks, not sits in a chair.

CONVALESCENCE

Appearance. A great morale booster is to look well; to look well implies that one feels well (Fig. 79). The older person may be neglectful of his appearance; hence, a bit of encouragement by the nurse may direct his attention to "how he looks" rather than "how he feels." An attractive hair-do brightens a woman's spirits; this may be done by simple brushing and combing, setting a wave or braiding long hair. A cleverly placed hair ribbon, flower or small ornament in the hair may bring compliments from those who come in contact with the elderly woman. Both men and women enjoy a new garment or a bit of color on their person. Even conservative men seem to like bright-colored pajamas. A small flower on the lapel of his kimono will brighten his spirits. A shave and a haircut do for a man what lipstick does for most women. Almost everyone finds the fragrance of certain dusting powders and cognes refreshing. This has special appeal if it is a scent that is in keeping with the individual's personality. Surely the nurse will be able to find some one thing that will help immeasurably to cheer her older patient.

Rehabilitation. Following surgery it is imperative to encourage in the older individual the desire to live

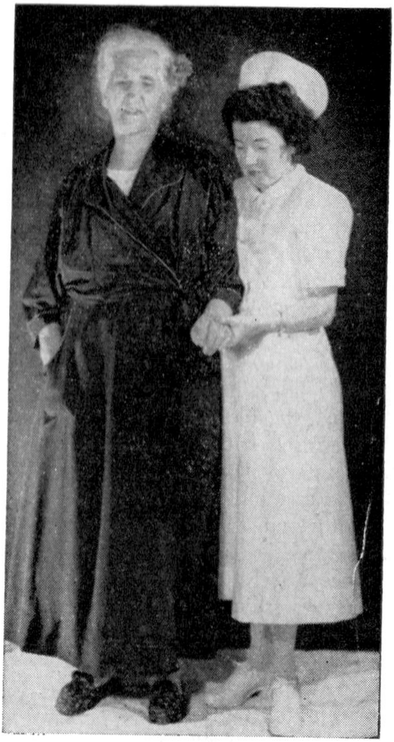

Fig. 79. A 70-year-old patient 5 days after a right colectomy for carcinoma, illustrating early ambulation and encouragement from the attending nurse.

and to regain activity. Convalescence may be difficult because strength is regained slowly. Above all, the elder one needs a great deal of patience. He has a tendency to fret about his limitations. Some authorities advocate that one day be allowed for each decade of one's age for convalescence from acute illness. Patients often find this difficult to accept.

Every attempt should be made to

maintain an interest in people or things. Diversional and recreational therapies are of invaluable help for the aged and deserve a generous part of the patient's time. All phases of the rehabilitative program must be within the realm of possibility. The older person must be encouraged to do things for himself in order to become self-sufficient. The nurse must refrain from becoming overly motherly in this respect.

It must be emphasized that old people can learn; the learning process is not limited to the young. Hence, the oldster can learn to care for himself and can learn absorbing and interesting hobbies. It is for the nurse and all other members of the health team to teach and direct this potential learner. Instructions must be clear and complete. They must be repeated frequently enough to allow the patient to grasp them. He should be aware of the reasons for doing prescribed activities; many times the patient misinterprets such activities as measures to release the nurse from her many duties rather than accepting them as a means essential for his recovery.

Throughout the entire convalescence complications may occur. The nurse needs to remember that symptoms may be insidious and overlooked easily. She should be suspicious of the slightest complaint. When complications do occur, they must be combated vigorously and rapidly, since delay may result in difficulties which never may be corrected.

No plan for rehabilitation will be successful unless it is continued beyond the walls of the hospital. Continuity of care can be planned with the visiting nurse programs and other community agencies as well as the patient's own family. In many instances, the geriatric patient does not have a family to whom he can return. Real adjustments may have to be made. The smoother the transfer, the more graceful will be the resumption of normal living for the elderly woman or man.

CHAPTER ELEVEN

Tumors and Cancer Nursing

The nurse is a very important member of any team fighting cancer. In the hospital her skill is a necessary adjunct to that of the surgeon, the radiologist and the internist. Within the community as a public health nurse, she regularly calls on the patient with cancer who is being treated at home. In industry, she not only must contend with illness of employees themselves but often worries about the health of their families as well. Directly or indirectly, her knowledge and influence supplement the doctor's plan of action for the diagnosis, the treatment, the rehabilitation or the terminal care of those who are cancer victims. (American Cancer Society, Inc.)

INTRODUCTION

Each cell in the human body is thought to have a definite function that it performs in conjunction with the other cells to form a useful machine. Thus, the skin cells protect the body surface; the cells of the breast secrete milk; the muscle cells contract, giving us movements. All these various groups of cells are held together by connective tissue. However, at times certain cells take on a new form of growth that is not useful. They cease to co-operate with their fellows of like nature to form a useful machine. They grow independently, often rapidly, taking nourishment from the body and giving nothing in return. Such a group of cells, similar in form to the normal cells but serving no useful purpose, is called a *neoplasm* or *tumor*.

The question, "What makes apparently normal cells adopt these strange forms of growth?" long has been asked, but a satisfactory answer has not been found as yet. Extensive studies seem to show that there may be certain hereditary tendencies toward tumor formation, and that irritation of long standing from any cause may excite cells to this abnormal development. The role of viruses, parasites and chemicals as potential causative agents also has been studied. These factors may play a part, but the real exciting cause has not been discovered as yet. Infection, as we generally speak of it, does not seem to play a role in tumor causation.

CLASSIFICATION OF TUMORS

Benign or Nonmalignant. Some tumors are surrounded by a definite capsule, remain localized in the tissue from which they spring, and disturb their host only by pressure on the surrounding structures and by robbing the normal tissues of their blood supply. These tumors usually grow rather slowly, and once removed they do not tend to recur. Such tumors are spoken of as *benign* or *nonmalignant.*

Malignant. Other neoplasms are not surrounded by a capsule, but grow by invasion into the tissues surrounding them. They invade the blood vessels or lymphatics and extend rapidly along these open channels. Often the tumor cells are broken off and carried bv the blood and the lymph to other parts of the body, where they set up a secondary growth. This property of these tumors is called *metastasis,* and the new or secondary growth is called a *metastatic growth.* The cells of these tumors grow rapidly and under the microscope resemble the rapidly growing cells found in the embryo. They invade the surrounding tissues in such a manner (they are crablike) that it is nearly impossible to remove all the tumor cells and, therefore, they tend to recur after the main body of the tumor has been removed.

The rapid growth of the tumor and its secondary growths sap the vitality of its host, with the result that there is a rapid loss of weight and strength. They bleed easily, producing a loss of the red cells in the blood—an anemia. The patient finally becomes thin, pale and weak, a shadow of his former self. This con-dition is spoken of as *cachexia.* Th course of the disease ends in deat These tumors are called *malignan*

We may summarize the character-istics of these two classes of tumo as follows:

Benign

Adult type of cell

Slow growth

Often incapsulated

Never grow into surrounding ti-sues

Always remain localized at orig-nal site

Do not tend to recur when re-moved

Harm the host only by pressure growth on surrounding structures

Malignant

Young type of cell

Rapid growth

Never incapsulated

Invade surrounding tissues wide

Form secondary growths by me-tastasis through lymph and bloc stream

Tend to recur when removed

Cause loss of weight and strengt anemia, cachexia and, eventuall death

At times a tumor that was at fi benign may take on malignant cha acteristics. For this reason it is we to remove all tumors as soon as th are discovered.

Subdivisions on Basis of Tissu

Neoplasms are subdivided furth according to the kind of tissue which they are formed. In embr onic life there are three divisions tissue from which all others a formed. These tissues are called (

endoderm, (2) mesoderm and (3) ectoderm.

Endoderm is the tissue from which the lining membranes (mucosa) of the respiratory tract, the gastro-intestinal tract and the genito-urinary tract are formed.

Mesoderm is the tissue from which muscles, bones, fascia and connective tissue are formed.

Ectoderm is the tissue from which come the skin cells and the cells composing its hair follicles, sweat glands and the entire nervous system.

The cells formed by the endoderm and the ectoderm are epithelial in type. Tumors arising from this tissue are composed of epithelial cells. They may be either benign or malignant.

A *benign epithelial tumor* is called a *papilloma* when it is a cauliflower-like growth springing from an epithelial surface. When the cells of the tumor come from the epithelium lining a gland, the tumor is called an *adenoma.*

A *malignant growth composed of epithelial cells* is called a *cancer* or a *carcinoma.* When it arises from skin cells, it is often spoken of as an *epithelioma. Melanoma,* a pigmented growth in the skin and in the eye, is extremely malignant. Myeloma and some forms of endothelioma also are in this group. When it springs from the glandular type cells, as of the mucosa of the gastro-intestinal tract, it is frequently called an *adenocarcinoma.*

Cancers tend to metastasize along the lymphatics; therefore, the secondary growths are looked for at the nearest lymph filter, the lymph nodes. Here cells are caught and begin to form an independent tumor like the parent or primary growth. Thus, in every case of cancer of the breast, the axilla is examined carefully for enlarged lymph nodes, because it is known that the lymph flow from the breast is through the axillary lymph nodes. Cancer usually occurs in patients past middle age.

Tumors arising from the mesoderm are called *connective-tissue tumors.* They also may be benign or malignant.

The benign connective-tissue tumors are composed of tissue much like that from which they arise, and they are named accordingly. Thus we speak of: *fibroma*—from fibrous tissue; *osteoma*—from bony tissue; *lipoma*—from fatty tissue; *enchondroma*—from cartilage; *rhabdomyoma*—from skeletal muscle; *myoma*—from uterine muscle; *endothelioma*—from the endothelium of the coverings of the brain; and *neuroma*—from nerve tissue. A *keloid* is a tumorlike overgrowth of fibrous tissue appearing in scars. (See pp. 409-410.)

Some of these types may become malignant.

A *malignant connective-tissue tumor* is called a *sarcoma.* It tends to metastasize via the blood stream and the tumor cells, being caught in the first blood filter, usually the lungs, set up metastatic growths there. These tumors are found most frequently in children and in young adults.

Some tumors, thought to arise from embryologic maldevelopment, contain more than one of the embryonal tissues. Those which contain two of the tissues, called *dermoids,* are not infrequently seen in opera-

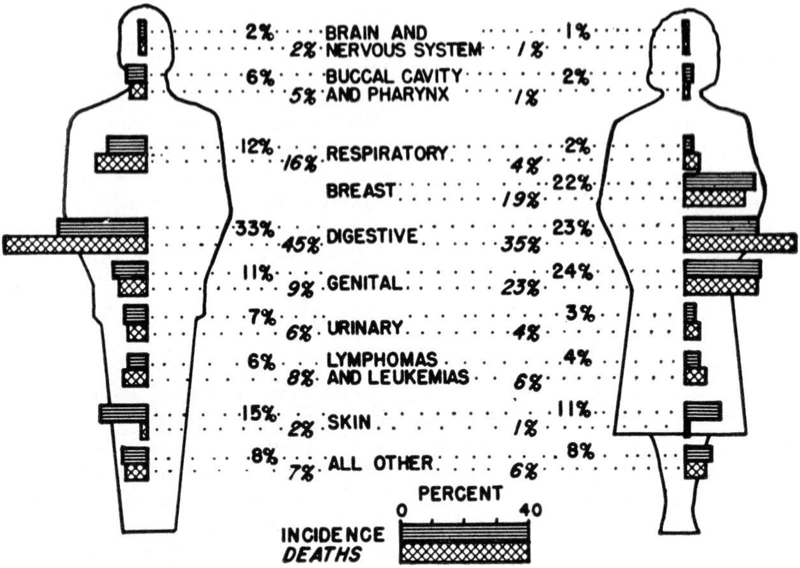

FIG. 80. Cancer incidence by sex and site, based on statistics from 10 major cities in the United States. (American Cancer Society)

tions on the ovary and the testicle. They may contain bone, teeth, muscle—all of which arise from the mesoderm and hair, skin and sebaceous glands—which develop from the ectoderm. When the tumor contains derivatives of all three embryonal tissues, it is called a *teratoma*.

New growths often are composed of more than one tissue and are named accordingly—fibro-adenoma, fibrolipoma, osteosarcoma and so forth.

INCIDENCE OF MALIGNANCY

The importance of malignant growth to the nursing and the medical professions can be understood if some of the facts concerning its incidence are reviewed. It is estimated that in the United States malignancy annually exacts a toll of at least 220,000 lives, ranking second as the principal cause of death, being exceeded only by heart disease. More than 1 out of 7 deaths that occur in adults is caused by malignancy. It is estimated that more than 70,000 cancer patients might have been saved last year had they recognized early symptoms and sought prompt treatment.

The most common malignancy of adult life is cancer. This dread disease affects men and women of all ages and of all races. No organ of the body is exempt.

TREATMENT OF NEOPLASMS

It has been learned that malignant neoplasms usually lead to certain death if untreated, and that benign tumors frequently become malignant without warning. Therefore, it must be realized that the patient who is the host to a tumor of any kind is the potential victim of a fatal disease. The only certain hope of cure lies in the possibility of surgical removal of the entire growth. In malignant tumors such treatment can be attempted only in the early stages, when the process is a local one.

When the growth has progressed to invade the surrounding tissues and distant metastases occur, any attempt to remove the tumor is without hope of success and the patient is doomed to slow, and often painful, death.

Treatment by radium and roentgen therapy has aided greatly in the cure of patients with malignant disease. This method is of special value in the treatment of external cancers, such as those of the skin, the lip, the mouth and the cervix of the uterus. Radiation also has proved to be of distinct value in the treatment of inoperable cases of malignant disease. As more experience with this form of treatment is obtained, the results improve constantly. However, surgical removal is the method of choice when there is any possibility that the entire growth can be removed.

In operating in malignant disease the surgeon removes the tissues for some distance about the original growth, and in the case of cancer he also removes the lymphatics that drain the area in which the growth is situated. Thus he attempts to remove the whole tumor with any small metastatic growths that have formed. Therefore, in operations for carcinoma of the breast, the overlying skin and the underlying muscles are removed with the breast, and the lymphatic channels of the axilla are dissected out carefully, along with any metastatic nodes that can be discovered.

THE NURSE AND THE CANCER PATIENT

In caring for patients with a malignant tumor, the nurse finds that the team of which she is a member never is limited to the surgeon, the patient and the nurse, but includes often the physician, the medical social worker, the nutritionist, the occupational and physical therapists, the psychiatrist and the clergyman. Over and above this, one cannot overlook the fact that the patient's family plays a significant role.

Early Detection. The hope of cure in malignant disease depends on the early recognition and treatment of the condition. Rapid progress is being made in the education of the public as to the dangerous consequences of untreated tumors. The intelligent nurse is one of the most effective agents in the dissemination of such information. Not infrequently her patients or their friends will question her concerning "a lump that has formed" or a rapid loss of weight with increasing "indigestion."

In order to answer such questions she should remember that these symptoms and signs suggest malignant disease: a swelling, usually painless, growing progressively larger; the abnormal appearance of blood from the stomach, the bowel or the pelvic organs; loss of weight; slowly increasing "indigestion"; or an ulcer that refuses to heal. If these symptoms occur in a person past middle age, they are especially suggestive, because cancer occurs most frequently at that time of life.

Knowing that only early treatment can cure, the nurse should urge an immediate examination by a good physician. The diagnosis is confirmed by the use of biopsy, cytologic test, endoscopy, roentgenogram, or blood tests.

Objectives of Nursing Care

The objectives are (1) to meet the fluid and the nutritional needs of the patient, (2) to assist in carrying out treatments of the malignancy itself, (3) to recognize the psychological and spiritual needs of the patient, (4) to assist in the rehabilitation and the convalescence of the patient and (5) to assist in planning for the care of individuals whose disease has not been terminated.

Fluid and Nutritional Needs. In the administration of fluids it may be necessary to administer fluids intravenously or subcutaneously in large amounts to overcome the existing dehydration. Blood transfusions often are necessary in the preoperative and the postoperative care of the patient. The nurse should not depend upon parenteral fluids when it is possible to give them by mouth. The diet for such patients should be especially selected to supply not only sufficient calories but also salts and hemoglobin-building materials. Although a high vitamin diet is not always recommended in malignancy, some attention should be given to this essential element in the diet. In some cases, as in malignancy of the mouth and the upper gastro-intestinal tract, solid food cannot be given easily, and it may be necessary to supply frequent small liquid feedings to maintain a sufficient caloric intake. So far as possible, the likes and the dislikes of the patient should be considered in arranging the diet.

Radiation Therapy. Frequently, inoperable lesions are treated by irradiation. This may have a marked systemic effect upon the patient and lead to nausea, vomiting, fever and a feeling of extreme malaise. Although this postirradiation upset may be only temporary, lasting from a few days to a week or more, it is during this period that good nursing care is most essential. The giving of sedatives, the careful selection of fluids and foods that will not induce or aggravate nausea and the constant reassuring attitude of the nurse are extremely helpful. Liver extract and vitamin B_1 are given hypodermically in many cases, and the administration of intravenous glucose is helpful. Pyridoxine given orally is helpful in minimizing nausea and vomiting. In skin reactions, the area usually is kept dry and free from irritation such as that produced by friction from clothing or adjacent structures. As a rule, the irradiation therapy is discontinued until the patient's reaction has subsided.

Radiation is obtained from the element itself (radium) and from radium emanation (radon), the gas resulting from the gradual disintegration of the element. Radium is applied commonly in needles or capsules of platinum. Radon is applied usually in the form of small gold tubes or "seeds" placed within the tissue.

The methods of applying radium or radon are as follows:

1. Contact Application. Tubes of radium or radon are placed in direct contact with the tumor.

2. Distance Application. A bomb of radium, heavily encased in lead, is applied at a distance from the skin for irradiation of internal lesions.

3. Interstitial Application. Needles containing radium, radon or radon "seeds" are implanted directly into tissues. Needles are removed after a definite time has elapsed.

A radon "seed" is placed in a special implanting needle. This resembles an ordinary hollow needle with a stylet and is about 8 inches long. To facilitate placing a "seed" in the hollow part of the needle, it is lubricated with petrolatum. This is done under aseptic conditions. When the needle is inserted at the site of tumor, the stylet forces the "seed" gently into the tissues and the "seed" remains there permanently.

4. Radioactive Salts. These have been used in the treatment of some malignancies, especially leukemias and malignancies of the thyroid. Radioactive iodine is used most frequently. It is given by mouth. When absorbed, it exerts its effect on the thyroid because iodine is absorbed by this gland.

Caution. In giving a patient radium treatment there are several precautions that the nurse should take for her own protection.

1. She always should use long forceps when she handles the element—distance is the best protection.

2. She should use a lead screen to protect her body.

3. She should work rapidly.

4. She should have a monthly blood count as a check against any onset of lymphopenia or anemia.

The nurse should know the exact time of removal of radium so that she may remind the physician when the time draws near. A sign or a tag on the bed indicating that the patient has radium will serve as a reminder that dressings and bedding must be inspected carefully before being discarded. When radium is removed, it is checked by the physician and the nurse to make sure that the total amount has been removed. No nurse should take the responsibility of removing radium or of changing or discarding any radium dressing: this is a physician's duty. Radium and its container should be washed in soapy water (never in a sink for fear of loss into the sewer), using long forceps, and returned to the radium department. Losses should be reported and attempts made to recover the missing pieces with a radium detector.

Psychological Aspects of Nursing the Cancer Patient. In modern cancer therapy it may happen frequently that extensive surgery and irradiation therapy may produce changes which are disfiguring or mutilating and not easily borne by the patient. The problems which are thus created may be almost overwhelming. These problems begin before operation, when the question is raised as to how much the patient should be told about the details of his disease and his operation; it must be handled differently in each patient. It is probably best that the nurse should not be called upon to divulge the details of diagnosis and treatment.

The adaption which has to be made to the therapeutic measures for the malignancy must begin in the preoperative period. The patients are particularly in need of support and reassurance in order to establish confidence in the skill of the surgeon and the hospital environment. When the patient approaches surgery with a sense of hopefulness and expectation, excellent results can be anticipated from a psychological point of view. If, however, he approaches surgery with the conviction that the operation is going to be painful, disfiguring and mutilating, it is almost to be expected that he should show depression and a marked sense of weakness postoperatively. Postoperative symptoms of depression may be sleep disturbance, loss of appetite and other manifestations, which may persist for an indefinite period. In their depression, patients may think there is hostility on the part of nurses, doctors and attendants.

Even when the physician is not blamed directly, often he is looked upon unconsciously as the injuring party; hence, resentment may appear particularly toward nurses in the immediate environment, social workers, and even members of the family. The symptoms often take more of a demanding attitude with complaints. The nurse must recognize this attitude as a part of the normal process of repair and should work through the anger and the resentment to win the patient over to a more normal attitude.

In other instances, patients may assume feelings of dejection accompanied by a sense of helplessness. Such anxiety often makes the patient turn to other people for help, advice, consolation and reassurance. This state is often only temporary, and the nurse, who is closest to him, can be of invaluable aid during this period of rehabilitation. Kindness and warmth give the patient the security he needs.

The nurse, of all medical personnel, has the most sustained and intimate contact with the patient during his hospitalization. Therefore, she is the person to whom the patient will turn most often for kindness and support during the early postoperative period. If the nurse is able to meet these needs, not only will the pressure and the anxiety be alleviated, but also the patient's perception of his hospital experience will be modified.

In summary, the psychology of cancer patients is the psychology of a person who is facing a fundamental struggle with security and his self-value. Such problems can be met best by professional persons. The nurse is in a very advantageous position to aid the patient in his efforts to overcome depression and anxiety and to resume normal function after surgery.

Terminal Nursing Care. Some authorities claim that the most important aspect in the care of the terminal patient is good nursing. Frequent changes of bed linen, cleanliness and keeping the patient warm are all comfort measures which can relieve a great deal of pain. During this care probably the most common emergency which the nurse should anticipate is hemorrhage. In some instances, the nurse can control bleeding by digital pressure. She should have on hand the necessary equipment for the physician.

Ambulation. The patient should be kept ambulatory as long as possible; however, the nurse must recognize when it is undesirable for him to get out of bed.

Nutrition and Hydration. The main limiting factor in attaining and maintaining a good nutritional level is anorexia. Specific food needs vary depending upon the location of the tumor. For instance, the needs of a patient with cancer of the stomach may be quite different from that of a patient with cancer of the liver or the lungs. Small, frequent feedings are more likely to be accepted, together with protein supplementation and parenteral vitamin administration. Dehydration and electrolyte imbalance have to be prevented by correcting inadequate fluid intake and output.

Skin Care. Good skin care is imperative. Tissues do not repair so easily as in the normal individual; therefore, preventive measures may eliminate much discomfort. Back and body massages are helpful; in addition, they are conducive to relaxation and help to relieve pain.

Pain. The nurse must be able to judge whether her patient needs a soothing treatment, a sedative or a hypnotic. Usually, drugs can be given sparingly at first and then gradually increased in kind and amount. One must be cognizant of the effects of drugs on the debilitated and the older patient. These individuals have increased sensitivity and may have a chain-type reaction to narcotics. First, they are drowsy, take less food, become dehydrated, retain urine, and have gastro-intestinal irritation, nausea and vomiting and ultimately develop a disturbed electrolyte and fluid balance. Of course, the treatment for such a condition would be to discontinue these medications or decrease their dosage.

Esthetic Factors. Facial tumors are often unsightly; the patient usually is very sensitive about his appearance. Such lesions should be covered if possible. Other features of the patient should be accented to detract attention from the tumor site. This can be done by careful grooming, attractive garments, etc. Bright lights in a room should be replaced by softer lights, inasmuch as shades of light and dark can tone down undesirable areas. The nurse should use her ingenuity in helping this individual to bear his burden more easily.

One of the most unpleasant features of cancer in exposed areas on the body is the foul odor that appears sooner or later. This is due to the sloughing of tissues. Every effort should be made to keep the patient and his room clean. Dressings should be changed frequently, removed quickly from the patient's room and deposited in a metal-covered container until they are sent to the incinerator. Bedclothes and the patient's clothing ought to be changed when soiled. The use of absorbent or oakum pads may help when drainage is present. The room should be ventilated properly. Deodorants may be necessary. Several of the essential oils, such as oil of geranium, oil of eucalyptus or oil of orange, will meet the situation. Neutroleum alpha is lasting and not unpleasant when one or two drops are applied to the dressing or to the bedclothing. Powdered charcoal in the dressing or potassium permanganate solution 1:2,000 as an irrigation often helps. Activated zinc peroxide is also effective in cleansing and deodorizing these wounds. Commercially prepared products are now available and can be disseminated from a bottle with a wick or by means of an electric deodorizer to absorb odors. These are quite successful.

The nurse should have a rational psychological approach toward death. She is often the person to whom the patient turns when he wants to talk about himself, his fears, his hopes, etc. To be able to listen and to offer encouragement are extremely important assets. Many times a patient demonstrates hostility and rebellion. In spite of this, the nurse must remain tolerant and show her patient that she stands by him in spite of his unpleasant actions. In this manner, eventually she will be able to discover the reason for his outbursts and then help him to resolve them. (See "Psychological Aspects of Cancer Patient Care," p. 201.)

Occupational and Recreational Therapy. Statistics reveal that the home is best suited for the care of this patient for several reasons. He is in a familiar environment and can see his friends and family. Many times, he can perform some household duties and thereby feel that he is helping. The financial burden on the family is reduced. The family knows what is happening to him, which often is not the case when he is in an institution. The home is more conducive for him to pursue his hobbies, such as caring for tropical fish, developing a miniature garden, etc. Much of the responsibility for his care rests with the family. The nurse and the physician can help them greatly in making the adjustment an easier one. For patients who do not have a home, the next best available environment should be sought. The nurse with sympathetic understanding can help her patient in making contact with the proper agencies for the adjustment of his social and economic problems.

CYSTS

A *cyst* is an abnormal collection of fluid within a definite sac or wall. Cysts may form in several different ways. When the outlet to a gland becomes blocked and the gland continues to secrete, a *retention cyst* is formed. The common sebaceous cyst or wen is an example. Remnants of fetal organs may secrete a fluid often forming a cyst of considerable size especially when springing from the pelvic organs of the female. After a time an extravasation of blood in the tissues may become surrounded by a definite wall and form an *exudation cyst.*

Cysts may be formed by parasites, especially the *Taenia echinococcus (Echinococcus granulosus)* or dog tapeworm. These cysts, spoken of as *hydatid cysts,* often are of considerable size and usually are found in the liver.

Treatment. Cysts should be removed when possible because occasionally they change into malignant growths. They often may become infected when incision and drainage are necessary.

UNIT I

BIBLIOGRAPHY

General

Cardew, E. C.: Study Guide for Clinical Nursing, Philadelphia, Lippincott, 1953.

Christopher, Frederick: Textbook of Surgery, ed. 5, Philadelphia, Saunders, 1949.

Cole, W. H., and Elman, Robert: Textbook of General Surgery, ed. 6, New York, Appleton, 1952.

Ferguson, L. K.: Surgery of the Ambulatory Patient, ed. 2, Philadelphia, Lippincott, 1947.

Harmer, Bertha, and Henderson, Virginia: Textbook of the Principles and Practice of Nursing, New York, Macmillan, 1943.

Homans, John: A Textbook of Surgery, ed. 6, Springfield, Ill., Thomas, 1948.

Mason, R. L., and Zintel, Harold: Preoperative and Postoperative Treatment, Philadelphia, Saunders, 1946.

Inflammation, Antisepsis and Asepsis

Berman, P., and Beckett, J. S.: Sterilizing surgical supplies, Am. J. Nursing **52**:1212-1214, 1952.

Broadhurst, J., and Given, L.: Microbiology Applied to Nursing, ed. 5, Philadelphia, Lippincott, 1945.

Johnson, A. E.: Penicillin therapy, Am. J. Nursing **48**:780-783, 1948.

Pratt, R., and Dufrenoy, J.: Antibiotics, ed. 2, Philadelphia, Lippincott, 1953.

Walter, C. W.: The Aseptic Treatment of Wounds, New York, Macmillan, 1948.

Witton, C. J.: Detergents, Am. J. Nursing **50**:410-412, 1950.

Preoperative Nursing Care

Anderson, C. M.: Emotional Hygiene, ed. 4, Philadelphia, Lippincott, 1948.

Dicks, Russell: Who Is My Patient?, New York, Macmillan, 1941.

Dripps, R. D.: The pharmacological basis for preoperative medication, S. Clin. North America, Dec., 1944.

Fetterman, J. L.: Practical Lessons in Psychiatry, Springfield, Ill., Thomas, 1949.

Gregg, D. E.: Anxiety—a factor in nursing care, Am. J. Nursing **52**: 1363-1365, 1952.

Levensen, S. M., and Lund, C. C.: Protein metabolism in surgical patients, Am. J. Nursing **48**:415-418, 1948.

Richardson, H. B.: Patients Have Families, New York, Commonwealth Fund.

Shorr, Nagle: The patient's spiritual needs, Am. J. Nursing **50**:64-67, 1950.

Van Schoick, M. R.: Emotional factors in surgical nursing, Am. J. Nursing **46**:451-453, 1946.

Anesthesia and Operative Care

Allen, F. M.: Refrigeration anesthesia, Trained Nurse & Hosp. Rev. **115**:174-177, 1945.

——: Refrigeration therapy, Trained Nurse and Hosp. Rev. **115**:265-268, 1945.

Bakutis, A. R.: Continuous spinal anesthesia, Am. J. Nursing **41**: 1254-1255, 1941.

Greisheimer, E. M.: The physiological effects of anesthesia, Am. J. Nursing **49**:337-343, 1949.

Griffin, N. L.: Preventing fires and explosions in the operating room, Am. J. Nursing **53**:809-812, 1953.

Owen, C. K., et al.: Twenty-six-gauge spinal needles for the prevention of spinal headache, Am. J. Surgery **85**:98-103, 1953.

Pratt, J. P.: Mental and emotional problems of anesthesia, Mod. Hosp. **70**:100-104, 1948.

Voorhees, I. W.: Anesthesia hazards in the operating rooms, Nursing World 418, Sept., 1950.

Postoperative Nursing Care

Bean, Helen: What a patient thinks about early ambulation, Am. J. Nursing **54**:169-171, 1954.

Carnahan, J. M.: Recovery room for postoperative patients, Am. J. Nursing **49**:581-582, 1949.

Cherkasky, M.: Hospital service goes home, Mod. Hosp. **68**:47-49, 1947.

Covalt, N. K.: Early exercise for the convalescent patient, Am. J. Nursing **47**:544-546, 1947.

Dade, L. S.: Diversional activities for patients, Am. J. Nursing **47**: 384-387, 1947.

Eastwood, D. W., and Mabrey, J. K.: Suction and the maintenance of an airway, Am. J. Nursing **53**:552-553, 1953.

Fine, J.: Care of the Surgical Patient, Including Pathological Physiology and Principles of Diagnosis and Treatment, Philadelphia, Saunders, 1949.

Frohman, I. P.: Demerol, Am. J. Nursing **53**:567-568, 1953.

Gigot, A. F., and Flynn, P. D.: Treatment of hiccups, J.A.M.A. **150**: 760-764, 1952.

Heifetz, C. J., Lawrence, M. S., and Richards, F. O.: Comparison of wound healing with and without dressings, Arch. Surg. **65**:746-751, 1952.

Ilgenfritz, H. C.: Preoperative and Postoperative Care of Surgical Patients, St. Louis, Mosby, 1948.

Jones, F. T.: The nurse's responsibility in rehabilitation, Am. J. Nursing **48**:74-76, 1948.

Lam, C. R.: What is "shock"?, Am. J. Nursing **51**:116-117, 1951.

Leon, Sister Agnes: Postanesthetic and postoperative recovery units, Am. J. Nursing **52**:430-432, 1952.

McAllister, S. E., and Pulaski, E. J.: A technic for dressing septic wounds, Am. J. Nursing **47**:396-398, 1947.

Morrissey, A. B.: Psychosocial and spiritual factors in rehabilitation, Am. J. Nursing **50**:763-766, 1950.

Poppe, J. K., and James, R. B.: Intratracheal suctioning, Am. J. Nursing **45**:538-540, 1945.

Rusk, H. A.: Implication for nursing rehabilitation, Am. J. Nursing **48**:74-76, 1948.

Seldon, T. H., Lundy, J. S., and Adams, R. C.: Nursing care as related to anesthesia, Am. J. Nursing **46**:377-378, 1946.

Sherfeg, M. J.: Psychiatry belongs at the bedside, Am. J. Nursing **47**: 682-685, 1947.

Woodruff, M. B.: To prevent and cure pressure sores, Am. J. Nursing **52**:606, 1952.

Fluid Therapy and Gas Therapy

Abbott, W. E., et al.: The danger of administering parenteral fluids by hypodermoclysis, Surgery **32**:305-315, 1952.

Bowen, A.: Intravenous alimentation in surgical patients, Mod. Med., March, 1946.

Cooke, R. E., and Crowley, L. G.: Replacement of gastric and intestinal fluid losses in surgery, New England J. Med. **246**:637-641, 1952.

Elman, Robert: Fluid balance from the nurse's point of view, Am. J. Nursing **49**:222-224, 1949.

Emerson, C. P., and Bragdon, J. S.: Essentials of Medicine, ed. 17, pp. 92-104 (fluids); pp. 106-120 (blood); pp. 120-126 (gas), Philadelphia, Lippincott, 1955.

Karp, M., and Sokol, J. K.: Intravenous use of alcohol in the surgical patient, J.A.M.A. **146**:21-23, 1951.

Kirby, C. K.: The clinical use of blood and blood derivatives, Am. J. Nursing **50**:88-90, 1950.

Lans, H. S., et al.: Diagnosis, treatment, and prophylaxis of potassium deficiency in surgical patients, Surg., Gynec. & Obst. **95**: 321-330, 1952.

Lawton, Curreri, and Gale: Invert sugar for parenteral nutrition in surgical patients, Arch. Surg. **63**: 561-567, 1951.

Newman, E. V.: The technic of venipuncture and intravenous infection, Am. J. Nursing **52**:418-424, 1952.

Technical instructions on the BLB mask, Hosp. Topics, pp. 71-72, April, 1953.

Unger, L. J.: Human blood plasma and plasma substances, Am. J. Nursing **54**:50-52, 1954.

Geriatric Nursing

Cherkasky, M.: The Montefiore Hospital home care program, Am. J. Pub. Health **39**:163-166, 1949.

Donahue, W. T.: Psychological aspects of feeding the aged, J. Am. Dietet. A. **27**:461-466, 1951.

Emerson, C. P., and Bragdon, J. S.: Essentials of Medicine, ed. 17, pp. 132-146, Philadelphia, Lippincott, 1955.

Ferderber, M. B.: Rehabilitation program for the aged, Pub. Health Nursing **44**:664-667, 1952.

Lawton, George: Aging Successfully, New York, Columbia, 1946.

Merritt, L. J.: Young ideas for elderly patients, Am. J. Nursing **52**:713, 1952.

Newton, Kathleen: Geriatric Nursing, St. Louis, Mosby, 1950.

Randall, O. A.: Grandma and grandpa live with us, Pub. Health Nursing **43**:26-30, 1951.

Sholtis, L. A.: Nursing the elderly surgical patient, Am. J. Nursing **51**:726-728, 1951.

Stieglitz, E. J.: Geriatric Medicine, ed. 3, Philadelphia, Lippincott, 1954.

Swartz, F. C.: A wider concept of geriatrics, Am. J. Nursing **53**: 1327-1328, 1953.

Thewlis, M. W.: The Care of the Aged, ed. 5, St. Louis, Mosby, 1946.

Worcester, A.: The Care of the Aged, the Dying and the Dead, ed. 2, Springfield, Ill., Thomas, 1940.

Tumors and Cancer Nursing

Best, N.: Radiotherapy and the nurse, Am. J. Nursing **50**:140-143, 1950.

Boeker, E. H., and Peterson, R. I.:

Nursing care of patients with advanced cancer, Pub. Health Nursing **44**:463-466, 1952.
Cherkasky, M., and Randall, M. G.: A community home care program, Am. J. Nursing **49**:650-652, 1949.
A Cancer Source Book for Nurses, New York, Am. Cancer Soc., 1950.
Cancer Nursing, A Manual for Public Health Nurses, Raleigh, N. C., Health Publications Institute, Inc., 1950.
Ferris, A. A.: Fifty grams of radium, Am. J. Nursing **53**:1080-1081, 1953.
Johnson, Dallas: Facing the Facts About Cancer, New York, Public Affairs Committee, 1951.
Handorf, L. L., and Pederson, T. E.: Nursing care in terminal cancer, Am. J. Nursing **50**:643-646, 1950.
Keller, C.: Raising the cancer patient's morale, Am. J. Nursing **49**: 508-511, 1949.
Quimby, E. H.: Safety in the use of radioactive isotopes, Am. J. Nursing **51**:240-243, 1951.
What should a patient with malignancy be told? (edit.), J. Indiana M. A. **45**:308-309, 1952.
Williams, Marvin: Precautions in working with radium, Am. J. Nursing **47**:226-228, 1947.

UNIT TWO

Nursing in Conditions of the Upper Respiratory Tract

CHAPTER TWELVE

Surgery of Nose, Throat and Pharynx

GENERAL CONSIDERATIONS

The respiratory system delivers oxygen to the lungs, where the blood, flowing through the pulmonary capillaries, picks it up and discharges carbon dioxide. With expiration the carbon dioxide is discharged into the air. The respiratory movements, inspiration and expiration, produce this interchange. These movements are brought about by the diaphragm and the intercostal muscles with help from certain abdominal muscles in an emergency. Air must enter and leave the lungs, and blood must be pumped through the lungs, for this mechanism to function properly.

Conditions that interfere with this mechanism result in an incomplete oxygenation of the blood (anoxemia). Arterial blood no longer has its bright red color; it is a dark purplish red. The patient's skin takes on a bluish pallor (cyanosis), which is best noted in the nail beds, the lips and the tongue.

Anoxemia may occur from circulatory difficulties, such as cardiac failure, congenital cardiac or vascular defects, pulmonary embolism and so forth. Certain drugs interfere with the oxygenation of the blood (sulfanilamide, carbon monoxide) and produce cyanosis.

Consideration is given in this chapter to the major and the minor lesions that interfere with the normal function of the respiratory system. This system begins with the nose and the throat and extends via the trachea to the bronchi and the lungs. It also includes the pleura, the bones and the muscles comprising the thoracic cage. Any disturbance of this system, such as obstruction of the air passages, paralysis of respiratory muscles, tumors or disease of the lungs or compression of the lung by fluid or air in the pleural cavity, may interfere in greater or lesser degree with the normal respiratory mechanism and produce various degrees of anoxemia and cyanosis.

SURGICAL CONDITIONS OF NOSE AND SINUSES

Epistaxis (Nosebleed)

Epistaxis or nosebleed may result from injury or from disease. Most often local or constitutional disease is the cause and, when the cause is removed, the attacks cease. The most common local causes are deviated septum, perforated septum, cancer and trauma. Such systemic diseases as hypertension and blood dyscrasias as leukemia also are causes of epistaxis. The bleeding usually occurs from a small artery or vein that runs upward on the septum near the nares.

Treatment. Mild attacks may be checked by snuffing iced water or by pressure. When the bleeding point can be seen, applications of adrenalin or silver nitrate stick usually suffice. Often, however, the origin of the bleeding cannot be found. In these cases, after spraying the nose with cocaine and adrenalin solutions, a rubber finger cot or the finger of a rubber glove may be inserted into the nostril, the open end being held with 3 or 4 hemostats while gauze packing is inserted. Pressure may be increased by moistening the gauze. The packing should be removed after 24 hours.

Nasal Obstruction–Sinusitis

Nasal Obstruction. Obstruction to the passage of air through the nostrils results frequently from a deflection of the nasal septum, hypertrophy of the turbinate bones or from the pressure of polyps–grapelike swellings that arise from the mucous membrane of the sinuses, especially the ethmoids. This obstruction also may lead to a condition of chronic infection of the nose and result in frequent attacks of nasopharyngitis. Very frequently the infection extends to the sinuses of the nose (mucus-lined cavities filled with air that drain normally into the nose). When sinusitis develops and the drainage from these cavities is obstructed by deformity or swelling within the nose, pain is experienced in the region of the affected sinus.

Treatment. The treatment of this condition requires the removal of the nasal obstruction, followed by measures to overcome whatever chronic infection exists. In many cases the underlying nasal allergy is the lesion requiring treatment. At times it is necessary to drain the nasal sinuses by radical operation. The operations performed depend upon the type of nasal obstruction found. Usually they are performed with local anesthesia. This is obtained by introducing into the nostrils pledgets of cotton soaked in 10 per cent cocaine solution with adrenalin. The nurse who assists the surgeon in operations on the nose and the throat must be extremely careful to identify the solutions of cocaine and procaine, for the toxic nature of cocaine when injected hypodermically would make the mistake a most serious one.

If a deflection of the septum is the cause of the obstruction, the surgeon makes an incision in the mucous membrane and, after raising it from the bone, removes the deflected bone and cartilage with bone forceps. The mucosa then is allowed to fall back in place and is held there by tight packing. Generally the packing used

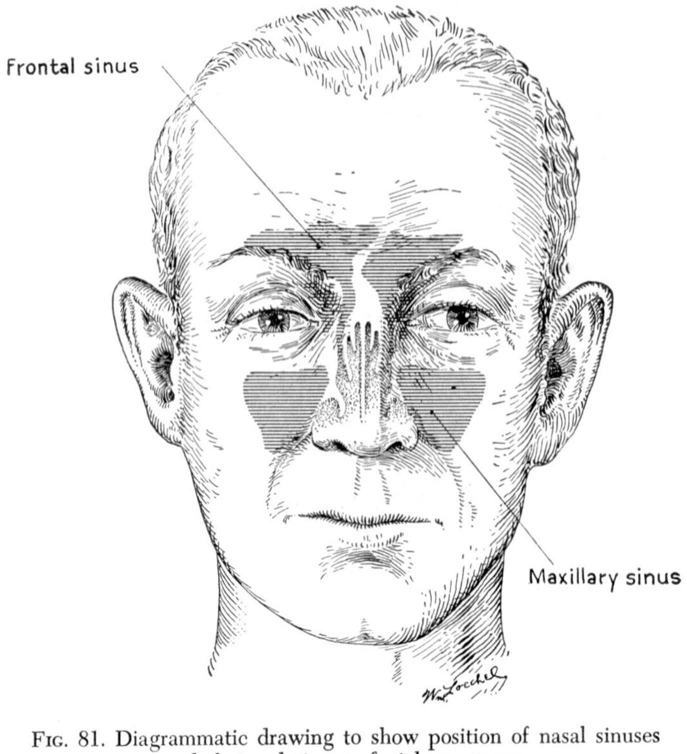

Fig. 81. Diagrammatic drawing to show position of nasal sinuses and their relation to facial structures.

is soaked in liquid petrolatum to facilitate its removal in from 24 to 36 hours. This operation is called commonly a *submucous resection.*

Nasal polyps are removed by clipping them at their base with a wire snare. Hypertrophied turbinates may be treated locally by astringent applications to shrink them up close to the side of the nose.

Sinusitis. The treatment of sinusitis usually is directed at first toward the removal of nasal allergies and infection. Cleansing and astringent sprays are given at frequent intervals and are supplemented often by drops of some mild antiseptic. Local heat applications give considerable measure of relief from pain, and appropriate antibiotics are given after culture and sensitivity tests are obtained. When drainage of the affected sinuses cannot be effected in this manner, more radical operation must be performed. The removal of turbinates, the enlargement of the opening leading from the sinus into the nose and irrigation of the cavities frequently are necessary.

In chronic sinusitis and sometimes in acute sinusitis, external drainage of the sinus with removal of polyps and diseased mucosa is necessary. For maxillary sinus, the incision is made along the upper gum line above the canine teeth (Caldwell-

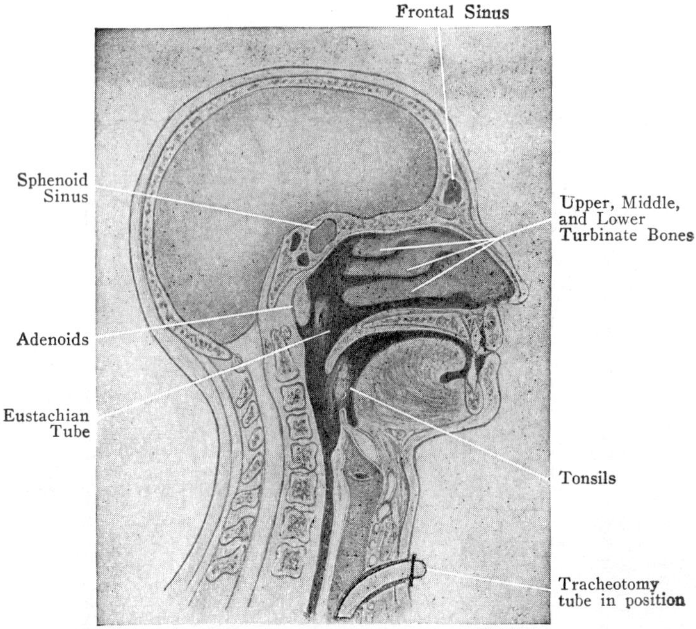

FIG. 82. Anatomy of head and neck. In addition, note the position of adenoids and tonsils and a tracheotomy tube in position.

Luc operation). To drain the frontal sinus an incision is made through the inner third of the eyebrow.

Fractures of the Nose

Fractures of the nose usually result from direct violence. As a rule, they do not produce any serious consequences, but the deformity that may follow often gives rise to obstruction of the nasal air passages and to facial disfigurement.

Immediately after the injury there is usually considerable bleeding from the nose, both from the nostrils and into the pharynx. There is marked swelling of the soft tissues adjacent to the nose and, frequently, a definite deformity.

Treatment. As a rule, the bleeding can be controlled by the application of cold compresses. A roentgenogram is helpful in determining the displacement of the fractured bones and in ruling out an extension of the fracture into the skull. With local cocainization of the nose or with intravenous anesthesia, it is possible usually to bring displaced fragments into alignment and then hold them by intranasal packing or external splints. The important points in the reduction of the fracture are to reform the nasal passages and to realign the bones so as to prevent disfiguring deformity. After reduction, the swelling that occurs may be decreased by the application of ice compresses with the patient in the sitting position.

Plastic Surgery of the Nose

The nose is such a prominent organ of the face that its deformity may cause the patient considerable embarrassment. The deformity may result from congenital causes, from disease or from injury.

Deformities resulting from congenital causes often may be corrected by simple operations in which the nose is straightened or lengthened by either removing offending bone or supplying new tissue (usually costal cartilage). The incisions are so placed as to be inconspicuous. In deformities resulting from injury or disease, various types of plastic surgery may be employed. Skin, tube or sliding grafts may be used to cover the defects left by scars, malignancy or injuries. In some instances, especially in older people with malignancy, artificial appliances may be modeled and held in place with the rims of glasses. (See Plastic Surgery, p. 411.)

Nursing Care

After operation the patient usually is placed flat on his back with the head slightly elevated. Ice compresses are used frequently after operation to reduce bleeding, swelling and pain. Hemorrhage is the chief postoperative complication, and it must be remembered that the spitting up or the vomiting of blood that has run back into the pharynx is as much a symptom of nasal hemorrhage as is the flow at the nares. Frequent swallowing, followed by belching, often is indicative of bleeding that results in an accumulation of blood in the stomach.

In cases in which local anesthesia has been used, the blood sometimes trickles down the throat, but the patient is not sufficiently aware of it to show a swallowing reflex. If the bleeding is excessive or continuous, or if any of the constitutional signs of hemorrhage appear, the surgeon should be called, and the nurse should get ready for his use fresh packing, a light, a head mirror, a nasal speculum and packing forceps.

These patients may have a liquid diet on the day of operation and whatever they prefer after that. Sedatives often are necessary on the day and the night of operation, but after that there is little need of them. The patient is tempted often to blow his nose because of a full feeling, but if it is explained to him that this is because of the packing in his nose, he will be more patient. Packing is removed usually after 24 hours.

SURGERY OF TONSILS AND PHARYNX

Peritonsillar Abscess (Quinsy)

Peritonsillar abscess, or quinsy, is an abscess that develops above the tonsil in the tissues of the anterior pillar and soft palate. As a rule, it is secondary to a tonsillar infection. The usual symptoms of an infection are present, together with such local symptoms as difficulty in swallowing (dysphagia), thickening of the voice, drooling and local pain. An examination shows marked swelling of the soft palate, often to the extent of half-occluding the orifice from the mouth into the pharynx.

Treatment. A considerable measure of relief may be obtained by throat irrigations or the frequent use of mouthwashes or gargles, using saline or alkaline solutions at a temperature of from 105° to 110° F. This treatment hastens the pointing of the process.

The abscess should be evacuated as soon as possible. The mucous membrane over the swelling first is painted with 10 per cent cocaine solution; then, after a small incision has been made, the points of a blunt hemostat are forced into the abscess pocket and opened as they are withdrawn. This operation is performed best with the patient in the sitting position, as it is easier then for him to expectorate the pus and the blood that accumulate in the pharynx. Almost immediate relief is experienced. After-treatment is warm gargles at intervals of 1 or 2 hours for from 24 to 36 hours.

Antibiotics, usually penicillin, are extremely effective in the control of the infection in quinsy. Given early in the course of the disease, the abscess may be aborted, and incision can be avoided. If antibiotics are not given until later, the abscess must be drained, but improvement in the inflammatory reaction is rapid.

Disease of Tonsils and Adenoids

Tonsils. The tonsils are two groups of lymphatic tissue situated one on each side of the oropharynx. They are frequently the seat of acute infectious processes and of chronic infection, constantly giving off toxins in small amounts. Therefore, they are looked upon as one of the most common sites of focal infection, producing chronic systemic diseases such as chronic arthritis, nephritis and so forth. Furthermore, they often grow to such a size as to interfere with normal respiration, a condition that is spoken of as hypertrophy of the tonsils. (See Fig. 83.)

Frequent acute infections, chronic infections, hypertrophy—all are regarded as indications for the removal of the tonsils.

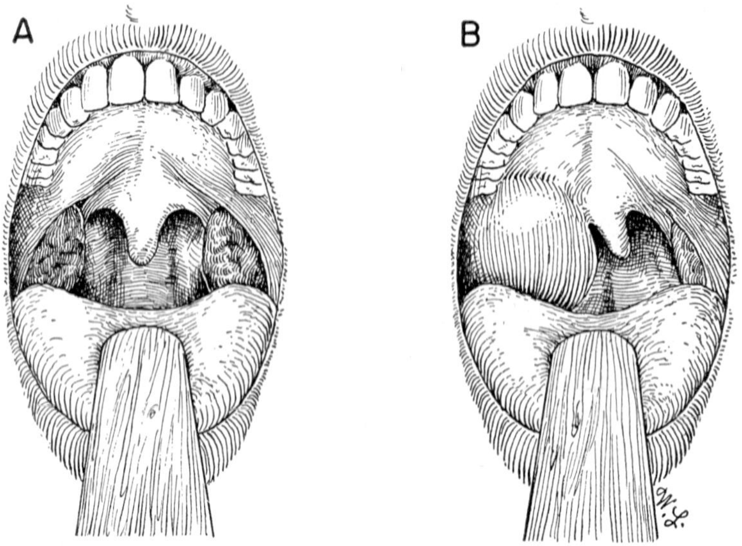

FIG. 83. Views of oral pharynx. (A) Showing enlargement of the tonsils. (B) Showing peritonsillar abscess on the right-hand side.

Tonsillectomy may be performed under local anesthesia with the patient in a sitting position or under general anesthesia with the patient in the dorsal position. The tongue is depressed and the tonsil is grasped with tenaculum forceps. The tonsil is freed by blunt, sharp dissection sufficient to allow the snare to encircle the remaining attachment, which is crushed and the tonsil is removed. Hemorrhage usually is controlled by pressure with small gauze sponges. Occasionally it is necessary to clamp and ligate the bleeding vessel. Often the blood is swallowed, or, if the patient is unconscious, it will run down into the stomach and not be recognized until the patient vomits copiously.

Adenoids. Adenoids are vegetations of lymphatic tissue that appear on the posterior pharyngeal wall during childhood. They frequently become large enough to prohibit normal respiration through the nose and, as a consequence, the children become "mouth-breathers." This condition produces deformity of the nose and the mouth and a general deterioration of health and physique. The treatment, of course, is operative removal, which is done usually in conjunction with a tonsillectomy.

Nursing Care for Tonsillectomy and Adenoidectomy

The chief danger after these operations is from hemorrhage; therefore, most surgeons require an estimation of the clotting time before operation. Furthermore, the nurse should notify the surgeon if the patient is menstruating. Atropine al-

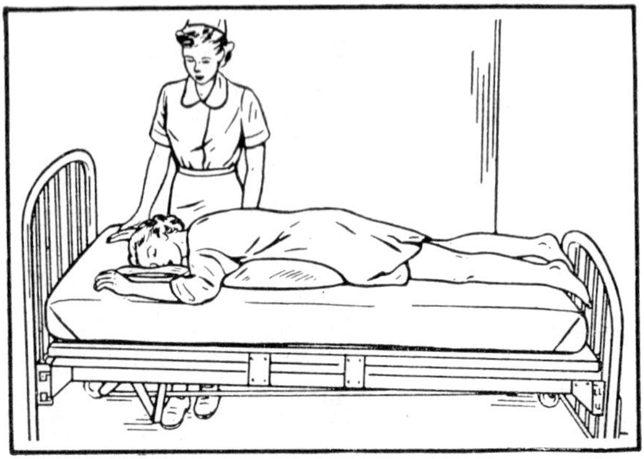

FIG. 84. Position following tonsillectomy which is comfortable and allows drainage of excretions from throat. (Winters, M. C.: Protective Body Mechanics in Daily Life and in Nursing, Philadelphia, Saunders)

ways should be given before operation under general anesthesia to decrease the amount of mucous secretion. After operation, the patient should be placed in the dorsal or the sitting position, according to the wishes of the surgeon. For patients who have had general anesthesia, the most comfortable position is prone, with the head turned to the side to allow for drainage from the throat (Fig. 84). An ice collar should be applied and a basin and gauze provided for the expectoration of blood and mucus. Children are treated best by placing them on the side, so that secretion may drain from the mouth and the pharynx.

Bleeding is the chief postoperative complication. The blood may be bright red if the patient spits it out at once. Often, however, it is swallowed and becomes brown in color immediately, due to the action of the acid gastric juice upon it. If the patient vomits large amounts of altered blood or spits bright blood at frequent intervals, or if the pulse rate increases gradually, the attending surgeon should be notified. The nurse should have in readiness for him a light, a head mirror, gauze, curved hemostats and a waste basin. Occasionally it may be necessary to suture or ligate the bleeding vessel. In such cases the patient must be taken to the operating room and given anesthesia.

If there is no bleeding, water and cracked ice may be given the patient as soon as desired. Acetylsalicylic acid, suspended in water as a gargle or given in chewing gum, sometimes is used to relieve discomfort. The diet should be liquid or semiliquid for several days, excluding orange or lemon juice and other acids. Ice cream is a very acceptable food, especially for children. The patient may be discharged from the hospital the day after the operation, but he should convalesce at home for several days.

Sulfonamides and Antibiotics. In all these acute infections of the pharynx the sulfonamides and penicillin are used. They are given prophylactically, as well as therapeutically, before and after surgical procedures on the pharynx and the larynx. (See p. 47.)

Aspirated Foreign Bodies

Foreign bodies frequently are aspirated into the pharynx, the larynx or the trachea, especially by children. They cause symptoms in two ways: by obstructing the air passages they cause difficulty in breathing that may lead to asphyxia; later they may be drawn farther down, entering the bronchi or one of their branches and causing symptoms of irritation, such as a croupy cough, bloody or mucous expectoration and paroxysms of dyspnea. The physical signs and roentgenograms confirm the diagnosis.

Treatment. In emergencies, when the signs of asphyxia are evident, immediate treatment is necessary. If the foreign body has lodged in the pharynx, it may be dislodged frequently by the finger. If the obstruction is in the larynx or the trachea, an immediate tracheotomy is necessary.

SURGERY OF THE LARYNX

Carcinoma (Cancer)

Cancer of the larynx occurs in both men and women. It may occur as early as the eighteenth year, but usually it is seen in men of middle age or older. The early symptoms are hoarseness or discomfort in the region of the larynx; later, there may be pain, obstructed respiration, difficulty in swallowing, bleeding or swelling of the neck by tumor growth.

Treatment. In the early stages it can be cured in more than 80 per cent of cases by proper surgical removal. The operation of choice is (1) laryngofissure for the early case and (2) laryngectomy for the more advanced case.

Laryngofissure. This operation is the splitting of the thyroid cartilage of the larynx in the mid-line of the neck and the removal of the portion of the vocal cord that is involved in the tumor growth. After bleeding has been controlled, the neck is closed and is allowed to heal. Sometimes a tracheotomy tube is left in the trachea when the wound is closed, in which event it is removed usually after a few days.

Laryngectomy. In this operation the entire larynx is removed. The trachea opens permanently on the lower portion of the front of the neck. The opening of the larynx into the pharynx is closed by sutures.

Nursing Care

Inasmuch as surgery of the larynx is done most commonly for a tumor that may be malignant, the nurse often has a patient who is worried for many reasons: Will the surgeon be able to remove all the tumor? Is it cancer? Will I die? Will I ever speak again? Therefore, the psychological preparation of the patient is as important as the physical. If he is going to have a complete laryngectomy, he should know that he will lose his natural voice completely but that, with training, there are ways in which he can carry on a fairly normal conversation.

Surgery can be done under local or general anesthesia. After operation the patient with a laryngofissure may have a tracheotomy tube. (See p. 219.) The physician may insert a naso-esophageal catheter (No. 16 French urethral catheter) and feedings are given under the same precautions that prevail in gastrostomy feedings. (See p. 307.) Oral feedings often are started on the first day after operation if acceptable to the patient. The tracheotomy tube is removed at the surgeon's discretion. This may be in 2 or 3 days.

In caring for a person with a total laryngectomy, it must be realized that the laryngectomy tube (which is shorter but has a larger diameter than the usual tracheotomy tube) is the only airway the patient has. The care of this tube is the same as for a tracheotomy tube.

Again, a naso-esophageal catheter is passed by the physician after operation and liquid feedings are given. Usually the nurse is permitted to remove and pass this tube after this, because there is no possibility of its getting into the trachea, the trachea now being sutured permanently to the skin as a tracheotomy. After a few days the patient can be taught to pass his own feeding tube. Good mouth hygiene must be followed rigidly. After about 7 days, when the incision has healed, the surgeon may allow the patient to begin oral feedings.

Chemotherapy often is a part of treatment, as there is a possibility of

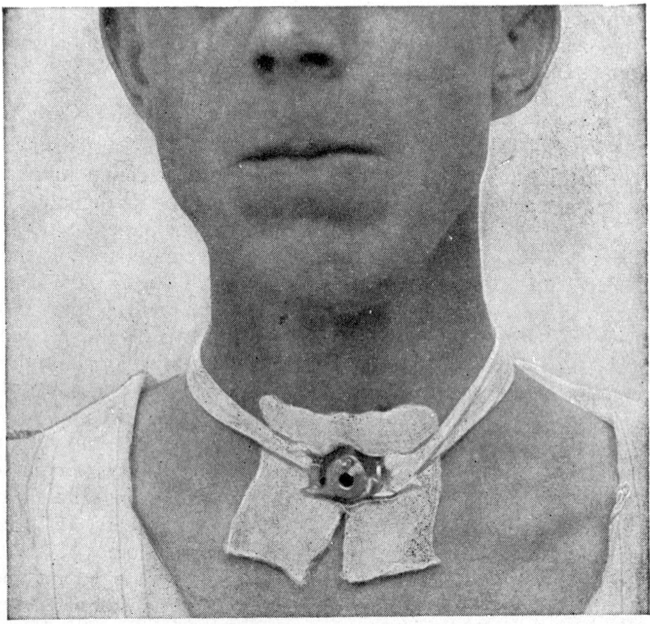

FIG. 85. Tracheotomy tube in use. After a few days the split dressing is changed to an unsplit one, and the tube is pushed through the dressing before it is inserted.

incisional contamination. Vitamins may be given as supplemental feedings, and infusions often are necessary to keep up fluid, electrolyte and nutritional balance.

With regard to the rehabilitation of such people, the partially laryngectomized patient has little difficulty, for in a matter of days his voice will improve. However, the completely laryngectomized patient often is depressed and needs encouragement. There are speech rehabilitation training programs in many large cities. The methods utilized are of two kinds:

1. The use of instruments, such as the artificial reed-type larynx. With other instruments the individual may have to carry a battery box or bellows to help amplify the tone. The chief disadvantages of them are that they do not produce natural voice sounds, and they are unattractive.

2. The use of esophageal speech. By this method the individual swallows air and, by proper muscle control, can produce sounds on the return "belch" of air. Laryngectomized patients make the best teachers for other laryngectomized patients. Results are fairly satisfactory, in that the patient is able to talk with no unnatural equipment. However, the voice produced is hoarse and similar to that of a person with laryngitis.

TRACHEOTOMY

A tracheotomy is an operation in which an opening is made into the trachea through which the patient may breathe. It is performed because of obstruction of the air passage in the larynx from any cause—tumors, foreign bodies, diphtheritic membranes, paralysis of the vocal cords and edema of the glottis; also for obstruction occurring during or after operations on the neck.

The patient is placed on the table with the head thrown back, a median incision is made through the skin of the neck, the muscles are separated and retracted and the trachea is opened in a vertical direction. A sterile tracheotomy tube then is inserted and held in place by tapes fastened round the patient's neck. Usually a square of sterile gauze is placed between the tube and the skin before the tape is tied. The tubes of proper size should occupy half the cross-sectional area of the trachea (Fig. 86). They should be made of sterling silver. Each tube consists of three pieces: an outer cannula, to which the retaining tapes are fastened; a pilot, an olive-tipped, curved silver rod that is used to guide the cannula into the opening in the trachea; and an inner cannula that is inserted into the outer cannula after the withdrawal of the pilot.

Nursing Care

Emergencies arise in which there is laryngeal obstruction and a tracheotomy must be done. The life of the patient is at stake, and strict observance of aseptic technic and the psychological preparation of the patient are of secondary importance. However, there are instances in which there is time to explain the purpose of such surgery to the patient, with the result that he will adjust better to his situation after operation. He should realize that he will lose his voice temporarily, and that he will breathe by means of a tube in his trachea.

Immediate Postoperative Care. This patient should have a nurse in attendance for at least the first 24 hours after operation. If this is impossible, he should be placed near the head nurse's station, where he can be watched closely. Surgery was done to relieve obstruction; it is the responsibility of the nurse to keep the newly made opening patent. Another objective in nursing care is to alleviate the apprehension of the patient. It is a new experience for him, and often he has a real fear of asphyxiation.

Slightly blood-tinged mucus usually is the first kind of secretion to come through the tracheotomy tube. As time passes, the amount of blood that comes through should diminish and disappear. If it does not, this may indicate hemorrhage, and it should be reported. All secretions should be wiped away carefully and

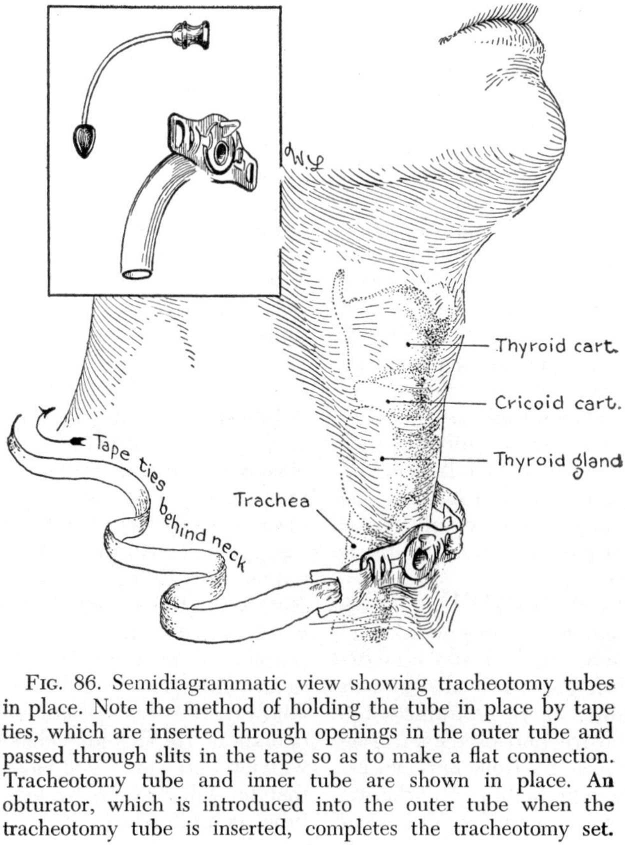

FIG. 86. Semidiagrammatic view showing tracheotomy tubes in place. Note the method of holding the tube in place by tape ties, which are inserted through openings in the outer tube and passed through slits in the tape so as to make a flat connection. Tracheotomy tube and inner tube are shown in place. An obturator, which is introduced into the outer tube when the tracheotomy tube is inserted, completes the tracheotomy set.

quickly before they are aspirated by the patient. An electric or a wall-suction apparatus should be on hand for aspiration. The receptacle for collecting secretions may have about 50 cc. of tap water in it to prevent tenacious mucus from adhering to the container, which would make it difficult to clean later. The rubber catheter connected to suction may be Size 8 or 10 for children and from 12 to 16 for adults. It should be cut diagonally at the tip and have 2 or 3 holes along the side. Suction should not be too strong to avoid injuring delicate mucous membrane. Catheter aspirations may have to be done every 15 minutes for the first day, but the needs of the individual patient will be the determining factor. The nurse usually is permitted to introduce the catheter up to 5 inches, but deeper aspiration may be done by the physician. The catheter should not remain in the tracheotomy tube longer than is necessary, for the amount of air intake will be lessened. If complete removal of mucus is not done at frequent intervals, the dried secretions may cause obstruction. A towel spread bib-fashion across the chest and below the tube may help when secretions are profuse.

The inner cannula is removed gently by the nurse about every hour for the first day and less frequently after that. It is important to keep this tube clean to prevent encrustations and clogging. If the secretion is thick, instill about 5 drops of sterile water into the trachea through the tracheotomy tube before aspirating. (Care of the tube is explained later.) Before the inner cannula is replaced, the patient should be aspirated. The outer cannula is not removed by the nurse. However, if the patient has a permanent tracheotomy, this may become her responsibility after about 10 days. Meanwhile, the surgeon changes the outer cannula as often as he feels that it is necessary.

A sterile dressing, 3 x 3 inches, is split to fit under the tapes and the shield of the tube so that the incision is covered (Fig. 85). This becomes soiled easily and should be replaced as often as is necessary. Care must be taken to prevent dislodging or moving the tube when this is done.

For a time after operation many surgeons cover the opening of the tube with a few layers of gauze moistened in warm saline solution. This tends to moisten the inspired air and to filter out dust, which function is performed in normal life by the nose and the pharynx. However, it will be more to the patient's comfort if the air in the room is kept moistened with steam or a croup tent than if moist gauze is used as mentioned, as this tends to prevent the evacuation of secretions.

The patient may have fluids during the day of operation and diet as tolerated after that if there are no other contraindications. Scrupulous mouth care is given before and after meals and whenever necessary. He may be placed in the semi-Fowler or sitting position. Morphine sulfate usually is not given as these patients are not in acute pain. Moreover, the drug is contraindicated because it depresses the cough reflex.

Paper and pencil should be kept near the patient so that he has a means of communication. He needs reassurance, especially during the first night, for he has a real fear that he will asphyxiate while he is asleep. A tap bell or electric cord signal should be within his reach.

Postoperative Complications. The nurse must realize that her responsibility to these patients lies not only in keeping a patent airway but also in recognizing untoward symptoms. Pulse and blood pressure should be checked at least every half hour during the first day to detect any signs of hemorrhage. This will not always be evident by oozing from the tracheotomy tube; bleeding may occur inwardly.

Increasing apprehension and restlessness may indicate anoxemia. Perhaps the airway is becoming blocked and suctioning may relieve the symptoms. If not, call the physician. The character of respirations can be suggestive of difficulty. Any changes from the usual type of breathing may indicate a problem. If they are increasingly more rapid and seem to have concomitant wheezing or crowing, there may be an obstruction. This also may be apparent if he has an indrawn appearance above the clavicles, in the suprasternal notch and in the epigastrium with each inspiration. Color change from pallor to cyanosis is a symptom of respiratory embarrassment. If aspiration does not help, call the physician immediately.

Emphysema is a condition in which air escapes into the tissues. A puffiness is noted near the stoma as air escapes from the trachea. This may extend to the upper chest, the neck and the face. A crackling sensation may be detected on gentle pressure. With absorption of air by the tissues, this disappears in a few days.

Wound infection can occur easily; therefore, good technic must be practiced in changing dressings and keeping the incision clean. If food or water leaks through the wound or the patient coughs or chokes immediately after eating or drinking, an esophageal fistula may have developed. This symptom should be reported to the surgeon at once. Occasionally, due to violent paroxysms of coughing or to insecure tying of the tapes, the tracheotomy tube may be expelled. The opening in the trachea will fall together and, unless immediate treatment is given, the patient may die from asphyxia. The nurse must remember in such an emergency that the Trousseau dilator or a hemostat will spread the tracheal wound and allow the patient to breathe until the duplicate tube can be inserted by another person.

Care of Tubes. Cold running water will remove much of the secretions from a tube. However, for more adherent mucus the following methods of cleaning are suggested:

Place the tube in a bowl with hydrogen peroxide. This will help to loosen secretions. Pipe cleaners are effective; they are soft and will not injure the metal, yet the inner wire gives a degree of firmness. A 2-inch bandage on a piece of folded wire also can be used. Small test tube brushes are effective. After a thorough cleaning, silver polish can be used to remove any tarnish. The cannula then is boiled or autoclaved and, finally, reinserted. Careful handling of tracheotomy tubes is important, because they are made of a soft metal and are damaged easily. A dented tube may fit poorly and cause trauma to the patient when an attempt is made to remove it. A part of one tube is not interchangeable with a similar part of another set of tubes. Therefore, each set of three parts must be kept intact.

In preparing tapes for a tracheotomy tube, ¾-inch twill tape makes a strong set of ties. Each tie should be 16 inches long. About 1 inch from the end, a horizontal slit should be made. This end of the tie can be inserted through the side opening on the outer cannula, and the opposite end of the tie then can be threaded through the slit end and drawn tightly. This is more effective than to tie a knot to anchor the tape to the cannula, because a sizable knot can cause a pressure area on the neck of the patient (Fig. 86).

Equipment at Bedside. The nurse who is caring for a tracheotomized patient should keep near at hand:

STERILE TRAY CONTAINING

Duplicate tracheotomy tubes with obturator.
Trousseau dilator.
Forceps.
Scissors.
2 retractors.
Hemostat.
Gauze sponges.
Pair of sterile rubber gloves.

TRAY CONTAINING:

A sterile bowl of saline (to flush catheter attached to suction).
A second rubber catheter.
A container of sterile split 3 x 3 gauze squares.

Tube cleaning equipment may be kept here or at a near-by sink.

Teaching the Patient. The patient is taught to care for his own tracheotomy tube as soon as feasible. The nurse can instruct him concerning the parts of the instrument and how they function. With the use of a mirror, she can show him how to remove and how to insert the inner cannula. The care of this delicate instrument must be explained and demonstrated in detail, and the patient should repeat the demonstration to the nurse. If the patient is unable to care for himself, some member of the family will have to be taught before he is discharged.

Sometimes the insertion of a tracheotomy tube is a temporary procedure to tide the patient over an acute respiratory obstruction. In such cases the patient must return gradually to normal breathing. This is accomplished by producing a partial obstruction of the airway in the tracheotomy tube by the insertion of partial corks. When they are first inserted the patient must be watched constantly for signs of respiratory obstruction. If the patient tolerates a small cork, the opening may be decreased further by the use of larger ones until eventually the entire opening can be plugged. When the patient tolerates complete obstruction of the tracheotomy tube, it may be removed and the opening permitted to heal. This process is known as *decannulation.* During this process the nurse must inspect the corks carefully to see that they are not broken. As a rule, they are fixed to the tracheotomy tube with braided silk threads. The most suitable corks are those made of pure rubber ground down to fit the tube. In learning to talk, the patient may be permitted to use a cork to close the opening temporarily so that voice sounds will be produced more clearly. Often merely the placing of a finger over the tracheotomy opening will aid him when he talks. However, this must be cleared with the physician, for talking may be contraindicated if the larynx is to be at rest following disease or edema.

If the tracheotomy is permanent, the patient should be instructed regarding the danger of aspirating water. Therefore, he must not swim and he must exercise caution in taking a shower. So far as appearance is concerned, women can wear filigree made specially by a jeweler or scarves, ties and so forth in such a way that the tracheotomy tube is not seen. Usually in a man the shirt will cover up the tracheotomy opening.

CLINICAL SITUATION: TRACHEOTOMY

Mr. Yomtob had a tracheotomy yesterday. As the nurse passed his room, she heard a gurgling sound with each inspiration through his tracheotomy tube.

1. The nurse should be aware that Mr. Yomtob
   ____(1) needed aspiration immediately
   ____(2) was breathing normally
   ____(3) was practicing an exercise used in speech rehabilitation
2. The best technic to use in aspirating Mr. Yomtob's tube is to insert
   ____(1) a snug fitting catheter up to 5 inches and allow it to remain there for 2 to 3 minutes
   ____(2) a No. 8 or No. 10 catheter up to 10 inches and draw it back and forth gently for short intervals
   ____(3) a loose fitting catheter up to 4 or 5 inches and draw it back and forth several times
3. The most effective agent for loosening secretions from the tracheotomy tube after it has been removed from Mr. Yomtob is
   ____(1) zephiran chloride 1:1,000
   ____(2) hypochlorite solution
   ____(3) alcohol
   ____(4) hydrogen peroxide
4. The best first step in teaching Mr. Yomtob to care for his own tracheotomy would be to allow him to
   ____(1) remove and insert the outer cannula
   ____(2) remove and insert the obturator
   ____(3) insert the catheter for aspiration
   ____(4) handle a tracheotomy set and become familiar with the tube
5. When Mr. Yomtob goes home, it is important for him to know that he should refrain from
   ____(1) swimming
   ____(2) taking a shower
   ____(3) drawing the bed covers up to his chin at night
   ____(4) eating foods and drinking fluids which are hot or cold

CHAPTER THIRTEEN

Surgery of the Chest

THE NURSE AND THE CHEST SURGICAL PATIENT

In this relatively young field of surgery, it is fascinating to follow the progress that has been made in recent years. The successful removal of a lung was unthinkable only a quarter of a century ago. As a result of the rapid progress of chest surgery, the demand for expert nursing care never has been greater.

In addition to the general principles of preoperative and postoperative care, the nurse who assumes responsibility for the care of a chest surgical patient needs to know certain aspects of his care. In general, these may be summarized as follows:

Preoperatively, the emphasis is on (1) assisting the surgeon with numerous special diagnostic studies, (2) reducing the number of organisms in the upper respiratory tract, (3) preparing the patient mentally and physically for the surgical program ahead and (4) acquainting the patient with some of the postoperative problems, such as requiring him to cough.

Postoperatively, the nurse is concerned with (1) maintaining a patent airway, (2) providing for maximum expansion of the remaining lung tissue, (3) recognizing early symptoms of untoward complications and (4) providing supportive and rehabilitative measures.

ANATOMY AND PHYSIOLOGY

The chest is the semirigid box, formed by the ribs and the muscles, that contains the lungs, the heart and the great vessels. The lungs and the inner chest wall are covered by a glistening membrane called the *pleura* that serves normally to prevent friction during movement of the lung in respiration. This act is brought about by the contraction and the relaxation of the strong muscle, the diaphragm. The pressure between the lungs and the thoracic wall (the intrathoracic pressure) is always negative (less than atmospheric pressure). This means that when an opening is made into this space, air rushes in to try to equalize it with atmospheric pressure and so upsets the normal expansion of the lung. The heart and the great vessels, the trachea and the esophagus occupy a space between the pleural cavities known as the *mediastinum.* Normally these tissues are held loosely in place because the pressure in the 2 lungs is equal but, if the pressure becomes unequal, the heart may be pushed to one side or the other, as in fluid in the pleura and atelectasis (collapse of the lung).

Essentially the function of the respiratory system is to provide a means of making a gaseous exchange. Oxygen is drawn into the pulmonary alveoli. Here it combines with the hemoglobin of the red corpuscles and in so doing displaces carbon dioxide, which passes through the capillary walls into the pulmonary alveoli and is pushed out with the expired air. In diseased conditions, it is important for the surgeon to know the adequacy of gas exchange and whether sufficient lung function will remain if surgery is done. This is determined by spirometric or ventilatory studies.

Great advances have been made in recent years in surgery of the chest, attributable to antibiotics and chemotherapy, better understanding of preoperative preparation, improved technic for the administration of anesthetic agents (endotracheal anesthesia) and improved operative technics.

DIAGNOSTIC STUDIES

Pulmonary Function Tests. These tests are done with a spirometer and are designed to determine how well the lung "ventilates," that is, its ability to take in oxygen and release carbon dioxide. In addition, tests are being perfected to determine how well oxygen and carbon dioxide are exchanged between the alveoli and the pulmonary capillary blood; this is called "diffusion." Several terms in common usage are of interest to the nurse:

Vital capacity is the maximum volume of air that can be expelled from the lungs by forceful effort following a maximum inspiration.

Residual volume is the volume of gas remaining in the lungs at the end of a maximum expiration.

Total lung capacity is the sum of the vital capacity and the residual volume.

Tidal volume is the amount of air inspired during each respiratory cycle when the patient is breathing naturally.

Minute volume is the amount of air inspired normally in one minute.

Maximum breathing capacity is the largest amount of air that can be breathed per minute by making the greatest possible voluntary effort.

These tests usually are done only on chest patients having borderline respiratory reserve. As a rule, no special preparation is required for these

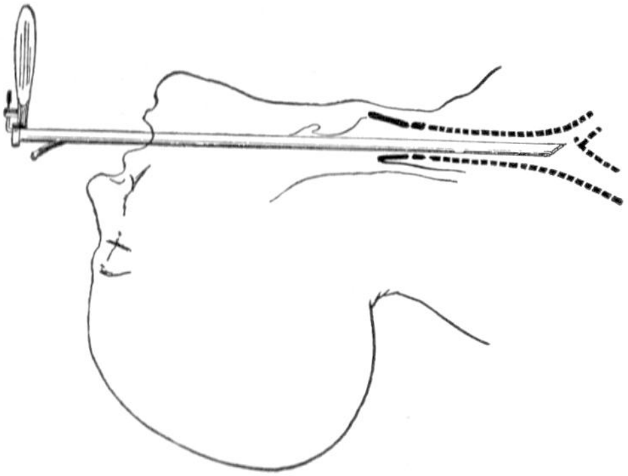

FIG. 87. Semidiagrammatic view shows the introduction of the bronchoscope.

tests; the nurse can tell her patient that he is to have a breathing test. He follows the instructions of the physician as to whether to breathe normally, inhale deeply, etc.

Roentgenograms *and sectional roentgenograms* (laminogram, planogram or strategram) are a real aid to the surgeon in recognizing lung function, the relationship of the vital structures and suggestions of pathology. Patience and co-operation on the part of the patient are desirable, and the nurse should endeavor to obtain them.

A **bronchogram** is an x-ray examination of the bronchial tree after a radiopaque dye is instilled. Before the procedure, a sedative and atropine are given, and usually a meal is withheld to prevent aspiration from regurgitation. Cocaine or pontocaine in the form of a spray through the nose and the mouth will help to prevent gagging and coughing when the tube is passed nasally. Following such a roentgenogram, food and fluids are withheld until the effects of the local anesthetic have worn off. The patient is placed on a regimen of postural drainage to allow the oily dye to be removed. Often because of the hazards of oil in the respiratory passages, he is sent home for two months before surgery is done.

Bronchoscopy and Esophagoscopy. When a foreign body enters the smaller air passages in the lungs, it may obstruct the bronchi with a resulting obstruction of air in the portion of the lung supplied by them. This produces a partial collapse of the lung with pulmonary symptoms of cough, expectoration and so forth. Secondary infection often occurs with resultant formation of chronic pulmonary suppuration or abscess.

In many cases it will be possible to remove the foreign body and to relieve the patient's symptoms by means of *bronchoscopy*. By this method of treatment, a lighted rigid tube is inserted through the pharynx and the trachea into the bronchus containing the foreign body. After aspiration of the secretions, the foreign body may be removed with forceps. Many brilliant cures have been effected by this method of therapy, which demands the highest degree of skill and adequate equipment (Fig. 87).

Bronchoscopy also is used in the diagnosis and the treatment of many intrathoracic diseases. By means of this lighted tube, tumors of the air passages can be viewed and biopsied, secretions can be aspirated for study and medication is applied at times. In the study of some diseases of the lungs, such as bronchiectasis, radiopaque liquids are injected to outline the air passages on the x-ray film (*bronchogram*).

Esophagoscopy is the viewing of the interior of the esophagus through a lighted tube. It is used to remove foreign bodies, to inspect lesions of the esophagus, such as ulcers, diverticuli and tumors, and often to make a positive diagnosis by removing small bits of tissue for microscopic examination (biopsy).

Nursing Care

Before bronchoscopy or esophagoscopy the patient must take nothing by mouth for at least 6 hours. Morphine sulfate or a similar drug usually is given adults. All removable dentures must be removed. The patient should be told what to expect so as to gain his co-operation. Many times, such a patient fears that he is to undergo real surgery. When he sees physicians and nurses garbed in operating masks and gowns, he may reasonably be upset.

When the patient returns from the operating room the local anesthesia used in the throat may interfere with swallowing and cause him to choke. After bronchoscopy, cracked ice may be given during the first 2 hours. After that, liquids may be given and, if the hypodermic does not cause nausea, the patient is permitted to return to the preoperative diet in about 6 hours. Difficulty in breathing, particularly in children, is looked for and reported promptly.

Until the local anesthesia has disappeared after esophagoscopy, care should be exercised in giving liquids; then they may be given, if they are tolerated, and the patient is permitted to return to the preoperative diet in about 6 hours.

Usually bismuth-subnitrate powder is given dry on the back of the tongue in order to coat the esophagus as the powder is swallowed. Some discomfort on swallowing may occur, but marked discomfort should be reported promptly.

Thoracentesis or the aspiration of chest fluid may be a therapeutic or a diagnostic procedure. It is necessary to place the patient in a position that is most comfortable for him and desirable for the surgeon (Fig. 88). The nurse can reassure her patient and explain the nature of the procedure.

Equipment is as follows:

STERILE TRAY CONTAINING:

Procaine ½ per cent with syringe and needles
Aspirating needle as desired by physician
30 or 50 cc. syringe
3-way stopcock with rubber attachment
Kelly hemostat
Gauze dressings
Lumbar puncture drape

IN ADDITION:

"Scrub-up" or "prep" tray
Sterile rubber gloves
Specimen tubes
Sterile wrapped glass graduate

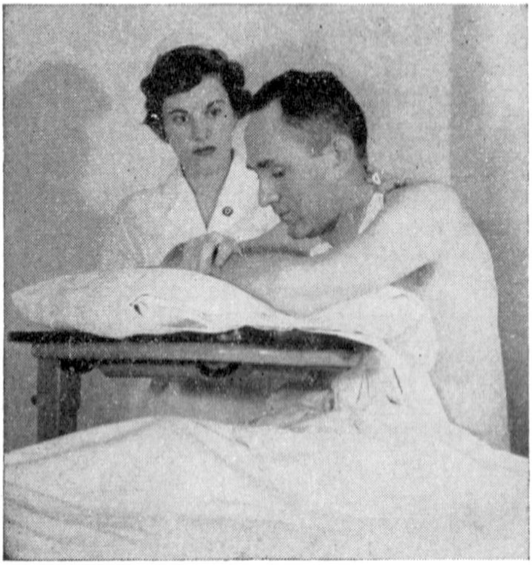

FIG. 88. Positions for thoracentesis. (*Top*) Patient in sitting position in bed with pillow over the bed table for support. (*Bottom*) Patient with feet over the side of the bed, using the bed table for support.

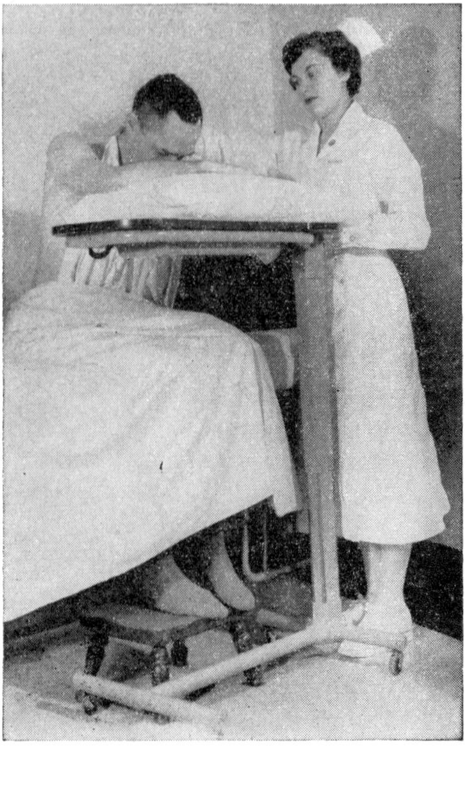

Often a physician will want to have penicillin available to inject into the chest after withdrawing fluid.

Sputum Studies. Of the laboratory tests, urine, blood and sputum studies always are done. For a sputum culture, the patient should be instructed to cough deeply so that a true specimen may be obtained for the sterile petri dish. Often a qualitative study is done to determine whether the secretions are saliva, mucus or pus. Usually they separate into layers that are seen readily when a conical glass container is used. For quantitative studies, the patient is given a waxed pasteboard container into which to expectorate. This is weighed at the end of 24 hours, and the amount and the character is described and charted. In disposing of

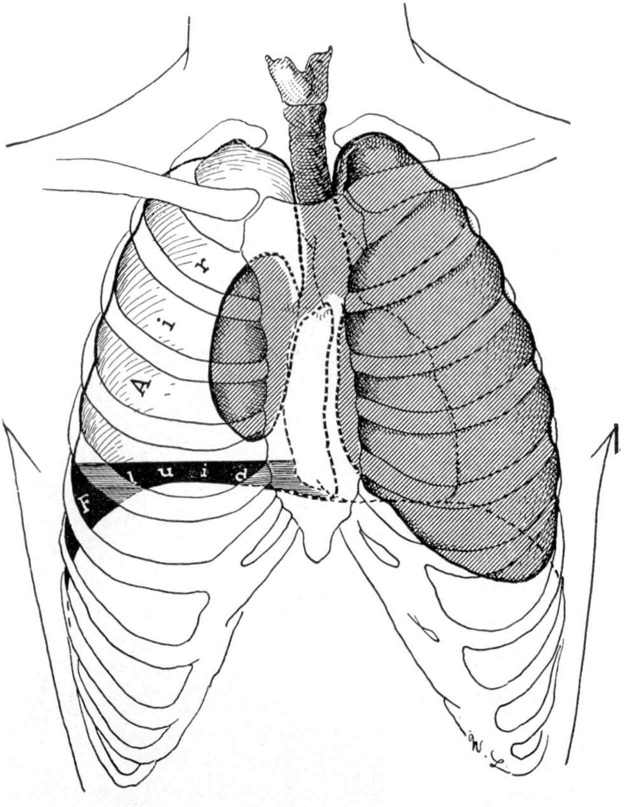

FIG. 89. Diagrammatic view of the chest cavity showing hydropneumothorax on the right side with atelectasis (collapse) of the right lung.

such a specimen, sawdust is added to the container in order to absorb and minimize the spread of organisms and then it is wrapped in paper until it is taken to the incinerator. To prevent odors, all sputum containers should be covered and concealed. Malodorous discarded mouth wipes should be removed, and there must be good ventilation in the room. Metal sputum containers should be cleaned thoroughly and sterilized frequently.

Exploratory Thoracotomy. The chest is opened surgically only as a last resort in attempting to establish a diagnosis after all other studies fail.

COLLECTIONS OF AIR AND FLUID IN THE PLEURAL CAVITY

Hydrothorax. Serous (nonpurulent) effusions may occur in such medical conditions as cardiac or renal failure, lung and pleural tumors and so forth. The presence of the fluid may so embarrass respiration as to require aspiration (thoracentesis). (See Fig. 88.)

Pneumothorax and Hemothorax. Air in the pleural cavity may occur spontaneously from rupture of a lung alveolus; it may be induced deliberately to collapse cavities and set the lung at rest, as in the treatment of tuberculosis; or it may arise from trauma, the air entering the pleural cavity through the resulting wound or from the injured lung. Bleeding usually accompanies such trauma, so that a hemopneumothorax results. Aspiration of the blood and air permits re-expansion of the lung and a return to a more physiologic state. In neglected cases or in those in which an infection has taken place, operation with removal of the clot and drainage is necessary.

Tension Pneumothorax. When the wound in the chest wall permits air to enter the pleural cavity but not to leave it with each respiration, or when lung wounds permit air to enter the pleural cavity and not escape, the trapped air produces an increasing pressure within the pleural cavity, collapsing the lung and displacing the heart and the great vessels toward the uninvolved side. This produces a rapid and a serious disturbance of respiratory and cardiac function that may end fatally. The chief symptoms are acute chest pain, dyspnea and cyanosis. Immediate relief may be given by the introduction of a large aspirating needle into the anterior upper chest. The trapped air escapes and the tension is relieved. Usually a sterile rubber tube is attached to the needle and led under water in a small bottle attached to the patient. This permits air to escape with each expiration but not to enter the pleural cavity with inspiration.

Chylothorax. Injury to the thoracic duct or to other lymphatic radicals in the chest may permit the escape of lymph into the pleural cavity. The lymph from the thoracic duct, rich in fat absorbed from the intestines, is called *chyle*, and the condition is called *chylothorax*. Injuries to the lymphatic radicals may arise from trauma or from operations in the posterior thorax, such as esophagectomies or sympathectomies. Small leaks may heal spontaneously, but thoracentesis may be required to relieve respiratory embarrassment. If the leak continues, operative intervention is required to suture or ligate the injured vessel. Continued loss of chylous fluid ends fatally.

CHEST WOUNDS

Wounds of the chest must be considered as among the most acute of surgical emergencies. These wounds may involve the chest wall only or they may involve the pleura, the lungs, the heart or the great vessels, and often the diaphragm and abdominal viscera. Should the wound involve only the chest wall, it should be handled as one would any other soft tissue injury.

When the wound enters the chest, air may enter the pleural cavity (pneumothorax). The lung is no longer held expanded by a negative pressure in the thorax, and it is said to "collapse." If the wound is large, air passes in and out of the thorax with each respiration, making a sucking sound. The disturbance of respiration and of the heart and great vessels produces shock and often death.

Other symptoms may be dyspnea and cough, with the spitting up of blood (hemoptysis). This last symptom indicates an injury to the lung, and, of necessity, the pleura, with a resultant entrance of air (pneumothorax) and blood (hemothorax) into the chest cavity. Should there be a wound of the diaphragm, abdominal symptoms suggesting hemorrhage or peritonitis complicate the picture further.

Treatment. The treatment of these patients should be begun by the first person who reaches them. The important thing to do is to stop the sucking wound. After applying antiseptics, the wound should be packed firmly with sterile gauze and covered with a tight adhesive strapping. The patient will improve almost at once.

After the surgeon has cared for the wound, the nurse should watch the patient carefully for signs of additional hemorrhage and shock. Morphine may be given generously for a few days until the wound is healed partly.

RESPIRATORY INFECTIONS

Infections of the pleural cavity often occur as a secondary disease. Bronchitis, bronchopneumonia, lobar pneumonia and pleurisy are encountered in surgical patients as complications of operations. For a discussion of these diseases the student is referred to the section on respiratory complications in Chapter 8, p. 140.

EMPYEMA THORACIS (PYOTHORAX)

Acute Empyema Thoracis

Empyema thoracis is a collection of pus in the pleural cavity. It occurs as a result of pneumonia or injury to the chest wall, and is most frequent in children. The usual history is of an acute pneumonia, in which a septic temperature persists or develops after the crisis has occurred. The patient is extremely ill, often with sufficient dyspnea to require a sitting posture (orthopnea) in order to obtain relief. Roentgenograms, which are of considerable aid to the surgeon, must be taken in the upright position.

Treatment. The causative organ-

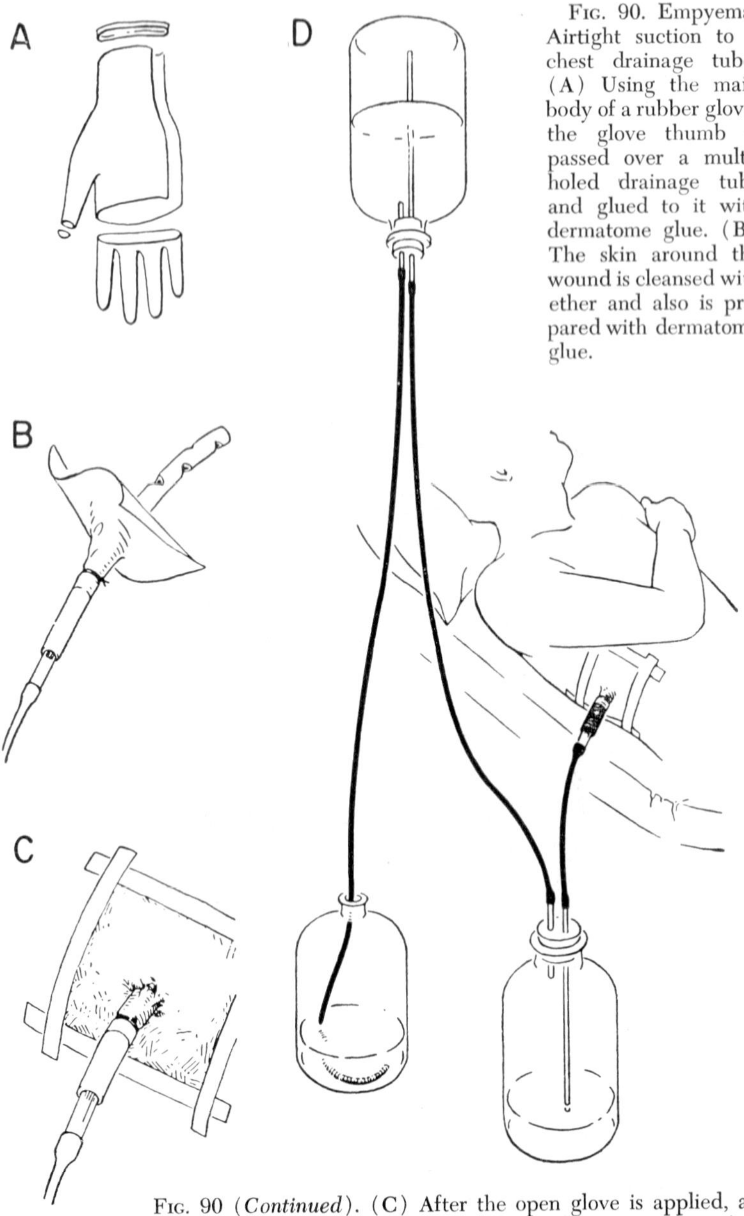

Fig. 90. Empyema. Airtight suction to a chest drainage tube. (A) Using the main body of a rubber glove, the glove thumb is passed over a multi-holed drainage tube and glued to it with dermatome glue. (B) The skin around the wound is cleansed with ether and also is prepared with dermatome glue.

Fig. 90 (*Continued*). (C) After the open glove is applied, adhesive strips prevent curling of the edges of rubber. (D) A Wangensteen suction is connected to the drainage tube. (Johnson, Julian, and Kirby, C. K.: Surgery of the Chest, p. 99, Chicago, Yr. Bk. Pub.)

isms are identified, and the appropriate antibiotic is administered. A regimen of intermittent aspiration and instillation of antibiotics is tried. The use of fibrinolytic enzymes such as trypsin, streptokinase and streptodornase seems to be effective in dissolving fibrin clots and decreasing the viscosity of pus. However, if the patient still has a temperature elevation after a week or 10 days, and the cavity is not well on the way to obliteration, surgical drainage is done.

Operations. The operations are of two types. In the first type, an effort is made to drain the pleural cavity without permitting the entrance of air into it. This is spoken of often as *closed drainage*. In the second type, drainage of the empyema cavity is accomplished by the removal of a section of rib, which permits an opening into the pleural collection. This is spoken of as *open drainage* or *thoracotomy*, and is used in cases with thick pus.

When the pus is thick, indicating an empyema of long duration, the pus cavity usually is fairly well

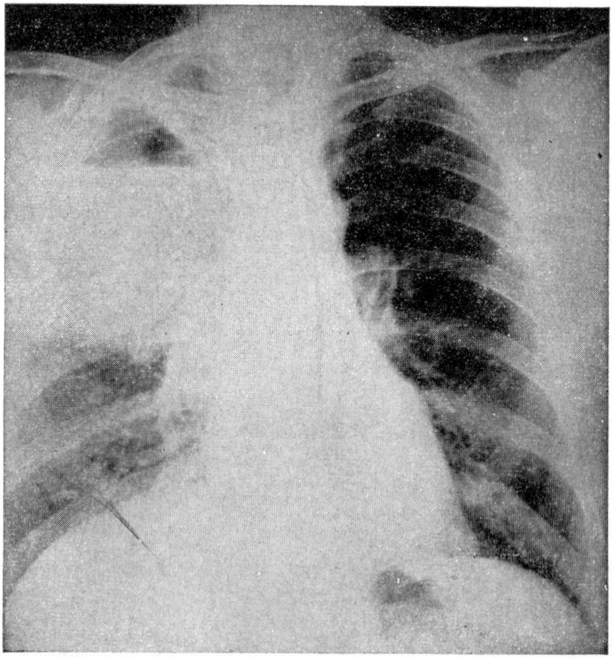

FIG. 91. Roentgenogram of chest showing abscess of the right lung. Note the large abscess cavity filled partly with fluid. This is indicated by the fluid level with air above the fluid in the upper part of the cavity. The left lung appears to be relatively normal.

walled off, and the danger of collapse of the lung is not so great. A simple and effective method of securing an airtight system is described in Figure 90.

After an operation for empyema, the chief consideration in the recovery of the patient is the collapse of the empyema cavity by expansion of the lung. To this end the patients are instructed to breathe deeply every hour; they are urged to blow into a spirometer or a blow bottle, using the increased intra-pulmonary pressure thus developed to expand the lung.

These patients should be allowed out of bed as soon as possible, usually after from 7 to 10 days. They may sit in a wheel chair and out of doors in the sun if this is possible. A high caloric diet is given, especially high in carbohydrates.

As soon as the drainage has decreased sufficiently, the tube may be removed from the chest and the wound is covered by simple gauze dressings. The convalescence should be passed as much as possible in the open air and sunlight.

Chronic Empyema Thoracis

When an empyema has been of long duration (months), the lung becomes covered by a tough exudate that prevents its expansion. In some patients the tough inflammatory exudate covering the lung may be removed to allow the lung to expand to its normal extent. This is called *decortication*. (See p. 253.) In other cases of chronic empyema, the cavity that remains must be closed. To this end, long sections of the ribs covering the cavity are removed to allow the soft tissue to fall inward against the lung. This operation is called a *thoracoplasty*. The same type of operation may be performed to collapse the cavities in the lungs produced by tuberculosis or bronchiectasis.

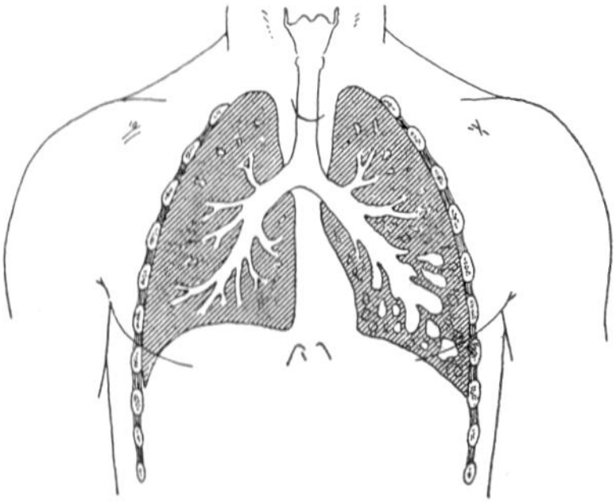

Fig. 92. Semidiagrammatic drawing shows marked dilatation of the air passages in the left lower lung, as found in bronchiectasis, and that the right lung appears to be relatively normal.

LUNG ABSCESS

Abscess of the lung occurs less often since the advent of chemotherapy. It produces cough with profuse foul expectoration, associated with a septic temperature and other signs of inflammation. It is found usually in patients with poor oral hygiene after general anesthesia, tonsillectomies and pneumonia. The nurse should try to prevent lung abscess by providing good mouth care, especially preceding general anesthesia, and by preventing aspiration of vomitus or infected material at all times.

Treatment. Lung abscess requires the same treatment as an abscess in other parts of the body; i.e., drainage. At times, when the abscess is near the center of the lung, drainage may be accomplished by the use of the bronchoscope, aided by postural drainage. The cavity is aspirated and treated with antibiotics at frequent intervals. The patient is kept in such a position, by elevation of the foot of the bed, so that the pus that forms may drain downward readily and be expectorated. When the abscess is located in the periphery of the lung, drainage must be accomplished through the chest wall. This operation usually is performed in several stages. Postoperative treatment is similar to that of a thoracotomy for empyema. In some cases the part of the lung containing the abscess may be removed (lobectomy).

Nursing Care

After drainage of an empyema or a lung abscess there is usually a somewhat prolonged period of drainage before the wound closes entirely. In many cases, it may be necessary for some person in the family to perform the simple dressings that will prevent excoriation of the skin and an offensive odor. Therefore, it is advisable frequently to give instructions in the method of dressing the wound and to demonstrate it. Often it is wise to see that these patients are placed under the supervision of a public health nurse or some community agency that will help the family to meet any problems that may arise as a result of the care and the needs of these patients.

BRONCHIECTASIS

Bronchiectasis is a pathologic dilatation of the bronchi. It occurs usually in one of the lower lobes or both of them. Often it develops from a chronic infection of the bronchial wall. The enlargement of the bronchi permits a collection in them of large amounts of exudate. The chief symptom of this condition, which may occur both in childhood and in adult life, is a chronic cough with large amounts of foul, purulent sputum. Often the sputum is blood-streaked and, as ulceration occurs in the infected cavity, hemorrhage may take place. As the disease goes on, a typical clubbing of the fingers is noted.

The diagnosis can be made on physical examination, but it is confirmed by x-ray examination of the chest made after radiopaque oil has been injected into the trachea. The dilated bronchial cavities are outlined by the injected material (bronchogram, p. 227).

Treatment. Conservative treatment such as postural drainage may give some measure of relief, but usually no permanent benefit can be expected except by surgical removal of the lung involved. It may be necessary to remove a segment of a lobe (segmental resection), a lobe (lobectomy) or an entire lung (pneumonectomy).

Segmental resection is the removal of an anatomic subdivision of a pulmonary lobe. The chief advantage is that only diseased tissue is removed, with greater conservation of healthy lung tissue. It usually is done for bronchiectasis. Bronchography aids in the delineation of the segment.

Postoperatively, 2 tubes from the chest of the patient are connected to water-seal controlled suction. Air from air leaks following segmental resection is removed by this method,

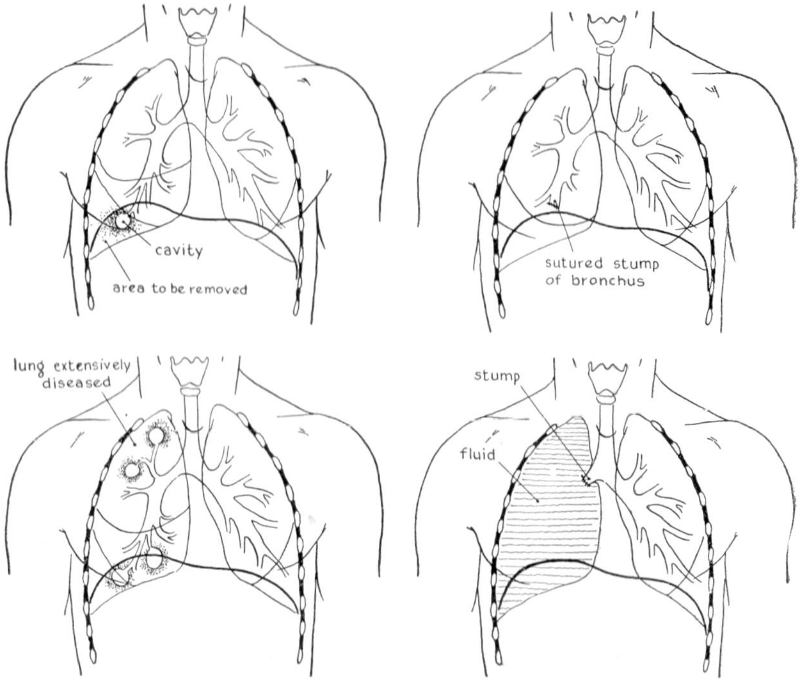

FIG. 93. Diagrammatic drawings show lobectomy and pneumonectomy for for lesions of the lung. The lesions shown are abscesses or tuberculous cavities, but the same operations may be done for bronchiectatic cavities or for lung tumors. (*Top, left*) Lesion in the lower lobe of the right lung and (*top, right*) appearance after lobectomy. (*Bottom, left*) Multiple areas of disease in the right lung. These may be tuberculous cavities, an abscess cavity, a bronchiectatic cavity, or a lung tumor. (*Bottom, right*) Appearance after removal of the entire lung–pneumonectomy.

and the remaining lung is maintained in a more expanded state. This is discontinued in 2 or 3 days. (Preoperative and postoperative nursing care for segmental resection is the same as for lobectomy and pneumonectomy, discussed later.)

CANCER OF THE LUNG

Tumors, both benign and malignant, are found in the lung, apparently with increasing frequency. These tumors appear to come from the lining membrane of the larger air passages and occur much more often in men of 40 years of age and beyond. Early symptoms are a cough and a wheeze. Then the tumor produces most commonly a chronic cough, often associated with pain or discomfort in the chest, some dyspnea on exertion and sputum that often contains streaks of blood. The diagnosis is made by a combination of diagnostic methods. Usually the roentgenogram shows a definite tumor mass, and by bronchoscopy one may remove sections of the tumor or examine the secretions for tumor cells.

Treatment. In the treatment of carcinoma of the lung, chronic diffuse suppuration of the lung, as in bronchiectasis, and sometimes lung abscess, it may be necessary to remove a lobe or all of one lung in order to remove the disease process. These operations are spoken of as *lobectomy* when only one lobe is removed or *pneumonectomy* when an entire lung is removed. (See Fig. 93.) Such operations are performed under endotracheal anesthesia; as a rule, a wide incision is made between the ribs to expose the pedicle of the lung. After the diseased tissue is removed, the chest wall is closed tightly and often a drainage tube is inserted into the pleural cavity. This tube may or may not be used for airtight suction or water seal drainage but, in any event, it must be kept airtight unless otherwise ordered. The surgeon may make an intrathoracic injection of penicillin and/or streptomycin in the postpneumonectomy patient for a few days.

NURSING CARE OF CHEST SURGICAL PATIENTS

Preoperative Care

In addition to a skillful operation, the success of chest surgery depends upon good preparation before operation and intelligent observation and nursing care after operation.

Psychological Aspects. Usually there are several days to the preoperative phase which provides time for the nurse to talk with her patient. By listening to him, she may be able to discover how he really feels about his illness and the proposed treatment. He may reveal significant reactions: the fear of hemorrhage because of bloody sputum, the discomfort of a chronic cough and chest pain, the social stigma attached to a foul-smelling sputum, the fear of death because of dyspnea —all contribute to his psychological make-up. The nurse can help him to overcome many of his fears by correcting any false impressions, by offering reassurance in the capability of the surgical team and by reporting special problems to the appropriate services available.

General Preparation. This is a general evaluation of the patient to determine and to correct any associated problems, such as metabolic disturbances, dehydration, cardiac impairments, etc. If he is malnourished and has a history of weight loss, naturally he will be placed on a high-caloric, high-protein diet reinforced with vitamins. He is encouraged to be up and about to maintain good muscle tone. Blood tests, including sedimentation rate, are done. The patient is told that he will be required to cough postoperatively and that it may hurt to do so. The nurse can emphasize the importance of bringing up secretions. She also can tell him that he may be receiving oxygen therapy and that this is routine to facilitate breathing. Also, blood transfusions may be given. He should know that such treatment does not necessarily mean that his condition is precarious.

Reduction of Organisms in Upper Respiratory Tract. MOUTH HYGIENE. Inasmuch as the mouth is a portal of entry for organisms into the respiratory tract, good oral care is a necessity. If the patient needs dental care, this should be reported to the physician. Brushing of the teeth must be done upon rising in the morning, after each meal and before retiring.

TOPICAL PENICILLIN. Penicillin in the form of a mist may be prescribed. Penicillin vapor can be produced by squeezing a rubber bulb of a glass or plastic nebulizer, or the nebulizer may be attached by means of a rubber tubing to an oxygen tank. The flow of oxygen is adjusted easily so as to produce the mist slowly. The patient must be instructed to keep his finger over the opening (through which penicillin is injected

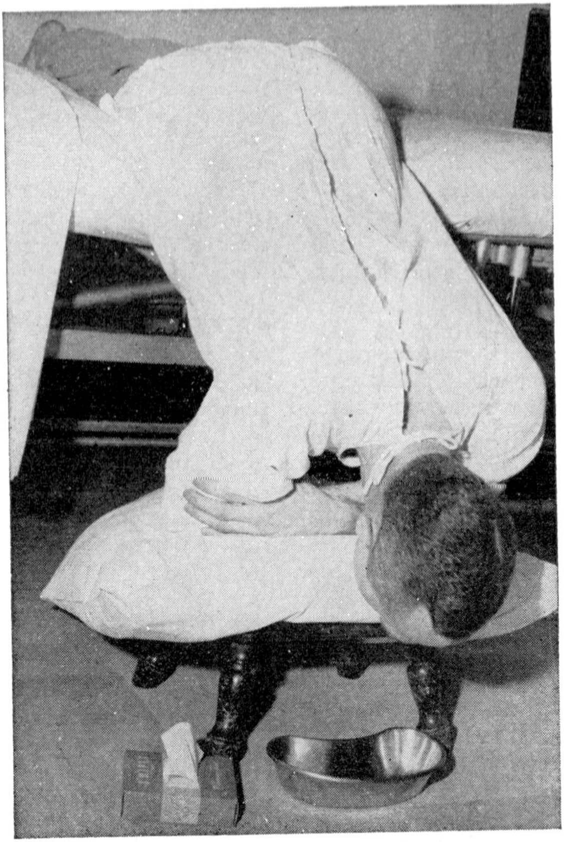

FIG. 94. Position for postural drainage: arms resting on pillow on footstool with thighs on bed.

into the nebulizer) while inspiring and to release his finger when exhaling so as to obtain the maximum effect.

Postural drainage may be indicated in bronchiectasis and other chest conditions to bring up excess secretions. A special tilt table can be used, or the patient may be placed in a prone position on the bed in such a way that the upper part of his body is over the edge of the bed. Postural drainage usually is done for about 5 to 10 minutes, 3 or 4 times a day, including immediately upon rising in the morning and before retiring at night. The patient should be encouraged to cough and expectorate as much sputum as possible into a receptacle in which it can be measured. The nurse should prevent the patient from becoming chilled or exhausted. If the sputum is foul-smelling, this procedure may well be carried out in a room away from other patients. Deodorizers should be used. Paper wipes and a bag for their disposition must be available. Following postural drainage, it is refreshing for the patient to brush his teeth and use a mouthwash; he then should rest in bed for a half hour.

Antibiotics and Chemotherapy. In addition to the above methods for reducing the number of organisms present, systemic antibiotic therapy and chemotherapy are used.

Immediate Preoperative Preparation. The night before surgery, the patient is given a mild sedative, after he has had the operative area shaved (see Fig. 11 B), and an enema, if ordered. The usual preparation immediately before surgery is done. In patients with suppurative diseases, atropine is withheld until postural drainage is done. Usually, chest surgical patients receive a larger amount of atropine than abdominal surgical patients, so that secretions are minimized.

The anesthetic is administered by the endotracheal technic, and one anesthetic or a combination of anesthetic agents is used.

Postoperative Nursing Care

Preparation of Room. While the patient is in the operating room the nurse has an opportunity to gather the equipment essential for postoperative care. The bed should be one that can be elevated to the Trendelenburg position. Oxygen by tent or nasal catheter should be ready. A thoracentesis set, as well as pneumothorax equipment, must be available.

If the patient is to have suction, this equipment should be ready and in working order. It is necessary that the drainage bottle and tubing to the patient be sterile, and that a minimum amount of tubing and glass connecting tubes are used. Paper wipes should be on the bedside table and a paper bag ready to be pinned to the side of the bed as a receptacle for soiled wipes. Mouth suction can be set up to remove secretions from the nose, the mouth and the throat.

Reception of the Patient. During transfer of the patient to the recovery room or the patient's unit, it is extremely important to note that a patent airway is maintained. The patient usually is supine with his head turned to the side to allow for secretions to drain. Blood pressure, pulse and respirations are taken every 15 minutes for 2 or 3 hours, then at 30-minute intervals for the next several hours. Usually, these vital signs are taken hourly during the first night. Oxygen therapy is administered by tent or nasal catheter. It is used only as long as necessary. Beyond this time, it retards early ambulation and discourages coughing.

Position of the Patient. Following the stabilization of the vital signs and the patient's return to consciousness, the head of his bed is elevated 30° to 45°. It is preferable not to use the Trendelenburg position because the elevation of the diaphragm may interfere with ventilation. Adequate blood replacement usually takes care of shock. On the other hand, some surgeons feel that the Trendelenburg position should be used not only to combat shock but to facilitate postural drainage. The best advice is to check with the surgeon responsible for the particular patient.

The pneumonectomy patient should be turned hourly from the back to the operated side and not turned directly onto his unoperated side. Turning to the unoperated side is contraindicated because of the possibility of the spread of infection and additional strain on the already overtaxed remaining lung.

The lobectomy patient usually can be turned from the back to either side; however, some surgeons prefer that the patient not lie on the operated side so that optimum lung expansion can take place on that side.

For individuals who have had a segmental or a wedge resection,

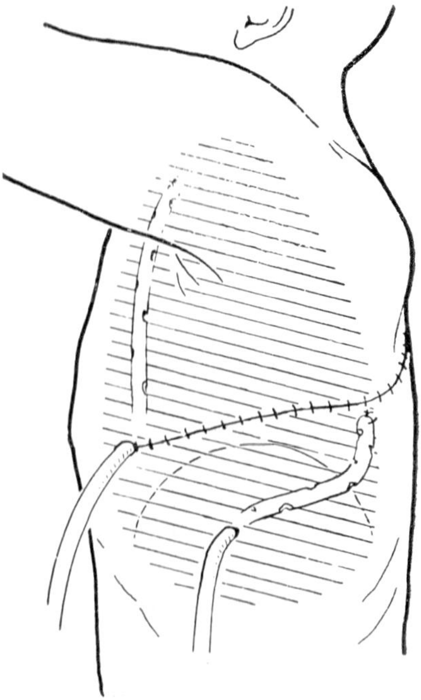

FIG. 95. Postoperative drainage of the chest. The upper drainage tube is used for the escape of air from leaks in the resected lung. The tip is anchored in the parietal pleura near the apex and brought out through the anterior end of the incision. The lower tube is usually for serosanguinous drainage. (Johnson, Julian, and Kirby, C. K.: Surgery of the Chest, p. 99, Chicago, Yr. Bk. Pub.)

lying on the operated side is contraindicated since it is desirable to have the remaining lung tissue on this side expand as much as possible. The use of a single Balkan frame, with hand trapeze, is a great help in moving the patient; it encourages

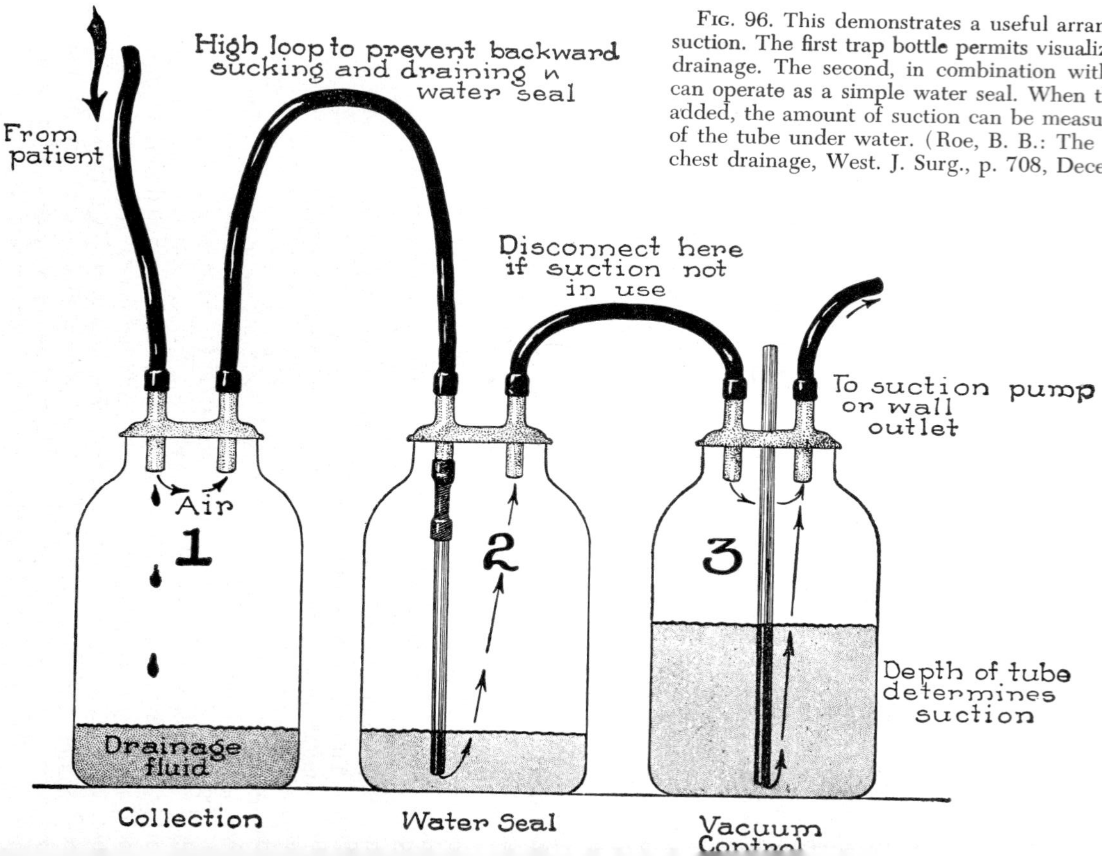

FIG. 96. This demonstrates a useful arrangement for chest suction. The first trap bottle permits visualization of the fluid drainage. The second, in combination with the first bottle, can operate as a simple water seal. When the third bottle is added, the amount of suction can be measured by the depth of the tube under water. (Roe, B. B.: The use and abuse of chest drainage, West. J. Surg., p. 708, December, 1953)

him to help himself and to move more frequently.

Pain and the Use of Narcotics. Narcotics are used judiciously for these patients. Certainly they must be individualized, for the threshold of pain varies from person to person. Many surgeons forbid the use of morphine in postoperative chest patients. On occasion, some of the intercostal nerves are injected or cut during the operation, thus reducing the problem of pain. The important point for the nurse to remember is that she wants her patient as comfortable as possible but does not want his cough reflex dulled.

Fluids and Nutrition. The patient usually receives a blood transfusion during the operation or immediately after it, and this is followed by an infusion. The rate of flow should not be greater than 50 to 60 gtt./min. (unless ordered by the physician) because of the danger of pulmonary edema. The early symptoms of such a complication are cyanosis, dyspnea, rales and bubbling sounds in the chest, as well as frothy sputum. Such a condition must be reported to the physician immediately. Clear fluids may be given when the patient has responded to treatment and when no nausea is present. The next day and thereafter he may have solid foods as desired.

Adequate Air Exchange. Immediately after operation, many of these patients receive oxygen as a supportive measure. This is essential because of his diminished respiratory reserve due to decreased lung volume, blood loss and reduced blood pressure. The quality of respirations must be noted by the nurse. Dyspnea, cyanosis and acute chest pain suggest a tension pneumothorax and they should be reported immediately. The treatment would be an aspiration of the chest or thoracentesis, for which the nurse should be prepared.

The use of the blow bottle can be dangerous to a patient who has had extensive surgery because of the fear of blowing out a ligated section of the bronchial tree. Therefore, a blow bottle should be used only when it has been ordered specifically by the physician.

Suction and Drainage. Catheters which are positioned strategically in the chest for postoperative connection to drainage bottles are placed there for two chief reasons: (1) to allow for the escape of air which otherwise might produce a pneumothorax, a shift of the mediastinum to the unoperated side or an emphysema and (2) to allow for the withdrawal of serosanguineous fluid (Figs. 95 and 96).

The important aspect of nursing attention is this: Be certain that the tubes are open. "Milking" the tubes will prevent plugging with clots or fibrin. Only enough suction tubing should be used to bridge the bottles and to extend to the wall and the patient, allowing leeway for the patient to turn. Excess tubing can be tripped over and often is caught behind the bed. The system should be airtight, with no kinks in the tubing. A safety pin or a clip is effective in securing drainage tubing to the draw sheet. A trough can be made with the draw sheet so that the tubing is nestled and the safety pin does not constrict the tubing. Abdominal pads or small pillows round the tube to make a trough also will help.

The color, the consistency and the amount of drainage should be charted at least every 24 hours. In closed suction it is important to clamp the suction tubing before removing the drainage bottle to measure the contents.

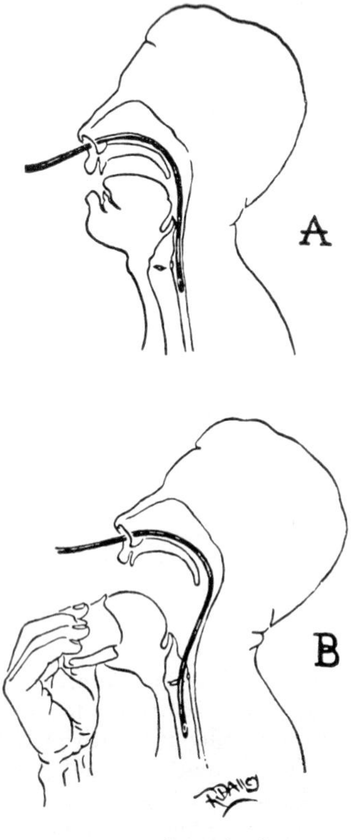

Fig. 97. Endotracheal aspiration. (A) Shows the tendency of the catheter normally to pass into the esophagus. (B) With the tongue and the epiglottis drawn forward, the plane of the glottic opening is more horizontally inclined, permitting ready passage of the catheter into the trachea. (Lindskog, G. E., and Liebow, A. A.: Thoracic Surgery and Related Pathology, p. 618, New York, Appleton)

Usually the catheters are removed in 2 or 3 days, providing that the remaining lung tissue is well expanded, that air leaks are eliminated and that the total fluid drainage is less than 75 cc. daily. Pneumonectomy patients usually do not have chest suction and drainage; however, if used, it is similar to that described.

When drainage tubes are removed, the surgeon withdraws the tube as the patient exhales. A 2 x 2 gauze sponge is applied quickly and made airtight with adhesive taped snugly. Some surgeons use petrolatum gauze rather than a dry dressing. Since the procedure is moderately painful, it is often done 30 minutes after morphine sulfate has been given.

The Removal of Retained Secretions. This is undoubtedly the most important aspect of postoperative nursing care in the chest patient. It is imperative that he cough strongly enough to bring up secretions. He usually is taught to do this preoperatively and knows that he will have pain. By splinting the chest anteriorly and posteriorly with her forearms or the palms of her hands, the nurse can give support to the wound. The danger in retaining secretions is that of atelectasis and pneumonia. When mucus is thick and tenacious, steam inhalations may help. If the nurse is unsuccessful in getting her patient to bring up secretions or if he refuses to cough, an

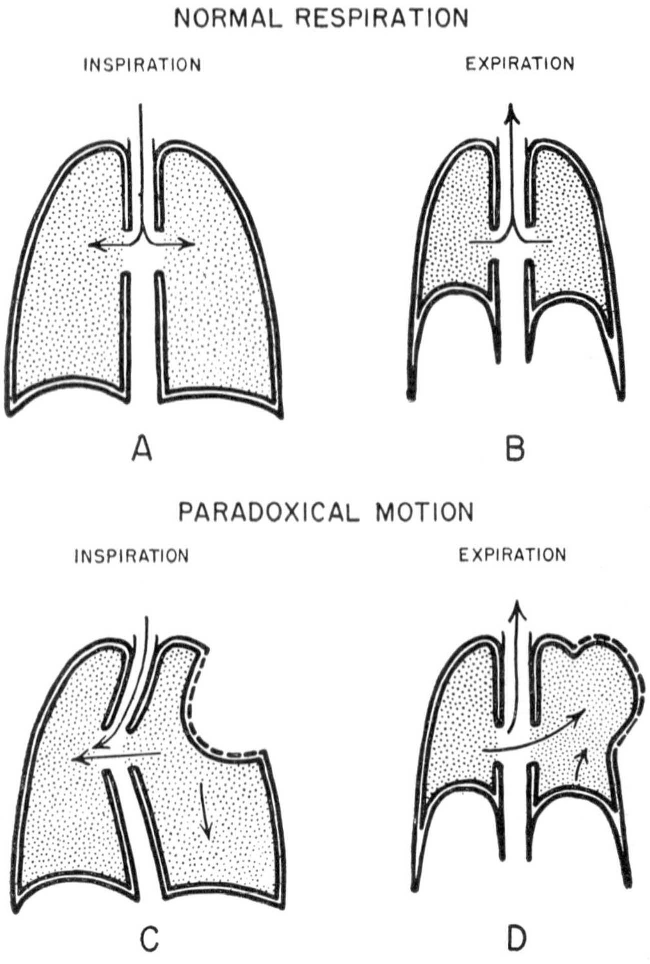

FIG. 98. (A and B) Normally, on inspiration all portions of the thoracic cage move outward, and the diaphragms move downward. Motion is in the opposite direction on expiration. (C and D) When a portion of the chest wall becomes flexible as a result of losing its bony support, motion of the flexible area is controlled by the changing intrapleural pressures and is in a direction opposite to that of the normal positions of the chest wall. (Johnson, Julian, and Kirby, C. K.: Surgery of the Chest, p. 21, Chicago, Yr. Bk. Pub.)

endotracheal aspiration must be done. Usually the surgeon does this; however, in many hospitals, this is becoming a nurse's responsibility.

ENDOTRACHEAL ASPIRATION. A No. 16 rubber catheter, wall or electric suction, a square of gauze, tissue wipes and an emesis basin are all that is required for this procedure. The patient is instructed to sit upright. When he protrudes his tongue, it is grasped with a dry piece of gauze and pulled forward gently. Then the tube is advanced through the nose until it reaches the glottis. Then the patient is instructed to inhale or cough, and the catheter is passed quickly into the trachea (Fig. 97). Inability of the patient to produce vocal sounds distinctly is the best evidence that the catheter is in the trachea. Then the catheter is connected to gentle suction. The catheter should be moved slowly up and down the trachea. The chief value of endotracheal aspiration is that it stimulates the cough reflex and produces violent coughing.

Complications. *Atelectasis, emphysema,* and *tension pneumothorax* have already been mentioned. In patients in which three or more ribs have been removed, there is a possibility of paradoxical chest motion.

Paradoxical chest motion can occur when the integrity of any portion of the thoracic bellows is lost, such as multiple rib fractures or removal of several ribs as in a thoracoplasty (Fig. 98). The nurse should observe chest movements of her thoracic surgical patients. Upon detecting paradoxical motion, she should report it immediately, for if uncorrected, it may result in serious respiratory and circulatory impairment. Treatment usually consists of firm adhesive strapping of the chest with the application of pads or a sandbag for further support. In some instances a type of skeletal traction may be employed to keep the chest wall from collapsing.

In general, the signs and the symptoms which should be reported to the surgeon immediately are cyanosis, dyspnea, pallor, acute chest pain, increase in pulse and respiratory rates, temperature elevation over 99° F., systolic blood pressure reading below 90 mm. and evidence of hemorrhage on the dressings.

Early Ambulation and Convalescence. If shock has been prevented adequately and the patient does not have heart disease or a limited cardiovascular reserve, he may get out of bed the evening of or the day after surgery. Drainage tubes and bottles may hinder this somewhat.

Breathing and postural exercises recommended by the surgeon and physical therapist are begun a day or two after surgery to produce better lung ventilation, to restore motion and muscle tonus in the shoulder girdle and trunk and to maintain normal posture.

Roentgenograms are taken frequently to determine the patient's progress. If air or fluid accumulates in the chest, it will be necessary to aspirate by means of a thoracentesis.

For patients who have had surgery for lung cancer, the nurse will refer to the chapter on cancer nursing, p. 195.

Rehabilitative plans are made by the surgeon, the nurse, the patient, his family, the physical therapist and

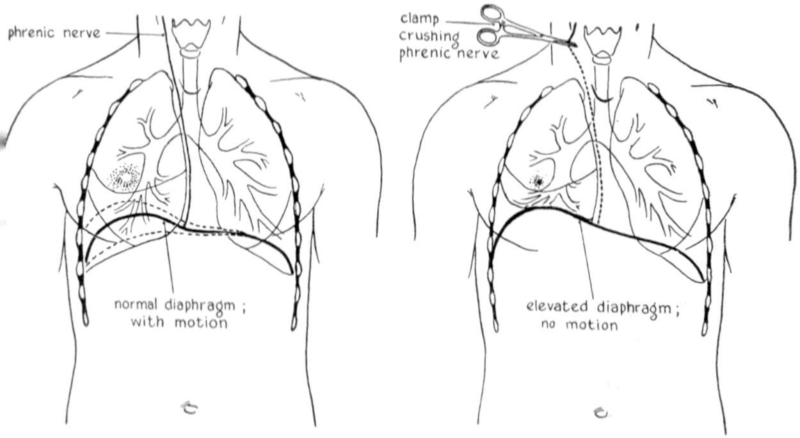

FIG. 99. Diagrams show tuberculous cavity in the right lung treated by phrenic crush. (*Left*) Cavity shown in the middle of the right lung. The dotted lines represent the excursion of the diaphragm. (*Right*) Result after crushing the phrenic nerve in the neck. The diaphragm is elevated on the corresponding side, thus collapsing the cavity and permitting healing by setting the lung at rest.

he medical social worker. The nurse vill find the following points helpful n her suggestions to the patient:

1. Practice deep breathing exer-ises for the first few weeks at home.
2. Practice good body alignment y standing up straight with shoul-lers held back [preferably in front f a full-length mirror].
3. Practice exercises that he did vhile in the hospital.
4. Practice good oral hygiene by rushing teeth well and visiting his lentist frequently.
5. Remain away from crowds dur-ng upper respiratory epidemics.
6. Seek medical attention at the nset of an upper respiratory infec-ion.
7. Avoid areas where the air is illed with dust, smoke, and irritating hemicals.
8. Avoid anything which may cause spasms of coughing.
9. Maintain good nutrition.
10. Obtain adequate rest.*

SURGERY OF THE MEDIASTINUM

The mediastinum, or the space in the chest between the two pleural cavities, often has to be attacked surgically for infections, tumors, cysts and, occasionally, an enlargement of the thyroid gland. As a rule, the approach to these lesions is through the chest wall; consequently, the pleura usually is opened. The preoperative and postoperative precautions and nursing care previously discussed should be observed.

* Adapted from Bickford and Budd: Pulmonary resection. 2. Nursing care, Am. J. Nursing **52**:43, 1952.

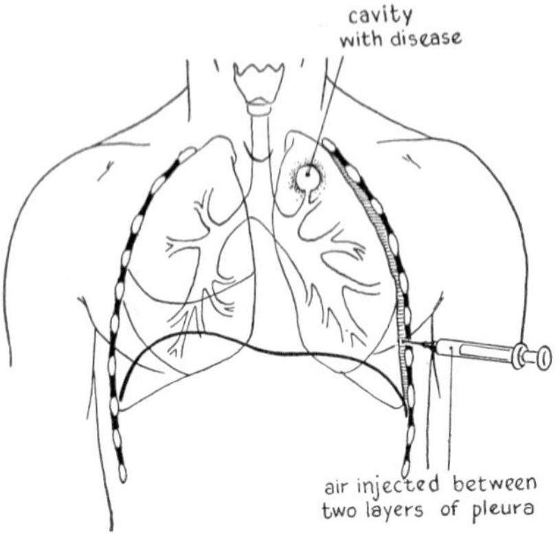

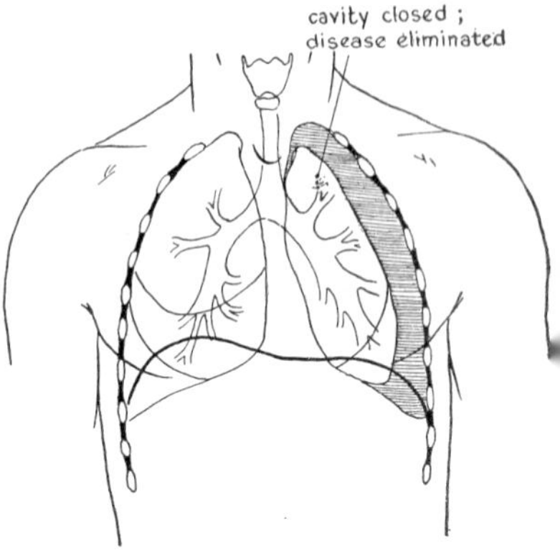

FIGS. 100 and 101. Pneumothorax. Semidiagrammatic drawing to show tuberculous cavity in the upper part of the left lobe.

FIG. 100 (*Left*). The needle is introduced between the ribs to inject air into the pleural cavity.

FIG. 101 (*Right.*) Collapse of the lung is effected by the introduction of air into the pleural cavity. Note that the cavity in the lung has been collapsed in this way, the lung is at rest and healing is permitted.

SURGERY IN PULMONARY TUBERCULOSIS

Pulmonary tuberculosis is more common than any other form of infection caused by the tubercle bacillus. Optimum benefits are obtained when the patient is rested, both physically and mentally. When this is achieved, defense mechanisms are better able to cope with the infecting organism. The treatment of this disease is predominantly medical. However, many times the disease has spread to such an extent that more drastic means of securing needed rest for the affected lung must be employed. For the most part, these are considered surgical procedures and they may have a temporary or a permanent effect. The usual temporary procedures are phrenic nerve paralysis, artificial pneumothorax and pneumoperitoneum. Permanent procedures are thoracoplasty and pulmonary resection. Drainage, such as cavernostomy, is used only in poor operative risks or in patients who have advanced, bilateral disease.

PHRENIC NERVE OPERATIONS

The lung involved may be placed partially at rest by paralyzing the diaphragm on the side involved. Temporary paralysis (6 to 15 months) is achieved by crushing the nerve (emphraxis), and permanent paralysis is produced by avulsion (exeresis) or partial excision of the nerve. The paralysis produced by blocking the nerve impulses to the diaphragm in this way causes this muscular structure to rise in the chest and to remain nearly motionless during the act of respiration. In this way the lung involved is placed at rest because tension on the lung tissue is lessened, and healing of the tuberculous process is favored (Fig. 99).

Artificial Pneumothorax

The same end is accomplished frequently by the introduction of air into the pleural cavity by a needle inserted through the chest wall (Fig. 100). The air is introduced carefully under sterile precautions in measured amounts and under measured pressure. Thus expansion of the lung is prevented by pressure from without, and a more or less complete collapse of the tuberculous cavities is produced. In this way the patient's cough and sputum are reduced, and the lung is kept at partial rest, thereby assisting in the healing process. At first, a small amount of air is injected (300 to 500 cc.) and thereafter it is increased until the desired collapse has been achieved to bring the disease under control. This procedure is known as *pneumothorax*. Since this is a temporary measure because the air is absorbed eventually, the patient returns for "refills."

Nursing Care

The patient usually has a sedative before the first pneumothorax. Some surgeons require that the chest be shaved. The skin is prepared with an antiseptic, and a blunt-pointed needle is inserted into the pleural space. The needle is attached to a syringe until the space is entered. Then the syringe is removed, and the pneumothorax machine is connected. A manometric pressure reading is noted and recorded by the nurse. In the common type of pneumothorax apparatus, 2 water bottles are connected by means of rubber tubing. As one bottle is elevated, fluid flows by gravity into the lower bottle. A measured amount of air in the lower bottle consequently is displaced and flows into the pleural space. Throughout the procedure, the nurse must observe the patient's color, pulse and general reaction. Any changes should be reported to the physician immediately. When the treatment is completed, he is moved carefully to his bed and turned on the affected side. Any signs of increasing dyspnea, discomfort or sudden pain, cyanosis or hemoptysis should be reported immediately, as they may indicate a spontaneous or tension pneumothorax. (See p. 231.)

Pneumoperitoneum

This is the injection of air into the peritoneal cavity to collapse a lung or the lungs. It is of most value in the treatment of bilateral tuberculosis. When used in unilateral disease, it may be combined with a phrenic emphraxis. In this combination, the injected air will accumulate under the relaxed paralyzed diaphragm, causing a collapse of the diseased lung. Pneumoperitoneum is not a procedure to replace all other forms of collapse therapy; rather, it is a technic that can be used successfully in selected cases.

The chief nursing problem is to teach patients and convince them that collapse therapies are given in addition to and not in place of bed rest. Ordinarily, after this procedure, patients do not complain of a sense of fullness in the abdomen. The sensation is not of a distended and tight

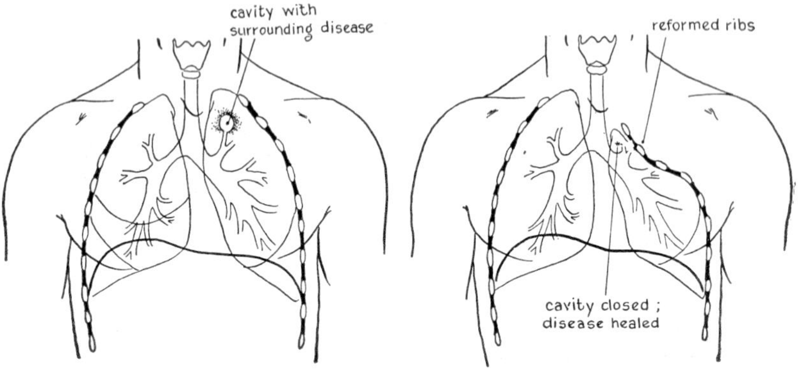

FIG. 102. Thoracoplasty. Semidiagrammatic drawings show method of collapsing the lung cavity by thoracoplasty. (*Left*) Cavity shown in the upper lobe. (*Right*) Collapse of the cavity effected by upper rib thoracoplasty.

abdomen as is true when air is within the intestinal tract. There should be no discomfort in breathing, moving about or walking. Occasionally, a patient may complain of nausea, dizziness, abdominal distention and pain in the shoulder.

Pneumonolysis and Apicolysis

Almost half of the individuals in whom pneumothorax is tried have an unsatisfactory collapse because of pleural adhesions. By using a thoracoscope, the adhesions can be cut by a cautery. This is called *pneumonolysis.* If the adhesions are confined to the apex of the lung, the procedure is called *apicolysis.* Following this procedure, which usually is done under local anesthesia, the patient is kept at complete rest. He is not to lie on the operated side. Coughing is to be discouraged because of the dangers of producing a traumatic pneumothorax. Subcutaneous emphysema may develop, which is uncomfortable but gradually disappears without further treatment.

Thoracoplasty

The collapse of the lung produced by the above-mentioned procedures is frequently of such temporary or partial nature that a more radical and complete attack must be made upon the diseased lung or section of the lung. This is accomplished by *thoracoplasty,* an operation in which the bony framework of the chest wall is removed over wide areas to permit a permanent collapse of the lung (Fig. 102). This operation often is performed in several stages. As a rule, 3 ribs are resected in each stage. These patients are selected carefully after submitting to studies to determine the adequacy of the remaining lung, the condition of the heart and the nutritional level of the patient. The number of stages necessary depends upon the patient's general condition, the extent of the lesion and the amount of collapse achieved with each. Usually from 10 to 14 days elapse between each stage because of the high mortality rate if extensive rib resection is done at one time.

Preoperative Nursing Care

An understanding of the mental problems of this patient is essential. When one realizes that he usually has a history of illness of a year or more, that he may have been in a sanatorium for a long while, and that he probably has had his hopes raised innumerable times only to be blasted when therapy failed, one is more tolerant of his reactions. He must be made to realize that a thoracoplasty is not an immediate cure, and that convalescence is slow. The socio-economic factors cannot be neglected. In addition to the preoperative and the postoperative care described on p. 238, the patient usually is on isolation precautions. Some physicians prefer to have their patients raise as much sputum as possible about one half hour before operation. This may be done by postural drainage or by coughing voluntarily. The shaving of the chest and the remaining preparation is the same as that for other chest surgical patients.

Postoperative Nursing Care

Postoperative care is directed toward preventing many possible

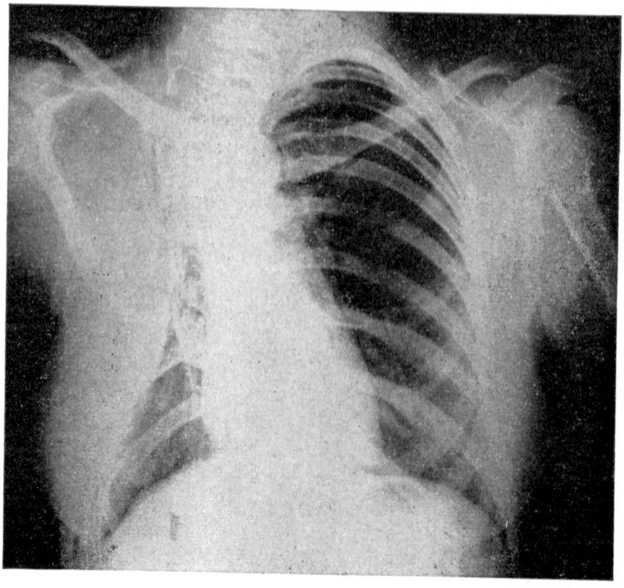

FIG. 103. Roentgenogram showing patient with right-sided thoracoplasty. Note the complete collapse of the right lung effected by the operation.

complications—for example, shock, hemorrhage, respiratory and circulatory collapse, paradoxical motion, the spread of infection, wound infection and deformity. The patient is kept in the Trendelenburg position until he is conscious and his vital signs are satisfactory. He should be turned from his back to the operated side every second hour and encouraged to cough in an effort to bring up secretions. Often the tight adhesive strapping is not sufficient to allay the patient's fears when he coughs, and it is necessary for the nurse to splint the wound with the palm of her hand or her forearm. During this postoperative period, the nurse must be on the alert for signs that suggest a retention of secretions such as "wet" inspirations and expirations after coughing, increasing dyspnea and a temperature elevation. If this occurs, the physician should be notified and an endotracheal aspiration tray made available. Every effort must be exerted to prevent atelectasis, not only because of the resultant obstruction of a portion of the lung but also because of the likelihood of spread of infection.

Paradoxical motion is one of the complications that can occur in the postoperative thoracoplasty patient (see Fig. 98). By applying external pressure, this phenomenon can be controlled. Sandbags that weigh about 5 lb. can be applied beneath the clavicle. Unfortunately, they are cumbersome and difficult to keep in place. Some surgeons prefer to apply thick gauze pads beneath the clavicle and in the axilla. They are held in place by 2-inch adhesive strips applied over the back and the shoulders so that skin tension will be distributed widely. Blistering from adhesive must be guarded against.

Physical Therapy and Convalescence. Passive and then active movements of the arm on the affected side should be started on the day of operation and continued after that on instructions from the physician and the physical therapist. Proper body posture with adequate support of the back, the shoulders and the arm must be maintained. A Balkan frame with a trapezelike bar provides an excellent means for the patient to move in bed with a desirable amount of exercise. Often the patient favors the operated side by lifting the arm with the opposite hand, by rotating the trunk instead of the head and by drooping his shoulder protectively. Without a doubt this leads to scoliosis and a crippling posture, and it must be prevented. In all efforts at rehabilitation, the patient must express a desire and a willingness to help himself. After the second or the third stage of thoracoplasty, a small, firm pillow may be placed in the axilla on the operated side. This will increase collapse of the thoracic wall and prevent scoliosis. Some physicians prefer to have the patient use a chest sling, which is a piece of canvas from about 12 to 15 inches wide and 3 feet long. A hammock is formed to encase the patient as he lies on his operated side. By counteracting weights (pulley system) he is lifted from the bed, thus utilizing body weight to produce further collapse. He remains in this position

:or only a few minutes at first, after which the time gradually is increased :o 30 minutes 3 times a day.

The successful care of this patient ncludes special emphasis on good nouth hygiene, plenty of fresh air, adequate nutrition, proper exercise and an optimistic frame of mind. Diversional occupational therapy :hat is prescribed carefully is essen-·ial because of the long period of essentially inactive convalescence. Usually this rehabilitative and "rest-ng" stage is spent in the sanatorium.

Pulmonary Resection in Tuberculosis

Pulmonary resection is gaining in-:reasing favor for several reasons. It s being recognized that reversible orms of collapse therapy are at-ended by a high incidence of serious complications, such as artificial pneu-nothorax. The results of thoraco-plasty are revealing that lesions do not heal and that sputum is not con-verted in many cases. Pulmonary esection is becoming increasingly safer as a result of improved anes-hesia, better operative technic and he effectiveness of streptomycin and para-aminosalicylic acid. The indica-ions for wedge resection, segmental esection, lobectomy or pneumonec-omy are dependent upon many fac-ors. When prescribed, the nursing care is the same as that described on pp. 238-247.

Thoracoplasty with Pulmonary Resection

When lobectomy or pneumonec-omy is performed for tuberculosis, ome surgeons prefer to do a thora-coplasty in 3 to 6 weeks. In unusu-ally good operative risks, these pro-cedures can be done at the same time. The purpose of doing a rib resection is to prevent overdisten-tion of the remaining lung tissue. The possibility of bronchopleural fis-tula and tuberculous empyema is lessened. Usually 4 ribs are removed following lobectomy and 6 or 7 fol-lowing pneumonectomy.

Streptomycin and Para-aminosalicylic Acid

Surgery for tuberculosis has been made safer with streptomycin and para-aminosalicylic acid (PAS). The limiting factors with regard to the use of streptomycin are its toxic manifestations and the development of resistance to the tubercle bacillus. Present-day therapy suggests that when 1 Gm. of streptomycin is given intramuscularly 2 or 3 times a week with 12 Gm. of PAS daily (oral), these limitations are reduced sig-nificantly. Dihydrostreptomycin can be substituted for streptomycin if toxic effects are produced by the latter. The length of therapy is 3 or 4 months before thoracoplasty or pulmonary resection, followed by 4 or more months postoperatively.

DECORTICATION OF THE LUNG

Decortication is the surgical re-moval of fibrinous deposit on the pleura which prevents re-expansion of the lung and has resulted from prolonged pneumothorax and tuber-culous empyema. It is done in se-lected cases when there is little like-lihood of reactivation of the disease and where healthy lung tissue can be re-expanded. The care preoperatively and postoperatively is the same as that described in "Nursing Care of Chest Surgical Patients," page 238.

REFERENCES AND SUGGESTED READING

Unit Two: Nursing in Conditions of the Respiratory System

Throat

Conley, J. J.: Tracheotomy, Am. J. Nursing **52**:1078-1081, 1952.

Emerson, C. P., and Bragdon, J. S.: Essentials of Medicine, ed. 17, pp. 162-164 (tonsils); pp. 164-165 (adenoids); pp. 166-167 (tumors), Philadelphia, Lippincott, 1955.

Greene, J. S.: Speech rehabilitation following laryngectomy, Am. J. Nursing **49**:153-154, 1949.

Hall, J. T., and Sadler, J. B.: Nursing care in tonsillectomy and adenoidectomy, Am. J. Nursing **47**:537-539, 1947.

Holmquist, E. W.: Nursing the adult tracheotomized patient, Am. J. Nursing **47**:310-314, 1947.

Martin, Hayes, and Ehrlich, H. E.: Nursing care following laryngectomy, Am. J. Nursing **49**:149-152, 1949.

Chest Conditions

general

Berlin, Ingebord: Lobectomy (a nursing care study), Am. J. Nursing **48**:720-723, 1948.

Bickford, E., and Budd, E.: Pulmonary resection. 2. Nursing care, Am. J. Nursing **52**:40-42, 1952.

Bugden, W. F.: Pulmonary resection, Am. J. Nursing **52**:38-39, 1952.

Emerson, C. P., and Bragdon, J. S.: Essentials of Medicine, ed. 17, pp. 187-188 (empyema); pp. 188-191 (lung abscess); pp. 191-19[illegible] (bronchiectasis); pp. 196-19[illegible] (lung cancer), Philadelphia, Lippincott, 1955.

Harris, H. W.: What do you know about coughing?, Am. J. Nursing **53**:162-163, 1953.

Johnson, A. F., and Heffernan, Harriet: Penicillin aerosol therapy, Am. J. Nursing **46**:834-837, 1946.

Johnson, J., and Kirby, C. K.: Surgery of the Chest, Chicago, Yr. Bk. Pub., 1952.

Lacy, M., and Hitchcock, M. O.: Retained secretions following thoracic surgery, Am. J. Nursing **51**:607-609, 1951.

Lindnuff, F. S.: Physical therapy and chest surgery, Physiotherapy Rev. **27**:94-100, 1947.

Lindskog, G. E., and Liebow, A. A.: Thoracic Surgery and Related Pathology, New York, Appleton, 1953.

Poppe, J. K., and James, R. B.: Intratracheal suctioning, Am. J. Nursing **45**:538-540, 1945.

Roe, B. B.: The use and abuse of chest drainage, West. J. Surg. p. 706, December, 1953.

Rothwell, B. C.: Nursing care in pulmonary edema, Am. J. Nursing **48**:700-701, 1948.

Smith, B. G.: Spontaneous pneumothorax, Am. J. Nursing **43**:553-557, 1943.
Taylor, B. I.: Taking food and fluids through a tube, Am. J. Nursing **53**:303-305, 1953.

SURGERY FOR TUBERCULOSIS

Arnason, T.: Tuberculosis in older persons, Am. J. Nursing **46**:317-319, 1946.
Bosworth, H. W.: The care and education of the tuberculosis patient, Am. J. Nursing **46**:764-766, 1946.
Ellison, B. M.: Nursing care in collapse therapy, Am. J. Nursing **50**: 473-475, 1950.
Emerson, C. P., and Bragdon, J. S.: Essentials of Medicine, ed. 17, pp. 792-814 (tuberculosis); pp. 794-804 and pp. 811-814 (pulmonary tuberculosis), Philadelphia, Lippincott, 1955.
Hetherington, H. W., and Eshleman, F. W.: Nursing in the Prevention and Control of Tuberculosis, pp. 112-140, New York, Putnam, 1950.
Hornbein, R., and Patterson, W.: Tuberculosis—a social and emotional problem, Am. J. Nursing **47**:376-381, 1947.
Keill, K.: The emotions in tuberculosis, Am. J. Nursing **47**:601-602, 1947.
Lincoln, L.: Thoracoplasty—nursing care, Am. J. Nursing **44**:1022-1027, 1944.
Lurie, M. B.: Control of airborne contagion of tuberculosis, Am. J. Nursing **46**:808-810, 1946.
Moyer, R. E., Sears, L. H., and Williams, M. H.: Pneumoperitoneum, Am. J. Nursing **53**:332-335, 1953.
Riley, A. O., and Longhurst, G. M.: Pulmonary decortication, Am. J. Nursing **52**:878-880, 1952.
Tebrock, H. E., Fisher, M. M., and Mamlok, E. R.: The new drug—Isoniazid, Am. J. Nursing **52**: 1342-1344, 1952.

CLINICAL SITUATION: PULMONARY RESECTION

Jennifer Wainscote passed her twenty-fourth birthday in the Westgate Sanatorium and now, 6 months later, is about to have a pulmonary resection. She has had pneumothorax and phrenic emphraxis on the left side for pulmonary tuberculosis.

1. The usual procedure for a pneumothorax is to

____(1) inject approximately 300 cc. of air beneath the diaphragm
____(2) aspirate fluid from the pleural cavity and replace volume per volume with air
____(3) inject a measured amount of air into the pleura under measured pressure

2. Postural drainage is most effective when the area to be drained is

____(1) high in the apex of the lung
____(2) in the lower part of the lung

3. Symptoms of tension pneumothorax are

____(1) elevated pulse rate, cyanosis, apprehension
____(2) dyspnea, acute chest pain, cyanosis

_____(3) increased pulse pressure, dyspnea, hemoptysis

4. The purpose(s) of a water seal in segmental resection is (are) to prevent

_____(1) emphysema
_____(2) pneumothorax
_____(3) atelectasis
_____(4) spread of infection

5. In paradoxical motion

A. the thoracic cage moves

_____(1) outward on inspiration
_____(2) inward on inspiration
_____(3) inward on expiration
_____(4) outward on expiration

B. the diaphragm moves

_____(1) downward on inspiration
_____(2) upward on inspiration
_____(3) upward on expiration
_____(4) downward on expiration

6. Postoperatively Jennifer should be

_____(1) encouraged to cough
_____(2) discouraged from coughing

7. The reason for the response in Question 6 is that coughing

_____(1) strains the vulnerable suture line
_____(2) produces pain and increases demand for narcotic
_____(3) produces greater exchange between carbon dioxide and oxygen in the alveol

8. A p.r.n. narcotic for Jennifer should be used

_____(1) liberally
_____(2) sparingly, if at all
_____(3) as frequently as for any postoperative patient

9. The reasons for the answer to Question 8 is that narcotics

_____(1) decrease respiratory frequency
_____(2) increase respiratory frequency
_____(3) decrease cough reflex
_____(4) increase cough reflex

UNIT THREE

Nursing in Conditions of the Circulatory System, the Blood and the Blood-forming Organs

CHAPTER FOURTEEN

Surgery of the Heart and the Blood Vessels

A number of important advances have been made during recent years in the field of cardiovascular surgery. Better anesthesia, a wider range of diagnostic methods and a more thorough understanding of the underlying physiologic mechanisms have been responsible largely for these improvements.

DIAGNOSTIC AIDS

Angiocardiography. By the injection of a radiopaque dye, about 40 cc. for adults, into the vessels of the arm, x-ray visualization of the right heart and the great vessels may be obtained. This is an excellent method of study of abnormalities of these vessels and is especially important in demonstrating congenital and acquired malformations of the right heart, as well as pericardial and mediastinal lesions.

Catheterization of the Heart and the Great Vessels. A radiopaque catheter may be inserted through the

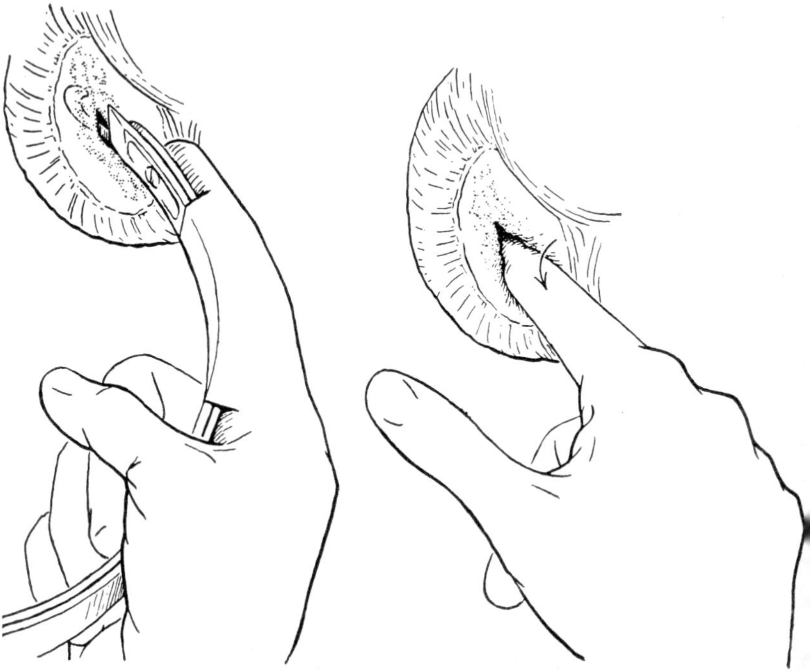

FIG. 104. Mitral Commissurotomy. (*Left*) A drawing of the special knife used in cutting commissures. The surgeon wears two gloves on his operating hand; the outer glove is cut in two places to accommodate the knife. (*Right*) Illustrates the finger fracture method of breaking the fibrous bands at the ends of the mitral valve. (Johnson, J., and Kirby, C. K.: Surgery of the Chest, p. 329, Chicago, Yr. Bk. Pub.)

veins of the arm and into the right side of the heart and the pulmonary artery. By this method, blood samples may be tested for oxygen, and other components and pressure readings may be taken. In addition, through catheters inserted into the various arteries (right and left brachial, left common carotid, femoral) radiopaque material may be injected to demonstrate abnormalities of the aorta and the other great vessels. Finally, direct injection through a needle into the aorta is carried out frequently in the lumbar region to demonstrate renal circulation and other abnormalities such as aneurysm and thrombosis of the lower aorta.

SURGERY OF THE HEART

Wounds of the heart, if they are large, may end rapidly in death from bleeding into the pleura or externally. Smaller wounds, such as stab or small caliber bullet wounds, may be less rapidly fatal, and death is due not so much to loss of blood as to interference with cardiac function by blood collected in the pericardial cavity. This is called *cardiac tamponade,* and it is characterized by a weak cardiac beat and consequent fall in blood pressure. Early recognition of the difficulty and prompt operative intervention—evacuating the blood in the pericardial cavity and suturing the heart wound—result often in prompt recovery.

Chronic constrictive pericarditis is a chronic inflammatory thickening of the pericardium with an obliteration of the pericardial space. Often the adherent pericardium may become calcified. The heart action is much embarrassed by this tough, unyielding enclosure, and edema, ascites and hepatic enlargement result. The fixation of the heart to the pericardium produces often a retraction of the chest wall with every heartbeat. Surgical removal of the constricting diseased pericardium is the only treatment of any benefit. This is done by cutting away the overlying costal cartilages and excising carefully the thickened covering of the heart.

Commissurotomy for Mitral Stenosis. In mitral stenosis due to rheumatic fever, often there is thickening and fusion of the commissures. In selected cases, it is possible to free these commissures surgically by fracturing them with the surgeon's index finger (finger fracture method) or by cutting them with a special knife (Fig. 104).

In doing this surgery, it is necessary for the pleura and the pericardium to be opened after making an incision through the third or the fourth interspace. Procaine is infiltrated around the base of the left auricular appendage, and a purse-string suture is applied. When the tip of the appendage is excised, the surgeon is able to insert his finger; by tightening the purse-string suture there is little blood loss while the surgeon fractures or cuts the commissures. When the surgeon withdraws his finger, immediately the purse-string suture is closed tightly.

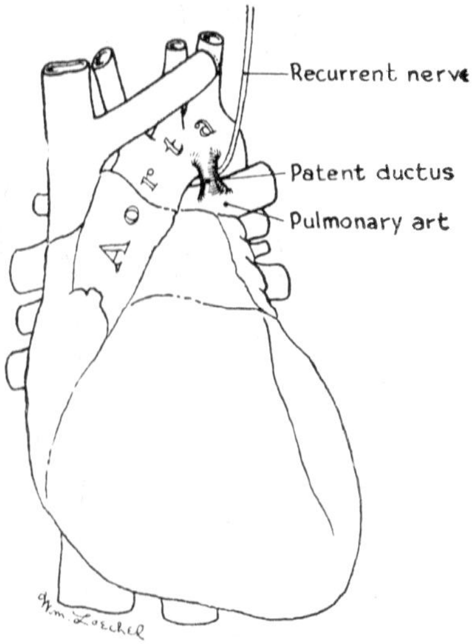

Fig. 105. Diagrammatic drawing of the heart and the great vessels, showing patent ductus arteriosus. This is a congenital communication between the aorta and the pulmonary artery. It closes as a rule. However, when it remains open, often it is necessary to close it surgically.

Nursing Care

Preoperatively and postoperatively, the nursing care is similar to

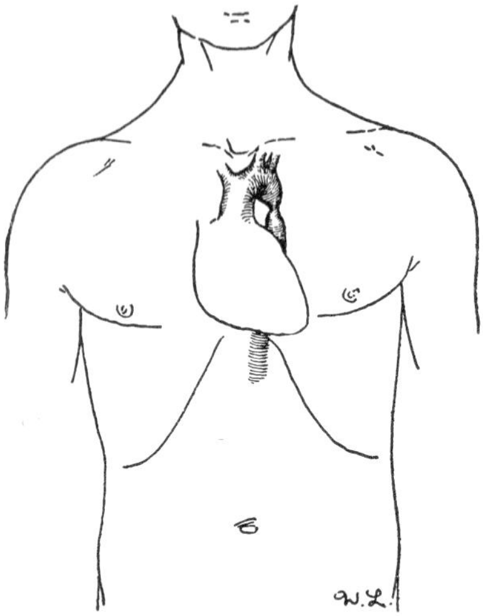

FIG. 106. Diagrammatic view to show the narrowing of the aorta in the usual position found in coarctation of the aorta.

that of chest surgical patients. Before surgery, the patient may be digitalized. Vital signs are recorded for postoperative comparison. Usually, this individual looks toward his proposed operation with optimism inasmuch as he has experienced a long session of restrictions, which may have included hemiplegia.

Postoperatively, oxygen therapy, blood transfusions and chest suction will be used. Vital signs are taken every 15 minutes until stable. A thoracentesis and tracheotomy set are available for emergency use.

Upon returning to consciousness, the patient is turned from his back to the unoperated side. The operated side is contraindicated because it will interfere with lung expansion and it may cause herniation of the heart from its pericardial sac. Coughing is encouraged to bring up secretions; the wound is splinted for support during this maneuver. Sedatives are given for the first 3 or 4 days because the patient has pain. Diet is increased as tolerated. Usually, the patient is out of bed by the fifth day and ready for discharge by the tenth day.

A striking postoperative reaction in many of these patients is an emotional depression accompanied by a definite personality change. The reason for its occurrence is not known, but gradually the patient "comes out of it."

SURGERY OF THE GREAT VESSELS

Patent Ductus Arteriosus (Fig. 105). Normally in fetal life the ductus arteriosus is open between the pulmonary artery and the arch of the aorta, such being essential to life in utero. This should close soon after birth but, if closure does not occur, the patient usually will show signs of abnormal existence in the form of retarded or seriously restricted growth, hypertrophic heart, a subsequent streptococcic endocarditis and, at times, aneurysmal dilatation, embolus and so forth. To prevent these occurrences, the duct may be closed by suture or ligature. The best time for such a ligation is between the ages of 4 and 12. The surgical approach for this must be through the chest and the pleural cavity; therefore, all preoperative, operative and postoperative nursing precautions for chest surgery must be observed. (See Chap. 13, p. 238.)

Pulmonary Stenosis. This is a congenital narrowing of the pulmonary artery at its exit from the heart. It leads to an inadequate flow of blood through the lungs with a resulting cyanosis. When pulmonary stenosis is accompanied by a defect of the interventricular septum, a shift of the aorta to the right side and a hypertrophy of the right ventricle, the condition is called *tetralogy of Fallot*. Children so affected are spoken of as *blue babies*. Two methods now are used in the treatment of tetralogy of Fallot. The Blalock and Taussig method of directing blood to the lungs is by an anastomosis between the pulmonary artery and one of the aortic branches, such as the left subclavian, the left common carotid or the innominate. The Potts method is a direct anastomosis between the aorta itself and the pulmonary artery. This will increase the flow of blood through the lungs and relieve the cyanosis.

Coarctation of the aorta is a congenital narrowing of the aorta. About one fourth of all patients affected live relatively normal lives; however, most patients begin to show symptoms as they approach adolescence. Hypertension is noted in the upper extremities and lower pressure in the lower extremities, often so low that a pulse is not palpable in the vessels. The chief difficulty is that as such an individual grows older, extreme hypertension can occur in the upper part of the body, causing headache, cerebrovascular accidents, rupture of the aorta and death.

This condition, which occurs twice as often in males as in females, can be corrected surgically in one of two ways. The coarctation can be removed, and the two ends of the vessel can be anastomosed. At times, this is impossible because of an inelastic aorta or because the defect may involve a long section of the aorta. In these cases, it is necessary to use a graft.* The ideal time for surgery is from ages 8 to 16. Before the age of 8 the vessel is too small, and after 16, degenerative changes begin to take place in the arterial walls.

Nursing Care

Preoperatively, the physical preparation is similar to that of general surgical patients. The emotional reaction of this individual must be observed, since apprehension usually exists whether it is expressed obviously or not. Blood pressure readings of all four extremities are taken and recorded; these are compared with postoperative readings.

Postoperative care is similar to that of chest surgical patients. Water-seal drainage is used, oxygen therapy is administered, and the patient is given antibiotics and sedatives. Often an indwelling catheter is used to assist in urinary output. Blood pressure readings are taken; usually, the pressure will take from 2 to 3 weeks to reach normal levels.

Every attempt is made to keep the patient quiet with narcotics and later with codeine and aspirin. When the patient is discharged, he still will be taking this latter combination of

* In hospitals where this surgery is performed, grafts are collected from young individuals within 5 hours after death. They are stored aseptically in special fluid at a temperature just above freezing or they may be kept in a deep freeze unit.

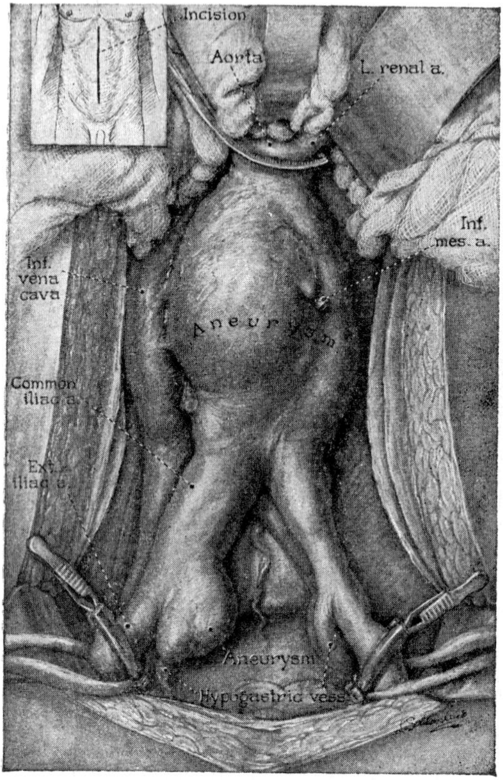

FIG. 107. Aneurysm as seen at laparotomy. The cyst caused by a previous spontaneous dissection of the aorta can be seen. There was a clotted aneurysm of the right common iliac artery and a calcified plaque at the bifurcation of the left common iliac. (Bahnson, Henry: Considerations in the excision of aortic aneurysms, Ann. Surg. **138**: 381)

medications. The reason for this is that chest pain is present, and he is entitled to medication relief. For the first several days after operation, he may favor one side when he turns and may be apprehensive about moving. The nurse can help him to overcome his fears by telling him that it is necessary to move from side to side and that he cannot hurt himself.

A normal diet is resumed as tolerated. Ambulation can begin when his chest and urinary catheters have been removed. If he has had a graft, he may have to remain in bed for a week before getting up.

Upon discharge, his activities can be extended gradually. Follow-up visits to his physician are necessary. By the end of 2 months, he should be leading a fairly normal life.

Aortic Aneurysms. *Aneurysms* are areas of weakness of the wall of the aorta, which appear as outpouchings from its wall. They usually occur in later life and may appear as a saccular bulge coming from the aortal wall or as a spindle-shaped swelling involving the entire wall of the aorta.

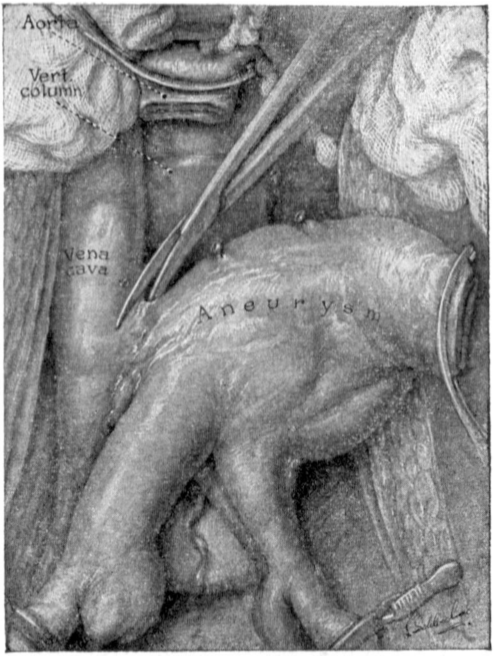

FIG. 108. The aorta and the external iliac arteries have been occluded, and the aneurysm is being removed. Adherence to the vena cava has been intimate in all such patients, and several tears usually are sutured. (Bahnson, Henry: Considerations in the excision of aortic aneurysms, Ann. Surg. **138**: 382)

Aneurysms appear in the aorta as a result of disease (usually syphilis), advancing age (arteriosclerosis) and occasionally of trauma. For many years these aneurysms were looked upon as incurable, and palliative procedures were employed in an effort to strengthen their wall, thereby preventing their enlargement and rupture. These measures included (1) the introduction of fine wire into the aneurysm through a needle, by means of which an electric current may be passed to bring about massive clotting in the aneurysm, (2) the wrapping of the aneurysm with cellophane, fascia, etc., to strengthen the wall of the aneurysm and prevent its enlargement and (3) at times, the ligation of the aorta itself.

More recently, as experience has been gained in great vessel surgery, the surgical attack on these aneurysms has become bolder. Now it is possible in many cases either to remove the aneurysmal sac and suture the opening in the aorta or to remove the entire portion of the aorta containing the aneurysm and restore the circulation by introducing an aortal graft.

Nursing Care

In caring for a child or an adult with a circulatory disturbance of the heart or the great vessels, the nurse will watch carefully his color, the quality of his pulse and variations in the pulse quantity in the extremities. She may note that he tires

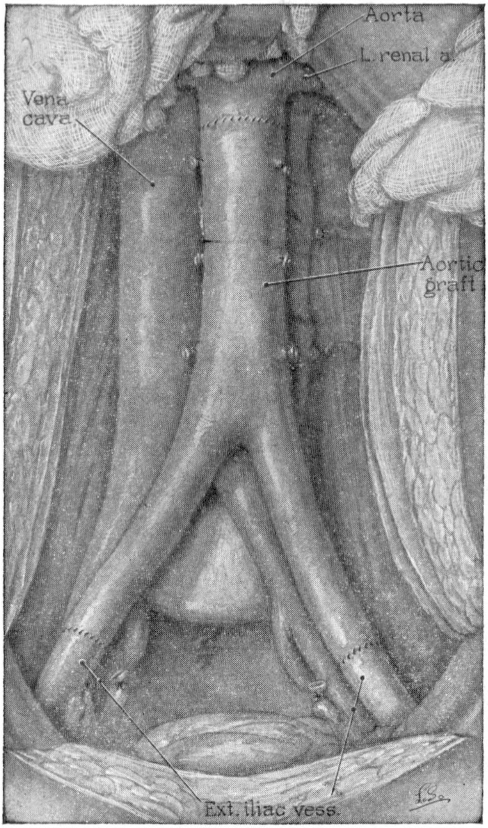

FIG. 109. The aortic homograft has been sutured to the aorta just below the renal arteries and to the two external iliac arteries. (Bahnson, Henry: Considerations in the excision of aortic aneurysms, Ann. of Surg. 138:382)

easily, that he appears to be underdeveloped and that he is subject to infections. Upon examining the patient the physician determines the activity to be undertaken by him.

In anticipation of surgery, the patient may have to undergo many diagnostic tests, such as electrocardiogram, fluoroscopy and blood tests. He will require reassurance, particularly if his problem is one of long standing, for then his fears and mental upsets are far greater than those of the patient with an acute appendicitis. An adequate fluid intake and a well-rounded diet are encouraged. Here, again, such a patient usually has a poor appetite and lingers quite a while over a tray. Attractive dishes and patience on the part of the nurse will encourage him to eat.

The family must be informed by the surgeon of the seriousness of cardiac surgery. The nurse can help by speaking reassuringly to the family and by giving support to the physician's statements.

There is nothing different in the immediate preoperative preparation of this patient from other chest patients. While he is in the operating room, oxygen equipment, an intravenous setup, suction and emergency drugs (cardiac stimulants) should be available in the patient's unit. He will receive oxygen for several days. Attention must be directed to preventing upper respiratory infections, to lessening pain and promoting comfort. Rest is very essential immediately after operation; therefore, a complete bed bath, which is exhausting, should not be attempted. Hourly changes of position, use of the blow bottle for lung expansion and observation for cyanosis or color change constitute initial postoperative care. The blood pressure and the pulse are checked frequently; the quality of the pulse, as well as variation from one extremity to another, is noted. The ability of the patient to move his extremities also must be observed, for a limited blood supply during surgery may predispose to a paralysis. Fluid and electrolyte balance must be maintained. Visitors must be limited so that the patient will receive his rest. Sometimes it is necessary to do a chest tapping on the first or the second day after operation to remove accumulated chest fluid. A thoracentesis tray should be available.

Gradual activity is begun the day after operation, and the patient advances from a liquid diet as indicated by his tolerance. Meanwhile, observation of the patient is continued for untoward signs of fatigue, dizziness, cyanosis and so forth. Getting out of bed is attempted after he has had proper preliminary preparation, such as sitting up in bed and "dangling." Patients who have been operated on for patent ductus arteriosus make a more rapid recovery than those who have had surgery for tetralogy of Fallot.

Depending upon the success of surgery, the patient will assume more normal activities as time progresses. Any limitations must be understood thoroughly by him and his family before he is discharged from hospital. The tendency is for the patient to overtax himself in his eagerness to return to normal activity.

SPLENORENAL AND PORTACAVAL ANASTOMOSIS

Cirrhosis of the liver and thrombosis of the portal vein lead to an obstruction of the portal venous system. This is characterized by ascites, by the appearance of varicose veins of the lower esophagus and the cardiac orifice of the stomach and often by hemorrhage from these vessels, with hematemesis. The control of the hemorrhage is a life-saving procedure. In some cases a direct attack is made on the varices in the lower esophagus by exposing the vessels through a thoracotomy incision, and the veins themselves are ligated. In many cases conservative therapy is advised, and after the emergency is over, some direct attack upon the portal hypertension is attempted. In cases in which a thrombosis of the portal vein is present, an anastomosis may be attempted between the splenic and the renal veins. By this method the portal blood is shunted into the caval system through the

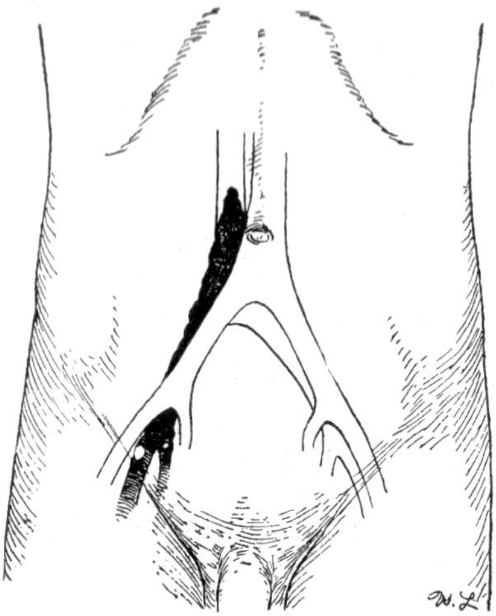

FIG. 110. Diagrammatic drawing shows a clot or thrombus in the right femoral vein extending upward to the vena cava.

renal vein. In other instances an anastomosis is made between the portal vein and the inferior vena cava. This is spoken of as a "portacaval shunt." In selected cases, especially those in which the liver function is not too abnormal, excellent results are obtained.

Nursing care for these operations is the same as for any abdominal or thoracoabdominal operation.

THROMBOSIS AND EMBOLISM

The clotting of blood in the heart or in an artery or vein is spoken of as *thrombosis,* and the clot is called a *thrombus* (Fig. 110). This phenomenon may be due to an injury of the vessel or the heart wall, to a slowing of the blood flow or to changes in the blood itself, especially dehydration. Any foreign body, such as a clot, floating free in the blood stream is called an *embolus.*

Thrombophlebitis and Phlebothrombosis. Two types of thrombosis may occur in the veins. One is due to trauma or infection of the vein wall and is associated with inflammatory changes in the vein and the surrounding tissues. This is called *thrombophlebitis.* Usually it is easy to diagnose by the presence of redness and tenderness along the course of the vein with edema and pain in the extremity. The patient's temperature usually is elevated 1 or 2 degrees, and the pulse rate also may be increased. Thrombophlebitis causes the so-called milk leg that sometimes is a sequel to many lower abdominal operations, especially those associated with infection, or it may follow various types of trauma (see p. 144).

The second type of thrombosis, *phlebothrombosis,* occurs usually in the deep veins of the leg. It is due mainly to stasis of blood in the extremities rather than to trauma or infection. It is more likely to appear in those patients who have a depressed circulation from cardiac disease, in older people, in patients with anemia or a blood dyscrasia, or in those patients who are required to remain in bed. In contrast with thrombophlebitis, the symptoms are "silent." There may be minimal signs in the legs of pain or tenderness, or there may be no signs. The leg usually is not swollen to any noticeable degree. The temperature is only slightly, if at all, elevated. The first sign of its presence may be a pulmonary embolus. An embolus is the greatest danger from this type of complication.

Treatment. The treatment of both complications is, first, preventive. Early ambulation or bed exercises are important factors in prophylaxis. However, when they do occur, the treatment of the two conditions is quite different. In thrombophlebitis, efforts are made to relieve the arteriospasm and the venospasm that cause the pain and the swelling. This may be achieved by producing sympathetic release to the part involved and consequent vasodilation. Local or systemic heat is one method of doing this. Another method, and one that is used more frequently, is procaine block of the sympathetic ganglia to the extremity involved. In addition, a tight bandage on the extremity involved and early exercise or walking will hasten the course of recovery and prevent to some extent late sequelae.

The treatment of phlebothrombosis is mainly the prevention of pulmonary emboli. There are two methods of attempting this. One is the administration of heparin and/or Dicumarol, which are anticoagulants. These drugs, with adequate concentration in the blood, prevent clotting and, therefore, may prevent the extension of thrombi in the leg and subsequent pulmonary emboli. When heparin is given, the blood-clotting time must be evaluated at frequent intervals to make certain that the clotting time is delayed sufficiently to be effective and that it is not increased to a level at which it may be dangerous. When Dicumarol is used, the same information is obtained by studying the prothrombin time of the blood. The other method consists of ligating the veins from the extremity, above the point of thrombosis, thereby blocking the channel of travel for clots that may break off and be carried to the heart and the lungs. The vein or veins usually ligated are the superficial femoral, although the common femoral, the common iliac or the vena cava may be ligated to prevent a fatality from pulmonary embolus.

While these two conditions are different fundamentally, often they appear together in some degree; therefore, one must be cautious in their management.

Arterial Thrombosis and Embolism. Arterial emboli arise most often from vegetations of the heart valves in subacute bacterial endocarditis. Occasionally in coronary arterial disease, a thrombus may form on the wall of the heart, from which emboli may enter the circulation and produce arterial embolism. When an embolus lodges in a vessel, there is an associated thrombosis at the site of the lodgment. Thrombosis may occur also in arteries without previous lodgment of an embolus. In either event, the blood flow distal to the thrombosis is shut off suddenly. The symptoms produced by an arterial embolus are due to tissue ischemia with development of acute pain, then numbness, loss of sensation and, eventually, gangrene, unless the collateral arterial vessels can provide an adequate blood supply.

Surgical Therapy. In the treatment of thrombosis and embolism, surgical therapy is of value from two points of view:

First, in arterial and venous thrombosis, a marked spasm of both arteries and veins brought about by a reflex vasoconstriction via the sympathetic nerves has been demonstrated. It has been found possible to relieve the pain in many of these cases and at the same time improve the circulation by blocking the sympathetic impulses with procaine. The injection is made round the sympathetic ganglia, usually in the lumbar region, because the thrombosis or embolism occurs most often in the vessels of the lower extremities.

Second, another method of surgical treatment is removal of the clot or of the segment of the vessel containing the clot. In the first instance, an attempt is made to re-establish the circulation. The vessel is opened, the clot is removed by suction and the vessel is closed. When the vessel with the clot is removed, one must depend on the collateral circulation for the maintenance of the nutrition of the part, the purpose of the removal of the segment being to remove the impulses that are causing the vasoconstrictive reflex.

In all these cases, the intravenous use of heparin or other anticoagulant is recommended in order to prevent subsequent thrombosis, either at the site of the operation on the vessel or elsewhere. A patient with an arterial embolus usually is extremely ill from a cardiac lesion and, therefore, the operation, as a rule, is performed under a local anesthesia. The prognosis is not good, and it is made poorer definitely if the operation is delayed.

Nursing Care

It is not unusual for a nurse to have a patient who during his convalescence complains of pain in the calf of the leg that is aggravated when the foot is dorsiflexed (Homan's sign). She must be aware of the fact that this may be a symptom of phlebothrombosis, and that she should not massage the part to avoid dislodging a thrombus. She should keep the patient in bed and notify the physician.

When a ligation is to be done or a clot is to be removed, the nurse must know what area or areas are to be prepared. A common method employed by some surgeons to indicate the site is to make an X on the skin with an applicator stick dipped in methylene blue. For a femoral ligation, the inguinal and, possibly, the pubic areas should be shaved on the side that is affected.

Postoperative care is according to the orders given by the surgeon. The operative dressing must be examined for signs of hemorrhage. In addition, the nurse must realize that the patient may have a serious circulatory difficulty. It is important to check the pulse and the blood pressure and also to pay attention to any mention of pain or numbness in an extremity or pain in the chest. In any circulatory problem the patient as a whole must be considered.

PERIPHERAL ARTERIAL DISEASE

Raynaud's Disease

Raynaud's disease is found most often in young people between the ages of eighteen and thirty; it affects the female more often than the male. It is characterized by a blanched, almost deathlike, appearance of symmetrical parts of the extremities—that is, both hands or both feet or all four members—or by local asphyxia, which produces a marked purplish color in the extremities involved. These phenomena are brought about by some disturbance in the vasomotor mechanism to the part which produces spasms of the arteries, and they seem to be initiated by exposure to cold. When they occur frequently, they cause nutritional changes in the part and gangrene appears in areas—most often the fingertips—and sometimes large parts of the member are involved. The disease occurs in an attack from which the patient may recover, but the recurrence of the attack is not infrequent.

Treatment. In mild cases without gangrene, conservative therapy, such as protection from cold, and at times fever therapy by intravenous typhoid vaccine, may be found to be helpful. In marked cases, however, an interruption of the sympathetic nerves by removal of the sympathetic ganglia or division of their branches is the only method of affording much improvement. These ganglia are located either in the upper part of the thorax and lower neck for the upper extremity or along the vertebral column behind the peritoneum for the lower extremity. The operation for removal of these ganglia is spoken of as a *sympathetic ganglionectomy.*

Thromboangiitis Obliterans (Buerger's Disease)

Buerger's disease is a recurring inflammation in the arteries and the veins of the extremities, usually of the lower extremities, and results in thrombus formation and occlusion of the vessels. The cause of the condition is not known, but it is believed by many to be of bacterial origin because of the acute stages of the disease.

It occurs primarily in men between the ages of 25 and 45, and there is considerable evidence that smoking is a factor, if not in the etiology at least in the progress of the disease. As a rule, the patient appears for treatment when the disease has affected so many of the vessels of the extremity as to reduce the peripheral arterial circulation. He complains of cramps in the legs after exercise which are relieved by inactivity; often there is considerable burning pain. As the disease progresses, definite cyanosis of the part appears when it is dependent, and ulceration with gangrene occurs, especially about the nails and the toes.

Treatment. The treatment of Buerger's disease may be divided into two classes, conservative and operative. In most cases, the conservative treatment is recommended until gangrene makes amputation advisable. It comprises rest, postural exercises to improve the circulation of the part and the use of various types of apparatus designed to exercise the blood vessels by producing an alternate congestion and anemia of the part. In addition, relaxation of the blood vessels by fever therapy, usually typhoid vaccine intravenously, is found to be helpful. Intravenous procaine and drugs that block the sympathetic (vasoconstrictor) nerves also are used.

Surgery is used in two stages of the disease. In the early stage in persons below 45 years of age, when there are still evidences of vascular spasm, removal of the sympathetic ganglia has been of value in some cases. In the late stages of the disease, after gangrene has appeared because of deficient circulation, amputation may be necessary. Occasionally, conservative measures may be practiced after desensitization of the part involved by injecting alcohol into the sensory nerves. However, the disease is a progressive one, and often the amputation of a single toe must be followed by amputation of another, until eventually it is necessary to amputate a foot or a leg (p. 568).

Arteriosclerosis—Gangrene

With advancing age there is a replacement of the muscular walls of the arteries by fibrous tissue and, eventually, even by calcium salts. With this change there is a decrease in the lumen of the vessels so that the blood supply to the distal portions of the extremities is reduced gradually. Sometimes a gradual gangrene of the toes results. Usually this is of the dry type, a mummification. Frequently, however, the gangrenous area becomes infected secondarily and produces marked systemic, as well as local, symptoms.

Treatment. Preventive measures, such as keeping the feet clean and wearing loose shoes, should be taken. There is rarely any treatment of any value for the arteriosclerotic with gangrene, except removal of the gangrenous parts. In such cases, in order to obtain a wound that will heal, it is necessary that a high amputation be performed, usually through the thigh. (See Amputation, p. 568.)

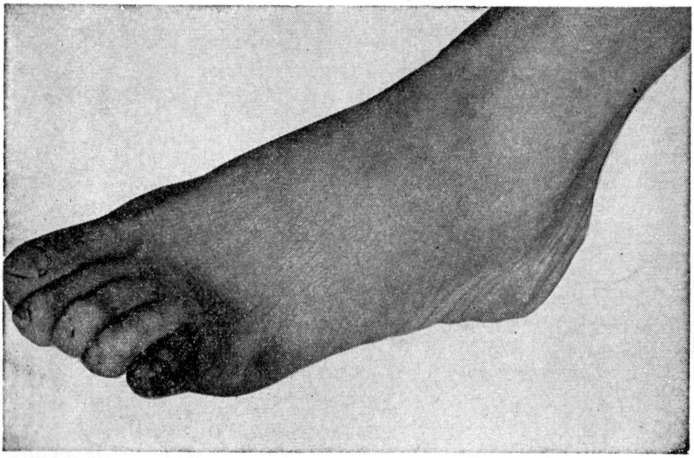

Fig. 111. Diabetic gangrene.

Mechanical Methods in Treatment of Peripheral Vascular Disease and Embolism

The Sanders Oscillating Bed. A method of administering passive postural exercises to allow of the intermittent filling and emptying of capillaries, venules and arterioles is the use of the Sanders oscillating bed. The bed is set upon a rocker operated by a motor so that it tilts on its long axis at regular intervals. The intervals may be adjusted according to the needs of the patient and the wishes of the physician. This method of administering passive postural exercises may be carried out day and night. It is claimed by some to have produced relief of the rest pain and of the pain associated with ulcers and gangrene. It may be used in arteriosclerosis and thromboangiitis obliterans and, in minor degree, of arterial embolism.

Diathermy. This method of treatment has been used to produce peripheral vasodilatation. Electrodes are applied to the lumbar region or to the thigh and, with the passage of the current, there is a definite increase in the temperature of the part, indicating an increased blood flow and vasodilatation.

Nursing Care

The attitude of the nurse in caring for patients with peripheral vascular conditions is important, for much of the progress made by such patients depends upon nursing care. Their problems may appear minor compared with those of other surgical patients and, as a result, often they are neglected; yet they may have long histories of circulatory difficulties and are depressed and greatly in need of help.

As a rule, tobacco in any form is denied these patients and the nurse should see to it that this proscription is enforced. This restriction is important especially in patients with Buerger's disease.

Care of the Feet. The nurse and the physician are responsible for instructing the patient in this connection. It must be realized that the chief objective is to protect him from foot trauma. Each night the feet should be washed with neutral soap and warm water. They must be dried thoroughly, but not roughly. Lanolin or petrolatum can be used to prevent drying and cracking of the skin. Lamb's wool placed between the toes helps to prevent irritation. Woolen socks can be worn in winter and white cotton socks in warm weather. A clean pair should be available every day. Bed socks may be worn, but hot-water bottles or electric heating pads should not be used. Comfortable socks that are not too loose should be worn. The patient must be instructed not to use strong antiseptics, such as tincture of iodine, lysol and so forth. Corns and calluses require expert care. The trimming of toenails is done best after a footbath; they should be trimmed straight across. The patient also should be instructed not to cross his knees when sitting. Any signs of blister, ingrowing toenail, infection and so forth must be reported to the physician.

If postural exercises are prescribed, the patient should elevate the extremities for a minute and then place them in a dependent position until the rubor or cyanosis becomes maximum, then lie with them in the horizontal position for a minute. These time intervals may be changed according to the disease, the condition of the patient and his ability to continue them. Again, it is important to emphasize that if the leg is to be elevated, the object (such as a bed cradle or an inverted chair) on which the part is resting must be padded to prevent injury to the limb.

Contrast baths may be used at times. These should be large enough to immerse both feet to the middle of the leg. Cold water at from 40° to 50° F. is placed in one and warm water at from 102° to 105° F. in the other. The feet and the legs are immersed alternately in the water in each container for one minute for a period of about 15 minutes. This procedure may be repeated 2 or 3 times a day.

Dressings. If it is desirable to treat an extremity with moist dressings and there are no open wounds, this can be done with surgically clean gauze and solution. However, if there is an ulcer or an open infection, strict asepsis must be followed. In this case it is easier often to use sterile gloves than to attempt to change or apply dressings with forceps. The extremity must be supported adequately when bandage dressings are removed or applied. Often the surgeon will débride necrotic tissue and irrigate the wound. Petrolatum gauze or plain dressings moistened with saline at room temperature may be applied. If only some parts of an extremity are to receive moistened dressings, the best way to prevent areas from becoming wet is to apply petrolatum. Rubber dam and plastic materials, such as pliofilm, are far more effective in acting as nonconducting and waterproof wrappings than waxed paper. Another advantage is that they can be autoclaved and are not torn easily.

Nutritional and Drug Therapy. Nutritional needs also must be met in people with peripheral vascular disturbances. High vitamin and high caloric diets are desirable. The diabetic requires especial care in this regard and, further, strict asepsis should be observed in his case in the event of hypodermic medication.

Often the extreme pain suffered by these patients necessitates the administration of narcotics, but this situation should be avoided if possible. Usually relief can be obtained by intravenous typhoid therapy or by repeated saline injections.

ARTERIAL HYPERTENSION

In a small group of cases of persistent elevation of blood pressure, the term *malignant hypertension* is applied because the disease is progressive and results eventually in death. Hypertension usually is regarded as a medical disease, but in cases of malignant hypertension surgery now is demanding a place in the therapy. In patients in whom the hypertension has not produced marked change in the vital organs, it may be possible to relieve the marked elevation of blood pressure and prevent further progress of this dangerous disease by the division of the sympathetic nerves. This operation is carried out on each side of the chest, a variable number of sympathetic ganglia in the chest and the first and the second lumbar ganglia being removed. In addition, the greater and lesser and least splanchnic nerves are divided (*thoracolumbar sympathectomy* and *splanchnicectomy*). Extremely high blood pressure may be reduced so much that the patient may be relieved of many of the symptoms of hypertension. In some cases the fall of blood pressure is so nearly complete that, when the patient stands, his vascular system is not adjusted to the low blood pressure and he may feel faint. In these cases, supporting elastic bandages and compression of the abdomen with sponge rubber and an elastic belt will be necessary for a time until the patient adjusts himself to the new blood pressure.

ANEURYSM

Aneurysm is a saccular dilatation of a blood vessel. Usually it is not looked upon as a surgical disease, but there are two types that may respond to surgical therapy.

Traumatic Aneurysm. This is produced by an injury to the wall of an artery. A stretching of the injured portion of the arterial wall occurs with the formation of a gradually enlarging sac. This type of aneurysm appears in the extremities, where injury is most frequent. It may be treated either by excision of the enlarged damaged portion of the artery or by repair of the arterial wall. The latter operation is known as *aneurysmorrhaphy*.

Arteriovenous Aneurysm. The second type of aneurysm that is treated frequently by surgery is known as *arteriovenous aneurysm*. This may result from a congenital communication between the veins and the arteries or from an injury in which healing results in a communication between them. The symptoms of this disease are due to this communication; the veins pulsate and become widely dilated. In the surgical treatment of this lesion, an attempt is made to divide the communication. It may be possible to sever it directly or it may be necessary in some cases to excise the entire segment of vessel containing the communication.

VARICOSE VEINS

The blood flow in the veins is maintained in a direction toward the heart by a series of cup-shaped valves. A deficiency of these valves may be produced by disease, as in phlebitis, or by long-standing distention, due to back pressure on the veins, as in pregnancy, or to long periods of being in the erect position. When the valves become deficient, the veins dilate gradually. This phenomenon occurs almost always in the lower extremities, and the veins most affected are those that lie in the subcutaneous fatty tissues, especially the long saphenous vein.

The dilatation of this vein produces a venous stasis with secondary edema, replacement fibrosis in the subcutaneous fatty tissue, pigmentation of the skin and, because of these changes, a lowered resistance to infection and to trauma. The symptoms produced most often are disfigurement due to the large size of the vein, easy fatigue of the part, a

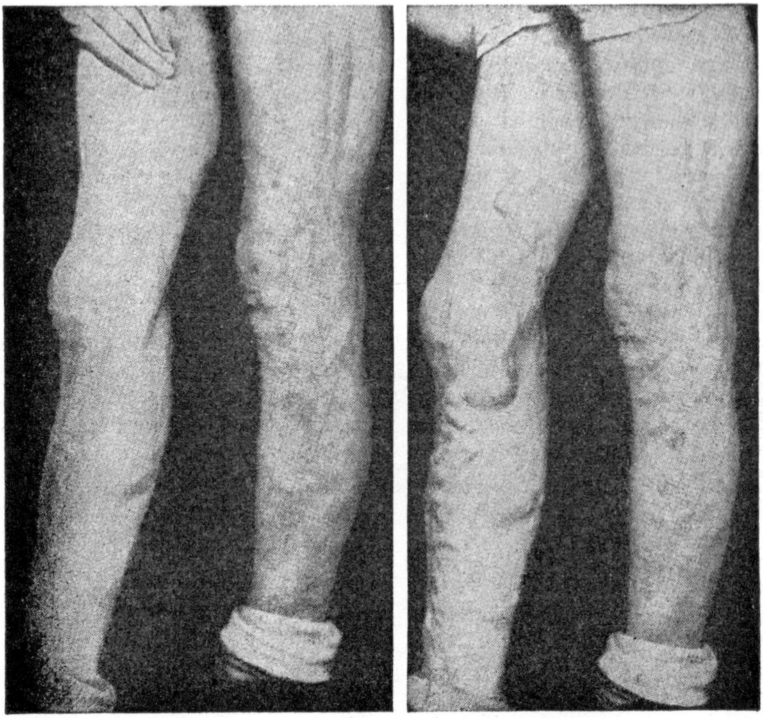

FIG. 112. A patient with varicose veins. (*Left*) The patient was placed on a bed with the leg elevated so as to drain the blood from the superficial veins. Manual pressure then was applied over the uppermost portion of the vein and the patient was asked to stand. Note that, with hand compressing the upper portion of the vein no veins are seen in the lower leg. (*Right*) Hand pressure has been removed from the upper portion of the thigh, and the veins have filled up rapidly. This indicates incompetence of the valves, which permits the backward flow of blood in veins.

heavy feeling, cramps in the legs at night and, often, pain during the menstrual period. The veins may occur at any age, but they appear most commonly in women after pregnancy. If varicose veins are untreated, the changes in the lower leg mentioned above may appear. Repeated attacks of inflammation are not uncommon and ulceration may develop.

Treatment. In the treatment of varicose veins, it is essential to remove the hydrostatic pressure of the column of blood in the veins. This can be done by a ligation of the saphenous vein in the upper part of the thigh.

Then the dilated saphenous vein with its incompetent valves is removed by a procedure called "stripping." A metal or plastic stripper is inserted into the lower end of the vein in the groin and is threaded down the leg toward the knee and the ankle. If the vein is not too tortuous it may be possible to thread the stripper through the entire vein down to the ankle. In other cases the stripper may be caught in vein pockets in the thigh or the leg. An incision is made at the lowermost point of the stripper, and the end of the stripper is pulled out of the vein. By tying the vein to the stripper and pulling downward, the vein is pulled out of its location in the subcutaneous tissues. Pressure along the course of the vein is all that is necessary to control bleeding. After several incisions are made, excision of tortuous veins may be necessary in addition. The legs are dressed with gauze and elastic adhesive bandages. The veins which then remain may be closed by the injection of sclerosing substances, such as sodium morrhuate. These produce a local chemical thrombosis that closes the veins and in most cases relieves the symptoms.

When varicose veins have progressed to ulceration, supportive therapy of some type is of value, in addition to the treatment of the veins themselves. This support may be given by elastic bandages or stockings, but can probably be accomplished best by the use of a gelatin paste (Unna's) boot. This is applied over the ulcer, involving usually the foot and extending upward as far as the knee. (See p. 273.) With this treatment most ulcers will heal.

The final word in the treatment of this crippling condition has not been said as yet. Injection does not always suffice, and often, due to the escape of the sclerosants, a slough of greater or lesser severity may result. Many surgeons are inclined to ligate and excise portions of the diseased veins in several areas. This treatment does not result in sloughing yet it is satisfactory.

Nursing Care

This patient usually is ambulatory following surgery; however, the nurse is expected to check circulation in the patient's operated leg occasionally. If edema or other circulatory disturbances are noted, the patient is put to bed, and his leg is elevated on a pillow.

The nurse can emphasize several points in her contact with these patients. Circular garters must be avoided. When sitting, the patient should not cross his legs, as this may impair circulation. The patient should avoid standing for long periods of time. If the extremities swell, the condition can be alleviated by proper elevation and support of the legs. He can be taught how to apply and to care for elastic bandages. Also, he should take precautions to avoid trauma, as leg ulcers and infections do not heal easily.

PHLEBITIS

Phlebitis is encountered frequently in surgery as a postoperative complication. It has been discussed in Chapter 8. However, it may occur also after trauma or disease. It is seen frequently in association with severe injuries such as fractures, especially of the lower extremity, and occurs after delivery as a complication of the puerperium. As a rule, the phlebitis involves the lower extremities, and the symptoms, the

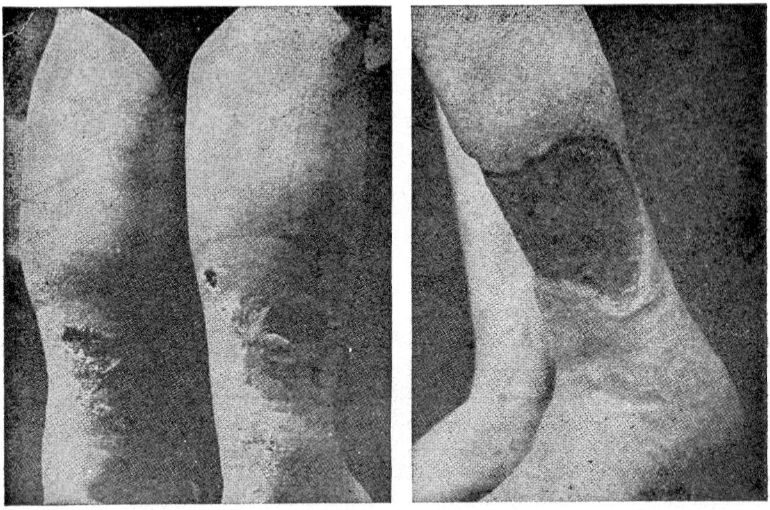

FIG. 113. (*Left*) Relatively early stage of the ulceration in a thrombophlebitic process. (*Right*) Late stage of ulceration following thrombophlebitic edema. Note the punched-out edges of the ulcer with marked induration and fibrosis round its edge.

signs and the treatment are similar to those described for postoperative phlebitis. (See pp. 144 and 146.)

THE POSTPHLEBITIC LEG

As a result of the block of the deep veins in phlebitis, the superficial veins often dilate to take over the return of venous blood from the leg. The clot in the deep vein is canalized and partly absorbed in time, so that the deep veins again may partly function. However, the valves of the vein usually are destroyed by the phlebitis; thus, blood may pass downward toward the foot when the patient is in the erect position. This results in a chronic venous stasis with associated changes: discoloration, swelling and ulceration. The treatment of this type of venous stasis is much more difficult than that resulting from varicosities of only the superficial veins. In some cases there may be no superficial venous enlargement visible or palpable.

Various measures have been suggested in the attempt to remove the venous stasis. These include ligation of the superficial femoral veins and ligation of the saphenous (long and short), if these are varicosed. Most often a more conservative method of therapy is applied, consisting largely of methods to prevent venous stasis by providing external pressure and gravity drainage of venous blood. In order to impress upon the patient the necessity for thwarting venous stasis and swelling of the legs, certain rules have been suggested for the patient with phlebitis. These are:

1. Prevent swelling by constant wearing of elastic stockings. These should be put on the first thing upon arising and worn until going to bed at night. The only time the stockings should be removed is when bathing.

2. Standing produces increased venous stasis; therefore, some slight exercise should be attempted, such as walking, moving the toes in the shoes, etc. In the year following the attack of phlebitis, the legs should be elevated to a horizontal position on a chair at least 5 minutes out of every 2 hours.

3. At least 2 or 3 times a day the legs should be elevated above the head by lying down. With the leg elevated on the back of a sofa or even against the wall while the patient is lying on his back, the venous blood is drained by gravity from the part. Whenever possible, the leg should be elevated on another chair when sitting down.

4. At night, the foot of the bed should be elevated 6 or 8 inches to permit venous drainage by gravity to take place.

5. Patients with irritation of the skin or the leg should apply bland, oily lotions to the skin to prevent scaling and dryness.

6. Finally, the patient should be careful to avoid all trauma, bruising, scratching or other forms of injury to the skin of the leg and the foot.

If these suggestions are carried out repeatedly, it is possible to avoid many of the complications that otherwise appear in the postphlebitic leg.

CLINICAL SITUATIONS

Coarctation of Aorta

Jake Kessler did not know he had a congenital anomaly of the aorta until a physical examination revealed an unusually high blood pressure (left arm), whereas the pulse in his lower extremities proved to be absent. The 17-year-old high school student submitted to a repair of his coarctation with the consent and the encouragement of his parents.

1. If untreated, coarctation of the aorta may cause

_____(1) cerebrovascular accidents
_____(2) a fusion of the commissures
_____(3) atresia of the aorta
_____(4) rupture of the aorta

2. Correction of a coarctation of the aorta can be done by

_____(1) anastomosing the pulmonary artery with one of the aortic branches
_____(2) cutting the fibrotic thickened area with a special knife
_____(3) introducing fine wire into the affected area
_____(4) excising the constricted area and repairing the defect with a graft

3. Postoperative chest pain which persists for some time is an indication

_____(1) that surgery has been effective
_____(2) that surgery has not been effective
_____(3) of postoperative complications
_____(4) that may be disregarded and will disappear.

Saphenous Ligation

Mrs. Leith, aged 42 and about 50 pounds overweight, has been bothered with "sore legs" ever since the arrival of Johnny. Since then she has had 3 more children. She had several injections for her varicosities but these failed to give relief. After the Trendelenburg test, the physician recommended a saphenous ligation.

1. The action of a drug used in injections for varicosities is
______(1) as an antiseptic; it flushes and sterilizes the inside of the vein
______(2) enzymatic; that is, it digests unhealthy tissue and restores normal lining
______(3) irritant to the extent that the walls of the vessel become swollen, a clot is formed and the vein is obliterated

2. A sclerosing drug is
______(1) trypsin
______(2) sodium morrhuate
______(3) protamin sulfate
______(4) Priscoline

3. For the Trendelenburg test, Mrs. Leith was requested to lie down and elevate her leg. Upon rising, the varicose vein probably would
______(1) fill rapidly
______(2) remain collapsed

4. Following the saphenous ligation, Mrs. Leith was up and about. When she complained of some pain and swelling in her operated extremity, the nurse should
______(1) put her to bed, elevate the leg on a pillow, give aspirin
______(2) tell her that this is expected and that it will improve in a few hours
______(3) have her sit down with leg elevated on a chair; gently but firmly massage the extremity

5. Points to be stressed in instructing Mrs. Leith about her care are:
______(1) cross the legs when sitting in order to rest the involved leg
______(2) apply pressure above the varicose veins by wearing circular garters
______(3) elevate legs when possible with support to the entire leg down to the heel

6. When Mrs. Leith was about to leave the hospital, she asked the nurse if her varicose veins would "come back again." The best reply is
______(1) "No, now that you have had surgery, the vein which caused you so much trouble has been removed."
______(2) "Perhaps, since there is no 100 per cent cure for varicose veins, especially in obese people."
______(3) "Much will depend on you. By following all our suggestions for proper rest, diet and hygienic care, you may have a complete cure."

CHAPTER FIFTEEN

Surgical Conditions of the Blood, the Lymphatic System and the Spleen

THE BLOOD

As a rule, the treatment of diseases of the blood, such as the various types of anemia and leukemia, do not concern the surgeon. However, these are encountered frequently as complications of surgical lesions. Secondary anemia is not at all uncommon in patients with malignant disease or with bleeding from ulcers or hemorrhoids, or in females with bleeding from the generative organs. The surgeon must recognize this very definite complication and take steps to remedy it by means of transfusion and appropriate therapy to build up the red blood cells. The methods and the technic of transfusion have been described in Chapter 7, pp. 173 to 178.

Septicemia and Pyemia

Infections of the blood stream, septicemia and pyemia are definite complications of surgical infections. These diseases have been discussed as a logical final step of an inflammation and the student is referred to page 20 for their symptoms and treatment.

Purpura (Subcutaneous Hemorrhage)

Purpura is the name given to subcutaneous hemorrhage, either minute or large. In addition, hemorrhage from the mucous membrane of the mouth and the intestinal tract occurs often. Several different types of purpura are recognized. One of these, so-called idiopathic thrombocytopenic purpura, is known to be associated with a decrease in the blood platelets. It occurs often in the acute form, in which case transfusion would seem to be the best method of therapy. In the chronic form with recurrent attacks of bleeding, very frequently removal of the spleen is of value (see Splenectomy, p. 284).

Hemophilia

Hemophilia is a hereditary disease. It is transmitted only by the female and appears only in the male children. It is characterized by a prolonged clotting time, so that such persons may bleed excessively from a minor wound; for instance, from a small cut or from the wound caused by the pulling of a tooth. When such patients develop surgical lesions that demand operation, it is of particular importance that the surgeon bring the clotting time to normal in order to avoid the possibility of serious hemorrhage.

Treatment. The most prompt and effective treatment is the transfusion of unmodified blood. Citrated blood appears to be equally as good, although the incidence of reaction after transfusion with it is somewhat higher than that seen in the normal. The intramuscular injection of whole blood, usually in amounts of about 20 cc., has been of benefit in some cases. As a local hemostatic, fresh serum or thrombin is valuable.

Because this disease appears only in the male, it was thought that female endocrine therapy might be of value in treatment. However, despite considerable work in this regard, the injection of female endocrine products in the treatment of the hemophiliac has not proved to be of value.

Ictero-anemia (Hemolytic)

This disease runs in families and is characterized by recurring jaundice, fever, anemia and an enlarged spleen. It is due to defective red corpuscles with increased fragility. Splenectomy gives symptomatic relief.

THE LYMPHATIC SYSTEM

The lymphatic system begins in the tissue spaces and extends via delicate lymph channels toward the trunk. In its course are located lymph nodes that act as filters, in which cells (tumor cells, bacteria) floating in the lymph may be caught. The lymphatics of the gastro-intestinal tract absorb products of digestion, chiefly fat, and this lymph is called chyle. The lymphatics drain eventually into the venous system via the thoracic duct, the large venous channel that passes upward in the posterior mediastinum and empties into the left subclavian vein.

Lymphangitis and Lymphadenitis

Lymphangitis is an acute inflammation of the lymphatic channels. It arises most commonly from a focus of infection in an extremity. Usually it is caused by the Streptococcus. The characteristic red streaks that extend up the arm or the leg from an infected wound outline the course of the lymphatics as they drain toward nodes in the elbow or the axilla in the arm or the knee or the groin in the leg. The presence of a lymphangitis indicates that the infection has not become localized, but is extending at least to the lymph nodes, and in some cases, it may progress and involve the blood stream (septicemia). The absorption of toxins produces high fever, often chills, in addition to the local symptoms of pain, tenderness and swelling along the lymphatics involved. The lymph nodes in the course of the lymphatic channels also become enlarged, red and tender (acute lymphadenitis), and often become necrotic and form an abscess (suppurative lymphadenitis). The nodes involved most often are those in the groin, the axilla or the cervical region. Also lymphadenitis occurs frequently without any signs of a preceding lymphangitis, due to bacteria that have lodged in the lymph nodes from lymph drained from a focus of infection. The same signs (redness and swelling) and symptoms (pain, tenderness and fever) as already mentioned for acute lymphadenitis are present. Here, again, abscess formation may take place.

Lymphangitis and acute lymphadenitis now are not of serious import, because these infections are caused nearly always by organisms (Streptococcus and Staphylococcus)

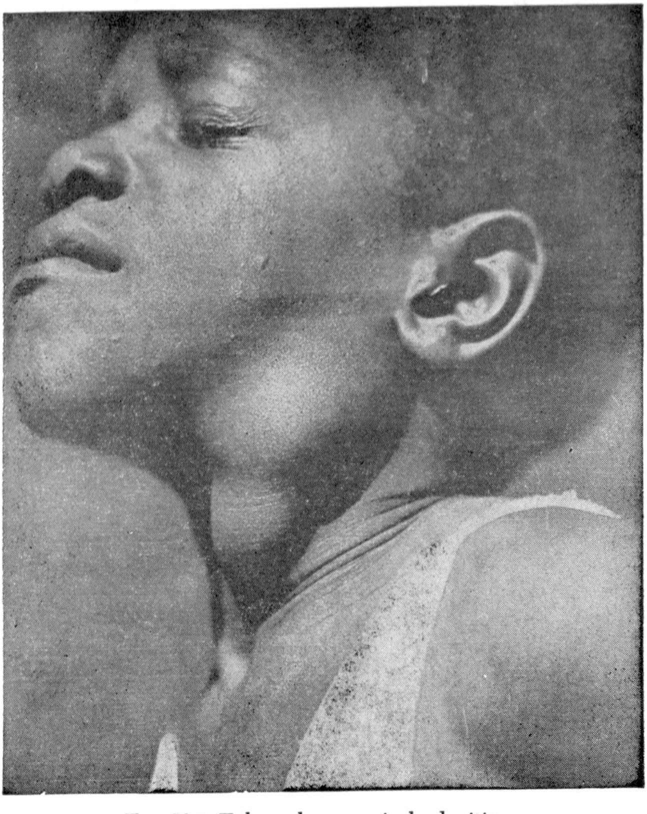

Fig. 114. Tuberculous cervical adenitis.

that are brought under control rapidly by the sulfa drugs and penicillin. The part affected is treated usually by rest, elevation and the application of hot moist dressings, but the rapid response to penicillin and/or sulfadiazine usually makes this treatment unnecessary after a very short time. If necrosis has resulted in abscess formation, incision and drainage become necessary.

ACUTE CERVICAL ADENITIS

Acute cervical adenitis is an acute infection of the lymphatic glands of the neck, usually secondary to an infection in the mouth, the pharynx or the scalp.

This condition occurs very frequently in children, and the prophylactic treatment should be directed toward preventing infection in these areas or removing it should it occur. School nurses and public health nurses especially should inspect the teeth and the tonsils of children under their care and should recommend appropriate prophylactic treatment. Pediculosis of the scalp (lice) is a very common cause of infection of the posterior group of glands. These parasites should be looked for in every case of "glands of the neck," and parasiticides should be applied in all positive or suspicious cases.

The patients develop a swelling of one side of the neck that is markedly tender and edematous. The systemic signs, which in the case of children usually are marked, are those of an acute infection. The process often goes on to abscess formation and spontaneous rupture if the swelling is not incised.

Treatment. The treatment in the early stages comprises attention to the focus of infection, the use of penicillin intramuscularly and the application of warm moist dressings or poultices. If an abscess forms, incision and drainage are required. Frequently the hot moist applications are continued for several days after operation.

TUBERCULOUS CERVICAL ADENITIS

Tuberculous cervical adenitis is a chronic infection of the lymph nodes of the neck. It occurs most commonly in children and in young adults. The nodes increase gradually in size and become slightly tender. At first they can be rolled under the skin as a separate "knot." Gradually, however, the nodes become fused and fixed in the neck tissues. Finally, cold abscesses (see pp. 588-589) form and, unless the swelling is incised and evacuated, it ruptures spontaneously and a sinus forms.

Treatment. The treatment comprises removal of the primary focus of disease, if it can be found, in the mouth or the pharynx; removal of the whole group of glands; and other measures (the exposure of the patient to sunlight and fresh air, the intake of good food and so forth) discussed under the hygienic treatment of tuberculosis (Chap. 26, p. 590). Streptomycin has proved to be extremely valuable in the treatment of this form of tuberculosis.

The patient with this form of tuberculosis usually does not demand long-continued hospitalization. Nevertheless, recovery depends upon the institution of good hygienic measures over a prolonged period of time. Frequently it is possible to place such people in the hands of a public health nurse or some other social agency in the community. In this way the proper hygienic therapy may be taught and supervised after the patient leaves the hospital.

Lymphedema—Elephantiasis

An obstruction to the lymph flow in the extremities produces a chronic swelling of the part, especially if it is in a dependent position. The obstruction may be in both the lymph nodes and the lymphatic vessels, and at times it is seen in the arm after a radical mastectomy for carcinoma, and in the leg in association with varicose veins or a chronic phlebitis (Fig. 113). In the latter case the lymph block usually is due to a chronic lymphangitis. Lymph block due to a parasite (filaria) is seen frequently in the tropics. When chronic swelling is present, there are frequent bouts of acute infection characterized by high fever and chills. These lead to a chronic fibrosis and a thickening of the subcutaneous tissues and hypertrophy of the skin. To this condition of chronic swelling of the extremity, which recedes only slightly with elevation, is given the name elephantiasis.

The swelling of lymphedema may be prevented by the application of elastic bandages or stockings. Often elephantiasis produces such marked disability that surgical relief is sought. The thickened fibrosed subcutaneous fat and much of the excess skin are cut away, along with the fascia overlying the muscles. The remaining skin is sutured back in place and pressure dressings are applied. These operations (Kondoleon) often are performed in stages.

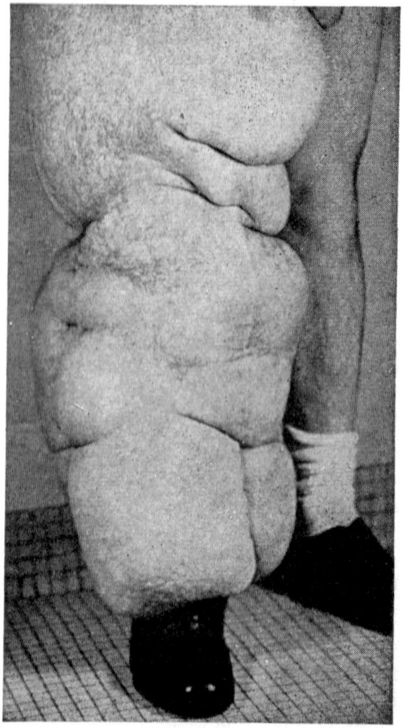

Fig. 115. An example of marked elephantiasis of the right leg. The scar denotes site of a previous attempt at operative reduction of the elephantiasis.

Nursing Care

A block to the lymphatic flow in an extremity means that the part involved may be traumatized easily. Before operation, the arm or the leg is supported on a pillow and bandaged. Some surgeons order diuretics to help in reducing edema. Sulfa drugs and penicillin may be given prophylactically. The part is washed carefully with soap and water prior to surgery. In the postoperative care of these patients, transfusions usually are necessary to prevent the shock that may arise from the long operative procedure and rather profuse blood loss. The extremity is elevated for at least two weeks and then is lowered gradually. If it is a leg, weight is borne only with support. Precautions to avoid injury must be observed carefully.

Tumors of Lymphoid Tissue—Lymphomas

Tumors of lymphoid tissue are called lymphomas. This term includes several types of lesions that are characterized by enlargement of lymph nodes and eventually end fatally. The leukemias, although really tumors of blood-forming organs, are included under this term because of the associated enlargement of lymph nodes. They are not treated surgically, except in occasional instances for biopsy of lymph nodes.

Hodgkin's disease is manifested by the enlargement of lymph nodes usually in the neck. It is associated with weakness and anemia, and eventually is fatal. Surgery is performed occasionally to obtain a lymph node to confirm this diagnosis.

Lymphosarcoma is a rapidly growing tumor of the lymph nodes that also is seen most commonly in the neck. Surgery is used only to obtain tissue for a microscopic diagnosis. The lymphomas are diseases that rarely require surgical treatment. As a rule, they respond temporarily to roentgen irradiation, and in some instances chemotherapy with nitrogen mustard may be used.

THE SPLEEN

The spleen, the largest lymphoid organ in the body, is situated in the upper left portion of the abdomen under the diaphragm. It becomes of interest surgically when it is injured or diseased. Not infrequently splenic rupture is produced with severe injury to the left loin and the upper left abdomen. In such cases, rapid hemorrhage from the highly vascular organ makes splenectomy necessary. In hemolytic jaundice and in some other diseases of the blood (purpura, splenic anemia, leukemia and so forth), removal of the spleen often is of value as a therapeutic measure.

Splenectomy. This is not a difficult operation when the spleen is small but, when the organ is hypertrophied and surrounded by many adhesions, its removal is more difficult. Hemorrhage and abdominal distention are the most frequent postoperative complications. The nursing care of such patients is the same as for those who have undergone laparotomy. It should be borne in mind that surgery for disease of the spleen is fraught with much danger because of the serious associated diseases of the liver and the blood. Rupture of the spleen is associated frequently with other severe injuries that increase the gravity of the case. After splenectomy, the majority of patients have a constant temperature that at times is as high as 101° for ten days or so. Occasionally deficient wound healing and dehiscence of the wound follow the operation.

Enlarged spleen (splenomegaly) often causes such discomfort or disability as to justify its removal. In these cases a snugly fitted abdominal binder helps to prevent postoperative overdistention of the stomach and the intestines. Prostigmine or Pitressin administered hypodermically is of value in this connection.

REFERENCES AND SUGGESTED READING

Unit Three: Nursing in Conditions of the Circulatory System, the Blood and the Blood-forming Organs

Heart and Great Vessels

Bahnson, H.: Considerations in the excision of aortic aneurysms, Ann. Surg. **138**:377, 1953.

Christensen, S. P.: Portal hypertension, Am. J. Nursing **53**:1206-1207, 1953.

Colt, J.: Care of the patient with an aortic graft, Nursing World **127**: 12-13, 1953.

Crystal, D. K.: The operable cardiac anomalies, Am. J. Nursing **49**:587-589, 1949.

Emerson, C. P., and Bragdon, J. S.: Essentials of Medicine, ed. 17, pp. 277-283 (valvular heart disease); pp. 283-286 (coronary heart disease); pp. 287-289 (congenital heart lesions); pp. 289-298 (cardiac failure), Philadelphia, Lippincott, 1955.

Holman, E., and Forrest, W.: The surgical correction of constructive pericarditis, Surg., Gynec. & Obst. **89**:129-144, 1949.

Janton, O. H., Glover, R. P., and O'Neill, T.: Indications for commissurotomy in mitral stenosis, Am. J. Med. **52**:621-625, 1952.

Johnson, J., and Kirby, C. K.: Surgery of the Chest, Chicago, Yr. Bk. Pub., 1952.

Owens, M.: Valvulotomy: a nursing care study, Nursing World **127**: 18-20, 1953.

Price, C. G.: Mitral stenosis, Am. J. Nursing **51**:72-74, 1951.

Smith, E. M.: A nursing staff prepares for cardiac surgery, Am. J. Nursing **49**:598-591, 1949.

Takayoshi, M.: Nursing care of patients with portal hypertension, Am. J. Nursing **53**:1208-1209, 1953.

Wallace, M.: Care of the child with tetralogy of Fallot, Am. J. Nursing **52**:195-198, 1952.

Whiteside, W. C.: Surgical treatment of patent ductus arteriosus, Canad. Nurse **45**:183-184, 1949.

Arteries and Veins

Bauer, G.: Combating thrombosis and pulmonary embolism, Am. J. Nursing **47**:589-591, 1947.

Emerson, C. P., and Bragdon, J. S.: Essentials of Medicine, ed. 17, pp. 253-257 (thrombosis and embolism); pp. 258-270 (peripheral arterial diseases); pp. 270-271 (phlebitis and varicose veins), Philadelphia, Lippincott, 1955.

Krause, G. L., and Vetter, F. C.: Varicose veins, Am. J. Nursing **53**: 70-72, 1953.

McDermott, J. B.: Patience and an

old-fashioned remedy, Am. J. Nursing **50**:86-87, 1950.

OTHER CIRCULATORY CONDITIONS

Blank, M.: Nursing care in Hodgkin's disease, Am. J. Nursing **48**: 563-564, 1948.

Emerson, C. P., and Bragdon, J. S.: Essentials of Medicine, ed. 17, pp. 262-264 (hypertension); pp. 233-238 (lymphomas); pp. 271-272 (lymphatic disorders); pp. 205-244 (blood), Philadelphia, Lippincott, 1955.

Fedder, H.: Nursing the patient with sympathectomy for hypertension, Am. J. Nursing **48**:643-646, 1948.

Lahey, F. A., and Norcross, J. W.: Splenectomy: when is it indicated?, Ann. Surg. **128**:363, 1948.

Palumbo, L. T.: Some recent advances in surgery of the autonomic nervous system, Am. J. Nursing **52**:700-702, 1952.

Smithwick, R. H., and Kinsey Dera: Surgical treatment of hypertension, Am. J. Nursing **47**:153-155, 1947.

Victor, Sister Mary: The oscillating bed—a therapeutic aid, Trained Nurse & Hosp. Rev. **110**:428-430, 1943.

Ward, A. S.: Frostbite, Am. J. Nursing **52**:68-69, 1952.

CLINICAL SITUATION: SPLENECTOMY

Bobby Thatcher, aged 8, was playing "cowboys and Indians" when he fell from a tree and landed on a wooden peg which served as a marker in a strawberry patch. He was rushed to the hospital, and an emergency splenectomy was done.

1. The function of the spleen is to

_____(1) participate in the formation of blood
_____(2) remove defective red blood cells from circulation
_____(3) secrete insulin
_____(4) produce lymphocytes

2. The chief danger from a ruptured spleen is

_____(1) hemorrhage
_____(2) blood stream infection
_____(3) production of a fatal hepatitis
_____(4) peritonitis

3. Postoperative care of Bobby will be

_____(1) similar to the care of a patient having abdominal surgery
_____(2) similar to the care of a patient having chest surgery
_____(3) similar to the care of a patient having cardiovascular surgery
_____(4) specific for this patient

UNIT FOUR

Nursing in Conditions of the Alimentary System

CHAPTER SIXTEEN

Surgery of Lips, Mouth, Tongue and Esophagus

SURGERY OF THE LIPS

Wounds

Wounds of the face and the lips rarely become infected because of the rich blood supply of that region. If an accidental wound is cleaned and sutured early, healing is rapid. This is the case also in the event of an intentional wound of the surgeon's making. Dressings are both unnecessary and conspicuous. The wounds are sutured best with silk or nylon and painted with Whitehead's varnish. Kindly healing occurs without much scarring.

Harelip and Cleft Palate

Harelip. Harelip and cleft palate are deformities that result from embryonal maldevelopment. Harelip may appear in any form from a mere notch on the lip border to a deep fissure that may extend up to the nostril. The deformity may be unilateral or bilateral. If the malformation is marked, the child should be operated on as soon as possible after birth. Operation is borne well at that early age, but if treatment is delayed the baby becomes a poorer surgical risk because of loss of weight and

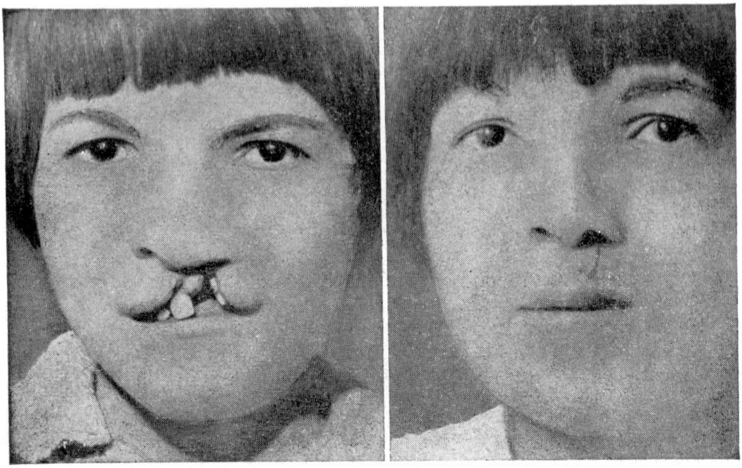

FIG. 116. Cleft or harelip and alveolus before and after repair. (Dr. R. H. Ivy)

strength due to his inability to nurse properly.

The operation is performed with the child on his back, the head being allowed to hang over the operating table and rest in the lap of the surgeon. In this way blood and mucus escape easily without being aspirated or swallowed. The easiest way to handle the baby is to roll him in a small blanket, binding the legs and the arms to his sides. The operation is a simple suturing together of the tissues of the lip to make it possible for the child to nurse.

After the operation, nursing should not be allowed for from 5 to 6 days, but mother's milk should be fed by a medicine dropper. The tip of the medicine dropper should be protected by a small rubber tube and placed in the corner of the infant's mouth. In this way there will be less strain on the suture line by sucking. The physical needs of the baby should be met so as to keep crying to a minimum: crying produces tension on the incision.

Cleft Palate. This deformity is associated frequently with harelip. The cleft may involve only the soft palate. However, it may extend through the hard palate and even involve one or both nostrils. Such children cannot talk or eat properly and an operation is required. This is done best in their second year. Flaps of periosteum and mucous membrane are formed and sutured together to close the defect. The harelip frequently is corrected at the same time. The excess of the red border is excised and the tissues of the lips are joined by one of several methods of plastic operations. The suture line is sealed with Whitehead's varnish and tension is removed from the sutures by the application across the lip of an adhesive strapping that tends to hold the cheeks together, or by adhesive strips placed round the lips.

Nursing Care

The success of the operation depends in large measure upon the care that these children receive both before and after operation.

In no circumstances is it advisable to operate on these patients in the presence of an infection of the nasopharynx or the tonsils.

Asepsis of the mouth cannot be attained, but a high degree of cleanliness is possible, and the extreme vascularity of these tissues usually ensures healing in spite of the bacterial flora that are present always. Both before and after operation the nose and the mouth should be sprayed or swabbed at frequent intervals with mild alkaline antiseptic solutions (liquor antisepticus alkalinus or Dobell's solution). Each feeding should be followed by a thorough cleansing of the mouth. The stitches on the inner and the outer parts of the lip may be swabbed carefully with a cotton applicator dipped in hydrogen peroxide to free the incision of milk or serum. If the wound is kept clean and free of infection, the cosmetic results are better.

Immediately after operation the danger is from asphyxia. To avoid this danger the child should be placed on his side with the head low, so that vomitus, blood and mucus may drain easily from the mouth. The tongue may fall back frequently and obstruct the pharynx. This may be prevented by affixing to the cheek, with an adhesive strip, the silk thread drawn through the tongue at the time of operation. As soon as the child has recovered consciousness, the thread may be removed.

Dyspnea may occur when the operation has brought about a considerable narrowing of the nostrils. The nurse should watch such children carefully and depress the lower lip with a strip of adhesive until the child becomes accustomed to the new condition. Arm restraints may be necessary to prevent him from touching his face and injuring the suture line. These may be made of padded splints and placed so that the elbow cannot be flexed. They should be removed every four hours to massage both arms. The child's position should be changed to avoid pulmonary complications.

If a child with both harelip and cleft palate has had only the harelip repaired, his mother must be instructed as to how to care for him until the second operation is performed. She should learn the most effective way of feeding her child and of protecting him from respiratory infections. The long-range postoperative care of a child who has had such repairs will include teaching him to enunciate properly. This calls for tact and patience all round.

Epithelioma

Cancer of the lip, usually called *epithelioma*, occurs most frequently on the lower lip in men as a chronic ulcer. It grows rapidly, develops into a foul crater and soon produces secondary growths in the glands of the neck.

Treatment. The treatment of this disease, if begun early, is wide excision of the growth, frequently with removal at the same time of the glands of the neck. If treated late, the lesion is removed locally by electrodesiccation, combined with radiation of the glands of the neck.

Nursing Care

The nursing care of the patient in the early stages is to give mouthwashes and keep the lesion or wound as clean as possible. Feeding often is a problem. Liquid and soft foods should be served attractively in amounts sufficient to enable the patient to gain strength and weight.

The inoperable cases are pitiable, both before and after electrodesiccation. The growth is painful and foul-smelling. Such people cannot eat, saliva drools over the lips or the lesion, and after months of suffering death comes usually from cachexia or secondary hemorrhage. The nurse should try to make the last days of such patients as comfortable as possible. They need kindness and understanding. They should have meticulous mouth care and the benefit of deodorants. The frequent use of sedatives is necessary.

SURGERY OF THE MOUTH AND THE TONGUE

Ludwig's Angina

Ludwig's angina is an acute septic inflammation of the tissues of the floor and the submaxillary region of the mouth and of the submaxillary region of the neck. Its onset is sudden: the patient has difficulty in talking and swallowing, he has pain and salivation and, finally, dyspnea. The patient is profoundly toxic, but does not exhibit the high temperature and the leukocytosis that might be expected. Death may occur suddenly, due to edema of the glottis that produces asphyxia or to intense toxemia.

Treatment. The treatment is early incision with drainage, then the application of hot wet dressings to the neck and the use of hot mouthwashes. If dyspnea develops, a tracheotomy must be performed. The nurse must watch these patients closely for respiratory difficulty, stertorous (noisy) breathing, cyanosis or rapid increase in swelling. These symptoms are the early signs of beginning respiratory obstructions. A tracheotomy often is required. Early treatment with penicillin often is able to abort the infection and to ward off serious complications.

Alveolar Abscess

Alveolar abscess usually is a sequela of dental infection. It begin with a moderate tenderness an swelling of the gums, which if un treated lead to a swelling of th whole side of the face with extrem tenderness and inability to open th mouth fully. Frequently the absces points on the cheek side of the in fected tooth, and pus may be ex pressed from that area by gent pressure.

Treatment. The abscess must b opened by an incision on the outsid of the gum that extends down t the jaw bone. A drainage tube usu ally is inserted for a few days. Th postoperative care is the administr tion of hot antiseptic mouthwash at 2-hour intervals, except when th patient is asleep. This treatme hould be continued until the swelling subsides. External heat also hasens the subsidence of the infection nd relieves pain and soreness to a arge extent. The patient should be ncouraged to expectorate and not o swallow the foul pus that collects n the mouth. A sputum cup or basin lways should be within easy reach.

Carcinoma of the Mouth

Carcinoma may arise in any part f the mouth. However, it appears nost frequently on tongue, cheek nd lip. Often the individual feels roughened area with his tongue. n tobacco chewers, the mucous nembrane of the cheek is the comnonest site. A jagged tooth may be ne source.

Carcinoma of the tongue occurs nost frequently in men past middle ge. The lesion is found usually on ne lateral margin. It begins as a nall ulcer that does not heal. The rowth spreads rapidly to the lymph odes of the neck. The earliest sympom is pain or soreness of the tongue n eating hot or highly seasoned ods. Later, pain develops on swalwing even liquids. Earache, face che and toothache become almost onstant. Speech becomes difficult nd salivation occurs. Unable to eat r sleep because of the pain, the atient loses weight and strength apidly. Death results usually from spiration pneumonia due to inability to swallow normally, from toxnia caused by septic absorption om the foul, ulcerating growth or om hemorrhage from the growth.

Treatment and Nursing Care

The only cure is surgery following early recognition of the condition. The enlargement of lymph nodes indicates metastases. This may necessitate more extensive surgical dissection combined with radium and x-ray therapy. When it is the tongue that is involved, it is necessary often to perform a hemiglossectomy or a glossectomy.

The care of the mouth is extremely important for the welfare of the patient. The type of nursing care given in these serious and often offensive conditions is an index frequently of the efficiency of the nurse. If the patient is conscious and able to help himself, the nurse can teach him how to keep his mouth clean. She must remind him and keep him supplied with a toothbrush or gauze-padded tongue depressor, as well as a mouthwash.

The general physical condition of a person often is reflected in his mouth. Therefore, good nutritional levels must be maintained. If the breath has a foul odor, the nurse must insist on good mouth care before and after each feeding. Often a bad taste in the mouth spoils the taste of food and limits the intake of nourishment. If the patient is a mouth-breather, he needs more mouth attention than the average person. The use of swabs of mineral oil with lemon juice is refreshing. Lanolin applied to dry and cracking lips is soothing.

In the case of patients with dentures, it is necessary that these be removed frequently and cleaned. Before they are replaced, the mouth also should be cleaned. Often care is given to the teeth, but the "furred" or coated tongue is neglected and bad breath continues. In the unconscious patient, the nurse is wholly responsible for maintaining good mouth hygiene. The use of a special mouth tray with all necessary applicator sticks, padded tongue depressors, mouthwashes, lubricants and so forth encourages frequent mouth attention.

Individuals with mouth lesions may have feeding problems. The use of a paper straw, a glass tube or a teaspoon may be effective. The Breck feeder, so frequently employed with children, may be of use. Food should be soft or liquid and nonirritating; that is, not too hot or too cold and not highly seasoned. It should be served attractively to tempt the patient to take it. Small, frequent feedings are more desirable than large, less frequent ones. The desires as well as the nutritional needs of the patient should be taken into consideration. If he is not able to take anything by mouth, it may be necessary to feed him by means of a nasal tube. The care of this is similar to that of a gastrostomy tube. (See p. 307.)

If the lesion is such that the patient salivates constantly, this may be relieved somewhat by inserting a gauze wick in the corner of the mouth. The saliva that drops from the end of the wick may be caught in a small basin. Another way of removing mouth secretions is by the use of a small rubber catheter attached to a suction apparatus. Mouth wipes, as well as a paper bag attached to the bed or the bedside stand to receive soiled tissues, always should be on hand. An effective way of holding dressings of the mouth or the lower jaw in place is by the use of a face mask. The strings can be tied at the top of the head.

To combat odors, the doctor may order such oxidizing agents for a mouthwash as potassium permanganate 1:10,000, hydrogen peroxide in half strength, sodium perborate and so forth. In addition, in the case of patients with malodorous cancer lesions, a room deodorant may be used. There are many effective kinds available. Good room ventilation must be maintained. In extensive mouth sores, a power spray can clean wounds effectively and necrotic tissue can be removed more easily. If radium is used, the usual radium precautions are observed. When radium needles are implanted, each needle has a thread attached to it. The patient should know upon waking that these are present and that they are not to be removed. The power spray is effective in cleansing the mouth when these are in place. Radium may be implanted in a moulage (molded dental compound), and this may be applied to some part of the mouth for a specific length of time. It is usually permissible to remove the mold for meals and at night. When it is reinserted, it is important for the nurse to note that it is in its proper position. (For care of radium, see p. 200.)

Speech often is interfered with or is difficult. Simply to supply the patient with a pad of paper and a pencil may make a tremendous difference in his depressed condition. Often these patients are reluctant to associate with other patients; they prefer to be alone. If there are two or more patients with a similar condition, they can help each other. It is easier for them, and for others, if they have their meals apart from other patients. Kindness, attention to cleanliness and keeping the patient comfortable are the keynotes of the nursing care of these patients. The doctor's orders regarding special treatments, diet and medications must be followed. In advanced malignant cases, the nurse should be on guard for hemorrhage.

DISEASES OF THE ESOPHAGUS

The esophagus is the mucus-lined tube that leads from the pharynx through the chest to the stomach.

Congenital Anomalies

The most common congenital malformation of the esophagus is *atresia* (absence or closure of the passage). The esophagus may end in a blind pouch and the remaining portion may be connected with the trachea and produce a tracheo-esophageal fistula. Many variations of malformation have been found. It is detected usually in the infant when he regurgitates on taking fluids, becomes cyanotic and chokes as the fluids escape from the nose and the mouth. The only treatment is surgical repair in the first few days of life. This usually includes a temporary gastrostomy. Besides the problem of caring for a very young infant after a thoracic operation, the nurse must recognize the importance of feeding and maintaining fluid balance.

Trauma

The esophagus is not an uncommon site of injury. Stab or bullet wounds of neck and chest often produce such injury. Swallowed foreign bodies—dentures, fish bones, safety pins and so forth—may injure the esophagus as well as obstruct its lumen. Usually, foreign bodies can be removed with the aid of the esophagoscope. The injuries to the esophagus are the more serious part of the problem, because they may lead to deep cervical or mediastinal abscess, or to stricture formations. Drainage of such abscesses requires a thoracic exposure.

Burns

Stricture of the esophagus also occurs usually in children after chemical burns.

The acute chemical burn of the esophagus has associated severe burns of the lips, the mouth and the pharynx with pain on swallowing and, sometimes, difficulty in respiration due either to swelling in the throat or a collection of mucus in the pharynx. Many are profoundly toxic. If the patient is able to swallow, fluids should be given in small quantities at a time. Secretions should be aspirated from the pharynx if respiration is embarrassed. The necessity for high fluid intake may require administration by the intravenous route.

When the acute stage subsides, the patient may swallow normally for a time, but usually multiple stricture levels form in the esophagus. These may be dilated by the retrograde bouginage method of Tucker. A gastrostomy opening is made and a braided silk string is inserted into the esophagus. One end is brought

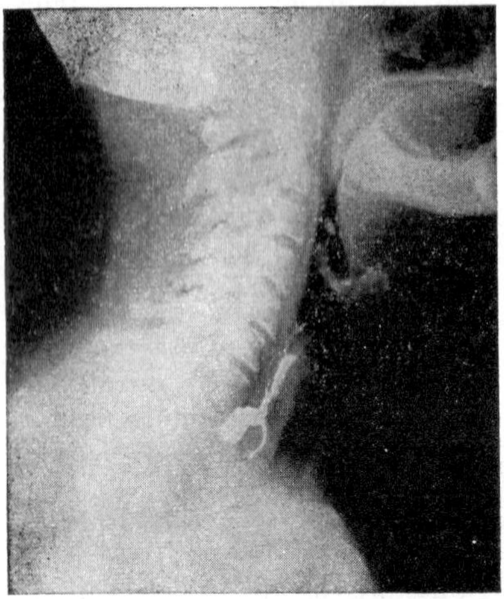

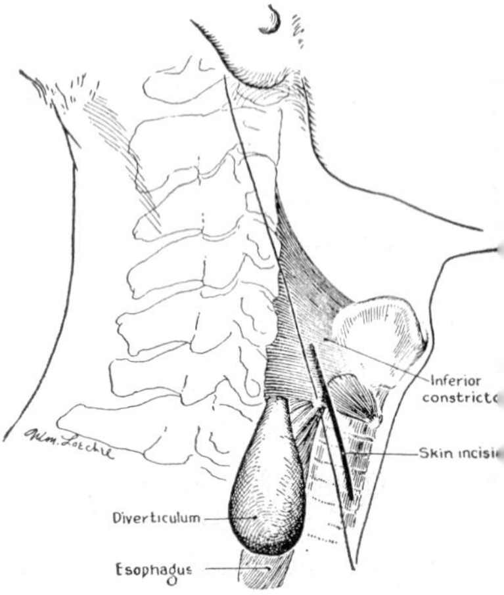

FIG. 117 (*Left*). Diverticulum of the esophagus. Roentgenogram showing the appearance of an esophageal diverticulum. Note the retention of barium in the diverticulum.

FIG. 118 (*Right*). Diagrammatic drawings show how diverticulum projects through the muscles of the upper portion of the pharynx.

out through the gastrostomy opening and the other end through the nose. The two ends are tied together and form a complete loop. Dilatation is obtained by pulling larger and larger bougies upward through the esophagus by means of the string. It is important that this string be left in place at all times. The gastrostomy is kept open by means of a gastrostomy tube, through which feedings may be given if necessary. Dressings round this tube should be changed whenever soiled. The tube should be changed daily to prevent irritation about the wound. (See Gastrostomy, p. 307.)

DIVERTICULUM

A *diverticulum* of the esophagus is an outpouching of the wall of this structure, usually in the cervical region and on the posterior aspect. The patients notice first a sensation of difficulty in swallowing, with fullness in the neck, and often they state that it feels as though their food stops before it gets into the stomach. The operable variety is due to a weakness in the wall, and the pouch appears on one side of the neck. It causes symptoms by becoming filled with food, which is regurgitated later.

These diverticula may be removed surgically. After operation, the nurse must feed the patient through a nasal tube that usually is inserted at the time of operation. The feedings may include any liquid, but a careful record of their kind, amount and character must be kept in order that the surgeon may know that the patient is receiving sufficient calories. After each feeding, the tube should be irirgated carefully with water. The wound also must be watched carefully for evidences of leakage from the esophagus and a developing fistula.

Nursing Care

When a patient has difficulty in swallowing, it is usual to limit his diet to those foods that pass more easily. Consequently, these patients often are the victims of unbalanced diets and unbalanced fluid levels. Often also, they express a fear of cancer. Preoperative preparation by the surgeon and the nurse is directed toward getting him into optimum physical and mental condition. Food and/or fluids high in vitamin and protein content are given. Diagnostic tests, such as esophagoscopy and x-rays, are carried out. The nurse should explain the procedure to the

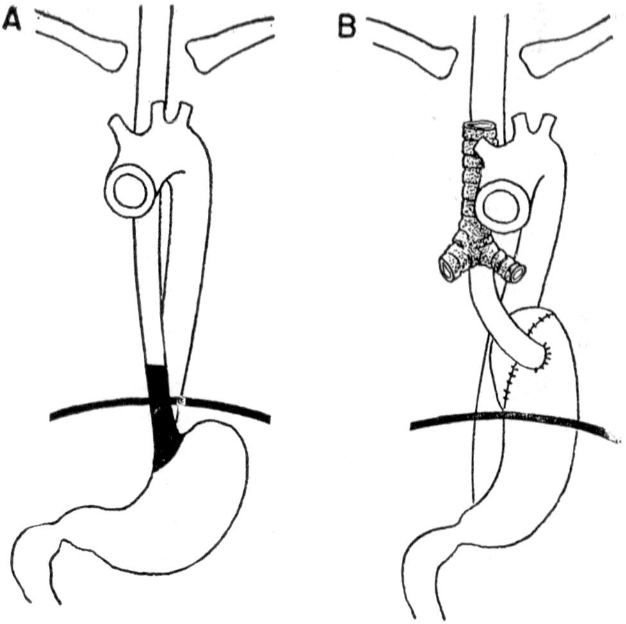

FIG. 119. (A) Black portion of esophagus indicates carcinoma. (B) Relations of the viscera after resection of a carcinoma of the lower fourth of the thoracic segment and the abdominal segment of the esophagus. The proximal esophagus is relatively long and a large segment of the stomach, including the lesser curvature, the cardia and the fundus, has been resected. The anastomosis lies in the lower portion of the mediastinum.

patient before he is taken for such an examination so as to allay his fears. After an esophagoscopy the patient may complain of a sore throat. This passes in a few hours with mild sedation. A day or two before the operation a silk string usually is swallowed by the patient. This enables the esophagoscopist to follow more readily into the esophagus with his scope and eliminates the danger of rupture of the diverticulum. The lighted scope makes the surgery much simpler. A Levin tube is threaded through the scope and into the stomach before the scope is removed. The anesthesia used may be local or inhalation. The patient often is out of bed on the day of operation. After operation for transthoracic esophagectomy, the patient may be given oxygen therapy to facilitate breathing and to prevent anoxemia. The nursing care in this most serious condition follows the general principles employed in thoracic surgery.

Carcinoma

Carcinoma of the esophagus is a disease that occurs in older people, and more often in males. It is characterized by a gradually increasing difficulty in swallowing. At first only solid food gives trouble but, as the growth progresses and the obstruction becomes more complete, even liquids cannot pass into the stomach. Regurgitation of food and saliva occur, and there is a progressive loss of weight and strength due to starvation. The diagnosis is confirmed by x-ray examination and by esophagoscopy. Bronchoscopy usually is performed also, especially in tumors of the middle and the upper third of the esophagus, to determine whether the trachea has been involved by the tumor and to help in determining whether the lesion can be removed.

Surgical removal of the growth is the only hope of cure. This can be accomplished by an approach through the thorax or through the abdomen and thorax for lower esophageal lesions. The portion of the esophagus containing the growth is removed, and the continuity of the gastro-intestinal tract is reformed by bringing the stomach into the chest and implanting the proximal end of the esophagus into it (see Fig. 118). The chest is closed after insertion in the pleural cavity of a drain that is led under water or is attached to a suction apparatus.

If the growth is found to be inoperable either before or at operation, a gastrostomy often is performed as a palliative procedure to permit the administration of food and fluids.

Nursing Care

Frequently it takes many days to prepare these patients for surgery. Numerous laboratory tests are required of blood protein, hemoglobin and so forth to determine the patient's physiologic status, and an effort is made to correct the deficiencies by the parenteral administration of blood, fluids, amino acids, electrolytes and vitamins. These measures, in addition to roentgenograms and esophagoscopic studies, may be somewhat troublesome to an older patient. A sympathetic and an understanding nurse can do much to make the patient understand the necessity and the value of the various procedures.

In the postoperative phase, the fundamentals of care are similar to those used in gastric and thoracic surgery. The patient usually is placed in an oxygen tent. He must be turned frequently and encouraged to take deep breaths. Even so, by the second day there may be an accumulation of blood and serous fluid in the pleural cavity that necessitates a thoracentesis. The fluid withdrawn often is replaced with a prescribed amount of penicillin.

In surgery of the esophagus, a nasal catheter usually is inserted in the esophagus as far as the esophagogastric anastomosis or through it. This must be attached to a continuous suction apparatus. It is removed within three to five days, and fluids may be given by mouth in increasing amounts. Soft foods are added gradually. Intravenous blood and fluids must be continued for several days after operation until the patient is able to take sufficient food and fluids by mouth. Penicillin usually is given prophylactically for several days preoperatively and after surgery.

CHAPTER SEVENTEEN

Surgery of the Abdomen

General Considerations. The gastro-intestinal canal begins with the lips and terminates at the anus. It is approximately 24 feet in length in the adult. Throughout its extent it has certain functions that are concerned with digestion of food. Any appreciable interference with these functions may cause indigestion.

It has been stated authoritatively that 60 per cent of the symptoms encountered by the physician arise from the digestive tract. These symptoms are enumerated as dyspepsia, heartburn, flatulence, pain, eructations, constipation, distress, distention, nausea, vomiting, bloating, gas and anorexia. Nine of these 13 complaints are gastric manifestations. This is the reason for the statement that the stomach is the spokesman of the body. Moynihan has said that the stomach is the biggest liar in the body, and this probably is true, for acute gastro-intestinal symptoms may be, and usually are, associated with lesions in the abdomen; yet, abnormal conditions in the head, the neck and the thorax can, and very frequently do, manifest themselves reflexly and mimic abdominal disease. The nausea, the vomiting and the borborygmi of brain lesions, the inordinate hunger, the diarrhea and the indigestion of the psychopathic patient, the so-called nervous indigestion and the diarrhea of the toxic thyroid, the abdominal pain and the rigidity secondary to pulmonary lesions and, lastly, the upper abdominal distress incident to cardiac decompensation and coronary disease —all are examples of this reflex phenomenon. Fright, shock and severe pain of any organ may cause cessation of peristalsis, nausea and vomiting. Even the physiologic condition of pregnancy is an offender with its hyperemesis. And yet, it is the irony of fate that when carcinoma invades the stomach it causes gastric symptoms so slowly that when the patient

PLATE 1

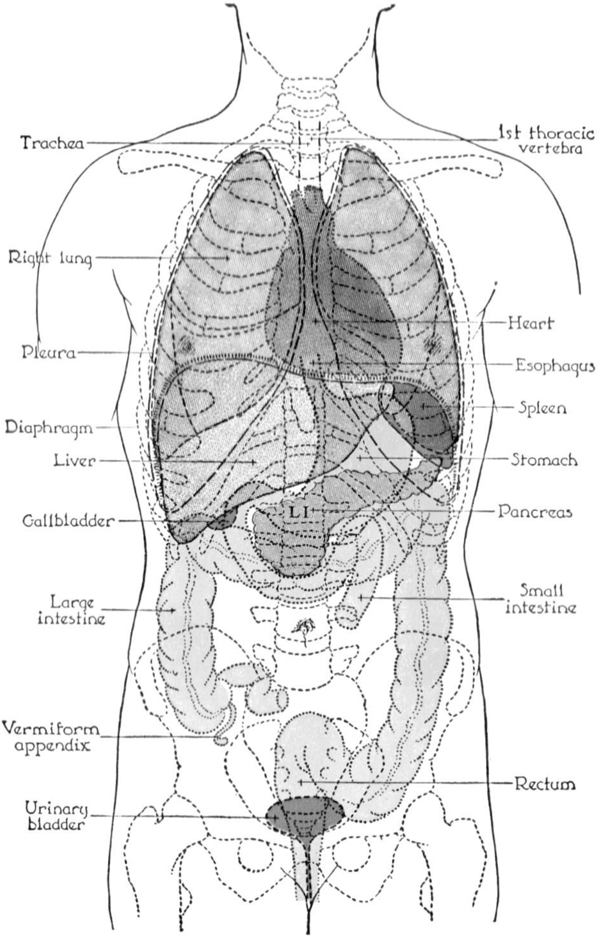

Location of the principal organs. This diagrammatic representation shows the position of the organs in relation to the surface of the body, as well as the skeletal framework. The kidneys (not shown) are behind the stomach, one on each side of the spine. (Eliason: First Aid in Emergencies, Philadelphia, Lippincott)

complains of indigestion it is often too late for complete removal, the only cure known at present.

Although there are many causes of indigestion that are amenable to medical and hygienic care, they should be considered surgical until proven otherwise if they persist for long periods of time (weeks).

Preparation of the Patient. Preparation for abdominal operations is no different essentially from that necessary for other operations. Because the surgeon never can be absolutely sure what incision will be necessary, the entire abdomen, from the symphysis to the costal arch, should be shaved and prepared. It is unwise to purge these patients before operation, but a thorough cleansing enema should be given in the morning before they are sent to the operating room. If the operation is to be performed on the lower abdomen, it is essential that the urinary bladder be emptied, either normally or by catheterization.

Abdominal Organs. Before studying individual diseases and operations, the nurse should be familiar with the prefixes denoting abdominal organs and the suffixes used to denote the diseases of or operations upon these organs.

Suffixes used to denote the names of disease and operations are:

itis—inflammation of—as *appendicitis,* an inflammation of the appendix.

otomy—to make a cut into—as *gastrotomy,* to make an opening into the stomach.

ostomy—to make a mouth or opening into—as *cystostomy,* to insert a tube into the urinary bladder.

ectomy—to cut or remove—as *salpingectomy,* to remove the fallopian tube.

pexy—to sew up in position—as *nephropexy,* to sew the kidney up in position.

orrhaphy—to repair a defect—as *herniorrhaphy,* to repair a hernial defect.

plasty—to improve by changing the position of the tissue—as *pyloroplasty,* an operation to enlarge the pyloric opening of the stomach.

(See also inside of book cover.)

ABDOMINAL TOPOGRAPHY

For purposes of convenience in description, the abdomen has been divided into nine regions by imagi-

Organs	Prefix	
Stomach	*Gastr*	*Gastritis*—inflammation of stomach
Pylorus	*Pylor*	*Pylorectomy*—removal of pyloric end of stomach
Liver	*Hepa*	*Hepatitis*—inflammation of liver
Gallbladder	*Cholecyst*	*Cholecystitis*—inflammation of gallbladder
Common bile duct	*Choledoch*	*Choledochitis*—inflammation of common bile duct
Small intestine	*Enter*	*Enteritis*—inflammation of intestine
Colon	*Col*	*Colitis*—inflammation of large gut
Appendix	*Appendic*	*Appendicitis*—Inflammation of appendix
Urinary bladder	*Cyst*	*Cystitis*—inflammation of urinary bladder
Fallopian tube	*Salping*	*Salpingitis*—inflammation of fallopian tube
Ovary	*Oophor*	*Oophoritis*—inflammation of ovary
Pelvis of kidney	*Pyel*	*Pyelitis*—inflammation of pelvis of kidney
Kidney	*Nephr*	*Nephritis*—inflammation of kidney
Rupture	*Herni*	*Herniorrhaphy*—repair of hernia
Loin or abdomen	*Lapar*	*Laparotomy*—incision in the abdomen

nary lines, as illustrated in Figure 120.

The abdominal cavity normally contains a small amount of fluid that lubricates the peritoneal surfaces. This cavity is lined with a thin, glistening membrane called the peritoneum. This structure covers all the abdominal organs, forming folds between which the coils of gut are located. Some organs (such as the liver, the pancreas, the kidney and the urinary bladder) are not covered completely by peritoneum; hence inflammations of these structures may not always involve the general abdominal cavity but may develop into retroperitoneal extensions or abscesses.

PERITONITIS

Peritonitis is inflammation of the peritoneal cavity. Usually it is due to bacterial infection, the organisms coming from disease of the gastrointestinal tract, the internal genital organs of the female and, less often, from outside by injury or by extension of inflammation from an extraperitoneal organ such as the kidney.

Symptoms depend, of course, on the location and the extent of the inflammation, and these in turn are determined by the disease causing the peritonitis. At first a diffuse, colicky type of pain is felt. This tends to become constant, localized and more intense near the site of the

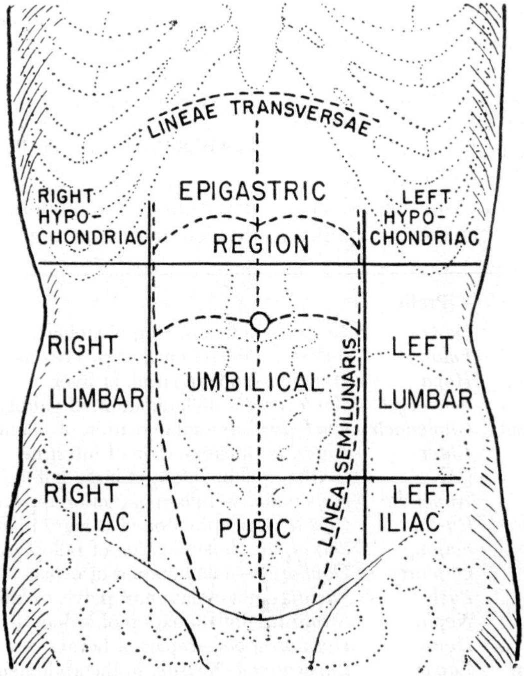

FIG. 120. Regions of the abdomen.

process. The area of the abdomen affected becomes extremely tender and the muscles become rigid. Usually, nausea and vomiting occur and peristalsis is diminished. The temperature and the pulse rate increase, and almost always there is an elevation of the leukocyte count. These early signs and symptoms of peritonitis also are the symptoms of the disease causing the condition.

Treatment and Nursing Care

Treatment is directed toward removing the cause: if this is an acutely inflamed appendix, an appendectomy is performed; if it is a ruptured duodenal ulcer, the opening in the duodenum is closed; and so on.

If the cause of the peritonitis is removed at an early stage, the inflammation subsides and the patient recovers. Frequently, however, the inflammation is not localized and the whole abdominal cavity becomes involved. The patient is acutely ill. He has severe pain and must be treated gently. Treatment and nursing care are concerned with combating the infection, establishing and eliminating the cause of the peritonitis, and making the patient as comfortable as possible.

Nothing is given by mouth; therefore, good mouth hygiene must be carried out by the nurse. Fluids of saline and glucose are administered by vein in an attempt to establish an adequate fluid level and to ensure an adequate urinary output both before and after operation. This is important, for many toxins are thrown off in this way. The effectiveness of this regimen can be attained only by the accurate recording of fluid intake and output by the nurse. This includes the measuring and the recording of vomitus. The antibiotics, especially penicillin and streptomycin or chlortetracycline or oxytetracycline, may be given parenterally. Usually penicillin and streptomycin are administered intramuscularly, whereas chlortetracycline or oxytetracycline may be given in intravenous solutions.

It is essential that the nurse observe and record symptoms accurately. Her description of the nature, the location and the shifts of pain in the abdomen is very important. She may do much in establishing confidence and hope in the patient, who realizes very often the seriousness of his condition.

When he has recovered from the anesthetic after operation, the patient is placed in the Fowler position to facilitate drainage. Nothing is given by mouth and he continues to receive fluids by vein. To prevent vomiting and distention, a gastrointestinal tube is passed through the nose into the stomach and/or the duodenum. This tube is connected to wall or Wangensteen suction and must be checked by the nurse to see that it works properly. Obviously, it will be necessary to give care to the nose and the mouth to keep the patient comfortable. Cotton applicators dipped in water or mineral oil are effective in cleaning the nose. The use of a toothbrush and a mouthwash by the patient is refreshing. Mineral oil with lemon juice is pleasant as a lubricant for dry lips.

Drains are inserted frequently during the operation, and it is essential that the nurse observe and record the character of the drainage. Care must be taken in moving and in turning the patient to prevent dis-

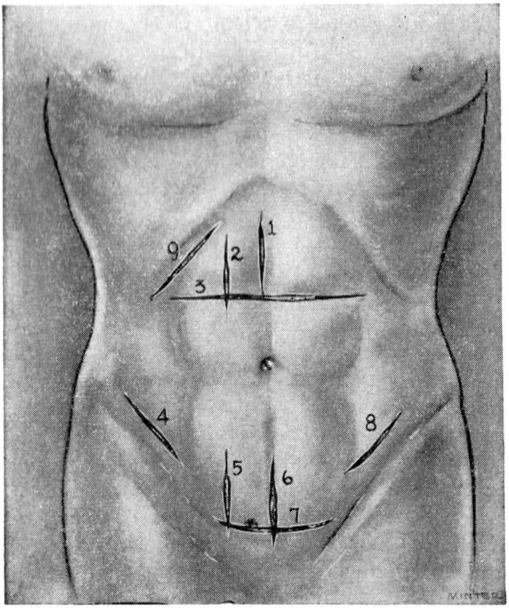

FIG. 121. Abdominal incisions. (1) Paramedian. (2) Upper right rectus. (3) Transverse. (4) Gridiron (McBurney). (5) Lower right rectus. (6) Suprapubic. (7) Pfannenstiel. (8) Left iliac gridiron. (9) Subcostal.

lodging or removing the drains accidentally. When the temperature and the pulse rate fall, the abdomen becomes soft, peristaltic sounds return and the patient begins to pass gas and have bowel movements, the peritonitis is subsiding. Food and fluids can be given by mouth in increasing amounts and parenteral fluids are reduced.

Two of the most common complications that must be watched for are wound evisceration and abscess formation. Any suggestion from the patient that an area of the abdomen is tender or painful or "feels as if something just gave way" should be reported to the surgeon.

SURGERY OF THE ABDOMEN

Incisions

Laparotomy or abdominal section are terms used to describe any operation that involves opening the abdominal cavity. The gridiron or the McBurney incision (Figs. 121, 137, 138) is the simplest. It opens the abdomen through a small wound made by spreading the fibers of the muscles through which it passes. This incision is suitable especially for operations upon the appendix, and, as it has the advantage of being closed without tension, it makes a firm wound in which hernias rarely form.

More widely useful, however, are the vertical incisions made in the midline or to either side of it. These are made to pass between or through the rectus muscles. Many other types of incisions may be made. These vary, depending upon the preference of the surgeon.

In making abdominal incisions,

the wound always is protected from skin contamination by the clamping of towels or gauze sponges to its edge. Bleeding points are caught and ligated as they appear, and the tissues are divided layer by layer as they are encountered.

In all operations on the gastro-intestinal tract, the surgeon makes an opening into a tube filled with many kinds of bacterial life. Because of the highly acid juices of the stomach, the upper intestine and the stomach are believed to contain less bacteria than the lower. Nevertheless, whenever the intestinal tract is opened, there is danger of the spread of infection from it into the peritoneal cavity unless strict precautions are taken. Moist sponges are placed round the portion through which the incision is to be made, and all tissues not directly implicated in the operation are covered as completely as possible. Rubber-covered clamps may be placed on the gut in order to prevent the escape of intestinal contents. When the incision in the gut has been made, the contents of the opened loop are sponged out and the sponges are discarded.

When the openings in the intestines have been closed, all instruments, needles, sutures, scissors and so forth that have been used are removed from the operating table. Soiled sponges are discarded after the suture line has been mopped off with moist gauze, and fresh sterile towels or covers are placed about the operative field. The surgeon's gloves and those of his assistants should be changed before the operation is continued.

These precautions are taken in every gastro-intestinal operation and are observed rigidly in operations on the large intestine, where infection is found most commonly. Closure is made in the reverse order, and each layer is united accurately until the wound has been closed. As a general rule, sutures are not placed in fat or muscles, but only in the firm aponeurotic layers, which are able to hold the wound closed until healing has taken place. Reinforcing, "stay" or tension sutures of heavy silk or wire often are employed to give added strength and to prevent the formation of dead space in the wound.

SURGERY OF THE STOMACH AND THE DUODENUM

Anatomy and Physiology. The stomach is a hollow muscular organ into which food and fluids pass from the esophagus. The digestive juices, pepsin and hydrochloric acid, act upon food, and it is passed in small quantities into the duodenum, where the digestive processes continue. The stomach, which is in the upper left abdomen, has the capacity to expand and contract as necessary. It is supplied by the vagus and the sympathetic nerves. Stimulation via the vagus produces an increase in gastric secretion and in the muscular contractions of the stomach.

Congenital Hypertrophic Pyloric Stenosis

This condition, which is characterized by hypertrophy of the circular muscle fibers of the pyloric sphincter at the outlet of the stomach, requires surgical treatment more frequently than does any other condition during the first few months of life. Its cause is not understood definitely, but spasm of the pyloric

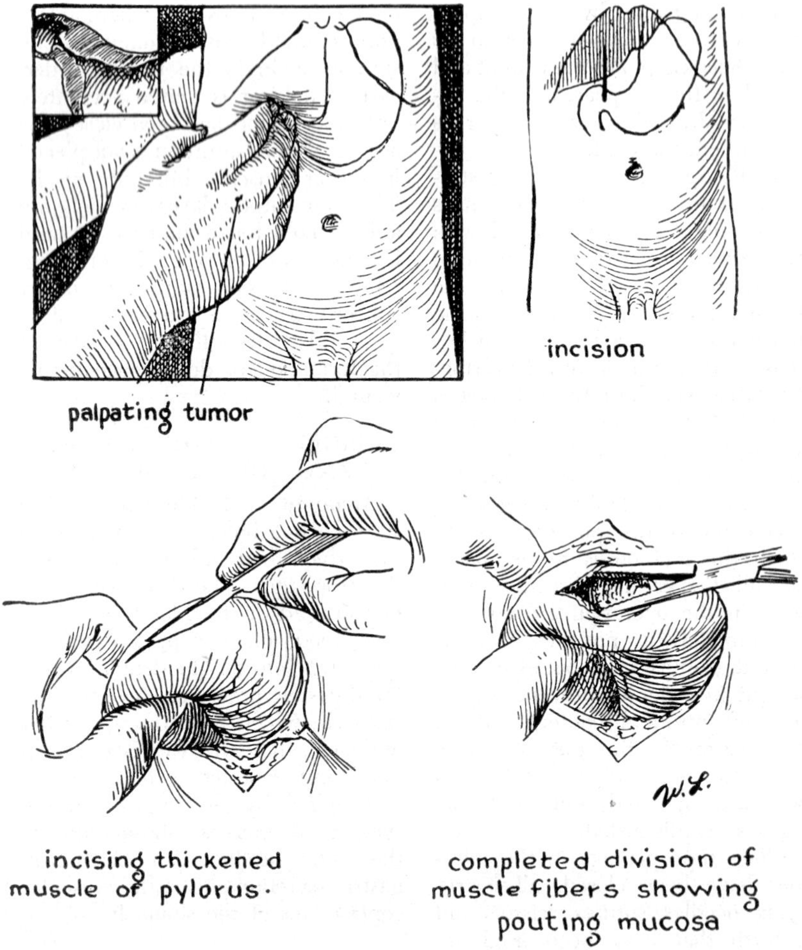

FIG. 122. Ramstedt operation for congenital hypertrophic pyloric stenosis.

muscle, in addition to edema of the mucous membrane from mechanical irritation of curds, would seem to be the main factors in its development. Heredity also appears to play a part in the etiology. The first-born male child is the one affected most frequently.

Diagnosis. Vomiting, which appears in the second or the third week of life, is the most constant symptom. As vomiting continues, the infant loses weight, dehydration appears and the stools become scanty. Peristaltic waves may be seen going from left to right across the upper abdomen during feeding. Palpation usually will reveal a small tumor mass in the right upper quadrant of the abdomen. The administration of a thin barium meal will show gastric retention and confirm the diagnosis.

Treatment and Nursing Care

The marked reduction in mortality in operative treatment of this condition during recent years is due largely to better preoperative care. Dehydration, acidosis, electrolyte imbalance and anemia must be corrected by adequate parenteral fluids, saline, glucose and blood. Transverse division of the hypertrophied circular pyloric muscle fibers to increase the diameter of the constricted area is the treatment of choice. This procedure is known as *pyloromyotomy* or the *Fredet-Ramstedt operation* (see Fig. 122). Prior to operation the stomach contents should be aspirated with a small rubber catheter passed through the nose. The catheter is left in place during the operation to keep the stomach deflated at all times. Body

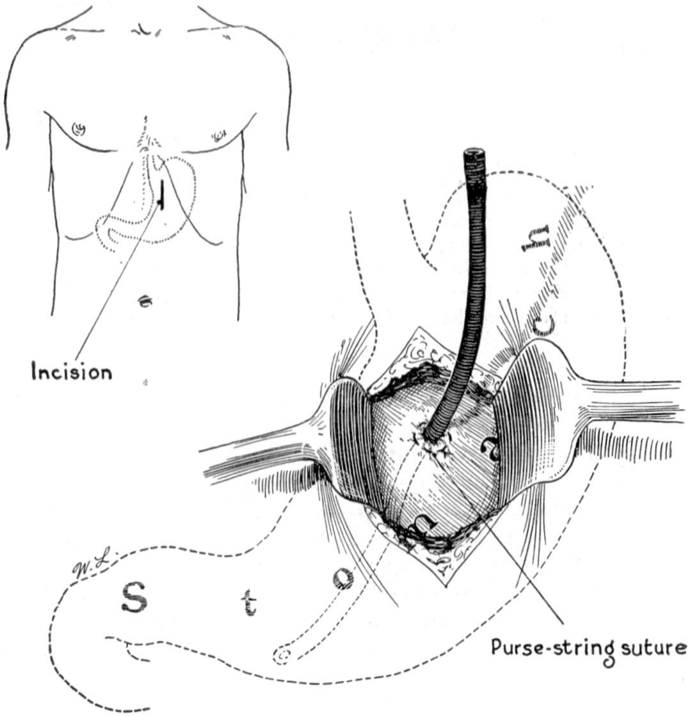

FIG. 123. Gastrostomy. Inset shows site of incision. A tube is inserted into the anterior gastric wall and held in place with several purse-string sutures.

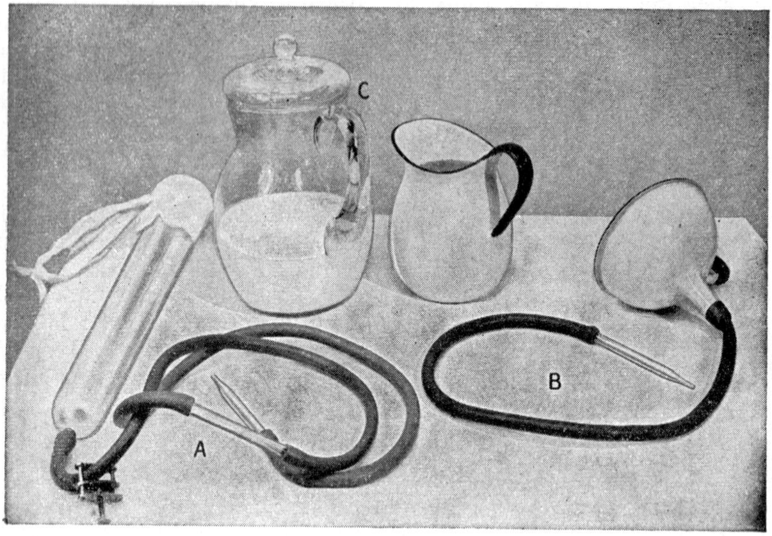

FIG. 124. Two types of equipment used in the feeding of patients with gastrostomy, jejunostomy and so forth. (A) This apparatus is used for the administration of feeding by the drip method. The rate of flow is regulated by the Hoffman clamp. Occasionally, a dropper is inserted into the tubing instead of the glass connecting tube. (B) The funnel used for a more rapid administration of the feeding. This type of apparatus generally is used when the patient feeds himself. (C) Note glass pitcher with feeding and pitcher containing water at body temperature for irrigating the tube and the apparatus after completion of the feeding.

heat of the infant must be conserved by keeping him well wrapped up while going to surgery. Preoperative medication consists usually of appropriate doses of atropine. Open-drop ether is the anesthesia of choice.

The postoperative care is important in the recovery of these severely ill infants. Feedings are begun as soon as the baby has recovered from anesthesia. Water is given first in 1-ounce quantities every two hours. This is followed by whey and increasing amounts of breast milk or formula, as indicated in the individual case. After from 10 to 14 days a normal feeding regimen should be attained. The nurse must observe her very young patient carefully for any signs or symptoms which might be suggestive of complications as otitis media, wound infection, evisceration and pneumonia. Fluid and electrolyte balance must be maintained and anemia corrected as indicated.

During hospitalization of the patient, the surgeon and the nurse should attempt to alleviate undue concern on the part of the parents.

A mother faces an emotional struggle which may be as difficult to treat as the organic disease of the child. These are situations in which the nurse can give assurance and encouragement. The results of surgery are very gratifying. Most large series of cases report a mortality of less than 1 per cent.

Gastrostomy

This operation, in which a permanent opening is made into the stomach, is performed for the purpose of administering food and fluids when an impermeable stricture of the esophagus exists. The esophageal stricture may be due to scar-tissue contracture. In children, it occurs often as a result of lye burns, and in older people it is due most frequently to a carcinomatous growth.

Preparation. The purpose of the operative procedure should be explained to the patient so that he will have a better understanding of his postoperative course. Fluids are administered by vein; the nature of the fluids is determined by the fluid, the electrolyte and the nutritional needs of the patient. (See p. 296, esophagus.)

Operation. The anterior gastric wall is grasped through the left rectus incision, and a tube is inserted into the stomach. This tube, usually a No. 20 or a No. 22 rubber catheter, is held in place by sutures placed round it. The end of the tube is brought through the wound to the anterior abdominal wall and clamped.

Postoperative Nursing Care

The psychological care of this patient is as important as his physical and nutritional care. The observing nurse will note his reactions and handle the situation accordingly.

The patient may be given fluids (10 per cent glucose solution is best) through the tube at once if he is much dehydrated. At first only an ounce or two at a time is given, but the amount is increased gradually until, by the end of the second day, from 6 to 8 ounces may be given at one time provided this quantity is borne well.

Liquid Feedings. Warm milk, cream, eggs, sugar, olive oil, broths and so forth may be given through the tube. The nurse may prepare a tray containing a glass buret, the barrel of a syringe or a funnel to which a rubber tubing and a glass adapter are attached. (See Fig. 124.) This would be attached to the gastrostomy tube at the time of feeding. Water at room temperature should be available and used to precede and follow the feeding. The feeding should be warmed by placing it in a basin of warm water. Feedings never should be given directly from the refrigerator. When fluid first is poured into the tubing, the receptacle should be tilted so that air will escape from the tubing and not enter the stomach and produce distention. The feeding should be allowed to flow into the stomach by gravity. The flow can be regulated by raising or lowering the receptacle. Force never should be used. If there seems to be an obstruction, stop the feeding and report the condition to the surgeon. The following diet has been found to be satisfactory:

	Calories
Milk, 300 cc.	336
Cream, 280 cc.	1,080
Eggs, 6	608
Sugar, 6 teaspoonfuls	120
Olive oil, 2 tablespoonfuls	360
Total	2,504

The mixture may be divided into 4 feedings for the day and 3 feedings for the night. They must be given very slowly. If the patient becomes nauseated, the fats must be decreased in amount and then increased gradually until the caloric requirement again is met. Water, 180 cc., should be given every second hour through the tube.

Feedings should be recorded carefully as to amount of fluid and contents, in order that the surgeon may know whether the patient is obtaining enough to satisfy his caloric, nutritional and fluid requirements. After each feeding, the tube should be irrigated with warm water and clamped. Neglect of this procedure may cause the catheter to become clogged. The nurse in charge of a patient with a gastrostomy always should have a duplicate tube sterilized and ready for use. After five or six days the tube may be removed if loose, and a fresh one, lubricated with petrolatum, inserted. Thereafter the tube is held in place by a thin strip of adhesive which first is twisted about the tube and then firmly attached to the abdomen. A small dressing is applied over the tube and the whole is held in place by a firm abdominal binder. Thereafter the tube should be changed every 2 or 3 days, and adults should be taught how to do this for themselves. The patient should learn also how to feed himself and should know what foods may be taken. Inexpensive strained baby foods are now available which can be used satisfactorily by these patients.

The skin about a gastrostomy opening requires special care. Soon or late it may become irritated due to the action of gastric juices which leak out round the tube. If uncared for, the skin becomes macerated, red, raw and painful. Daily dressing of the wound will avert this in large measure. However, it is well to apply some bland ointment, such as zinc oxide or petrolatum, to the area about the tube.

After several weeks, the tube may be removed and inserted only for feedings. Between times, the gastrostomy opening may be protected by a small gauze pad held in place by adhesive.

Peptic Ulcer

Symptoms. Ulcers appear in the stomach and the duodenum; occasionally they are found in the jejunum following operation. These ulcers are the result of the digestive action of the gastric acid pepsin. In most instances, they are treated medically. However, in a certain percentage of cases the ulcers may develop complications such as perforation, bleeding or obstruction to the pyloric outlet of the stomach or they are said to be intractable, that is, they do not respond to medical therapy. In such cases, surgical therapy must be carried out in an effort to rehabilitate the patient and to relieve him of his recurring attacks of pain and discomfort.

The periodic attacks of pain mean that the ulcer is healing and reforming alternately, a process that is accompanied by the formation of scar tissue. As these lesions usually are situated near the pylorus in the gastric or, more often, the duodenal wall, the scar tissue and the irritation of the ulcer cause disturbance in the function of the pylorus. A pyloric obstruction results and gastric retention occurs, as is evidenced by *vomiting* and *belching* after meals.

Diagnosis of these lesions is made more certain by the fluoroscopic and roentgenographic examination of the stomach after it has been filled with a radiopaque material. The outline of the stomach and the duodenum thus can be visualized, and the ulcer appears as a deformity in the roentgenogram. Gastric retention due to scar tissue formation at the pylorus is indicated by an enlarged stomach that empties slowly.

As the ulcer deepens, it may erode into a blood vessel and cause acute intestinal hemorrhage associated with foul tarry stools and the signs of internal hemorrhage described on page 139. For this reason the stools of these patients are examined frequently for blood, and, as any animal protein in the stools may confuse the chemical reaction, a meatless diet is given for at least three days before the stools are collected.

Perforation. The ulceration may progress rapidly, before scar tissue has time to form, and cause a perforation through the duodenum or the stomach. Patients complain of sudden stabbing pain in the epigastrium, a symptom often associated with shock. They have a chemical peritonitis—this is due to the acid secretion of the stomach—and on examination they show a rigid epigastrium so firm that it is usually described as boardlike. Any movement whatever causes excruciating pain; therefore, the first phase of treatment is the administration of morphine sulfate, Gm. 0.016 (¼ gr.). Ruptured ulcer should be considered to be the most urgent of emergencies, and the patient must be prepared for operation at once. Experience has taught that operation within 6 hours in such cases usually is successful but that after more than 12 hours very often it is fatal.

Preoperative Nursing Care

Often the cause of the ulcer will not be removed by surgical intervention alone. Constant fear or worry may be disturbing the individual. Only when this factor is eliminated can the best results be looked for. The surgeon and the nurse must realize that the "psyche" has much influence over the "soma," and all efforts to allay the apprehension and the fears of the patient should be employed. Perhaps an immediate preoperative worry is fear of the anesthesia or of malignancy. As these patients have a long illness, they are discouraged frequently and often are helped by spiritual therapy. Economic and social factors may have influenced the patient to such an extent that long hours of work, no recreation, tension, fatigue, etc., have contributed in good measure to his illness. The nurse might seek these factors tactfully in an effort to aid the physician as he directs treatment so that a recurrence of the patient's ulcer might be eliminated.

The patient has laboratory analyses, x-ray series and a general physi-

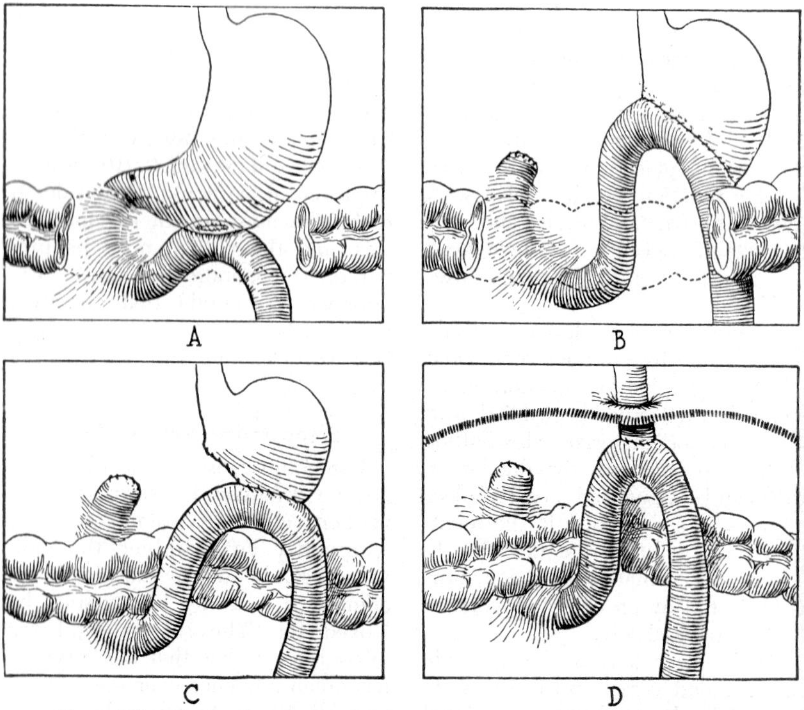

FIG. 125. Diagrammatic drawings to show types of gastric operations. (A) Posterior gastrojejunostomy. The jejunum is sutured to the stomach behind the colon, which has been cut away to show the anastomosis. (B) Subtotal gastric resection with posterior gastrojejunostomy. The resected portion includes the first part of the duodenum, the pylorus and from two thirds to three quarters of the stomach. The stump of the duodenum is closed by suture, and the side of the jejunum is anastomosed to the end of the stomach (Polya) posterior to the colon. (C) Subtotal gastric resection with anterior gastrojejunostomy (Hofmeister type). The resection is as in B. The anastomosis is made anterior to the colon, the side of the jejunum is anastomosed to part of the cut end of the stomach, and the rest is closed by sutures. (D) Total gastrectomy. The entire stomach is removed and the esophagus is anastomosed to a loop of jejunum under the diaphragm.

cal check-up before surgery is attempted. The function of the nurse is to prepare her patient for each of these diagnostic measures by explaining their nature and significance to him. Specific physical preparation will be prescribed by the physician.

Before operation is begun on the upper intestinal tract, special care should be paid to the hygiene of the mouth. The teeth of these patients usually are bad, and the nurse should urge frequent mouthwashes and a thorough brushing of the teeth at least 3 times daily.

The nutritional and fluid needs of the patient are of major importance. In those patients with pyloric obstruction, there usually is prolonged vomiting with resultant weight and fluid loss. Every effort must be made to restore an adequate nutritional level and to maintain an optimal fluid and electrolyte balance. Again, the nurse plays a key role in helping her patient achieve a satisfactory preoperative status so that postoperative hazards are kept at a minimum.

Occasionally, it is necessary for the patient to have a gastric lavage to remove retained food in the stomach. Wangensteen suction also may be used preoperatively. At any rate, a Levin tube often is inserted before the patient goes to the operating room and is left in place for operative and postoperative use. It is important that the colon be empty when the patient comes to surgery. Usually this is insured by an enema the day before operation. If gastrointestinal roentgenograms have been made shortly before the day of operation, it is most important that the patient have enemas to remove completely the barium that may remain in the colon. The nurse should report it when the enema returns still show the whitish color of barium in the fecal material. The patient usually has full fluids only during the 24-hour period preceding surgery. The abdomen should be prepared from the costal arch to the symphysis (see Fig. 11 C), although the incision usually is made in the upper right quadrant or the midline.

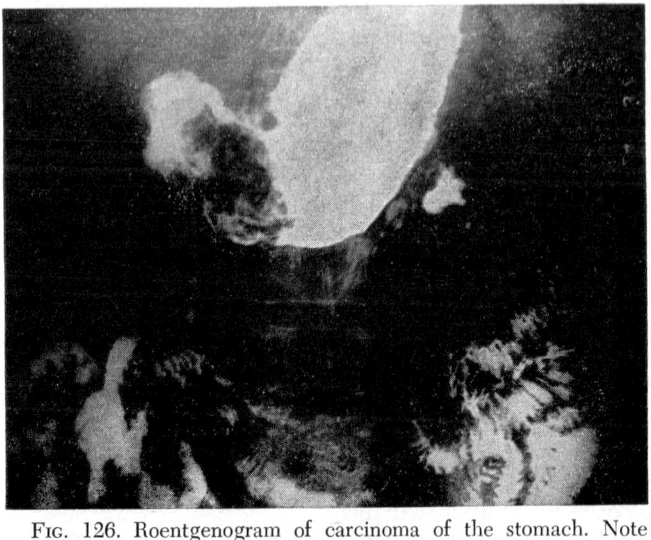

Fig. 126. Roentgenogram of carcinoma of the stomach. Note how the normal outline of the stomach is deformed by displacement of barium meal at the site of large gastric carcinoma.

Operative Treatment

In those cases in which bleeding is the outstanding symptom, there usually is a period of transfusion in preparation for the operative procedure. This is especially important in older patients in whom recurrence of hemorrhage often ends fatally. In these cases, the ulcer-bearing area is removed and the vessels leading to the area are ligated. As a rule, this entails a subtotal gastrectomy with removal of the ulcerated area in the duodenum. An end-to-side type of anastomosis is performed between the end of the stomach and the jejunum.

An almost immediate operation must be performed on those patients who reach the hospital with ulcers that are perforated and draining gastric or intestinal contents into the abdominal cavity. The abdomen is opened and the perforation through the ulcer is sutured and overlaid with omentum. In a few cases it may be necessary also to perform an anastomosis between the stomach and the jejunum. Ulcers complicated by a gradually increasing closure of the pyloric opening of the stomach occur usually in older people. In these cases, a conservative type of operation—posterior gastrojejunostomy—may be used. (Fig. 125 A.)

It is difficult to distinguish ulcers of the stomach from cancer of the stomach. Therefore, many surgeons are of the opinion that most large gastric ulcers should be treated by operation.

Usually the operation consists of an excision of the entire pyloric portion of the stomach, as much as three-fourths of the stomach proper often being removed with the ulcer. The end of the duodenum is close The opening in the stomach then sutured partially and the remainin opening is sutured to the side of th jejunum. (See Fig. 125 B and C.

In the case of intractable ulce not amenable to any type of medic nal or other conservative treatmen the foregoing operation is advise In this type of operation it is hope in both gastric and duodenal ulcer not only to remove the ulcer-bearin areas in both the duodenum and th stomach but to reduce the acid pep sin secretion of the stomach to level that will prevent the appea ance later of ulcers on the margin c the stoma or even in the jejunun

Vagotomy now is being performe in many of these cases. In this opera tion, both vagus nerves are sectione just before they enter the stomac thus abolishing the nervous factor i acid pepsin secretion. Vagotomy usu ally is performed with a gastr enterostomy or a gastric resection.

Carcinoma of the Stomach

Carcinoma of the stomach is foun most frequently in adults past mic dle life who have suffered for som time with indefinite indigestion. A the disease progresses there usuall is a loss of weight and strength, ass ciated with an increasing anemi Not infrequently the vomiting c blood occurs. A mass becomes pa pable in the upper abdomen an roentgenograms taken after a bi muth meal show marked deformit of the gastric outline. A gastroscop examination often confirms the dia nosis of a carcinoma. This involv the passing of a metal instrume with a light on the end of it throug the mouth and the esophagus in the stomach to enable the surgeon to see the stomach. (See Chap. 11 and page 227.)

Preparation for Operation. These patients should receive preparation similar to that for operation on peptic ulcers. Blood transfusions often are needed; gastric suction drainage usually is employed to empty the stomach before and after operation.

Operations Performed. Cure is effected often in the early stages by a resection of the part of the stomach containing the cancer; the continuity of the tract is restored by anastomosis. Complete gastric resection may be performed and the jejunum sutured to the esophagus (Fig. 125 D). Transfusions often are indicated during and after operation. Some of the complications that may follow these operations are shock, hemorrhage, vomiting, peritonitis, obstruction, hiccough, parotitis, pulmonary embolus and phlebitis. For a full description, see pages 136-158.

Nursing Care After Surgery on the Stomach and the Upper Gastro-intestinal Tract

In the operating room the administration of fluids is begun by transfusion and infusion, as much as from 2,500 to 3,000 cc. being given daily for the first two or three days. This is one of the best methods of warding off postoperative shock, a condition especially prone to develop in patients who have undergone operation for bleeding, perforated ulcer or cancer.

When recovery from anesthesia is complete, the patient is placed in the Fowler position, as this favors drainage of the stomach. Change of position from one side to the other at frequent intervals tends to prevent postoperative pulmonary and vascular complications. Nothing is given these patients by mouth for at least 24 hours. This precaution is taken to allow the suture line to seal off thoroughly and thus minimize the danger of leakage and peritonitis. Antibiotic and vitamin therapy are instituted parenterally. To relieve dryness of the mouth during this period, mouthwashes should be given at frequent intervals. To allow the patient to moisten his lips with ice that is enclosed in a piece of gauze often is refreshing. The nurse also can use an applicator stick dipped in mineral oil and lemon juice to swab dry lips. Very often a nasal tube attached to a Wangensteen apparatus is used to remove mucus, liquids, blood, gas and materials that accumulate in the stomach during the first 24 to 48 hours after operation. Repeated irrigation of the tube with syringe and salt solution may be needed to keep the tube open. The amount of solution used should be charted. With the nasal tube it is important for the nurse to give care to the nostrils. An applicator stick moistened with water and followed by an applicator stick dipped in mineral oil can be used to clean the nostril.

When the surgeon orders fluids, they should be given warm or hot and sparingly at first. Beginning with a dram or two every half hour, the amount is increased gradually until 3 or 4 ounces is being taken. Hot tea with sugar and lemon is very acceptable. Cold fluids usually cause distress. If the patient does not vomit, more fluid may be given by mouth. On the third or the fourth day, milk and other bland liquids may be added to the diet, and on the fifth day a routine diet should be instituted. Should the patient vomit, eruct or hiccough at any time, the intake should be stopped and instructions requested.

Patients who have been operated on for peptic ulcer often need instruction as to their diet for months and even years after operation, because, even though the ulcer has been removed, secondary ulcers sometimes occur. The best way to prevent these is to reduce the amount and the acidity of the gastric juice and to avoid coarse foods. Therefore, patients are instructed to avoid foods that tend to stimulate acid secretion in the stomach. Such foods are as follows:

All acids, i.e., vinegar, pickles, sour foods.

Raw fruits, i.e., apples, grapes, lemons, oranges.

Meat-stock soups, i.e., bouillon, consommé.

Condiments and spices, i.e., excess of salt, pepper, mustard, horseradish.

Concentrated sweets, i.e., honey, molasses, candy.

Coarse foods, i.e., nuts, corn, cabbage.

For the first six months, the patient may require six small meals a day because of his reduced gastric capacity. He must avoid overeating.

Merely to hand a patient awaiting discharge from hospital a diet list is not sufficient preparation. He should be brought to realize that emotional factors have a definite effect on food digestion. The need for peace of mind is so important; both he and his family should know this. If some of his problems remain unsolved, perhaps the medical social worker can help. The patient must realize that he is a responsible partner in his own treatment.

Complications After Operations on the Stomach

Shock has been mentioned as a complication, especially in very ill patients. The restoration of normal temperature and the administration of fluids are the prophylactic measures necessary in every case. For symptoms and treatment of shock, see Chapter 8, Postoperative Complications, page 136.

Vomiting nearly always occurs at least once or twice after operations on the stomach. The vomitus usually is composed of a dark, bloody fluid. Usually, nausea and vomiting disappear after 8 or 10 hours. If vomiting continues after the first 24 hours, it is due probably to blood retained in the stomach. A change of position or the giving of a glass of warm water or sodium bicarbonate solution may aid in the drainage of the stomach or induce vomiting. The nasal tube often is inserted to provide continuous gastric drainage by the Wangensteen apparatus.

Hemorrhage is occasionally a complication after gastric operations. The patient exhibits the usual signs (Chapter 8) and continues usually to vomit bright blood in considerable amounts. Treatment is the administration of morphine and the placing of an icecap on the abdomen. Adrenalin hydrochloride solution may be given in water or saline by mouth for its effect in producing vasoconstriction. The nurse should be prepared for the intravenous injection of saline or blood.

Pulmonary Complications. These

frequently follow upper abdominal incisions because of the tendency to shallow respiration. Therefore, the nurse should urge the patient to breathe deeply several times each hour when awake in order to obtain full aeration of the lungs. A change in position, turning the patient from side to side, also is an aid in preventing these complications.

Parotitis sometimes follows operations on the upper intestinal tract because patients may not have solid food for periods of almost a week and, consequently, the salivary flow is reduced markedly. Therefore, it is wise to pay special attention to the hygiene of the mouth and attempt to stimulate the flow of saliva by the use of chewing gum or small hard candies. (See Parotitis, Chap. 8.)

SURGERY FOR INTESTINAL OBSTRUCTION

Intestinal obstruction really is a symptom—it may be caused by many diseases—but obstruction to the intestinal flow is such a serious condition of itself that treatment often must be directed toward relief of the symptom before the cause can be removed. The commonest causes are postoperative adhesions, hernias, intussusception, volvulus and cancer.

The symptoms and the treatment of acute postoperative intestinal obstruction have been discussed in Postoperative Complications, Chapter 8, page 136. The type associated with hernias will be found described in connection with strangulated hernia (p. 355).

Intestinal obstruction may be only partial, causing colicky pain, noisy peristalsis, constipation, distention and, at times, nausea and vomiting. This state may continue for an indefinite period without getting any worse and then, unexpectedly, the symptoms of complete obstruction may appear. The patient develops sudden severe colicky pains. Vomiting of the forceful projectile type occurs, consisting at first of stomach contents mixed with bile. There is absolute constipation, although an enema may be effective in evacuating the lower bowel of fecal matter, which may have collected before the obstruction took place. Initially, temperature and pulse are normal; if the obstruction continues, vomiting becomes fecal or stercoraceous in type, pain continues, the abdomen becomes tender, the pulse rate increases and peristalsis is loud and tumultuous. If relief is not forthcoming, paralysis of the bowel results with marked distention, the skin becomes cold and moist and the outcome certainly will be fatal.

The gravity of this condition demands immediate action. Many patients who have lost much fluid and electrolytes from prolonged vomiting demand a period of preparation before any operation can be performed. The dehydration and the electrolyte loss must be overcome by fluid replacement, usually physiologic saline in large amounts. One of the most important phases of nursing care for this patient is the keeping of an accurate intake and output chart. During this period of preparation for operation, the intestinal tract is decompressed by the use of a Miller-Abbott, a Cantor or a Harris tube. Treatment depends upon the cause of the obstruction and the condition of the patient. If the obstruction has been of several days' duration and the patient obviously is very ill, the surgeon will attempt to relieve the obstruction in the quickest way possible. Under local anesthesia, the abdomen is opened and an enterostomy (ileostomy, cecostomy) or a colostomy is performed by suturing a tube into the distended bowel. After the patient has recovered sufficiently from the effects of the intestinal obstruction, the surgeon may perform a second operation to remove the primary cause.

If the intestinal obstruction has been of short duration and the patient is a good operative risk, the surgeon may attempt to remove the cause at the primary operation. If an abdominal band or adhesion has strangulated a portion of the bowel, the band may be cut; if an intussusception has occurred, it is relieved by the appropriate operation and so forth.

Intussusception is a telescoping of one portion of the gut into another. It occurs most frequently in children under ten years of age. The child, who up to the time of onset was well apparently, suddenly develops abdominal pain associated with vomiting. Bloody mucus passed by rectum is characteristic, and very often a mass may be palpated in the lower right part of the abdomen. If operation is performed early, the invaginated portion of the bowel often may be withdrawn. If, however, the intussusception cannot be reduced, or the bowel has been so damaged as to make it no longer viable, resection of the gut must be performed.

Volvulus is a condition in which a loop of intestine or colon becomes twisted on itself. It occurs most commonly in older persons and is associated with shock and extreme pain in the lower left quadrant of the abdomen. The operation is to untwist the bowel.

Cancer. Intestinal obstruction resulting from cancer of the large bowel occurs usually in a patient past middle life. The symptoms are slower in making their appearance than in obstruction of the small gut, distention is more marked and vomiting is a later symptom. A colostomy usually is performed. Later the growth may be removed.

Paralytic Ileus. Occasionally after abdominal operations, after operations on the kidney and, frequently, in cases of peritonitis, peristaltic movement becomes paralyzed due to traumatic or toxic affection of the nerves that have to do with the intestinal movement. This results in a distention of the intestine with gas, produced by decomposition of the intestinal contents or by the swallowing of air. The lack of peristalsis results in an accumulation of this gas in the gut, causing distention. Few or no peristaltic sounds can be heard, and the patient may be extremely uncomfortable, if not in marked pain. This condition is spoken of as *paralytic ileus* to distinguish it from *organic ileus,* which is caused by an organic obstruction of the intestine.

In the treatment of paralytic ileus, relief of the distention often is obtained by the introduction of a double lumen tube (Miller-Abbott tube). This is inserted through the nose into the stomach and, with the patient on his right side, enough of the tube is administered to permit its end to pass through the pylorus into the duodenum. After the tube is passed through the first portion of the duodenum, the rubber balloon near its tip is inflated by the introduction of air through the smaller portion of the double lumen tube. The inflated balloon is carried down the intestinal canal as the intestine is deflated by sucking out the gas through the larger portion of the double lumen tube, the Wangensteen apparatus being used. As soon as the intestine is deflated, peristaltic action appears to return.

Gastric and Intestinal Intubation

Tubes inserted into the stomach and the intestine are used to aspirate the contents of these organs in the active and the prophylactic treatment of many intra-abdominal lesions. The nasal catheter or so-called short tube is introduced through the nose or the mouth into the stomach. By aspiration, the gas and the fluids that collect in the stomach may be removed. It is especially valuable in the postoperative care of many patients after abdominal operations and especially in the treatment of vomiting postoperatively. The long tubes or double lumen tubes are rubber tubes which are introduced through the stomach into the intestinal tract. They are used to aspirate the intestinal content and so to prevent gas and fluid distention of the coils of gut. The long tubes are the Miller-Abbott, the Harris and the Cantor tubes. These are used in the active treatment of intestinal obstruction, especially that of the small intestine. They also are used prophylactically, being inserted the night before operation to prevent obstruction after abdominal operation. By their use the intestine is threaded upon the tube and so shortened and held together compactly, making it relatively easier to pack off the intestine at the time of operation upon the colon. Usually, the tubes are allowed to remain in place after operation until peristalsis is resumed, as shown by the passage of gas per rectum. Intubation usually is practiced in the treatment of all forms of intestinal obstruction, but it is especially effective in paralytic ileus and in postoperative obstruction. These patients can be given liquid nourishment by mouth with the tube still functioning.

Types of Gastro-intestinal Tubes

Miller-Abbott Tube. This is a double lumen, No. 16 Fr. 10-ft. tube: one lumen of the tube is used to inflate the balloon at the end of the tube; the other, entirely independent, is used for aspiration (Fig. 127). Before inserting the tube, the balloon should be tested, its capacity measured and then deflated completely. The tube should be lubri-

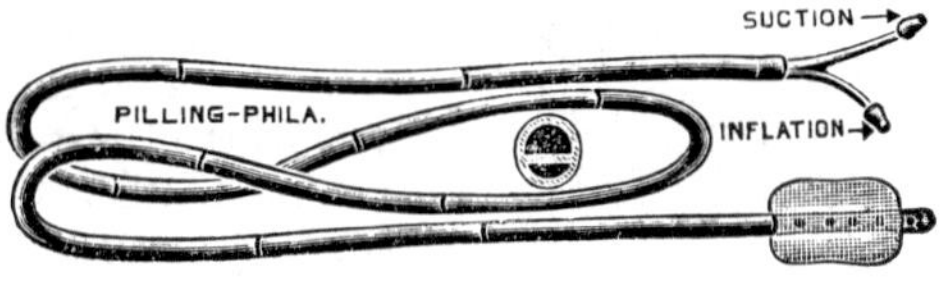

Fig. 127. Miller-Abbott tube.

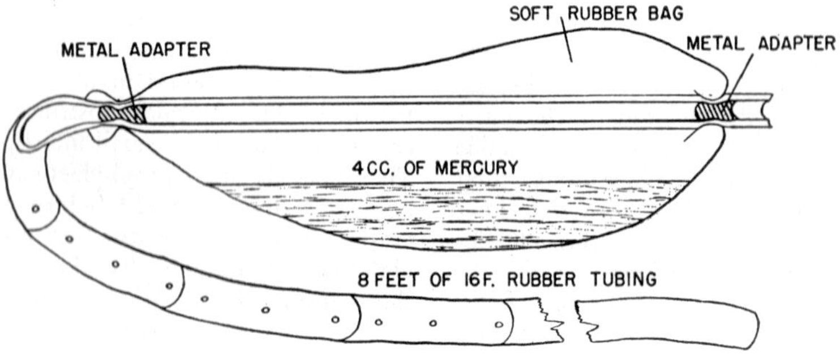

FIG. 128. Harris tube.

cated sparingly and chilled well before the doctor inserts the tip through the patient's nose. Markings on the tube indicate the distance it has been passed.

Harris Tube. This is a single-lumen, mercury-weighted tube of about 6 ft., and a lumen of 14 on the French scale. This tube has a metal tip that is introduced first into the nostril after having been lubricated. The mercury-weighted bag follows. The weight of the mercury carries the bag by gravity. As this is a single lumen tube that is used wholly for suction and irrigation, there is no difficulty in irrigating it. Usually a Y-tube is attached to the end of the tube, so that the suction apparatus is attached to one side, and an outlet with a clamp is available on the other side for irrigating purposes (Fig. 128).

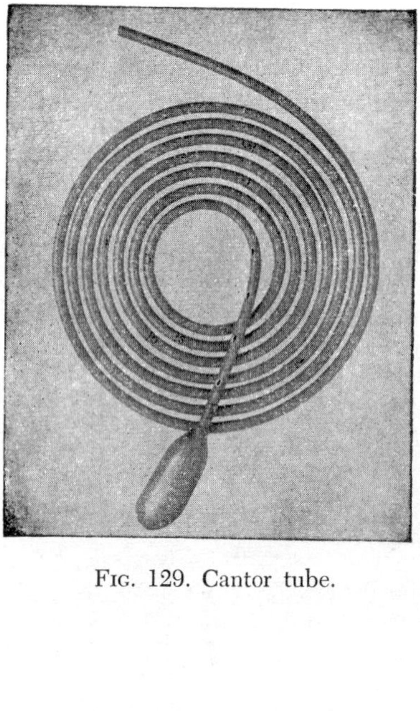

FIG. 129. Cantor tube.

Cantor Tube. The Cantor tube is 10 ft. long and No. 18 Fr. Its distinguishing feature is that it is larger and has the mercury-filled bag at the extreme end of the rubber tubing (Fig. 129).

Wangensteen Apparatus. PRINCIPLE. The flow of water from the siphon bottle (Fig. 130, d) to the waste bottle (Fig. 130, f) produces a vacuum or negative pressure in the uppermost portion of the siphon bottle. To permit this flow of water, only a short glass tube should be in the siphon bottle and attached to the tubing that empties into the waste bottle. The long glass tube in the siphon bottle should be connected with the tubing to which the section is to be applied.

The amount of negative pressure, when no trap bottle is used and the drainage flows directly from the patient into the siphon bottle, is equal to the distance between the end of the nasal tube in the patient's stomach (or wherever placed) and the level of the water in the waste bottle (Fig. 130, f). This negative pressure will vary with the amount of gas present in the nasal tube, for at this time the water distance is lessened and the suction accordingly is increased. When a trap bottle (Fig. 130, b) is used, the amount of negative pressure is equal to the distance between the levels of the water in the siphon and the waste bottles. Therefore, the amount of suction in both set-ups can be increased if the waste bottle is low-

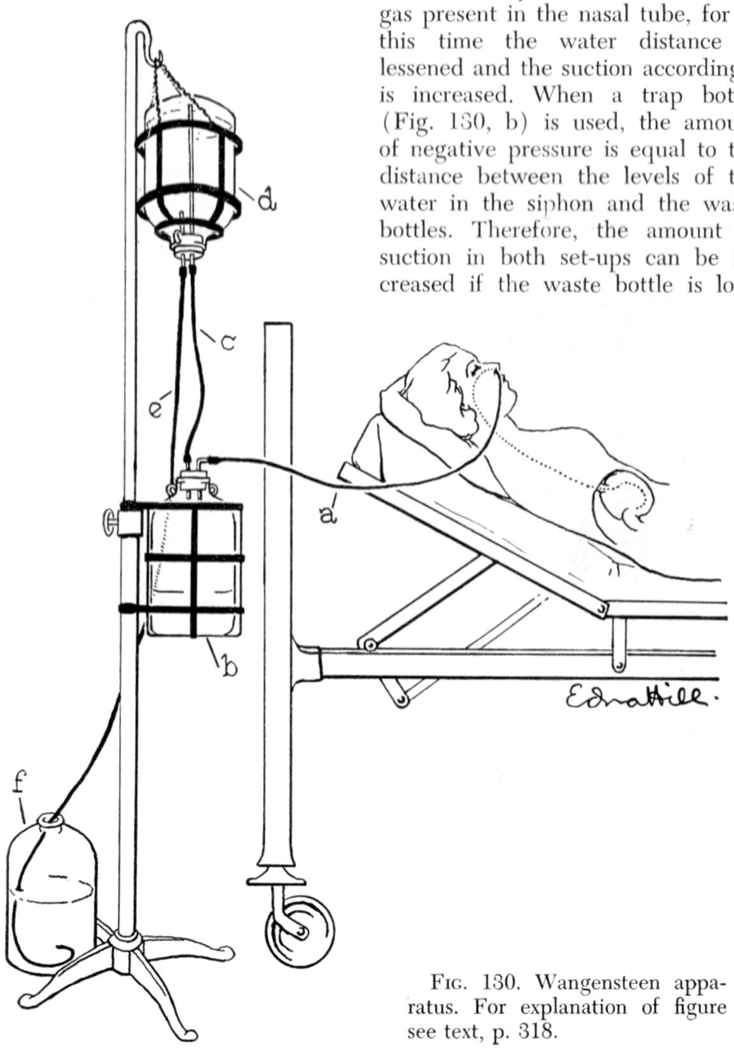

FIG. 130. Wangensteen apparatus. For explanation of figure see text, p. 318.

ered. As this bottle often is placed on the floor, this is the limit to the amount of negative pressure that can be obtained in the 2-bottle method (Fig. 131), and generally it is sufficient. In the 3-bottle method (Fig. 130), the suction at the end of the nasal tube also can be increased by raising the siphon bottle.

Purpose. The purpose of this type of suction is (1) to remove from the stomach and the upper intestinal tract gas and fluid materials that may accumulate there due to intestinal obstruction or to the irritation of the intestines, as found in peritonitis, and so to relieve nausea and vomiting; (2) to evacuate the stomach; (3) to detect bleeding in cases of hemorrhage from ulcers of the duodenum or the stomach; and (4) as a prophylactic measure in many postoperative conditions. This method of relief of upper intestinal obstruction and distention and evacuation of the stomach was proposed by Wangensteen and has been modified by many others. Miller and Abbott have introduced a tube that may be inserted not only into the stomach but also into the intestine for considerable distances to evacuate materials from distended loops of intestine, as well as the stomach (Fig. 134).

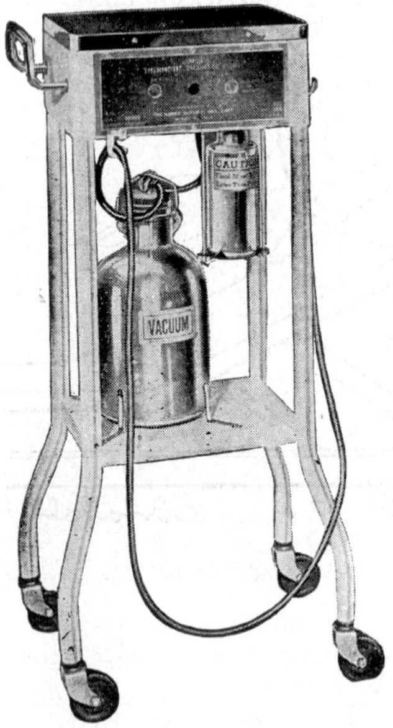

Fig. 131. An apparatus for gastric suction drainage that is operated electrically. Care must be taken to see that aspirated fluid does not enter the machine. (Gomco Surgical Manufacturing Corporation, Buffalo, N. Y.)

1. **To Start Suction Drainage:**

A. Fill the siphon bottle (Fig. 130, d) with water nearly to the top. (In some hospitals the amount of water used must be measured and recorded in order to measure the gas evacuated by the siphon.)

B. Put a small amount of water into the waste bottle (measured if required).

C. Place the cork tightly in the siphon bottle and secure it by ties and clamp, if necessary. The tubing (e) from the short glass tube in the siphon bottle should be placed into the waste bottle (f) so that it reaches the bottom and its end is under the surface of the water in the waste bottle.

D. Clamp the siphon tube (c) that leads to the long glass tube in the siphon bottle. Hang the siphon bottle on a standard. (If no trap bottle is used, test the siphon at this time and attach to the nasal tube, a.)

E. Set the trap bottle (b) in place and insert the cork snugly into it

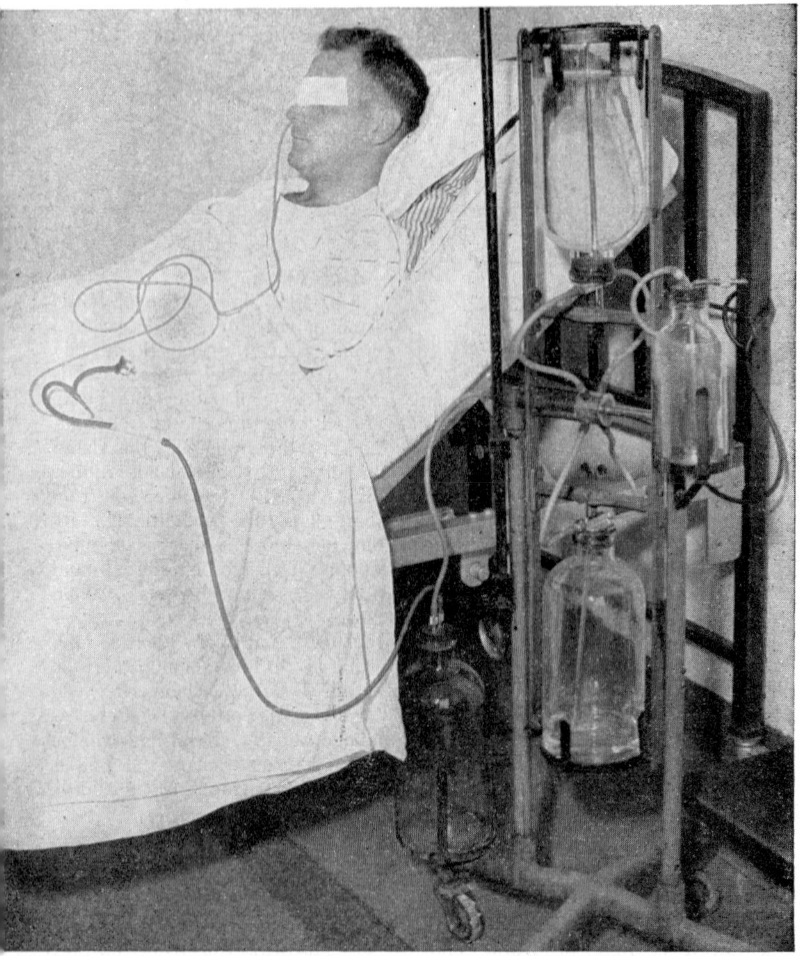

FIG. 132. Gastric suction using the Miller-Abbott tube and mechanical type of suction using bottles that can be rotated. Passage of the water from the upper to the lower bottle produces suction. When the upper bottle is empty, the entire apparatus can be rotated and suction started over again without emptying or changing bottles.

Clamp the siphon tube (e) and open the clamps on tubings (c) and (a). See that suction is properly functioning by releasing the clamp on the siphon tube (e) for a moment.

2. **To Introduce Nasal Tube and Attachment of Suction Apparatus:**

A. The nasal tube is prepared for use by sterilizing and placing it in a basin containing cracked ice for at

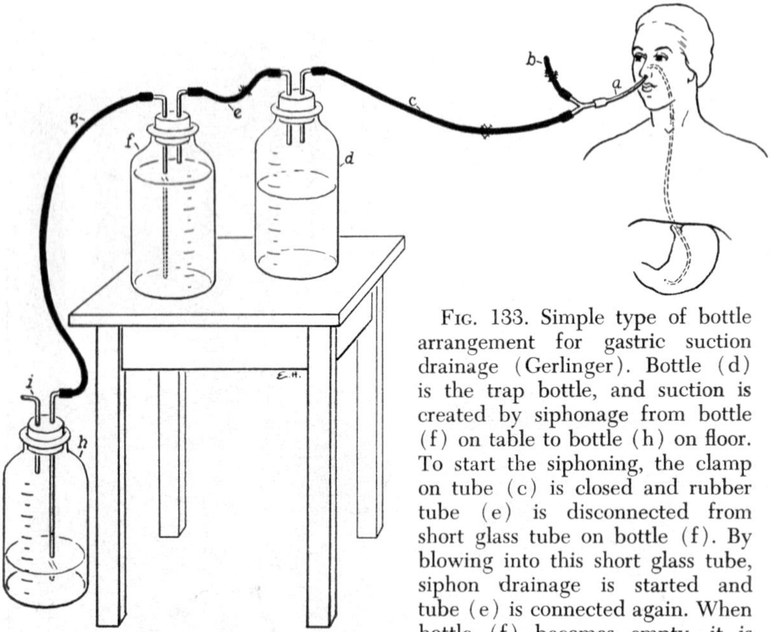

FIG. 133. Simple type of bottle arrangement for gastric suction drainage (Gerlinger). Bottle (d) is the trap bottle, and suction is created by siphonage from bottle (f) on table to bottle (h) on floor. To start the siphoning, the clamp on tube (c) is closed and rubber tube (e) is disconnected from short glass tube on bottle (f). By blowing into this short glass tube, siphon drainage is started and tube (e) is connected again. When bottle (f) becomes empty, it is replaced simply by bottle (h), which now is full, and, after blowing into tube (i) to begin siphonage, tube (e) is attached and suction drainage is continued. If the exchange between bottles (f) and (h) is made before the water level in bottle (f) gets below the level in the long glass tube, the siphonage already established will be maintained and will not have to be restarted. During exchange of bottles (f) and (h), the clamp on tube (e) is closed. When emptying trap bottle (d), clamps on tubes (c) and (e) are closed.

least 5 minutes. The tube then is introduced through the nostril, usually without a lubricant, although liquid albolene may be used. The introduction of the tube is the duty of the surgeon, but the nurse should provide the adhesive fixation for use when the tube has been inserted the required distance.

B. The nasal catheter is attached to the tube leading to the trap bottle (c), usually by a Y tube. The other end of the Y tube is attached to a small piece of rubber tubing closed by a clamp. Through this tube irrigations of the nasal catheter may be accomplished (Fig. 133).

C. The tube line from the nose to the trap bottle is fixed in position on the bed so that there will be no pulling upon it. This may be accomplished by a safety pin through the bed sheet or by adhesive-tape loops that may be tied or pinned to the bed.

3. To Maintain Constant Suction:

A. The siphon bottle must be refilled before it empties. When refilling, both tubes (e and c) leading from it should be clamped before the cork is removed. The fluid added to the bottle should be measured if required, the cork reinserted snugly in the bottle, and the bottle suspended again from the standard. Suction is reinstituted by opening the clamp on tube (e) leading to the waste bottle and then the clamp on tube (c) leading from the trap bottle. The siphon bottle (d) and the waste bottle (f) may be exchanged when water in the siphon bottle is low if a trap bottle (c) is used.

B. Inspect all tubes and corks to see that there are no kinks or leaks.

C. Keep the nasal catheter open by the injection of a measured small amount of water or saline through the Y tube connection, using a Luer tip or Asepto syringe. When fluid is injected, the tubing on the other side of the Y connection leading to the trap bottle should be clamped. Suction should not be made with a syringe unless ordered.

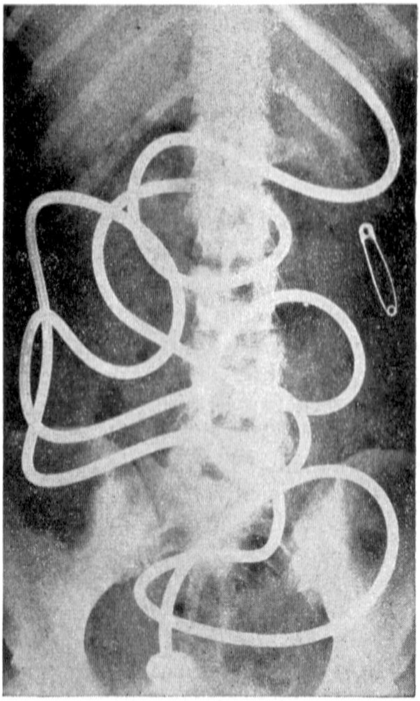

FIG. 134. Miller-Abbott tube in use. Note the balloon at the end of the tube, which has been distended with mercury. The tube has threaded its way down the intestinal tract and, by suction on the end of the tube, the intestine has been decompressed.

4. To Care for Apparatus:

A. The waste bottle should be emptied or exchanged with the siphon bottle as necessary, clamping tube (e) before removing the bottle. A small amount of water should remain in the waste bottle when it is returned for use again. The nurse should not forget to open the clamp on tube (e) after the waste bottle is replaced.

B. The nasal catheter should be inspected frequently, and no adjustments should be made in it without the permission of the surgeon.

5. To Maintain Adequate Intake:

While gastric-suction drainage is in use, an adequate parenteral intake should be maintained. The amount and the type of fluids are prescribed by the surgeon.

6. To Keep Accurate Records of:

A. Drainage, amount and type, every 12 hours.

B. Amount of fluid instilled by irrigation of the nasal catheter and the amount of water taken by mouth.

C. Amount and character of vomitus, if any.

D. Duration of any period in which the suction apparatus did not appear to function.

E. Effects produced by the treatment.

7. **To Care for Apparatus at End of Treatment:**

All tubing and bottles should be washed carefully, first with cold water and then with warm water and soap. After careful rinsing they should be returned to the central supply room. The nasal catheter should be boiled or autoclaved before being used again.

Nursing Care of Intubated Patients

Before the patient is intubated, it is wise for the nurse or the doctor to explain the treatment and its purpose. A co-operative patient adds much to the success of the procedure. He may be allowed to sit up, and a towel can be spread bib-fashion over his chest. Tissue wipes should be available. The patient ought to be screened from other patients, and the doctor should have adequate light. Often the physician will swab the nostril and spray the throat with pontocaine to dull the nasal passage and gag reflex and make the procedure more tolerable. Encouraging the patient to breathe through his mouth often helps, as does swallowing of water if permitted.

When the tube is passed to the desired distance, the nurse should fasten the catheter to the nose with adhesive tape. A minimum amount of adhesive for the maximum effect should be used. The tube then is connected to the suction apparatus. Enough leeway should be allowed to permit the patient to turn without risk of dislodging the tube. Rigid mouth and nostril hygiene must be followed in caring for these patients, as these tubes may be in place for several days. The use of applicator sticks dipped in water can be used to clean the nose. This can be followed by mineral oil. Frequent mouth attention is comforting.

When it is desirable to remove the tube, it is necessary to deflate the balloon and withdraw it gently and slowly for about 6 to 8 inches at intervals of 10 minutes until the tip reaches the esophagus, when the remainder is withdrawn rapidly out of the nostril. Should the tube not come out easily, force should not be used—the physician should be notified. When the tube is withdrawn, it should be done in such a way that the patient does not see it as it comes out. It is not a pleasant sight and may cause the patient to vomit. The use of a towel in which to wrap the tubing is effective. After this is done, the patient will be grateful for good mouth care.

Gastro-intestinal tubes must be cleaned thoroughly with plain water, then by soapy water. The balloon should be removed and discarded. A syringe can be used to force the solution through the tube. Organic solvents, such as alcohol or benzine, should not be used—they weaken rubber. The entire tube should be immersed in zephiran chloride for 10 minutes. After a thorough rinsing, the tube should be hung to dry in such a way that there are no angulations in it. As rubber tubing may retain an unpleasant odor, the tube can be soaked in lavender water for a few minutes if necessary. Before the tube is used again, a new balloon or bag should be attached. Some are attached by rubber cement and others are tied with black silk. Instructions for replacement of bags come with the tube.

Nursing Care for Intestinal Obstruction

The nursing care is a most important part of the treatment. Preoperative preparation is the giving of a small enema and the shaving of the entire abdomen. These measures often are supplemented by decompression of the intestine by the use of a Wangensteen suction attached to a Miller-Abbott, a Cantor or a Harris tube. The tubes frequently become clogged and must be irrigated by the nurse at frequent intervals. Extreme care must be exercised in irrigating the Miller-Abbott tube, in that the irrigating solution

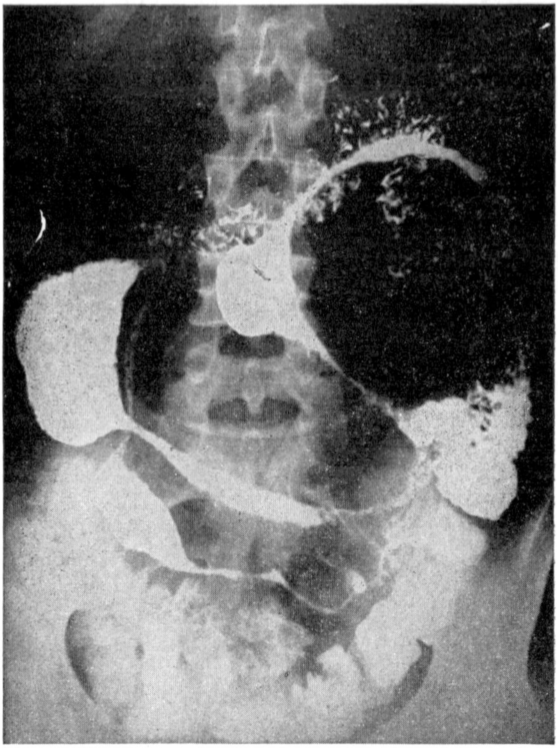

FIG. 135. Roentgenogram of a patient with marked regional enteritis. Note the extreme narrowing of the small intestine produced by the inflammatory process in the gut.

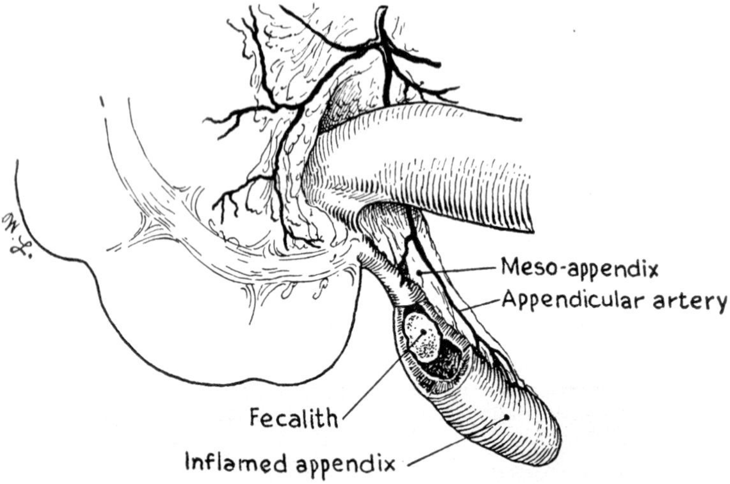

FIG. 136. Diagrammatic view showing how a fecalith obstructing the appendix can produce appendicitis.

must be introduced into the portion marked "Suction." The other lumen leads to the distensible rubber bag and serious accidents have occurred (rupture of the intestine) when, by mistake, nurses have introduced into the bag fluid meant for irrigation.

After operation, fluids must be given these patients in large amounts. An accurately kept intake and output record is essential, since it is information that the surgeon must have if the nutritional needs of the patient are to be met. If an enterostomy has been performed, a bottle should be attached to the side of the bed and a tube connected with the enterostomy tube, inserted in it. If peristalsis is active and the tube has been placed properly in the bowel, a considerable amount (from 500 to 1,000 cc.) of fecal fluid should drain away in the first 12 to 15 hours after operation. Frequently the fenestra of the enterostomy tube becomes clogged by fecal masses and obviously, the drainage will cease until the tube is cleared. The nurse should observe the amount of drainage accumulating in the collection bottle and, if there is no increase in the quantity of fluid for several hours, she should regard it as an indication that the tube has clogged. Many surgeons make sure that the fenestra remains open by having the nurse inject a half ounce of warm saline solution into the enterostomy or colostomy tube at intervals of from two to three hours. The skin about the enterostomy is protected by strips of petrolatum gauze, aluminum paint or zinc ointment. An accurate fluid record must be kept in these cases.

REGIONAL ENTERITIS

Chronic cicatrizing regional enteritis is an inflammatory narrowing of the small intestine. It appears mostly in young adults and causes symptoms in two ways: because of the inflammatory process, there is an irritability of the intestines that results in frequent movements, fluid loss, anemia and weight loss; the narrowing of the small intestine, usually in the lower ileum, produces an almost complete intestinal obstruction with attacks of colicky pain.

The disease is treated surgically in its more advanced stages by removing the diseased gut and anastomosing the small intestine to the large. At times the diseased gut is not removed, but an anastomosis is made between the ileum above the diseased portion and the transverse colon. The nursing care is the same as that for operations on the colon (p. 332).

APPENDICITIS

Anatomy and Physiology. The vermiform appendix is attached to the tip of the cecum. In length it varies from 6 to 10 cm. and is about 0.8 cm. in diameter. It is a rudimentary organ in man that serves no useful function, and is a common site of inflammation and obstruction. The position of the appendix is variable. This accounts for variations in the symptomatology of appendicitis.

Appendicitis is the commonest of the surgical diseases of the abdomen. It may occur in two forms, acute and chronic. The chronic form is caused most frequently by interference with the peristalsis of the appendix due either to adhesions or kinks or to fecal concretions within the lumen of the appendix. Chronic appendicitis is characterized by recurring short-lived attacks of lower right-sided colicky pain, often accompanied by nausea and tenderness over the appendix. Signs of inflammation usually are few, but at any time an acute condition may supervene.

Acute Appendicitis

Acute appendicitis usually begins as an inflammation of the wall of the appendix, due to bacterial invasion or to obstruction of its lumen by hardened fecal masses (fecaliths). In either case, the small channel of the organ becomes closed, and the bacteria always present form pus. If the inflammation continues, it may produce necrosis of the appendiceal wall with resulting perforation and peritonitis. The result is the same if the infection shuts off the blood supply to the appendix, producing gangrene. If the process is well walled off by omentum and gut, an abscess may form about the appendix but, if the whole abdominal cavity is infected, a general peritonitis results.

Symptoms. The usual symptoms of acute appendicitis are, first, abdominal pain, then nausea and vomiting. The pain settles later in the lower right abdomen and is accompanied by slight fever, leukocytosis, tenderness and rigidity over the region of the appendix. Because the location of the appendix varies slightly in different people, these clinical symptoms show many variations.

Before the patient is admitted to the hospital, it is imperative that nothing be taken by mouth. No laxative of any kind ever is given because of the great possibility of causing a

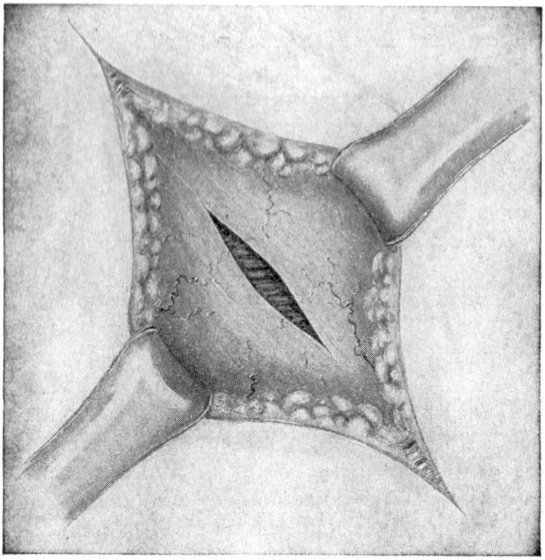

FIG. 137. Gridiron (muscle-splitting) incision, in line of fibers of external oblique aponeurosis.

rupture of the appendix. An icebag on the abdomen and rest in bed are the care advised before the patient is seen by the doctor.

Without doubt, in many instances of acute appendicitis recovery will take place without operation, but no surgeon can tell whether serious symptoms will develop and, if they do, whether they will subside safely without surgical intervention. As mortality after operation for appendicitis in the early stages is less than 1 per cent, it is safest to operate in all cases as soon as the diagnosis is made. To delay the operation involves the risk of peritonitis, abscess formation or intestinal obstruction, and these complications increase the mortality from 5 to 10 per cent.

Operative Treatment

Preparation for Operation. This depends entirely on the length of time spent in the hospital before operation. If an emergency operation is necessary, shaving of the abdomen, voiding by the patient and the administration of the prescribed hypodermic injection are required. Usually an enema is not given but, if one is ordered, it is given low and slowly. Chemotherapy and/or antibiotics are administered before and after surgery.

If the patient has been suffering from acute abdominal pain, he accepts the operation as a means of relief. This acceptance of surgery makes his anesthetic and postanesthetic course a relatively easy one. The operation may be performed under nitrous oxide, ether, spinal or local anesthesia. The usual incisions are the McBurney, the muscle-splitting or the gridiron (Figs. 137 and 138) and the lower right rectus incision (Fig. 121, 5). After the

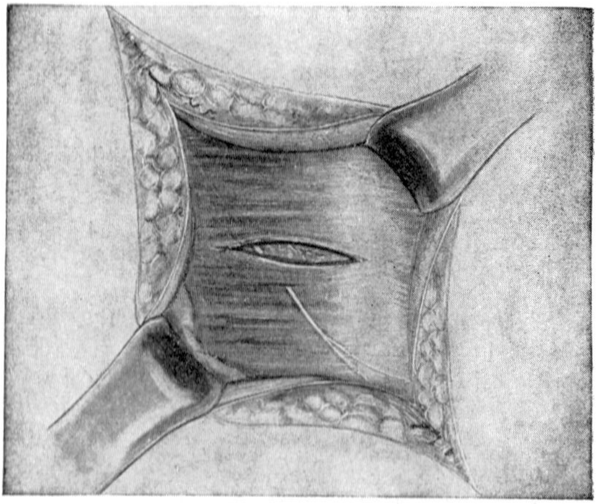

FIG. 138. Gridiron (muscle-splitting) or McBurney incision, a traverse incision in the direction of fibers of muscles.

peritoneum has been opened, the appendix is brought into the wound and its mesentery is ligated with a catgut ligature. The appendix is freed and a purse-string suture of catgut or silk is inserted round its base. After cutting through the organ at its base between clamps or ligatures, using the electrocautery or a knife followed by pure phenol and alcohol, the stump is inverted and the purse-string is tied. The appendix, the knife, the hemostats and the forceps used when the appendix was severed no longer are sterile, and they should be discarded. Sponges used to protect the wound and gut also should be removed from the table. If the appendix has perforated and caused an abscess or a peritonitis, drainage tubes must be inserted.

Postoperative Nursing Care

Appendectomy Without Drainage. As soon as the patient recovers from the anesthesia he should be placed in the Fowler position. Morphine, from 0.016 Gm. to 0.011 Gm. (gr. ¼-⅙), may be given at intervals of 3 or 4 hours. Fluid should be given by vein for the first 12 hours but, if there is no nausea at the end of from 6 to 8 hours, water or hot tea may be given by mouth in increasing amounts. Fluids and food may be given as desired the day after operation. An enema is given on the morning of the third day. The stitches are removed from the incision between the fifth and the seventh days.

After removal of the appendix a complication that at times is annoying is the inability to void. The patient may be allowed to stand with support or to sit on the edge of the bed with the feet on a chair. In this manner, the necessity for catheterization may be averted.

Appendectomy with Drainage. The treatment of patients after an appendectomy requiring drainage is complicated by local or general peritonitis. They should be placed in strict Fowler position as soon as they recover from the anesthetic and

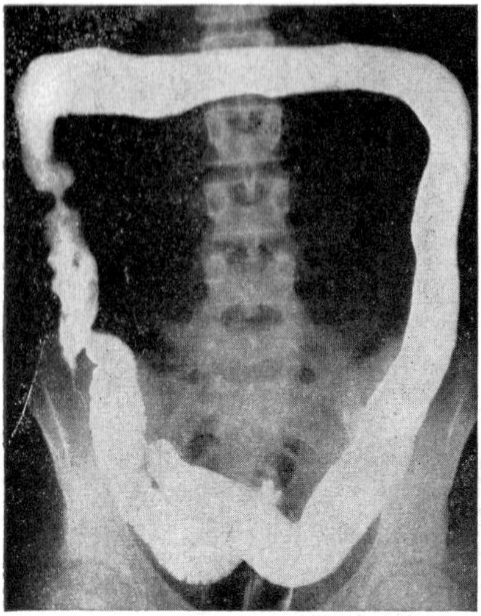

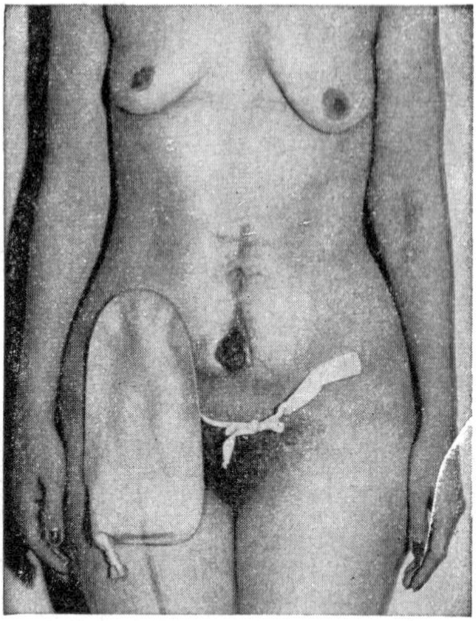

FIG. 139 (*Left*). Roentgenogram of colon in ulcerative colitis. The bowel has become a semirigid tube as a result of the long-standing inflammatory process.

FIG. 140 (*Right*). Patient with ileostomy wearing a Rutzen bag. This patient has had a subtotal colectomy. Because of ulcerative colitis, the colon has been removed from the cecum to the sigmoid. The sigmoid is seen implanted in the mid-line wound. The secretions of the ileum are caught in the rubber bag, which is cemented to the skin. The rubber band closes a spigotlike extension at the lower end of the bag. Removal of the band permits drainage of the secretions into the toilet. See also Fig. 146.

treatment for peritonitis should be instituted as described fully on page 300. These patients should be watched carefully for many days for signs of intestinal obstruction and secondary hemorrhage. Secondary abscesses may form in the pelvis, under the diaphragm or in the liver. These cause an elevation of temperature and pulse rate with an increase in the leukocyte count. A fecal fistula, with the discharge of feces through the drainage tract, develops at times. This complication arises most often after the drainage of an appendiceal abscess. The attention of the surgeon should be drawn to feces on the dressings.

SURGERY OF COLON, RECTUM AND ANUS

IDIOPATHIC ULCERATIVE COLITIS

Idiopathic ulcerative colitis is an inflammatory disease of the colon that results in the frequent discharge (from 8 to 20 per day) of watery, purulent, often bloody, stools. The disease is characterized by diffuse ulceration of the mucosal surface of the colon, with an inflammatory thickening of the wall of the gut as the disease progresses. At times there may be marked hemorrhage or perforation of the gut wall.

Depletion due to the frequent stools results in a marked loss in weight, anemia, dehydration and an evident nutritional deficiency. Often tenesmus associated with the disease confines the patient to the house, and weakness may make him bed-

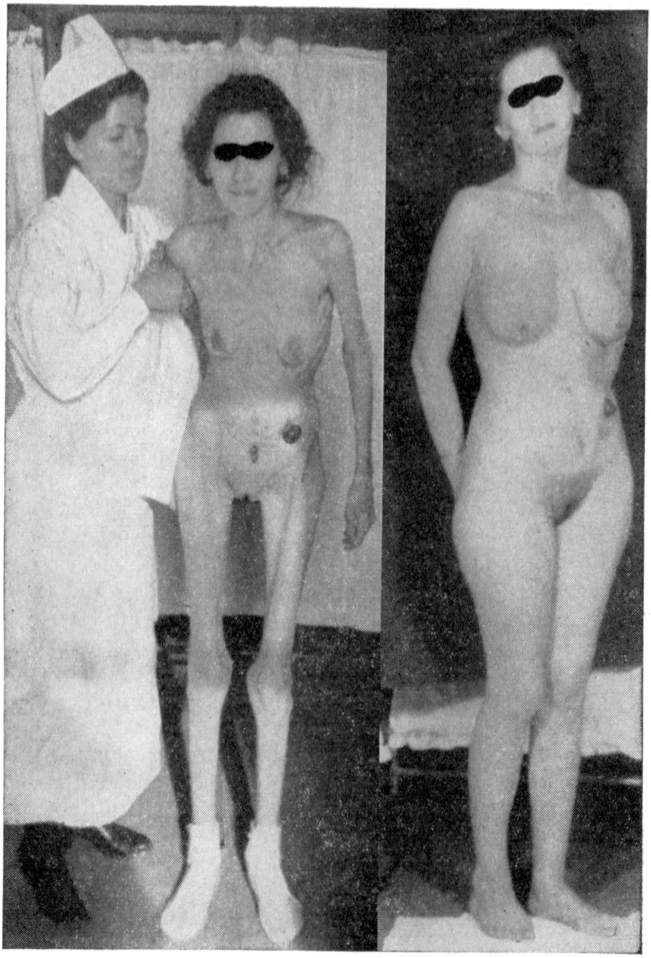

FIG. 141. (*Left*) Patient 3 weeks after ileostomy and partial colectomy. (*Right*) Same patient one year later. (Elsom, K. A., and Ferguson, L. K.: Am. J. M. Sc. **202**:59-68)

fast. Patients in a less advanced state may be treated medically, but the progressive narrowing of the bowel due to the inflammatory disease, hemorrhage, perforation and chronic invalidism make surgery necessary.

A prolonged period of preparation, with intensive fluid, blood and protein replacement, is necessary before operation is attempted. Chemotherapy and antibiotics are useful adjuncts.

The operations performed are directed toward diverting the flow of the intestinal contents from the diseased portion of the colon. If the disease involves only the distal colon, a colostomy in the transverse colon may be performed. If the whole colon is involved, an ileostomy (opening of the terminal ileum on the abdominal wall) must be performed. Usually it is necessary to remove the diseased colon (colectomy) at a later operation.

Nursing Care

The nursing care and the complications are much the same as those in carcinoma of the colon (pp. 335-337), the chief difference being the care of the ileostomy. The opening of the small gut on the abdomen discharges continuously the liquid contents of the small intestine. Because these discharges contain digestive enzymes, they are highly irritating to the skin of the abdomen.

During the first day or two after operation the discharges from the ileum are collected through tubes which are drained into a bottle at the side of the bed. However, as soon as possible, all tubes are removed, and the ileostomy bag is cemented to the skin surrounding the intestinal opening. The rubber cement so closely attaches the facing of the collecting bag that the secretions do not come in contact with the skin and are collected in the bag. This avoids the skin irritation which the enzymes of the ileostomy drainage may produce if they come in contact with the skin.

Because these patients lose much fluid and food in the early postoperative period, an accurate record of fluid intake, urinary output and rectal discharges is necessary to help the surgeon to gauge the fluid needs of the patient. Fluids, blood and amino acid are given in large amounts until the patient becomes accustomed to the new digestive arrangement.

Such patients probably are the most difficult of all to nurse. Their prolonged illness makes them irritable, weak and, at times, psychopathic. The nurse must recognize that this behavior often is a result of complex socioeconomic pressures. She must be consistent in expressing sincere friendliness and exhibiting a nonjudgmental attitude. Operation often results in an almost immediate change in their mental outlook and, as soon as they learn to care for their ileostomies, they become normal, affable and attractive people. A patient, sympathetic and tolerant nurse is most important in the recovery of these patients.

Carcinoma of Colon and Rectum

The chief surgical disease of the large intestine is cancer. This dread disease occurs not infrequently in the colon, especially in the sigmoid and the rectum. Unfortunately, the symptoms may be few until the growth has become very extensive. The patients, usually past middle age, complain of "intestinal indigestion" or other vague symptoms, often with a sort of diarrhea characterized by the frequent passage of small amounts of bloody mucus. The early morning evacuation of foul, watery mucus is characteristic. As the process develops, a gradually increasing constipation occurs, alternating at times with diarrhea. Finally, the obstruction to the bowel becomes complete, and the patient develops abdominal distention from the dilatation of the large gut with fecal contents. Colicky pains increase in severity, vomiting becomes incessant and surgical relief is imperative.

Diagnosis. This is established frequently by digital examination of the rectum, by proctoscopic examination and by roentgen-ray examination with a barium enema.

Preparation for Operation. This includes the shaving of the abdomen and the perineum and rectal irrigation that is continued until the fluid returns clear. Usually a high caloric, low residue diet is given for several days before operation if time and the patient's condition permit. If an emergency does not exist, these patients are prepared for several days by being given intestinal antiseptics of the sulfa group (sulfasuxidine or sulfathalidine) or the antibiotics (streptomycin, Aureomycin, Terramycin, neomycin). These are given by mouth to reduce the bacterial content of the colon and to soften and decrease the bulk of the contents of the colon. The nurse should pay attention to any mention of pain and its location. She also should record fluid losses, such as would occur by vomiting and diarrhea. This will aid the surgeon in regulating the fluid intake and maintaining proper balance. In the event that there is any possibility of a permanent colostomy, the patient should be informed of it by the surgeon, and he should be assured that it can be handled easily and need not interfere with his usual social and business life. He should be assured further that he need not develop into a dependent person. This mental preparation of the patient is an extremely important part of his preoperative care.

The patient is sent to the operating room with an indwelling (Foley) catheter in place.

Operative Treatment

Operative treatment depends upon the position and the extent of the cancer.

When the tumor can be removed, the involved colon is excised for some distance on each side of the growth to remove the tumor and the area of its lymphatic spread. If distant (liver) metastasis has occurred, the tumor may be excised for palliation but without hope of cure. The gut may be reunited by an enterocolostomy or by an end-to-end anastomosis of the colon. When the growth is situated low in the sigmoid or the rectum, the colon is cut above the growth and brought out through the abdominal wall, forming thus an abdominal anus, called a *colostomy*. The growth then is removed from below by a perineal incision. (*Abdominoperineal resection*, Fig. 142.)

In the event that the tumor has

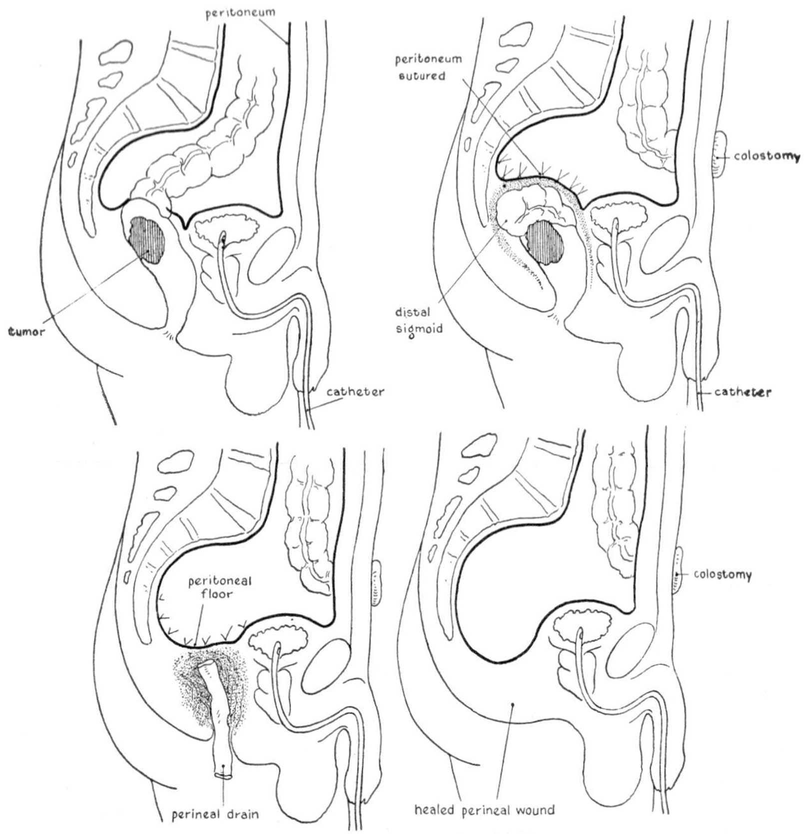

FIG. 142. Diagrammatic representation of abdominoperineal resection for carcinoma of rectum. (*Top, left*) Tumor in rectum. (*Top, right*) At operation, the sigmoid first is divided and a colostomy is established. The distal bowel has been dissected free to a point below the pelvic peritoneum. The pelvic peritoneum is sutured over the closed end of the distal sigmoid and rectum. The perineal resection includes removal of the rectum and free portion of the sigmoid from below. (*Bottom, left*) The perineum is closed loosely about drains placed beneath the peritoneum in the hollow of the sacrum. (*Bottom, right*) The final result after healing.

spread and involves surrounding vital structures, it is considered to be inoperable. When the growth in the rectum or the sigmoid is inoperable, and especially when symptoms of partial or complete obstruction are present, a colostomy may be performed. A loop of the colon, near the junction of the descending colon and the sigmoid, is brought out of

A

B

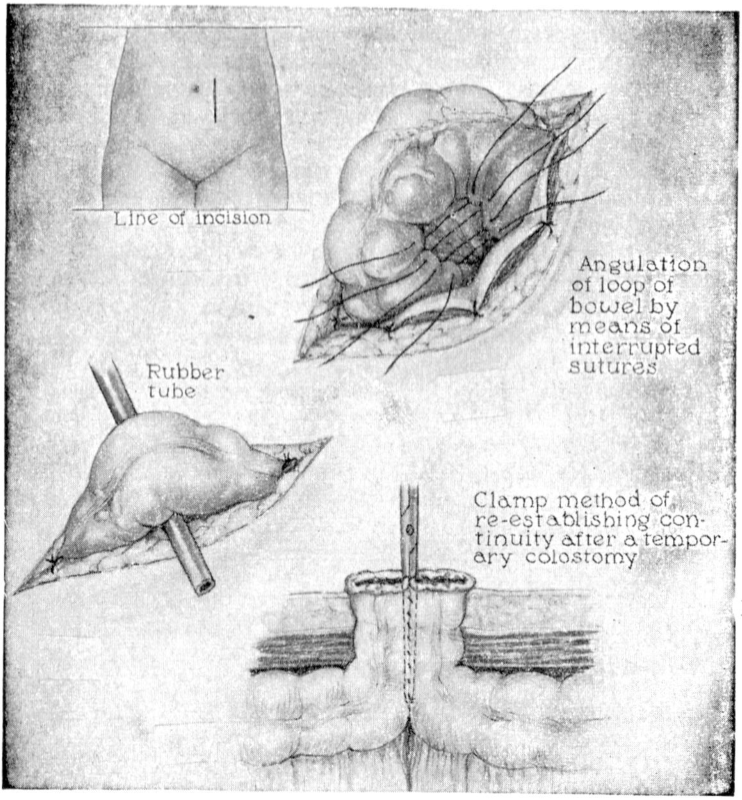

C

D

FIG. 143. (A and B) Steps in simple loop colostomy. (C and D) Steps in a Mikulicz temporary colostomy. After the latter procedure the colostomy is closed.

the abdomen through a lower left rectus incision and maintained in place by a glass rod or rubber tube inserted underneath the loop. If the obstruction is complete, the loop may be drained by the insertion of a rubber tube or by the use of a right-angled glass tube called a Paul's tube, which is held in the gut by a purse-string suture. When the obstruction is incomplete, the colostomy loop is allowed to remain unopened for several days to permit the peritoneal cavity to become thoroughly sealed off. During this time the patient is given liquids only. The gut is opened by electrocautery, as hemorrhage is slight after its use.

Nursing Care After Operations on Large Intestine

The usual immediate after-care for patients with abdominal operations is carried out. These patients are

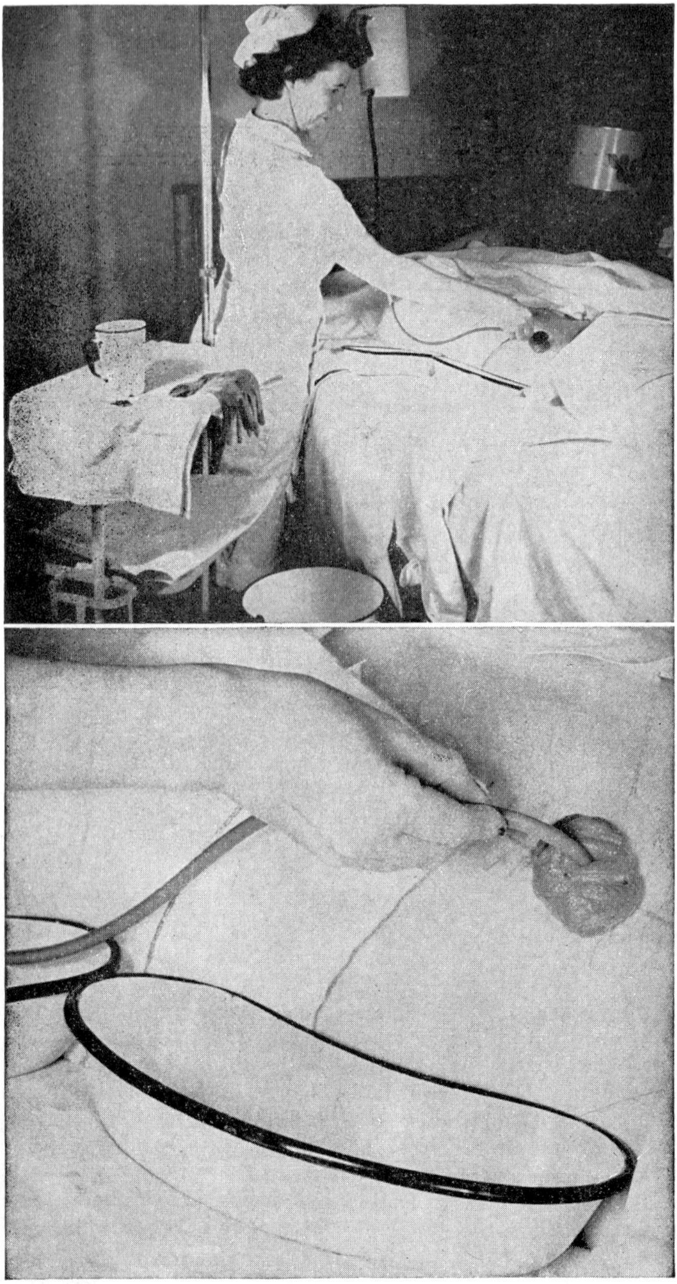

Fig. 144. (*Caption on facing page.*)

weakened considerably by an extensive operation and they should be watched carefully for symptoms of shock. Fluids and blood are given intravenously in amounts of about 3,000 cc. daily for the first few days.

In most cases a long (Miller-Abbott) intestinal tube has been inserted preoperatively. This needs irrigation at intervals to see that the openings are not clogged. The usual care of intestinal tubes is followed (see p. 317). Usually nothing is given by mouth for 24 to 48 hours, at which time peristalsis begins to return. As soon as peristalsis becomes active and gas is passed, liquid and then soft diet is given.

When an anastomosis has been performed after resection of a growth in the colon, a rectal tube very frequently is inserted through the anal canal to prevent distention of the gut by gas. The nurse should protect the end of the tube with a pad of cotton and gauze, as there may be some drainage of bloody material from the colon.

If a colostomy has been performed, the primary abdominal wound must be protected from the colostomy drainage. The colostomy loop is dressed with sterile petrolatum gauze and gauze dressings. The skin about the colostomy opening should be protected with a layer of petrolatum gauze or an ointment such as zinc oxide or boric acid. Montgomery straps, scultetus or laced adhesive should be used to facilitate the frequent change of dressings necessary.

Retention of urine is the rule after resection of the rectum. This is overcome by the use of a retention catheter for several days until muscle tone of the bladder is regained.

Colostomy Care. The surgeon may order irrigations through the colostomy opening. The doctor may prefer to do the first irrigation; after that it is the nurse's responsibility. A No. 16 or a No. 18 catheter may be used with the enema can. The patient may sit up in bed or, if permissible, he may sit in a chair before the toilet in the bathroom. A rubber sheet can be used as a trough leading into the toilet bowl. The patient is encouraged to watch the procedure as performed by the nurse. She should do it slowly and answer his questions. The catheter is inserted from 2 to 3 inches at first and the solution is allowed to run in. The catheter then can be inserted gently up to from 6 to 8 inches. At first, only about 500 cc. of solution is given, and this may be increased gradually every day up to 1,500 cc., or until the return flow is clear. The temperature of the solution is about 105° F., and the irrigating can is placed about 2 feet above level of

FIG. 144. Irrigation of a colostomy. (*Top*) The nurse is irrigating the colostomy with fluid from an enema can. Note the articles that are necessary: enema can with large rectal tube; fluid pitcher; emesis basin; bucket. The bed has been protected by a rubber sheet covered with a sheet or a towel. (*Bottom*) Shows the introduction of the rectal tube into the colostomy. This should be done with the fluid running. The fluid distends the gut and permits the advancement of the rectal tube with more ease and safety.

the colostomy opening. The purpose of the irrigation is to empty the distal bowel of fecal material. As distention of the colon is an effective stimulus for bowel evacuation, the irrigating solution should be introduced in such amount and with such pressure as to distend the bowel and give the patient a feeling of fullness. If the patient complains of cramps, the level of the can may be lowered to lessen the force of the flow. Solutions may be soap solution, plain water or saline. The irrigation may be given daily, every other day or every three days, according to the experience of the patient. Nothing but flatus should escape from the colostomy between irrigations. Attention should be paid to the time of day the procedure is carried out. It should fit into the posthospital routine of the individual. For a businessman, perhaps the most convenient time would be in the evening; for a housewife, it may be the middle of the morning. The establishment of definite habits will be appreciated by the patient.

As soon as he is able to do his own irrigation, the patient should be en-

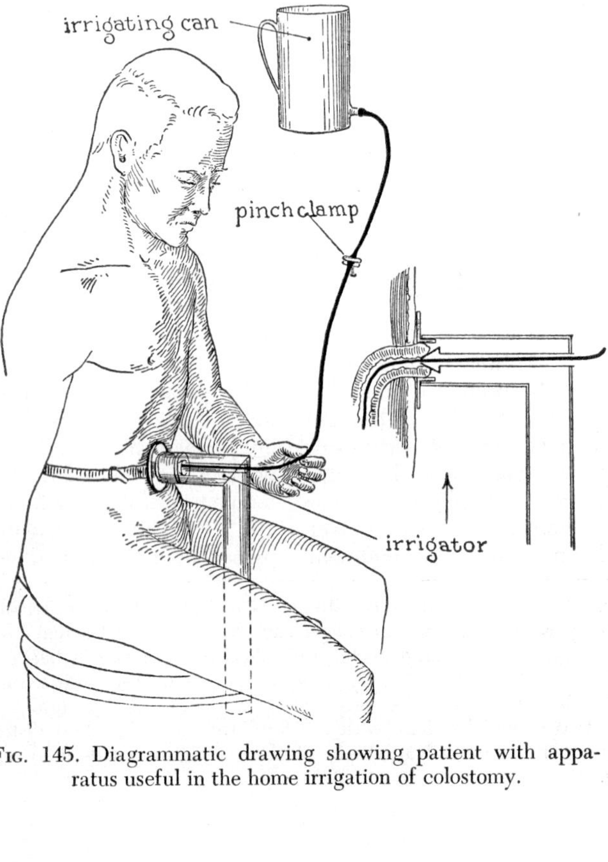

Fig. 145. Diagrammatic drawing showing patient with apparatus useful in the home irrigation of colostomy.

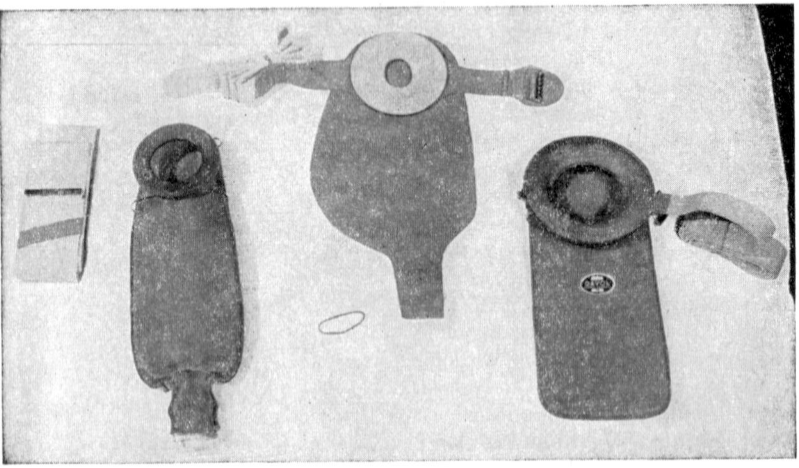

FIG. 146. Various types of bags that collect intestinal secretions. The bags on the left and on the right are the common types of colostomy bags. The bag in the center is the Rutzen type, which is cemented to the skin. This is used when the secretions are more liquid, as in the case of an ileostomy or an ascending colostomy.

couraged to do so. The doctor, the nurse and the patient's family want him to be an independent, self-sufficient person. Various types of irrigating sets are available. They are made of plastic material and rubber that permit the patient to insert a catheter through a cup-shaped transparent plastic cover directly into the colostomy. When fluid returns, it is directed downward through a rubber tube into a pail or into the commode. This makes it possible for the patient to care for himself at the toilet in the bathroom.

Colostomy bags may be worn immediately after irrigation, then a change to a simple dressing may be effective. Patients are instructed in the care and the cleaning of equipment so as to prolong its life and keep it free of odors. Cleaning by soap and water and exposing it to fresh air usually is sufficient to keep colostomy equipment clean. When the bowel is so regulated, the colostomy bag may be dispensed with and a simple pad and elastic belt substituted for it.

Skin care is very important, for it takes little to produce a painful excoriation. Again, soap and water should be used to clean the skin, and a lubricant such as petrolatum or zinc oxide ointment can be used.

It is well, in case the cancer has not been removed, to irrigate the lower loop, from anus to colostomy, every 2 or 3 days, to remove the irritating mucus that collects. If the growth has been removed by the perineal route, the wound should be watched carefully for signs of hemorrhage. The close proximity of the wound to the sacrum necessitates a frequent change of dressings in order to keep the area clean and dry.

The perineal wound usually contains a drain or packing that is removed gradually so that on about the seventh day all drains are out. There usually are sloughing bits of tissue that must come away for the following week or ten days. This process is hastened by mechanical irrigation of the wound. An irrigating can with 1:5,000 potassium permanganate solution and a soft rubber catheter at the tip facilitates this procedure, which should be carried out at least once daily until the wound is clean. The nurse often is taught to give these irrigations. During the procedure it is important to protect the bed with an extra rubber sheet and absorbent pads, and it may be well to time the irrigation so that it can be performed before the patient receives morning care.

In addition to the local care, the nurse must not forget that the patient, after an operation for cancer of the colon or the rectum, is extremely ill, and that the usual precautions must be taken to prevent the development of postoperative pulmonary complications, parotitis, phlebitis, and so forth. Also, careful watch must be kept for the development of intestinal obstruction, which is one of the most frequent postoperative complications. Colicky pain after eating and vomiting are the usual symptoms that make one suspect the development of this complication. Frequent change of position can prevent this.

Diet for Colostomy Patients. In order to control a colostomy, the diet must be regulated. It is necessary to begin with a strict diet, but later it can be more liberal:

Diet No. 1—Used in hospital while first gaining control and at any time later when loose movements occur.

Breakfast

Large portion of cream of wheat with boiled milk, sugar if desired
2 hard-boiled eggs
Dry toast
1 glass of boiled milk

Lunch

Creamed soups (creamed lettuce soup 3 or 4 times a week)
Creamed fish or meat
Baked or mashed potato
Boiled rice or custard

Dinner

Meat or fish, creamed whenever possible
Escalloped vegetable—no spinach or carrots
Soft pudding, custard or junket

Diet No. 2—Used after gaining control in the hospital (2 weeks) and continued for 2 months at home.

Cream of wheat, puffed wheat or puffed rice
Eggs—boiled, poached, baked or scrambled
Oven broiled bacon
White bread, plain or toasted
Plain white crackers or saltines
Butter, cheese, milk, tea, coffee, cocoa
Boiled rice, baked macaroni or spaghetti
Baked custards
Soups of all kinds except tomato or corn
Potato—baked, mashed or riced
Roast beef, lamb or chicken
Broiled steak or lamb chop
Fish—broiled, boiled or creamed
Sponge or angel cake

Diet No. 3—Added to No. 2 after 2 months if control is still effective.
Raw lettuce and celery

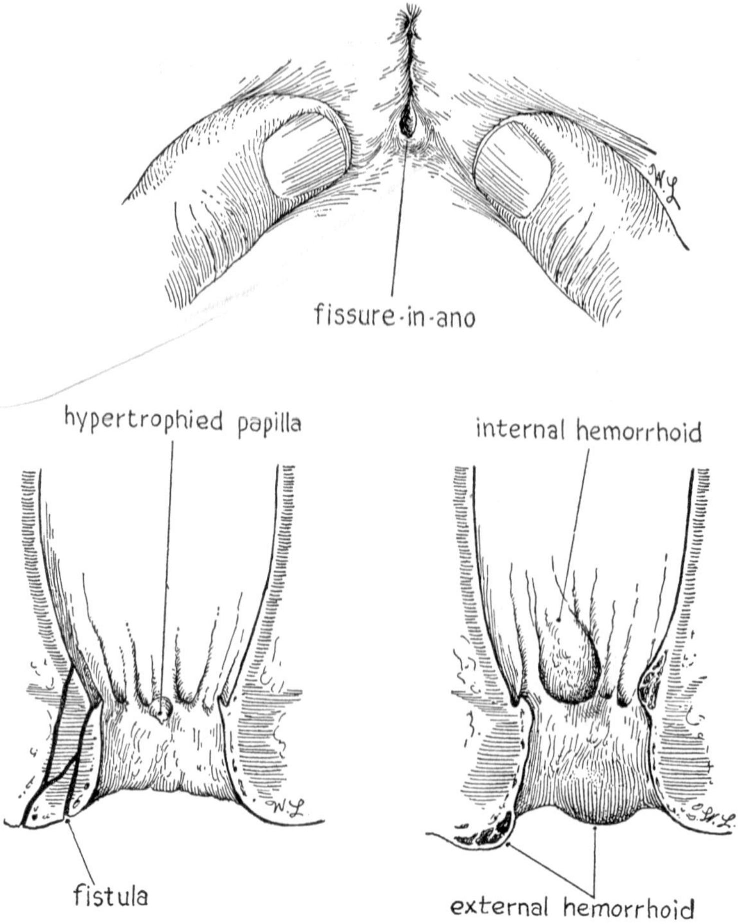

FIG. 147. Various types of anal lesions.

Cooked string beans, peas, carrots, beets, winter squash, cauliflower or asparagus
Cooked fruits
Orange juice

The patient will be able to tell that certain foods interfere with control and that these should be eliminated. Most patients with colostomy have trouble with green corn, baked beans and fried foods.

Other patients who have mastered their colostomies can help by visiting and talking with him. Often this form of psychological therapy is highly successful. His place in society can be a normal one. His degree of success depends upon the effectiveness of the teaching given by the doctor and the nurse.

Operations on Lower Rectum and Anal Region

Ischiorectal Abscess

Ischiorectal abscess is located in the fatty tissue beside the anus. Usually it is caused by infection from the rectum. Treatment consists of incision and drainage. Packing is inserted, and this demands daily changing. The dressing of these wounds is extremely painful; therefore, it is well to protect the edges of wounds with petrolatum gauze and to loosen the packing before removing it by soaking it with peroxide of hydrogen. These wounds are allowed to heal by granulation. Bowel movements should be kept soft by the administration of an ounce of liquid petrolatum morning and evening.

Fistula in Ano

Fistula in ano is a tiny tubular tract that has its skin opening beside the anus and goes from there by a tortuous route into the anal canal. Pus is leaking constantly from the cutaneous opening, making it necessary for the patient to wear a protective pad.

Three or 4 hours before operation, the perineum should be shaved and the lower bowel evacuated thoroughly, several warm soapsuds enemas being used. The patient should be allowed to evacuate the enemas on a commode. The last enema should return clear and should be evacuated entirely.

For operation, the patient usually is placed in the lithotomy position and the sinus tract is identified by inserting a probe into it or by injecting the tract with methylene blue solution. The fistula then may be dissected out or laid open by an incision from its rectal opening to its outlet. The wound is packed with gauze.

Postoperative treatment and complications are the same as those following hemorrhoidectomy (page 344).

Fissure in Ano

Fissure in ano is a longitudinal ulcer in the anal canal. It is associated frequently with constipation, and its most pronounced symptom is excruciating pain when the bowels move. The same preoperative preparation as for fistula in ano is indicated. Several types of operations may be performed: in some cases the anal sphincter is dilated and the fissure is excised; in others, a part of the external sphincter is divided. This gives a paralysis of the external sphincter with consequent relief of spasm and permits the ulcer to heal. When there is a large overhanging sentinel pile, excision of the ulcer and of the pile is performed.

After operation, the stools are kept soft or liquid for several weeks to permit healing to take place.

Hemorrhoids

Hemorrhoids or piles is the name given to masses of skin or mucosa over dilated veins in the anal canal. They occur in two locations. Those occurring above the internal sphincter are called *internal hemorrhoids* and those appearing outside the external sphincter *external hemor-*

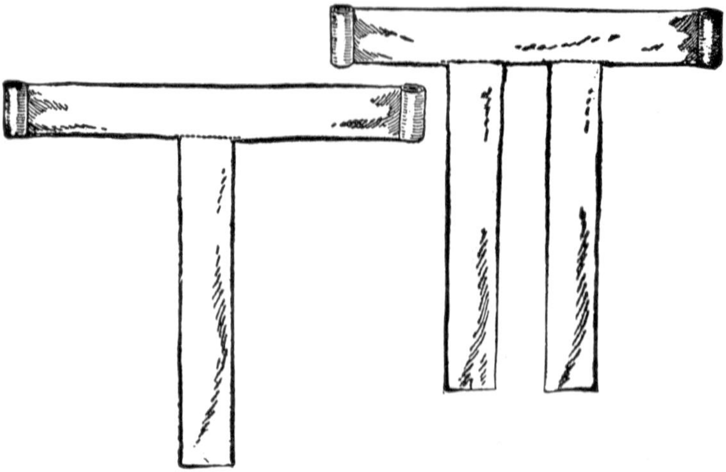

FIG. 148. (*Left*) T-bandage or T-binder. (*Right*) Four-tailed bandage.

rhoids. They cause itching, bleeding at stool and pain. Internal hemorrhoids prolapse frequently through the sphincter and cause considerable discomfort. If the blood within them clots and becomes infected, they grow painful and are said to be *thrombosed.*

Preoperative Treatment. The preoperative treatment is that described for fistula in ano.

Operation. The operation usually is digital dilatation of the rectal sphincter and removal of the hemorrhoids by the use of a clamp and cautery or by ligation and excision. After completion of the operative procedures, a small rubber tube, often covered with petrolatum gauze, may be inserted through the sphincters to permit the escape of flatus, and also of blood if there should be any hemorrhage. Instead of the rubber tube, some surgeons place pieces of gelfoam or oxycel gauze over the anal wounds. Dressings in such cases are held in place by a T binder.

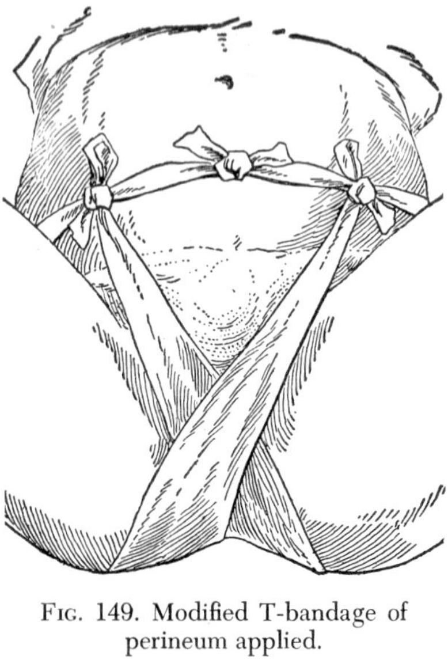

FIG. 149. Modified T-bandage of perineum applied.

Nursing Care in Rectal Surgery

Unusual finesse is required of the nurse in caring for patients with rectal problems. Such people often are sensitive and embarrassed and need someone on whom they can rely. The effect of emotional upset is seen when such a patient is to have a rectal examination by the doctor. He is not relaxed and co-operative. When the nurse and the physician secure the confidence of the patient, he is helped easily.

Position. The patient may be placed in the dorsal recumbent position with the knees flexed. An effective drape can be made by using a sheet or a bath blanket. A corner of the sheet is used to cover one leg and the opposite corner the other leg. Of the remaining 2 corners, one covers the torso and the other falls over the perineum and can be lifted easily at the time of the examination. Such draping prevents undue exposure, which is appreciated by the patient (Figs. 261 and 262).

Another comfortable position that is used frequently is Sims's lateral. The upper leg should be flexed sharply and the lower leg flexed less sharply for best positioning. Also, it is most desirable to have the buttocks well over to the side of the bed. The anus may be exposed by folding back a small section of the sheet. The knee-chest position allows the best exposure, but it is not the most comfortable one. The patient rests on his knees and chest with thighs vertical. The arms usually are above the head and give partial support. The patient's head should be turned so that the side of the face rests on the bed. Draping may be done with two sheets, one for the upper and one for the lower part of the body, or with a large sheet with an opening in the center. For any digital rectal examination, the physician needs a rubber glove or a finger cot and lubricant.

Special Care. The perineum is shaved carefully before surgery. This may vary with the nature of the operation. Usually a lower bowel irrigation is ordered, which should be given at least two hours prior to surgery. The skin area should be cleaned as thoroughly as possible.

After operation, the nurse should see to it that the perineum is irrigated with warm water after each bowel movement and after each voiding in the case of female patients. Liberal use of narcotics for the first 24 hours may be necessary. Voiding can be a problem; therefore, all methods to encourage voluntary micturition should be tried before resorting to catheterization.

Caution. After hemorrhoidectomy, hemorrhage may occur from the veins that were cut. If a rubber tube has been inserted through the sphincter after operation, evidence of bleeding should be apparent on the dressings. If, however, the patient feels faint, restless and anxious, and the pulse rate increases, the nurse should recognize internal or concealed hemorrhage and give appropriate treatment until the surgeon can be obtained.

After operation, rectal patients are kept in bed for the rest of the day of operation, and sometimes the second day. The prone position may be the more comfortable one, or the patient may prefer to be on his back with an airfoam pillow at his buttocks. Rectal temperatures are not taken. Pain is relieved greatly in these cases by the application of moist heat. This may be applied in the form of hot compresses or hot sitz baths 3 or 4 times daily, and especially after each bowel movement. Mineral oil may be ordered. Some surgeons prefer that a warm oil retention enema be given when the patient feels a desire to defecate; a soapsuds enema given through a catheter may be prescribed if there has been no bowel movement by the third day after operation. The food preferred by the patient is given usually.

Discharge. When it is time for the patient to be discharged from the hospital, he should know how to take sitz baths and how to test the temperature of the water. Sitz baths may be given in a bathtub, which necessitates the application of very warm water 3 or 4 times a day. If this tends to make some postoperative patients weak, sitz baths may be given by employing a bath basin or some large container with enough water to cover the perineum. The patient should be informed about his diet and made aware of the significance of proper eating habits. Also, he ought to know what cathartics he can take safely and why exercise is important. The surgeon usually outlines a schedule in detail to cover the daily routine. This can be reviewed for the patient by the nurse.

Pilonidal Cyst

A pilonidal cyst is found in the intergluteal cleft on the posterior surface of the lower sacrum. It is thought by some to be formed by an infolding of epithelial tissue beneath the skin, which may communicate with the skin surface through one or several small sinus openings. Hair frequently is seen protruding from these openings, and this gives the cyst its name—*pilonidal*—a nest of hair. The cysts rarely give symptoms until adolescence or early adult life, when infection produces an irritating drainage or an abscess. Trauma appears to play a part in producing the inflammatory reaction in these cysts.

In the early stages of the inflammation, the infection may be controlled by antibiotic therapy. Once an abscess has formed, as in cases of a hair-containing sinus, surgery is indicated. When an abscess is present, incision and drainage are performed. Usually, however, because the abscesses tend to recur or form secondary sinuses that cause irritating drainage, radical excision of the cyst is necessary. In patients with hair-containing sinuses without marked inflammatory reaction, operation is necessary for the same reason. The entire cyst and the secondary sinus tracts are excised. In many cases the resulting defect may be sutured, but in some the defect may be so large that it cannot be closed entirely and it is allowed to heal by granulation.

Nursing Care

The nursing care of these patients presents no problem. In those with abscess, hot moist applications are used frequently. After excision of the cyst, the care is that of any superficial wound. For the first few days, this patient often is more comfortable lying on his abdomen. Most patients may be allowed out of bed a few days after operation, and their

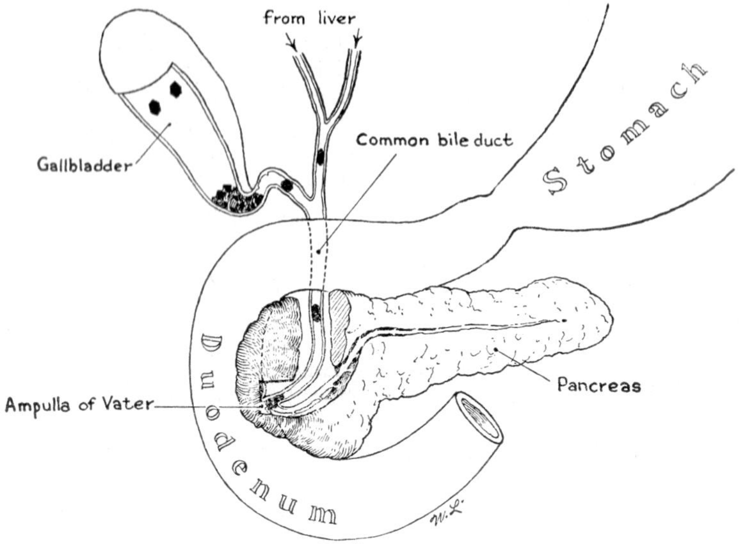

FIG. 150. Diagrammatic drawing showing the biliary ducts and the gallbladder. The diagram indicates, in black, common areas in which stones are found. It is evident that stones lying in the gallbladder and the cystic duct do not cause an obstruction of the flow of bile from the liver into the duodenum. Stones that lodge in the common duct or the ampulla of Vater obstruct the common bile duct and thus are associated with an absorption of bile pigment that produces jaundice.

postoperative care is carried out in the doctor's office.

SURGERY OF LIVER AND BILIARY PASSAGES

The liver, which is the largest gland in the body, is a most important organ in metabolism. The blood from practically all the abdominal organs passes through its capillaries before reaching the general circulation.

Many chemical reactions occur within its cells, preparing the various foodstuffs absorbed from the intestine for use by the body. The liver forms a secretion called *bile,* a brownish-yellow fluid that is carried to the duodenum by the bile ducts. This duct system has extending from it a small sac, the *gallbladder.* The ducts leading from the liver are called *hepatic ducts,* the duct from the gallbladder is called the *cystic duct,* and the duct formed by the junction of these two is called the *common bile duct* or *choledochus.* Bile plays a large part in the process of intestinal digestion and gives the normal brown color to the feces.

GALLBLADDER DISEASE

The diseases that need most frequent surgical attention are those that are associated with gallstones (cholelithiasis). These calculi form

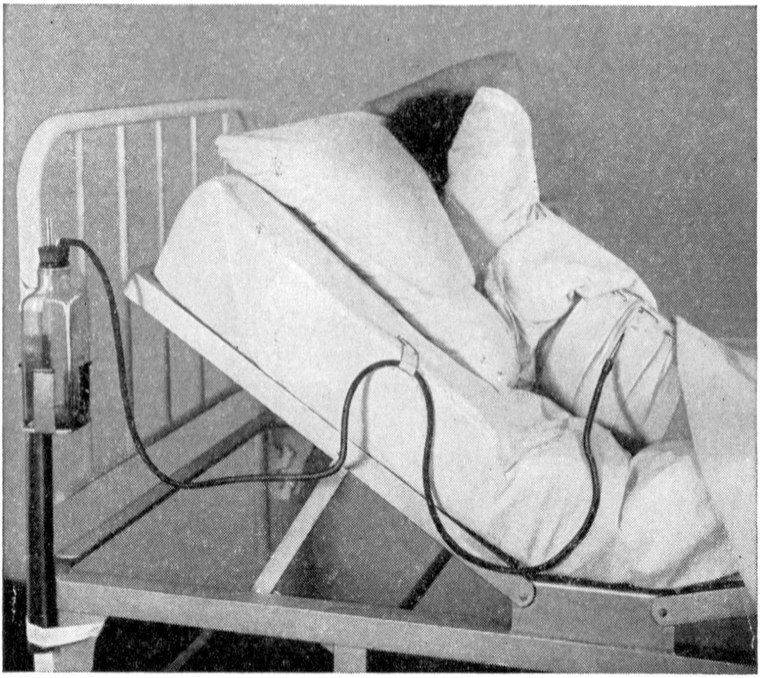

FIG. 151. Cholecystostomy. Note the drainage bottle attached to bedpost and also the drainage tube anchored to the bed by adhesive. The height of the bottle is adjusted as ordered by the surgeon. The height of the drainage bottle is determined by the rapidity of decompression desired.

ery commonly in the gallbladder lue to infection or to the precipitaion of bile constituents (bile salts ınd cholesterol). They appear to orm most frequently in women who ave borne children and usually in he fat type of individual. The presnce of the stones generally means ome dysfunction of the gallbladder, nd the disease is spoken of as hronic gallbladder disease.

Symptoms. Gallbladder disease ives rise to two types of symptoms: hose due to disease of the gallladder itself, with indigestion, chronic pain in the upper right abdomen and distention after eating; and those due to obstruction of the bile passages (especially the cystic duct) by a gallstone. This occurrence causes excruciating upper right abdominal pain that radiates to the back or the right shoulder and usually is associated with vomiting and nausea. These symptoms generally are so severe as to require morphine hypodermically. Such attacks are given the name of *biliary colic*.

Diagnosis. In the diagnosis of these "chronic" forms of gallbladder

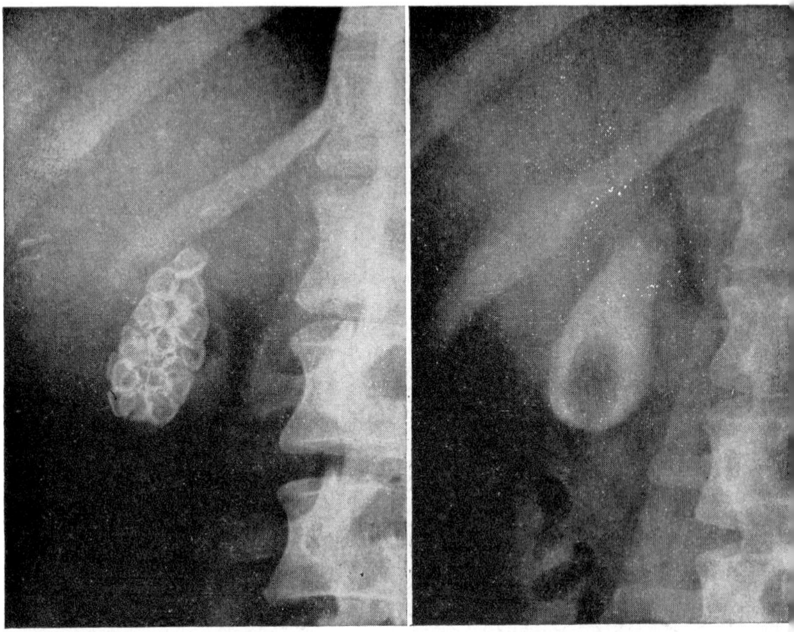

Fig. 152. (*Left*) Gallstones that show in a roentgenogram, due to calcification in their content. (*Right*) Single nonopaque gallstone shown as a negative shadow by displacing dye in cholecystogram.

disease, considerable information may be obtained by the *cholecystogram.* A dye is given, either by mouth or intravenously, which is excreted in the bile by the liver. Normally, the gallbladder shadow, as outlined, may be seen on the roentgenogram, and the shadow gradually decreases in size and becomes more dense as the dye is concentrated by fluid absorption. Finally, the normal gallbladder is able to empty part of its contents if a fatty meal is taken. The diseased gallbladder is indicated by a very faint shadow, which does not become concentrated and does not empty when a fatty meal is eaten (Graham-Cole test). A *duodenal drainage* with examination of the bile for crystals and pus cells is another diagnostic procedure.

At times the gallbladder may be the seat of an acute infection that causes acute pain, tenderness and rigidity of the upper right abdomen associated with nausea and vomiting and the usual signs of an acute inflammation. This condition is spoken of as *acute cholecystitis.* If the gallbladder is found to be filled with pus, there is said to be an *empyema* of the gallbladder.

Treatment. Surgical treatment is demanded for the relief of long-continued symptoms, for removal of he cause of biliary colic, and in ases of acute cholecystitis.

Preparation for a simple gallbladder operation is the same as for any ipper abdominal laparotomy. Paients may be placed on the operatng table with the upper abdomen aised somewhat by an air pillow or andbag in order to make exposure asier. (See Fig. 25.)

CHOLECYSTOSTOMY. This is an peration performed for the relief f certain cases of acute cholecystitis nd of chronic gallbladder disease. The gallbladder is opened, the stones nd the bile or pus are removed, and tube is sutured in the opening for lrainage. As soon as the patient is eturned to bed, the nurse should onnect this tube to a drainage bottle laced at the side of the bed. Failure o perform this duty may result in he leakage of bile round the tube nd its escape into the peritoneal avity.

CHOLECYSTECTOMY. This is the peration by which the gallbladder s removed after ligation of the cystic luct and artery. This operation is erformed in most cases of acute nd chronic cholecystitis.

BILIARY OBSTRUCTION

Not infrequently a gallstone may ass from the gallbladder through he cystic duct and lodge in the comnon bile duct; or the head of the ancreas, through which the comnon duct passes, may be the seat of carcinoma. Either condition may bstruct the flow of bile into the luodenum and result in the followng three characteristic symptoms.

The bile, no longer carried to the luodenum, is absorbed by the blood nd gives the skin and the tissues a yellow color known as *jaundice*. The bile pigments are excreted in some measure from the blood by the kidneys and gives the urine a very dark color. The feces, no longer colored with bile pigments, are grayish, like putty, and usually are spoken of as clay-colored. There frequently is marked itching of the skin, and nausea occurs after eating fatty foods because there is a marked disturbance of the digestion and absorption of fats when bile does not flow into the duodenum. Various laboratory tests of the blood (icteric index, van den Bergh, serum bilirubin, etc.) indicate the degree of pigment retention and therefore the depth of jaundice.

Operations upon patients with obstructive jaundice are most serious, because there is always marked damage to the liver and there is the added danger of hemorrhage. Therefore, these patients should receive special preparation. The diet should be low in fats and high in protein and carbohydrate. Frequently it is wise to administer protein solution intravenously for a day or two before operation.

It is well known that the hemorrhagic tendency in jaundice is due to a deficient formation of the prothrombin. This is an important factor in the clotting of blood, which becomes deficient in jaundice because of inadequate absorption of the fat-soluble vitamin K. Often the blood prothrombin may be raised adequately by administration of vitamin K, or a new supply may be added to the patient's blood by transfusion. Carbohydrates are given in large amounts by mouth and intravenously in order to build up the glycogen stores in the liver. The nurse should note the color of the urine and the stools and send specimens of these excreta to be examined for bile pigments. The operations performed depend upon the cause of the biliary obstruction.

Choledochotomy. In this operation an incision is made into the common duct for the removal of stones. After the stones have been evacuated, a tube usually is inserted int the duct for drainage. The gallblac der also contains stones as a rul These are removed and a cholecysto tomy or a cholecystectomy is pe formed. If a cholecystostomy is don one end of a drainage tube is suture in the gallbladder and the other en is connected to a bedside bottle.

When the common duct is ob structed due to the pressure of a

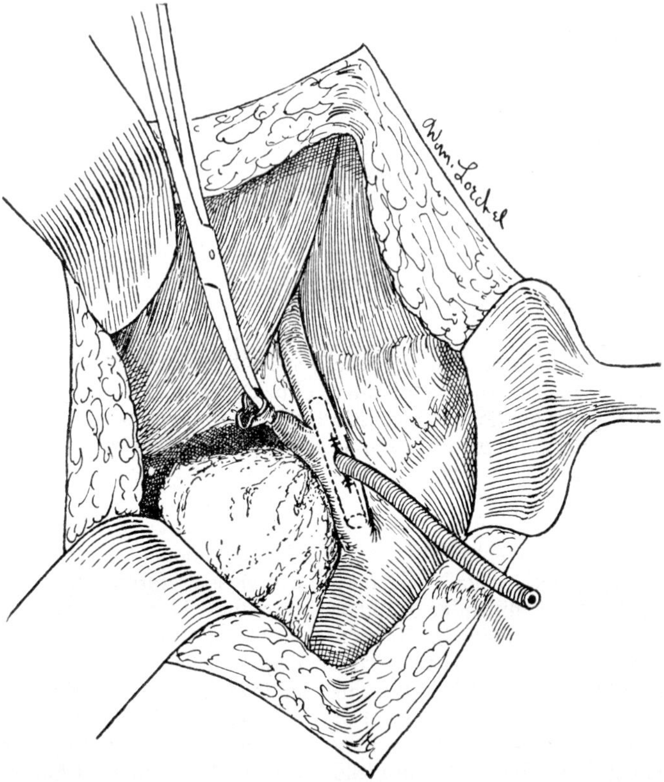

Fig. 153. Diagrammatic drawing showing the situation after an operation in which the gallbladder has been removed and a T-tube introduced into the common duct. A hemostat holds the ligated end of the cystic duct. The tube has been sutured in place in the common duct and led out through the wound.

ıoperable carcinoma of the head f the pancreas, an operation is •erformed that will lead the bile ıto the intestinal tract by a differ- nt route. (See p. 354, Carcinoma f Pancreas.)

Nursing Care After Operations on Biliary Tract

As soon as recovery from anes- ıesia has occurred, the patient is laced in the Fowler position. The sual treatment for any laparotomy : indicated, viz., fluids by vein; astric-suction drainage (Wangen- :een) if vomiting occurs; water and ther fluids may be given in 24 hours, nd an enema and a soft diet after 2 hours.

As mentioned before, in cases of ıolecystostomy or choledochostomy, ıe drainage tubes must be con- ected immediately to a drainage ottle or bottles. In addition, tubing ıould be fastened to the dressings r to the bottom sheet with enough eway for the patient to move with- ut dislodging it (see Fig. 151). In rder to prevent total loss of bile, ıe drainage tube or collecting bottle ıay be elevated above the level of ıe abdomen so that bile will drain ırough the apparatus only if pres- ıre develops in the duct system. 'he bile collected should be meas- red and recorded every 24 hours, s color and character being charted. fter 5 or 6 days of drainage, the ıbes may be clamped for an hour efore and after each meal, the pur- ose being to deliver bile to the uodenum to aid in digestion. The urse must exercise special care in ırning or lifting these patients in rder not to dislodge the tubes. Vithin 12 to 14 days, the drainage tubes are removed from the gall-bladder or common bile duct. Bile may continue to drain from the drainage tract in considerable quantities for a time and necessitate frequent change of the outer dressings and protection of the skin from irritation.

In all cases of biliary drainage, the stools should be observed daily and their color recorded. At frequent intervals specimens of both urine and feces should be sent to the laboratory for examination for bile pigments. In this way the surgeon is able to tell that the bile pigment is disappearing from the blood and is draining again into the duodenum. A careful record of fluid intake and output should be kept and totaled for each 24 hours.

After operations for biliary obstruction, patients are especially liable to secondary hemorrhage, which usually occurs as a general ooze from the operative field, but which may be concealed in the viscera. The local and the constitutional signs(p. 139) makes the diagnosis evident. The surgeon in charge should be called at once, and a dressing and transfusion tray should be provided.

The diet of these patients should be low in fats and, therefore, high in carbohydrates and proteins. The patients themselves usually will refuse to eat fatty foods because of the nausea that follows.

These patients are especially prone to pulmonary complications, as are all patients with upper abdominal incisions. They should be taught to take ten deep breaths every hour to aerate the lungs fully. Activating these individuals by getting them out of bed as early as permissible will reduce the likelihood of phlebitis, atelectasis, and so forth, which heretofore were common in these heavier patients.

SURGERY OF THE PANCREAS

The pancreas is one of the most important glands of the body. It lies transversely across the posterior wall of the abdomen, behind the peritoneum. It produces a secretion that enters the duodenum; also it produces insulin, which is the hormone concerned with the utilization of carbohydrates in the body. The latter secretion enters directly into the blood, and in this respect the pancreas belongs to the group of ductless glands.

Acute pancreatitis may be due to regurgitation of bile into the pancreatic ducts, or it may be hematogenous in origin.

The severer types of this infection may produce marked local hemorrhage, and the enzymes liberated may cause marked necrosis of the gland and of the fat in the adjacent parts of the abdominal cavity. The disease usually comes on suddenly, with severe abdominal pain and vomiting. The pain often extends across the back. The temperature may be marked, but in fulminating cases the patient may develop typical shock. This condition is responsible often for the diagnosis of "acute indigestion."

Chronic pancreatitis is a less common disease, occurring usually as a sequela of attacks of acute pancreatitis. The resultant fibrosis, calcification of the gland and obstruction of the ducts by calculi produce recurring painful attacks that even morphine does not relieve. These attack are associated with vague indiges tion, loss of weight and, at times jaundice. Surgical relief often i sought and attempted. In some cases relief of pain may be given by divi sion of the nerve pathways trans mitting the pain impulses (splanchni cotomy). Those with jaundice ma be treated by drainage or diversio of the bile flow, and in a few case complete excision of the pancreas ha been performed.

Tumors of the Head of the Pancreas

Tumors in this region are de tected by the fact that they ob struct the common bile duct wher it passes through the head of th pancreas to join the pancreatic duc and empty at the ampulla of Vate into the duodenum. Obstruction t the flow of bile produces jaundice clay-colored stools and dark urine This disease usually occurs in olde thin men. It must be differentiate from the jaundice due to a biliar obstruction caused by a gallstone i the common duct, which usually i intermittent and appears typically i fat individuals, most often wome who have had previous symptoms o gallbladder disease. The tumors pro ducing the obstruction may aris from the pancreas, from the com mon bile duct or from the ampull of Vater.

Operation is indicated in thes patients, first to be sure that th jaundice is not due to an impacte gallstone, which can be remove with relative ease. If a tumor i found, it may be removed if it ha not invaded many of the importa structures adjacent to it (portal vei

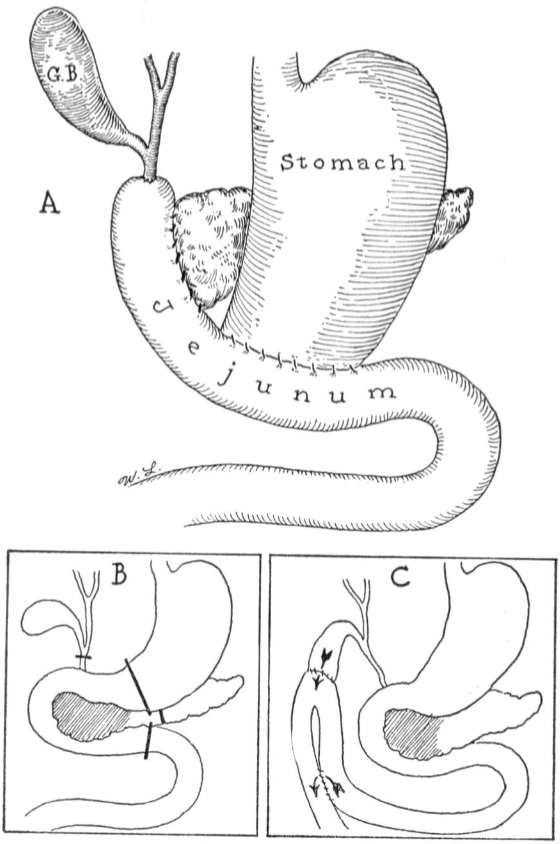

FIG. 154. Drawings which show types of operations for carcinoma of the pancreas. (A) Indicates the end result for resection of the carcinoma of the head of the pancreas or the ampulla of Vater. The common duct is sutured to the end of the jejunum, and the remaining portion of the pancreas and the end of the stomach are sutured to the side of the jejunum. (B) Shows lines that indicate the amount of tissue removed. (C) An alternate method of treatment when an inoperable tumor of the head of the pancreas has been found. In such cases the bile may be permitted to flow again into the intestine by anastomosing the jejunum to the gallbladder. In addition, an accessory operation between the loops of jejunum has been performed.

superior mesenteric artery). The operation entails removal of the head of the pancreas, the duodenum and adjacent stomach and the distal part of the common bile duct. The stomach, the cut end of the pancreas and the common bile duct then are anastomosed to the jejunum. This operation, first suggested by Whipple, may be done in one or two stages. It has resulted in cure in many cases of cancer of the ampulla and the bile ducts, but it is apparently only palliative in most cases of carcinoma of the head of the pancreas. When excision of the tumor cannot be performed, the jaundice may be relieved by diverting the bile flow into the jejunum. This is done by anastomosing it to the gallbladder (cholecystojejunostomy).

Nursing Care

When these patients come to the hospital, they are in such a poor nutritional and physical state that a fairly long period of preparation is necessary before operation can be attempted. Various liver and pancreatic function studies are carried out, vitamin K is given to restore the coagulability of the blood, and diets high in protein often are given with pancreatic enzymes. Blood transfusions frequently are used as well.

Because of the extensive surgery performed, much depends upon the nursing care after operation. This differs little from that after any upper abdominal operation, except that these patients are poor surgical risks and, therefore, they need intensive nursing attention in the immediate postoperative period.

Islet Tumors of the Pancreas

In the pancreas are located the islands of Langerhans, small nests of cells which secrete directly into the blood stream and which are, therefore, part of the glands of internal secretion (endocrines). The secretion, insulin, has to do with the metabolism of sugar, and a deficient secretion produces diabetes. Tumor of these cells produce a hypersecretion of insulin, so that the body suga is used up too rapidly. The fall of blood sugar (hypoglycemia) produces symptoms of weakness, mental confusion and even convulsions. These may be relieved immediatel by taking sugar by mouth or b intravenous glucose.

Once the diagnosis of a tumor o the islet cells has been made, sur gical treatment with removal of th tumor usually is recommended. Th tumors may be benign adenomas o they may be malignant. Complet removal results usually in a mos dramatic cure. In some cases th symptoms may not be produced b an actual tumor of the islet cells, bu by a simple hypertrophy of thi tissue. In such cases a *partial pan createctomy*—removal of the tail an part of the body of the pancreas— is performed.

Nursing Care

In preparing these patients fc operation, the nurse must be on th watch for symptoms of hypoglycemi and be ready to give sugar, usuall orange juice with sugar, should the appear. After operation, the nursin care is the same as that followin any upper abdominal operation.

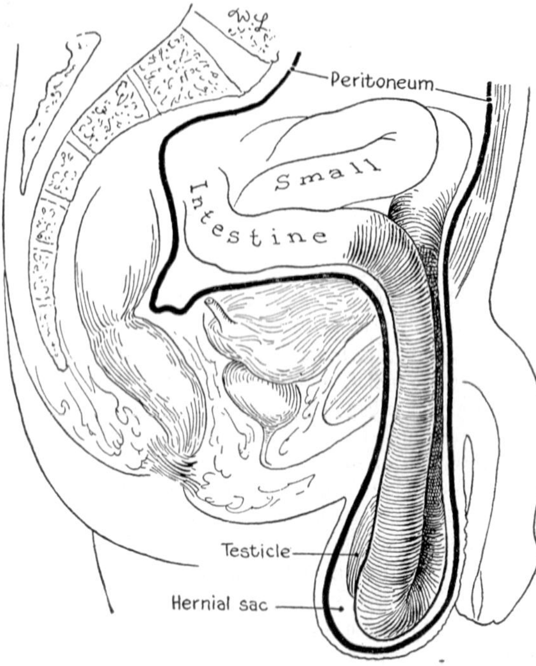

FIG. 155. Diagrammatic drawing that shows a hernia. Note that the sac of the hernia is a continuation of the peritoneum of the abdomen and that the hernial contents are intestine, omentum or other abdominal contents that pass through the hernial opening into the hernial sac.

ABDOMINAL HERNIA

A *hernia* (spoken of by the laity as rupture) is a protrusion of a viscus through the wall of the cavity in which it is naturally contained. This definition may apply to any part of the body; for instance, the protrusion of the brain after a subtemporal decompression is called *cerebral* hernia. However, in general, the term is applied to the protrusion of an abdominal viscus through an opening in the abdominal wall. The weakness may be congenital, i.e., a failure to close of one or more of the openings in the abdominal wall normally found in the fetus; or the weakness may be acquired, due to prolonged strain on the abdominal muscles or after illness or operation.

The hernial sac is formed by an outpouching of the peritoneum, and may contain large or small intestine, omentum and, occasionally, the bladder. When the hernia first is formed, the sac is filled only when the patient is on his feet, the contents returning to the abdominal cavity as soon as he lies down.

Types. There are four types of abdominal hernia. The most common type is the *inguinal*. This hernia is due to a weakness of the abdominal wall at the point through which the spermatic cord emerges in the male and the round ligament in the female. Through this opening the hernia extends down the inguinal canal and often into the scrotum or the labia. It is common in the male, and it may appear at any age.

Femoral hernia appears below Poupart's ligament (i.e., below the groin) as a round bulge. It is more frequent in women.

Umbilical hernia results from failure of the umbilical orifice to close. It is most common in fat women and in children as a protrusion at or slightly below the umbilicus.

Ventral or *incisional* hernias occur due to a weakness of the abdominal wall. They are due most frequently to previous operations in which drainage was necessary, complete closure of the tissues being impossible. Weakened by infection, only a slight bulge results at first, but this increases gradually in size until a definite hernial sac is produced.

There are many other forms of hernia, some of which occur inside the abdominal cavity. Such a hernia is spoken of as *internal* hernia.

Complications. As times goes on adhesions form between the sac and its contents, so that the hernia becomes *irreducible*. Any hernia, whether previously reducible or not, may at any time become incarcerated or strangulated. An *incarcerated* hernia is one in which the intestinal flow is obstructed completely. In a *strangulated* hernia the contents not only are irreducible, but the blood and the intestinal flow through the gut in the hernia are stopped completely. This condition obtains when the loop of gut in the sac becomes twisted; swelling occurs and a constriction is produced at the neck of the sac. The result then is an acute intestinal obstruction, plus the added danger of gangrene of the bowel. The symptoms are pain at the site of strangulation, followed by colicky abdominal pain, vomiting and swelling of the hernial sac.

Treatment

Surgical. In most cases the hernia should be repaired by operation; otherwise, the patient is in continual danger of strangulation. When this occurs, operation becomes imperative, and it is attended invariably by considerable risk.

The operation comprises removal of the hernial sac after dissecting it free from surrounding structures, replacing its contents in the abdominal cavity and ligating it at the neck. The muscle and the fascial layers then are sewed together firmly over the hernial orifice to prevent a recurrence. When it is impossible to approximate tissue in an effort to produce a strong wall, fascia lata grafts may be taken from the patient's thigh. In the repair of large hernias, tantalum gauze mesh has been implanted. Tantalum is an inert element which when woven into a gauze or a screen is malleable and strong and produces minimum tissue reaction. When a strangulation has occurred, the operation is complicated by the intestinal obstruction and injury to the bowel.

Mechanical. In infants, a hernia may at times be helped by the application of a truss, an appliance having a pad which is held snugly in the hernial orifice, and which should keep a reducible hernia reduced. A truss also may be used in the treatment of a hernia in adults when because of age or disease, it seems inadvisable to subject the patient to the risk of an operation. A truss does not cure a hernia; it simply prevents the abdominal contents from entering the hernial sac.

Preoperative Nursing Care

In emergency conditions of strangulated or incarcerated hernia, the nurse will prepare her patient as in any other acute surgical problem. However, most patients are individuals who are in good physical condition and are having a herniorrhaphy as elective surgery. The patient may be prompted by the knowledge that an unrepaired hernia may become a serious emergency or he may have difficulty securing employment because of this condition.

The suprapubic region and the anterior surface of the upper thigh should be shaved carefully. It is important for the patient not to have a cold or a cough. Such a strain may break the stitches and defeat the purpose of surgery. When he goes to the operating room, his bladder must be empty to prevent accidental injury during the surgical repair.

Nursing Care After Herniorrhaphy

Prolonged bed rest is not necessary after such operations, and in many cases patients are allowed out of bed a day or two after operation. In the event of edema and swelling of the scrotum, bed rest may be prolonged somewhat and a suspensory bandage or a jock strap may be necessary to give support and to provide pressure. (See p. 392.)

The chief complication to be watched for in connection with the repair of a hernia is the retention of urine. When these patients cannot be allowed to stand or to sit up, and if conservative measures fail to give relief, catheterization must be performed. Infection, or at least an imperfect healing, is all too frequent in these wounds. The elevation of temperature several days after operation or soreness in the operative region should lead to the discovery of the trouble. If early remedial measures are taken, the patient's convalescence is not delayed.

After most herniorrhaphies, the patient is instructed as to his activity after leaving the hospital. As a rule after a herniorrhaphy, athletics and extremes of exertion are not permitted for at least 6 or 8 weeks after the operation.

REFERENCES AND SUGGESTED READING

Unit Four: Nursing in Conditions of the Alimentary System

GENERAL

(See also those for Unit One, p. 205.)

Christian, T.: Nursing care in abdominal surgery, Am. J. Nursing **50**:797-800, 1950.

Emerson, C. P., and Bragdon, J. S.: Essentials of Medicine, ed. 17, pp. 309-390, Philadelphia, Lippincott, 1955.

Penberthy and Grover: Acute abdominal injuries, Surg., Gynec. & Obst. **94**:626-628, 1952.

Weiss, Edward, and English, O. S.: Psychosomatic Medicine, ed. 2, Philadelphia, Saunders, 158-251, 1949.

MOUTH

Emerson, C. P., and Bragdon, J. S.: Essentials of Medicine, ed. 17,

pp. 320-325 (mouth); p. 325 (tumors), Philadelphia, Lippincott, 1955.
Flood, J. A.: Nursing in cancer of the mouth, Am. J. Nursing **43**: 536-539, 1943.
Miller, C. J.: Cancer of the mouth, Am. J. Nursing **43**:531-535, 1943.
Phair, W. P.: Are you up to date on dental health?, Am. J. Nursing **53**: 183-186, 1953.
Welborn, J. F., and Water, M. H.: Nursing care for the patient having oral surgery, Am. J. Nursing **51**:74-77, 1951.

ESOPHAGUS

Adams, Herbert: The surgical aspects of obstructing lesions of the esophagus, S. Clin. North America **26**:3, 1946.
Battersby and Greve: Modern treatment of atresia of esophagus, Am. J. Nursing **50**:158-161, 1950.
Diller, Doris: Nursing care in esophageal operations, Am. J. Nursing **47**:811-813, 1947.
Emerson, C. P., and Bragdon, J. S.: Essentials of Medicine, ed. 17, pp. 327-328, Philadelphia, Lippincott, 1955.
Longmire, W. P.: Esophageal conditions and their treatment, Am. J. Nursing **47**:807, 1947.

STOMACH AND DUODENUM

Barrett, K.: Intubation in gastric surgery, Am. J. Nursing **43**:17-22, 1943.
Dragstedt, L. R.: Gastric vagotomy, Am. J. Nursing **48**:278-281, 1948.
Emerson, C. P., and Bragdon, J. S.: Essentials of Medicine, ed. 17, pp. 331-336 (peptic ulcer); pp. 336-339 (tumors), Philadelphia, Lippincott, 1955.
Heger, C.: Surgical nursing care of patients with duodenal ulcer, Am. J. Nursing **52**:861-862, 1952.
Mitchell, H.: The social sciences in nursing education (a study of a hemorrhaging gastric ulcer patient showing the influence of socio-economic factors), Am. J. Nursing **50**:179-181, 1950.
Palumbo, L. T.: Surgical treatment of duodenal ulcer, Am. J. Nursing **52**:857-861, 1952.
Panico, F. G.: Improved abrasive balloon for diagnosis of gastric cancer, J.A.M.A. **149**:1447-1449, 1952.
Saft, I. D.: Your stomach through the gastroscope, Am. J. Nursing **43**:162-164, 1943.
Wilson, Helen A.: Nursing care in gastric vagotomy, Am. J. Nursing **48**:282-283, 1948.

INTESTINAL TRACT, RECTUM AND ANUS

Agnew, J. W.: Abdomino-perineal resection, Am. J. Nursing **51**:225-226, 1951.
Carmel, A. G.: Proctologic nursing, Am. J. Nursing **48**:626-629, 1948.
Coller, F. A., and Vaughan, H. H.: Treatment of carcinoma of the colon, Ann. Surg. **121**:395-411, 1945.
Dericks, V. C., and Robeson, K. A.: Problems of colostomy patients, Pub. Health Nursing **41**:16-25, 1949.
Emerson, C. P., and Bragdon, J. S.: Essentials of Medicine, ed. 17, pp. 339-360, pp. 349-354 (appendicitis); p. 354 (regional enteritis); pp. 358-360 (peritonitis), Philadelphia, Lippincott, 1955.
Galetz, M. J.: An intestinal rehabili-

tation clinic, Am. J. Nursing **53**: 686-687, 1953.

Hirshfeld, J. W., and Sutton, H. B.: A new colostomy protector, Am. J. Surg. **84**:126-128, 1952.

Jaffe, L.: The patient and his ileostomy, Am. J. Nursing **54**:68, 1954.

Kaufman, Bel: Care of skin in ileostomy and colostomy, Am. J. Nursing **45**:354, 1945.

Lyons, A. S., and Garlock, J. H.: The relationship of chronic ulcerative colitis to carcinoma, Gastroenterology **18**:170-178, 1951.

Priest, P. I.: Teaching patients to take care of themselves, Am. J. Nursing **52**:1492-1494, 1952.

Streuben, E. M.: Nursing care for the patient with an abdominoperineal resection, Am. J. Nursing **51**:226-228, 1951.

Thompson, Bernice: Colostomy care. II. Use of the Binkley colostomy irrigator, Am. J. Nursing **48**:235-237, 1948.

Waples, Genevieve: Colostomy care. I. The use of the Lamson appliance, Am. J. Nursing **48**:233-235, 1948.

Hernia and Intestinal Obstruction

Bartle, H.: Strains and hernia, Am. J. Nursing **42**:1393-1397, 1942.

Blodgett, J. B., and Sheldon, N. S.: Intestinal suction, Am. J. Nursing **46**:90-92, 1946.

Emerson, C. P., and Bragdon, J. S.: Essentials of Medicine, ed. 17, pp. 345-349, Philadelphia, Lippincott, 1955.

Ferguson, L. K., et al.: Intestinal obstruction in the aged, Geriatrics **4**:341-352, 1949.

Gale, J. W.: Intestinal obstructions, Am. J. Nursing **48**:486-488, 1948.

Lemmer, K. E., and Watson, S. R.: Inguinal hernia, Am. J. Nursing **53**:1471-1475, 1953.

Throckmorton, T. D.: Tantalum gauze in the repair of hernias complicated by tissue deficiency, Surgery **23**:32-46, 1948.

Watson, S. R.: Nursing care in intestinal obstruction, Am. J. Nursing **48**:489-491, 1948.

Gallbladder and Pancreas

Brunschwig, A.: One stage pancreatoduodenectomy, Surg., Gynec. & Obst. **85**:161-164, 1947.

Buckley, M. E., and Crenshaw, V. P.: Nursing care of a patient with cholecystitis, Am. J. Nursing **46**: 812-815, 1946.

Eliason, E. L., and Welty, R. F.: Pancreatic calculi, Ann. Surg. **127**: 150-157, 1948.

Emerson, C. P., and Bragdon, J. S.: Essentials of Medicine, ed. 17, pp. 377-382 (gallbladder disease); pp. 383-387 (pancreatitis and tumor of pancreas), Philadelphia, Lippincott, 1955.

Finney, J. M. T., and Johnson, M. L.: Primary carcinoma of the gallbladder, Ann. Surg. **121**:425-434, 1945.

Frechette, B. E.: The surgical treatment of biliary disease, nursing care, Am. J. Nursing **53**:1064-1065, 1953.

Lowman, R. M., and Stanley, H. W.: An evaluation of Telepaque, a new cholecystographic medium, Connecticut M. J. **16**:591-593, 1952.

Mackay, A. G.: The surgical treatment of biliary disease, Am. J. Nursing **53**:1062-1064, 1953.

CLINICAL SITUATIONS

Abdominoperineal Resection

Ken Swartz, aged 55, was proud of his perfect health record during his service as bus driver. However, he now was experiencing peculiar bowel habits which varied from bouts of constipation to episodes of diarrhea. A barium enema and x-ray examination confirmed the suspicion of early carcinoma of the rectum. An abdominoperineal resection was planned.

1. Shortly after admission, Mr. Swartz complained of distention. In preparing a Miller-Abbott tube for insertion, the nurse should

_____(1) inject 4 cc. of mercury into the bag
_____(2) apply a fresh rubber balloon to the end of the tube
_____(3) lubricate the tube generously with petrolatum
_____(4) sterilize and place tube in a basin containing cracked ice

2. In withdrawing a gastrointestinal tube, the best procedure is to

_____(1) withdraw it slowly for about 6 to 8 inches at intervals of 10 minutes; when it reaches the esophagus, withdraw it rapidly
_____(2) withdraw the tube rapidly
_____(3) allow the patient to pull out the tube very slowly

3. Mr. Swartz should know that his colostomy

_____(1) requires that he wear a bag at all times
_____(2) demands aseptic care of the surrounding skin
_____(3) can be regulated by proper diet and exercise

4. Following a perineal resection, it will be impossible for the nurse to

_____(1) take a rectal temperature
_____(2) perform a perineal irrigation
_____(3) administer a colonic irrigation

5. Groups of foods which Mr. Swartz should avoid after his operation are:

_____(1) coarse cereals, hot breads, pastry
_____(2) raw fruits and vegetables
_____(3) American, cream or cottage cheese
_____(4) rice, cornmeal, macaroni

Cholecystectomy

Mrs. Molly Ranson was carrying a large bag of groceries when she experienced a sharp, stabbing pain in the right upper abdomen. She managed to get home, where she stretched out on a couch. The pain persisted, and she felt very nauseated, so she called her physician. The physician administered a sedative and made arrangements for hospitalization for an acute biliary attack. The admission orders included an order for a cholecystogram.

1. Preparations for the cholecystogram include:

a. The evening preceding the test

_____(1) a nonfatty meal
_____(2) a fatty meal
_____(3) nothing by mouth
_____(4) fluids only

b. The morning of the roentgenogram

_____(1) a fatty breakfast
_____(2) a nonfatty breakfast
_____(3) no breakfast
_____(4) fluids only

c. After the first roentgenogram and preceding the second roentgenogram
_____(1) a fatty meal
_____(2) a nonfatty meal
_____(3) nothing by mouth
_____(4) fluids only

2. Recording for all patients with biliary disease should include a notation of the color of the
_____(1) pupils of eyes
_____(2) whites of eyes
_____(3) gums
_____(4) lips
_____(5) tongue
_____(6) nail beds
_____(7) urine
_____(8) feces
_____(9) skin
_____(10) biliary drainage

3. The surgeon planned to remove the gallbladder and a stone from the common duct. This operation is called
_____(1) cholecystectomy and choledochotomy
_____(2) cholecystostomy and cholelithectomy
_____(3) excision of cholelithiasis and cholecystectomy
_____(4) a Whipple operation

4. Mrs. Ranson seemed more upset about leaving her husband with no one to take care of him than she did about facing major surgery. The nurse should
_____(1) determine whether Mr. Ranson is capable of caring for himself during this period
_____(2) assure the patient, but quietly notify the city welfare department
_____(3) convince the patient that she is the important person in this situation
_____(4) divert the patient's thoughts

5. Surgical risk of patients with jaundice is increased by the tendency of these patients to
_____(1) hemorrhage
_____(2) pulmonary infections
_____(3) intestinal obstruction
_____(4) wound infections

6. Preoperative treatment of jaundiced patients is directed toward
_____(1) elevation of blood prothrombin
_____(2) decrease of body weight
_____(3) increase glycogen store in liver
_____(4) decrease glycogen store in liver

7. Mrs. Ranson weighs more than 200 lbs. This fact should indicate to the nurse that during the first few postoperative days, she must be especially alert to use nursing measures designed to
_____(1) prevent decubitus ulcers
_____(2) decrease the weight rapidly
_____(3) prevent pulmonary complications
_____(4) prevent wound disruption

8. The following order was written: "Out of bed tomorrow. Apply Scultetus binder."

a. The binder should be applied while the patient is
_____(1) lying in bed
_____(2) standing with both feet flat on floor

b. The tails of the binder should be overlapped
_____(1) from below upward
_____(2) from above downward

UNIT FIVE

Nursing in Conditions of the Urinary Tract—Male Urology

CHAPTER EIGHTEEN

Surgery of the Urinary Tract and the Male Reproductive Organs

THE NURSE AND THE UROLOGIC PATIENT
ANATOMY AND PHYSIOLOGY
METHODS OF STUDY OF THE URINARY TRACT
SURGERY OF THE KIDNEY
DISEASES OF BLADDER, PROSTATE AND URETHRA
MALE GENITO-UROLOGY
ANATOMY AND PHYSIOLOGY OF MALE REPRODUCTIVE SYSTEM
DISEASES OF EXTERNAL GENITALIA
DISEASES OF TESTES AND ADJACENT STRUCTURES

THE NURSE AND THE UROLOGIC PATIENT

The patient with a genito-urinary problem deserves an understanding and dignified approach by the nurse in all her contacts with him. In many instances, he is sensitive and embarrassed and sometimes even possesses a sense of guilt. His dignity, sensitivity and confidence can be maintained on a wholesome plane by the proper response and conduct of the nurse.

The successful nurse needs to know male psychology. She should be aware of the position her patient occupies in his family and community. Early in her contact with him, she should note all evidences of the aging process, such as hearing, chewing, habits and posture, especially in bed. By careful observation, the nurse is able to determine his attitude toward life and toward his incapacity. Then from her evaluation, she is able to know and help him as an individual. At the same time she is equipped better to interpret the needs of the patient to the physician.

ANATOMY AND PHYSIOLOGY OF THE URINARY TRACT

The urinary tract is composed of the kidneys, the ureters, the urinary bladder and the urethra. Its function is the formation and the excretion of urine. The kidneys are two bean-shaped organs which lie embedded

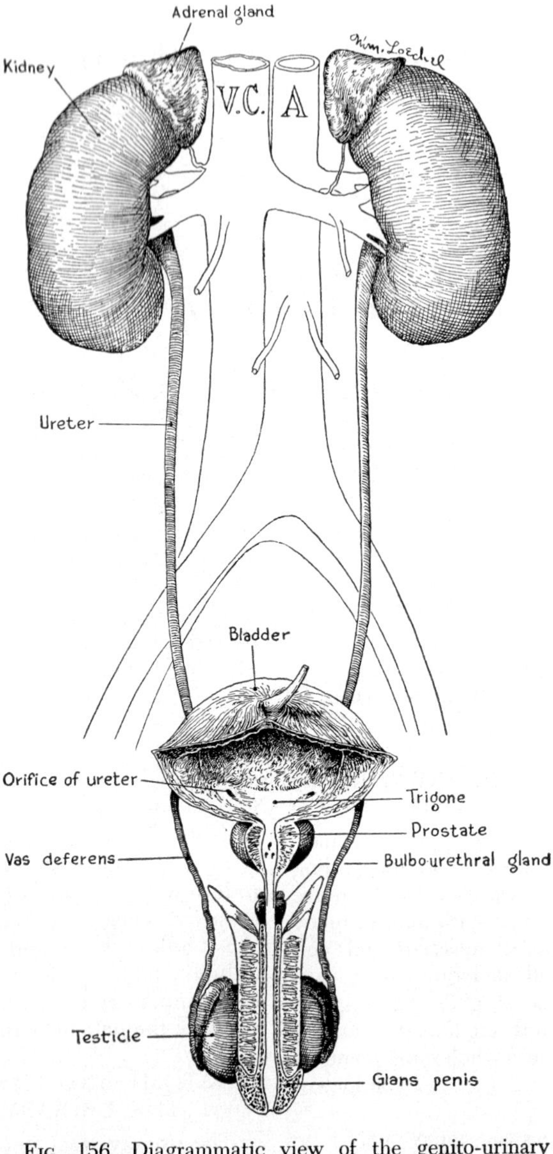

FIG. 156. Diagrammatic view of the genito-urinary tract and the male reproductive system. Note the position of the adrenal gland in relation to the kidney. The pelvis of the kidney lies somewhat obscured by the renal vessels. (V. C.) Vena cava. (A) Aorta.

in fat behind the peritoneum, one on each side of the spinal column opposite the last thoracic and the upper lumbar vertebrae. They act as selective filters for the blood that passes through them, removing various waste products of nitrogenous metabolism, such as urea, uric acid and excess salts, and yet preventing the loss, under normal conditions, of sugar, proteins and cells. The urine is a watery solution of these excretory products, the amount varying from 500 to 1,500 cc. per day, depending upon the fluid intake (oral or intravenous) and the fluid loss by other ways (perspiration, vomiting, diarrhea).

The urine is collected in a funnel-shaped structure called the pelvis of the kidney, to be emptied into an epithelial-lined tube called the *ureter*. The ureters have muscular walls which by peristaltic action transport the urine to a collecting reservoir, the bladder.

The urinary bladder receives urine drop by drop; by a sphincter mechanism under voluntary control, it collects and holds this fluid until its normal distention, usually about 300 to 400 cc., produces the urge to urinate. The bladder is evacuated by a voluntary relaxation of bladder sphincter through the urethra.

The urethra is short in the female, but in the male it passes through the prostate gland and the entire length of the penis.

METHODS OF STUDY OF THE URINARY TRACT

In most surgical lesions of the urinary tract, several methods of study are employed to detect abnormalities of its function and structure. The simplest study is of the urine. Besides the routine analysis of the urine, studies of renal function may be made by the urea clearance test and by tests to determine the ability of the kidney to concentrate the urine or to excrete dyes.

Urinalysis and Catheterization. Injury to or disease of the urinary tract usually produces some change in the composition of the urine. In many instances, the quantity of urine is significant. Normally about 1,500 cc. is excreted daily and specific gravity averages about 1.015 to 1.025. It is ordinarily pale yellow to amber in color, clear, and has an aromatic odor. Urine is acid in reaction and is negative for albumin, sugar and acetone.

Inasmuch as urine specimens are of diagnostic importance, it is necessary for the nurse to be as conscientious in collecting such a specimen as she is in giving medication. In a routine urinalysis of males, a freshly voided specimen is usually sufficient. In females, it may be necessary to have a catheterized specimen to avoid a possible mixture of vaginal secretions.

When specimens are collected for culture, a catheter always should be used in females. For a male urine culture, it is usually sufficient to have the patient void into a sterile receptacle, provided that the meatus is cleansed with soap and water followed by a nonirritating germicide. The reaction of urine is determined by the use of litmus paper or the more sensitive nitrazene paper.

Phenolphthalein Test. Another common method of estimating kidney function is by the use of the phenolphthalein test. This dye is known to be excreted rapidly by the kidney after intravenous or intramuscular injection. Delay in excretion is usually an indication of renal disease. The test is carried out on all patients with disease of the urinary tract.

From 20 to 30 minutes before the test is done, the patient is given several glasses of water to drink. He is then instructed to void. Then 1 cc. of phenolsulfonephthalein is injected intramuscularly. The time of giving the dye is noted, and at the end of an hour and 10 minutes the patient is instructed to void into a receptacle. A second glass of water is given. At the end of the second hour the urine is collected in a second receptacle. The above method of collecting the urine in this test is known as the medical technic.

When there is obstruction to the urethra, the bladder empties itself incompletely. Therefore, the urine is collected by catheter to make the test accurate. In order to avoid trauma to the urethra, it is customary to leave the catheter in place for the duration of the test. This procedure is known as the surgical technic. Accuracy and attention to details of technic and analysis are paramount.

Each hourly specimen obtained is made alkaline by the addition of 10 per cent sodium hydroxide (a pink to cerise color develops) and diluted accurately in a graduate to 1,000 cc. Specimens from the resulting pink solutions are compared in a color box with standard solutions. The normal dye estimation after intramuscular injection should yield 50 per cent for the first hour and 20 per cent for the second.

Blood Chemistry. More definite knowledge of the degree of impairment of the function of the kidneys may be obtained by estimating the amount of urea, creatinine and uric acid in the blood. Many other detailed blood analyses are made, which makes it necessary for the nurse to explain to the patient the necessity for blood specimens. The normal values for the more important blood constituents are as follows:

Blood urea nitrogen
(B.U.N.) 12-15 mg. per 100 cc. blood
Nonprotein nitrogen
(N.P.N.) 25-35 mg. per 100 cc. blood

Visualization (X-rays). X-rays are used to study the urinary tract in many ways. The direct examination ("flat plate") is used to determine the size and the position of the kidneys and to visualize stones in kidney, ureter and bladder (Fig. 159). Various organic compounds of iodine, when given intravenously, are excreted rapidly by the kidney in the urine. The presence of these compounds makes the urine-containing parts of the urinary tract opaque to the x-rays so that they can be delineated on the x-ray film (intravenous pyelogram, urogram or occasionally mentioned as K.U.B., kidney-ureter-bladder). (See Fig. 158.) This is not only a method of outlining the urinary passages but also a test of kidney function. The position of the ureters is often marked by taking an x-ray film with ureteral catheters in place. Less frequently the kidney pelvis and the ureters are studied by the injection of radiopaque solutions through ureteral catheters (retrograde pyelogram) or into the bladder through urethral catheters (cystogram).

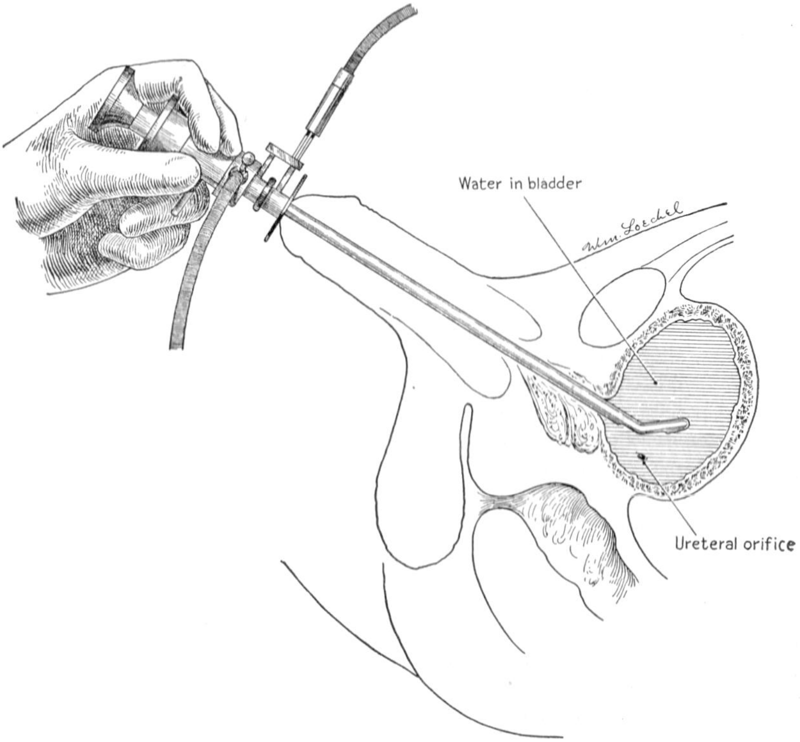

FIG. 157. Diagrammatic view of cystoscope introduced into the bladder in the male. The upper cord contains electricity for the light at the distal end of the cystoscope. The lower tubing leads from a reservoir of sterile water that is used to inflate the bladder. Of course, the entire procedure of cystoscopy is a sterile one.

By direct **palpation** it is frequently possible to determine the size and the movability of the kidneys. By rectal examination in the male, the prostate gland may be palpated digitally as a part of the study of the urinary difficulty that occurs as it hypertrophies in older men.

Cystoscopy. A direct method of study is by direct vision and catheterization of the ureters. This is performed through a cystoscope, which is inserted through the urethra into the bladder. By distending the bladder with sterile water, illumination from a small electric bulb permits visualization of the bladder wall and of the ureteral orifices. Small catheters may be threaded through these orifices into the ureters up to the kidney pelves, to collect urine from each kidney separately for analysis and bacteriologic study. They also outline the course of the ureters in x-ray studies.

Often it is the nurse who is called upon to explain the meaning of a cystoscopic examination to her patient. This is a real part of preparation, because if he has no idea of the type of procedure which is to take place, his fears will undoubtedly make him tense. The preparation usually includes his drinking one or two glasses of water before going to the examining department. Often a sedative plus the instillation of a local anesthetic into the bladder may be sufficient; however, depending upon the patient, it may be necessary to use spinal or general anesthesia. Since this is a sterile procedure, complete aseptic technic must be carried out.

The cystoscope is a delicate, expensive instrument which has many lenses and a small light bulb. It must be handled carefully; most cystoscopes cannot be sterilized by heat, but recently heat-resistant scopes have been made. In selecting a chemical for disinfection, one must be sure that it will not react with the cement which holds the lenses in place. An aqueous germicide, such as Zephiran Chloride 1:1,000, is effective if the scope is clean and dry before immersion. Ureteral catheters which are made of plastic material can be sterilized by autoclaving. If they are made of French woven fabric, they must be disinfected with a germicide. Thorough rinsing after chemical disinfection must be carried out.

When a cystoscopy is performed, sterile water or saline may be used as an irrigating fluid to distend the bladder. Following such an examination, most patients prefer to remain in bed for the rest of the day. If there is any pain, a sedative may help. The application of a hot-water bottle to the lower abdomen is soothing. Fluids should be taken liberally.

SURGERY OF THE KIDNEY

Congenital Anomalies

Congenital anomalies of the kidney are not uncommon. Occasionally there is fusion of the two, forming what is called a horseshoe kidney. One kidney may be small and deformed and often nonfunctioning. Abnormal vessels to the kidney may kink the ureter. Not infrequently there may be a double ureter or congenital stricture of the ureter. The treatment of these anomalies is necessary only if they cause symptoms, but it goes without saying that before renal surgery is attempted it is important to know that the other kidney is present and functioning.

Kidney Trauma

Various types of crushing injuries of the loin may injure the kidney, producing tears in its structure. The appearance of blood in the urine following an injury to the loin is highly suggestive of an injury to the kidney; therefore, a urinalysis always must be made.

In minor injuries to the kidney, healing may take place with conservative measures, such as the application of cold and firm adhesive support to the loin. When the kidney is injured sufficiently to cause hemorrhage of considerable amount, operation may be necessary. The damaged kidney usually has to be removed, although on occasions it is possible to repair it.

Kidney Infections

The infections of the kidney are classified as pyelitis, pyelonephritis and pyonephrosis, but they are usually stages of the same disease process. The infecting organism is usually the colon bacillus; less commonly the streptococcus or staphylococcus is the offender.

Pyelitis, an inflammation of the renal pelvis, may be seen as a childhood disease, especially in girls, and in adult life. It rapidly improves with bed rest, fluid administration and chemotherapy and antibiotic therapy. The persistent pyelitis of adult life usually is associated with an inflammation of the kidney (pyelonephritis), and, as the disease progresses, the entire cortex becomes involved, abscesses appear in the parenchyma, and the kidney becomes a bag of pus (pyonephrosis). This disease process most often follows some obstruction to the urinary flow.

The symptoms produced are at times very acute with fever, chills, nausea and vomiting, and pain in the loin, radiating to the thigh and the genitalia. Less often there is an insidious onset, with weakness, loss of weight and fever. The urine is loaded with pus cells and bacteria and usually red cells.

Treatment of renal infections consists of bed rest, intake of fluids in large amounts (3,000 cc. per day) and the administration of chemotherapy or antibiotics. Gantrisin (sulfisoxazole) has proved to be the most effective sulfonamide, and streptomycin and/or other antibiotics are widely used. When the infection is associated with an obstruction of the ureter, a ureteral catheter may be inserted through the cystoscope to provide drainage. When the obstruction cannot be relieved by ureteral catheterization, drainage of the kidney may be employed (nephrostomy); or, if the kidney function is entirely lost, nephrectomy may be necessary.

Carbuncle of the Kidney

Carbuncle of the kidney is an infection of hematogenous origin which is caused usually by the staphylococcus. It usually follows a cutaneous boil or carbuncle and is characterized by a fever, malaise and dull pain in the region of the kidney. This type of infection, if recognized, usually subsides with chemotherapy and penicillin.

Perinephritic Abscess

Perinephritic abscess is an abscess in the fatty tissue about the kidney which may arise secondary to an infection of the kidney or as a hematogenous infection originating in foci elsewhere in the body. The symptoms are often acute in onset with chills, fever, high leukocytosis and other signs of suppuration. Locally, there is tenderness posteriorly in the loin.

Treatment. The treatment consists of incision and drainage of the abscess by a lumbar incision.

In the postoperative care, the nurse should place the patient in the dorsal position. Because the drainage is often profuse, frequent changes of the outer dressings may be necessary.

Tuberculosis

Tuberculosis of the kidney is usually secondary to tuberculosis elsewhere in the body. It is a chronic infection, and at first the symptoms are mild. There is usually a slight afternoon fever and a loss of weight and appetite. The urine passed is often tinged with blood and contains many pus cells. In establishing the diagnosis, the urine may be examined for tubercle bacilli, or some of the urine may be injected into a guinea pig. If the organisms are present in the urine, in a short time the animal will die with tuberculosis. If the disease progresses, secondary infection usually occurs in the kidney,

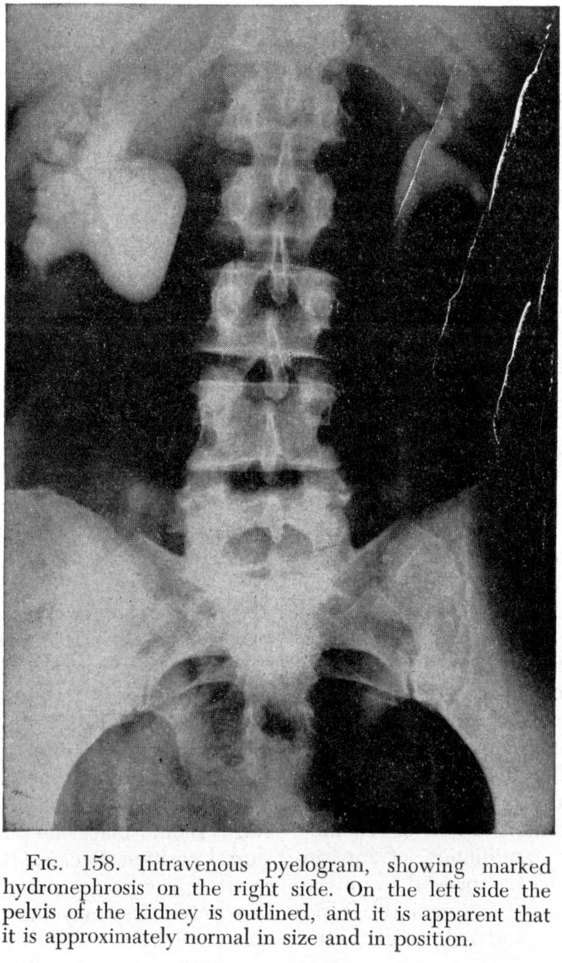

Fig. 158. Intravenous pyelogram, showing marked hydronephrosis on the right side. On the left side the pelvis of the kidney is outlined, and it is apparent that it is approximately normal in size and in position.

and the tuberculosis spreads to other parts of the urinary tract. The ureter and the bladder become infected by direct transmission from the kidney, and symptoms of bladder irritability (viz., frequency of urination, nocturia) are a later manifestation of the disease.

Treatment. This depends upon the extent of the disease. If the infection involves only one kidney and the other functions normally, the diseased one may be removed. If both kidneys are involved, surgery is out of the question, and hygienic measures must be employed. Streptomycin is used both with and without surgery as a therapeutic and prophylactic measure.

Nephroptosis

Nephroptosis, or movable kidney, is a condition found chiefly in thin, long-waisted women from 30 to 50

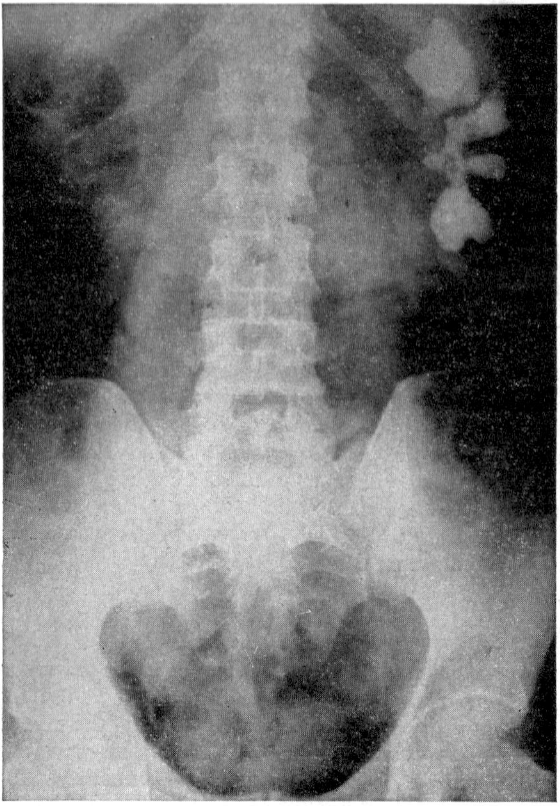

Fig. 159. Flat plate of the abdomen, showing a large calculus in the left kidney.

years of age. The pad of fat which normally surrounds the kidney is absent. The posture is usually poor, and the abdominal muscles are relaxed, the result of which produces a weakness and a dragging pain in the loin. At times the kidney may sag so that it almost reaches the pelvis when the patient stands (floating kidney). This abnormal movability may produce torsion or kinks in the ureter; acute pain, nausea and vomiting and at times chills and fever may be produced by this obstruction to the ureter. These attacks are known as Dietl's crises. The attack may often be relieved by having the patient lie down with a pillow placed under the hips or by manipulating the kidney.

Treatment. The treatment of the condition is directed toward building up the general health of the patient by rest in bed with the foot of the bed elevated, with forced feedings in order to build up a pad of fat which will hold the kidney in position. Belts are often applied to give abdominal support. One attack of Dietl's crisis warrants a complete urologic study (cystoscopy, pyelography, urography). If operative intervention is found to be necessary, the kidney may be fixed in position by sutures, by an operation called a *nephropexy*.

Hydronephrosis

Obstruction to the normal flow of urine will produce a damming up of urine with a resultant back pressure on the kidney. If the obstruction is in the urethra or bladder, the back pressure affects both kidneys, but if the obstruction is in the ureter, due to stone or kink, only one kidney is damaged. When the obstruction is of long duration, it produces a dilatation of the ureter above the obstruction (hydro-ureter), and the kidney becomes a mere shell filled with fluid. This condition is called hydronephrosis. If both kidneys are so diseased, their function of eliminating waste products from the body is markedly impaired, and there is danger of death from uremia (Fig. 158).

Treatment. When the cause of the obstruction can be removed (e.g., stone in the ureter and stricture of the urethra) of course the treatment must be in that direction. When one kidney only is involved, and its function is nil, nephrectomy may be performed.

Urinary Calculi

Stones are formed in the urinary tract due to the deposits of the crystalline substances (uric acid, calcium phosphate and oxalate) excreted in the urine. They may be found anywhere from the kidney to the bladder and vary in size from mere granular deposits, called sand or gravel, to stones as large as an orange found in the bladder.

When the stones block the flow of urine, hydronephrosis develops, and the constant irritation of the stone may be followed by a secondary infection, causing pyelitis, cystitis and so forth.

Stones in the kidney may produce few symptoms; usually, however, there is a dull ache in the loin, and the patient passes increased amounts of urine containing blood and pus cells. If the pain suddenly becomes acute, and if the loin is exquisitely tender and nausea and vomiting appear, the patient has an attack of *renal colic* (Fig. 159).

When stones lodge in the ureter, acute shocking colicky pain is experienced, referred down the thigh and to the genitalia. There is usually a frequent desire to void, but very little urine is passed, and it usually contains blood, because of the abrasive action of the stone as urine is passed. This group of symptoms is called *ureteral colic*. The diagnosis is confirmed by catheterization of the ureters and by x-rays.

Urinary calculi must be removed in order to relieve recurring attacks of pain and because their presence may lead to more serious secondary disease (hydronephrosis, secondary infection). If the stone is in the kidney, the operation performed may be a *nephrotomy* (simple incision into the kidney with removal of the stone), or nephrectomy, if the kidney is functionless due to infection or hydronephrosis. Stones in the kidney pelvis are removed by a *pyelotomy*, in the ureter by *ureterotomy*, and in the bladder by *cystotomy*. Sometimes an instrument is inserted through the urethra into the bladder, and the stone is crushed in the jaws of this instrument. Such an operation is called a *litholapaxy*. (See Fig. 154.)

Treatment and Nursing Care

Active treatment must be instituted for renal and ureteral colic; hot baths, sweats, morphine and atropine to allay spasm must be given, in addition to large amounts of fluid by mouth. No time should be lost by the nurse in carrying out these treatments, because at times the pain suffered by these patients is so excruciating that shock and coma result. A patient will be grateful for any relief. Cystoscopic examination and passage of a small ureteral catheter past the obstructive stone, whether in ureter or renal pelvis, will immediately relieve back pressure upon the kidney and alleviate the intense agony. Whether this is done or not, the nursing care of cases with calculi require constant watchfulness for the spontaneous passage of a stone. A glass urinal should be employed, and all urine should be strained through gauze or a fine strainer. When stones are recovered, the physician will have them analyzed and then will prescribe a suitable diet to prevent further stone formation. Most stones consist of calcium oxalate or phosphate, and in such cases an acid ash diet is given. Clots should be crushed and the sides of the urinal inspected for clinging stones. The lodgment of a stone in the ureter may at times cause complete suppression of urine, a condition termed *calculous anuria*. Unless this condition is relieved, uremia develops, and death rapidly follows. If no urine is excreted within 36 hours, immediate operation is indicated. If the location of the stone is known, it may be searched for and removed; otherwise, the diseased kidney is incised and drained, and the stone is removed at a later operation when the patient is in better condition.

Renal Tumors and Cysts

Malignant tumors of the kidney may arise from embryonal rests of adrenal tissue in the kidney, hypernephroma, or from malignant degeneration of renal tissue. The usual

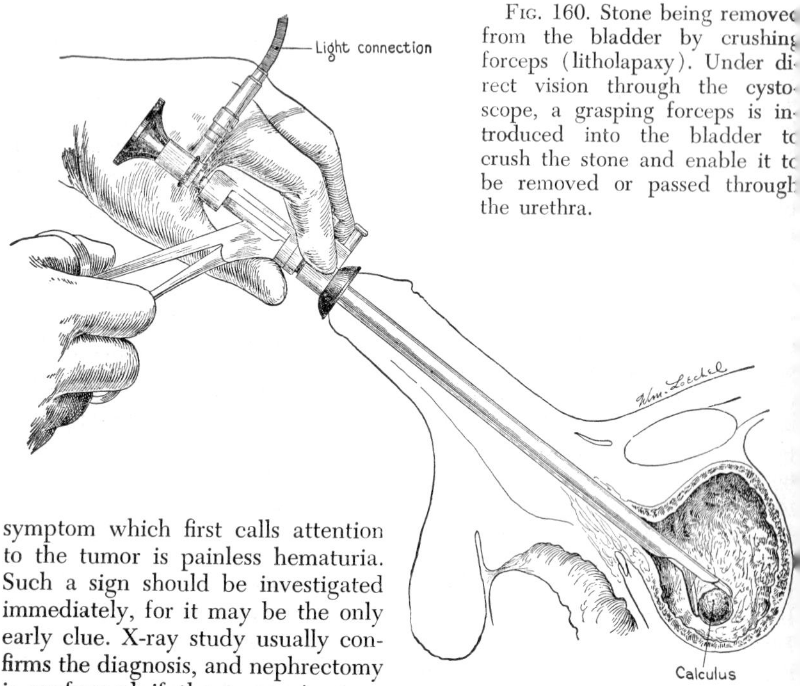

FIG. 160. Stone being removed from the bladder by crushing forceps (litholapaxy). Under direct vision through the cystoscope, a grasping forceps is introduced into the bladder to crush the stone and enable it to be removed or passed through the urethra.

symptom which first calls attention to the tumor is painless hematuria. Such a sign should be investigated immediately, for it may be the only early clue. X-ray study usually confirms the diagnosis, and nephrectomy is performed if the tumor is operable. Often x-ray therapy is used in addition and as a palliative measure in inoperable tumors.

Cysts of the kidney may be multiple, polycystic kidney, or single. Polycystic disease is usually congenital and involves both kidneys; therefore, it is treated only by surgery if infection occurs within the cysts. Solitary cysts often attain large size and are removed; the defect in the kidney is repaired.

Nursing Care Before and After Operation

As outlined above, all operations on the kidney should be attempted only after a period of study and preparation. Fluids should be given in large amounts to promote increased excretion of waste products before the time of operation.

Preoperative Care. The preparation is described on page 58. Usually the incision is made in the loin, and the shaving should extend past the spine posteriorly and beyond the midline anteriorly, above the rib margin and well below the iliac crest. Apprehension should be allayed by gaining the confidence of the patient. Often the loss of a kidney may give the impression to him that he will be an invalid the rest of his life. This is not true in most instances because normal function may be maintained by a single kidney.

Operation. The patient is placed on the operating table with a sand or air pillow under the loin of the unaffected side. The upper extremity corresponding to the side to be operated upon is extended to increase the size of the loin space. The lower extremity is flexed (Fig. 29, p. 90). The kidney is first exposed by an oblique incision, then delivered into the wound, and the appropriate operation is performed.

Postoperative Care. The general nursing care after operation is much the same as that after a laparotomy. It is important for the patient to move to prevent chest and peripheral vascular complications. Adequate fluids should be given by vein, and by mouth when nausea ceases. An accurate "intake and output chart" should be kept. A normal diet may be given to these patients as soon as peristaltic activity is present. This is best indicated by passage of gas. Following such operations as nephrotomy, pyelotomy and ureterotomy, urine may drain from the wound for a time. This should not be mistaken by the nurse for hemorrhage. Often following these operations, drainage tubes have been placed directly in the kidney, the pelvis, or the ureter; these will naturally divert the urine and keep the wound drier. The nurse should watch these tubes carefully after operation to see that there is no blockage, as from blood clot. Often following a nephrostomy, a surgeon will request periodic irrigation of the drainage tube. This is usually about 10 cc. of saline, inasmuch as the area to be irrigated is a small one. The nurse must be cautious in turning the patient on the operated side when a drainage tube is in place. A small pillow placed on either side of the tube will make a trough so that the tubing will not bend on itself. The character of the drainage and the number of cubic centimeters eliminated should be tabulated every 12 to 24 hours. Frequent changing of these dressings is necessary to prevent maceration of the skin and the offensive urinous odor which is embarrassing to the patient and all concerned. The Montgomery strap dressing is conveniently used in this connection. (See Fig. 45.)

Occasionally, clamps are left in the incision following nephrectomy, because it may be impossible to ligate the renal vessels. On examination of the operative site the nurse may see the handles of these instruments extending from the dressings over the wound. In no circumstances should the clamps be dislodged. Obviously, such a patient is not permitted to lie on the operative side. Pillows placed strategically add to the comfort of this patient.

Following a nephropexy, the patient is usually placed in such a position that his chest is lower than his hips to facilitate the adherence of the kidney to its new position.

Drug therapy to combat infection will include the sulfonamides, penicillin and streptomycin. The nurse is expected to be able to recognize the toxic manifestations of these agents and to report such an occurrence to the physician.

When a patient who has had a kidney operation is ready for discharge it is important that he know what his posthospital care should be. If he still has drainage tubes in place which must be irrigated, as is true of a nephrostomy, he or some member of his family should be taught the care of this dressing and treatment. For postoperative nephrectomy, it is imperative that he refrain from lifting heavy objects for the first year.

Complications

Hemorrhage. Following nephrotomy and nephrectomy, the patient should be watched carefully for signs of hemorrhage. When inspecting the dressings, the nurse should remember that the ooze usually collects at the back and not on the anterior dressings. The constitutional signs of hemorrhage—increase in pulse, restlessness and sweating—have been mentioned in Chapter 8. Because of the large vessels ligated, hemorrhages due to slipping of a ligature may be rapidly fatal. Therefore, the nurse should not hesitate to call the surgeon should the slightest suspicion of this complication arise.

Abdominal Distention. This complication occurs not infrequently after operations on the kidney and the ureter, and is thought to be due to a reflex paralysis of intestinal peristalsis. In a weakened patient, the symptom may become very distressing, even causing embarrassment of the heart and respiration.

For relief of the abdominal distention, decompression by the use of a Miller-Abbott or Cantor tube gives rapid relief. The tube may be removed as soon as normal peristalsis and passage of gas are apparent.

Pain. Pain similar to renal colic is often a distressing symptom after operations on the kidney and the ureter. It is due commonly to the passage of clotted blood down the ureter. This symptom is usually of short duration but demands adequate doses of narcotics for its relief.

DISEASES OF BLADDER, PROSTATE AND URETHRA

The bladder is a muscular sac lined with mucous membrane, lying behind the symphysis pubis and covered above by peritoneum. It receives the urine from the ureters and when it is sufficiently distended (the normal bladder capacity is about 500 cc.), sensations of discomfort are experienced. When the sphincters of the bladder are relaxed (voluntarily) urine is discharged via the urethra. This channel is short in the female, not more than 4 cm. (1½ in.) long, so that infection of the bladder by this route is not uncommon. In the male the urethra is much longer, passing through the prostate gland and the penis. (Fig. 166.)

Congenital Malformations. These occur occasionally in this region, resulting in the absence of the anterior wall of the bladder. This condition, known as *exstrophy* of the bladder, is often associated with other congenital defects, hernia and deformities of the urethra and the penis in the male (epispadias). Two methods have been used in the treatment of exstrophy. In one a plastic operation attempts to form a bladder, and in the other the ureters are severed at a point above their entrance into the bladder and are implanted into the rectum or the sigmoid. In either case, an ascending kidney infection often causes death in early life.

Bladder Injuries. Injury to the bladder may occur with a fracture of the symphysis pubis, and occasionally in drunken individuals from kicks or blows in the lower abdomen when the bladder is full. The immediate result is extravasation of urine into the retropubic space or the peritoneum with pain, shock and an inability to void. What urine is obtained either by voiding or catheter contains blood. If a rupture of the bladder is suspected, a measured amount of sterile saline is often introduced per catheter. Inability to recover the fluid injected confirms the diagnosis. Early operative repair of the injured bladder is indicated.

Cystitis. This is an inflammation of the urinary bladder which may be introduced from without or from the kidneys via the urine. A very frequent cause of infection from without is unsterile catheterization. In hospital practice, cystitis occurs more frequently in women, probably due to the short urethra and to the fact that catheterization is performed with an improper technic. The latter factor may be avoided by careful attention to the details of sterility and asepsis.

The cardinal symptoms of cystitis are three in number: pain in the region of the bladder, which may be constant or only during urination; frequency of urination; and changes (pus and often blood) in the composition of the urine.

Treatment. Pain and burning on urination may be alleviated somewhat by making the urine alkaline by the administration of sodium bicarbonate or sodium citrate gr. 20 (1.3 Gm.) 3 or 4 times daily. Urinary antiseptics are often employed. These are usually sulfa drugs (Gantrisin, specifically), streptomycin, Aureomycin, Terramycin and Chloromycetin, depending upon the organism.

These measures, combined with a bland diet and a large amount of fluids, usually suffice to relieve the ordinary case.

In more protracted cases, warm bladder irrigations are employed, using such solutions as potassium permanganate 1:8,000 solution and silver nitrate 1:5,000 solution. The irrigations are best performed with the patient on her back and the fluid injected slowly through a small soft rubber catheter. After 100 cc. have entered the bladder, the flow should be stopped and the fluid allowed to flow out through the catheter. Repeated injections should be made until the fluid returns clear.

When the cystitis is caused by stone in the bladder, or by some obstruction to the urethra, as a hypertrophied prostate or a stricture, frequently an operation is necessary to drain the bladder (cystostomy).

Bladder Tumors

Tumors of the bladder occur commonly in older individuals. They arise as a cauliflowerlike growth in the bladder mucous membrane. Bleeding occurs when the tumor is traumatized by the contraction of the bladder in urination. A tumor is suspected when large amounts of blood are passed in the urine, and the diagnosis is confirmed by direct examination of the bladder wall through the cystoscope.

Treatment. Most tumors are small and are treated by electrocoagulation of the growth through a cystoscope. After irrigation of the bladder, it is distended with water or saline, and the coagulating needle is placed in the growth. Excellent results are reported by this method of treatment. Radical surgery is often indicated. This may consist of a total

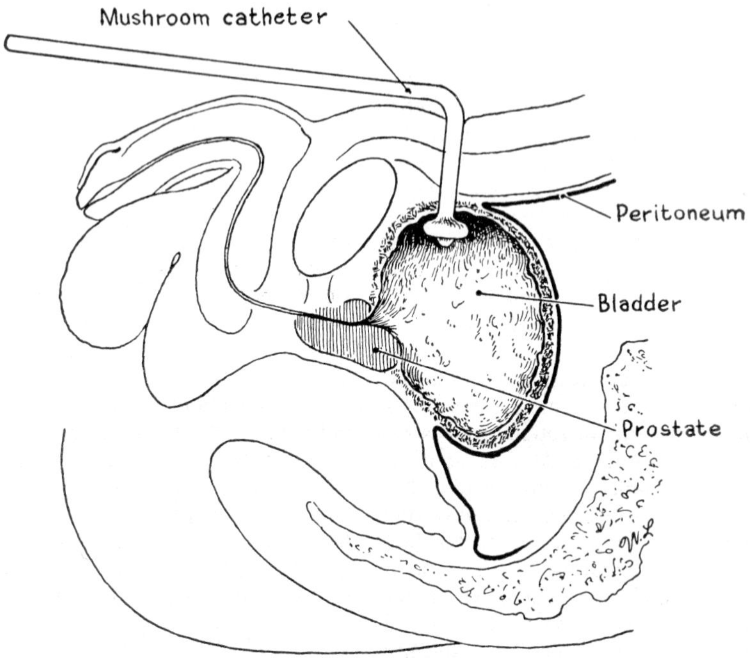

FIG. 161. Cystostomy with angled mushroom catheter in bladder.

cystectomy and implantation of the ureters into the colon. In extensive tumors which are not amenable to coagulation, irradiation therapy gives relief from continuous bleeding, but it is looked upon as only palliative and not as a curative treatment.

Nursing Care

Psychological preparation of the patient with bladder malignancy is important. The usual preoperative regimen is followed, and in addition the patient may be on a liquid diet for about five days preoperatively so that the colon is kept clean. Sulfathalidine, sulfasuxidine or streptomycin may be given to lessen the number of intestinal organisms. The patient should be told that hereafter he will be voiding per rectum.

Postoperatively, a drainage tube may be in place in the rectum. Irrigations of this tube may be ordered at frequent intervals. Force never should be used because of the danger of introducing an infection into the newly implanted ureters. Occasionally, magnesium sulfate solution is used as the irrigation fluid in order to lessen edema. Reassurance and encouragement should be a part of his care, for this is a new experience. When the rectal drain is removed, the patient will begin to learn to control his rectal sphincter. At first, urination will be frequent, and bedding may have to be changed. With patience, greater control will be gained, and he will be able to ask for the bed pan "just in time." An understanding nurse can help this patient greatly.

Cystostomy

An operation whereby the bladder may be drained through an abdominal wound (suprapubic cystostomy) is indicated in the treatment of diseases causing obstruction of the urethra (prostatic hypertrophy, occasionally stricture), for the removal of calculi and tumors from the bladder.

In preparation for the operation the abdomen and upper thighs should be shaved. This is the one abdominal operation in which it is not necessary to have the patient void immediately before operation. The patients are often aged and weakened by disease; hence, the operation is frequently performed under local or spinal anesthesia. The bladder is filled with fluid to carry the peritoneum upward and the patient is placed in the head-lowered position of Trendelenburg. An opening is made into the bladder below the peritoneum, and the appropriate operation is performed within the bladder. A drainage tube is then inserted into the bladder, and the bladder wall is closed round it (Fig. 161).

Nursing Care

The postoperative nursing care has much to do with the success of the operation. Especially in cases of prostatic hypertrophy, the patients are usually aged and rather poor operative risks. Pulse and blood pressure must be checked every half hour for the first two hours and then less frequently if stable. Shock is not an uncommon postoperative complication. Fluids must be given by vein and by mouth until at least 2,500 to 3,000 cc. are taken daily. The diet should be soft at first and increased accordingly. Since old patients are prone to pulmonary complications, the nurse should turn the patient frequently from side to side and urge him to take deep breaths every hour. After 24 hours the head and the shoulders should be elevated. Skin care is an important adjunct to good nursing care in these patients. Frequent washing of the skin with soap and water and the application of petrolatum or zinc oxide ointment will prevent excoriation.

The chief attention of the nurse, of course, should be directed toward keeping the bed and the patient dry. Many ways of accomplishing this purpose are in use. When a tube has been inserted into the bladder, it may be attached to a bottle at the side of the bed and so collect a large part of the urine. After a time, however, the urine tends to leak round the tube. Then suction drainage may be used. A metal cup which fits snugly on the abdominal wall is held over the cystostomy opening. Often it is provided with a central projection, which is placed in the bladder opening. With constant suction, the urine which collects in the bladder is removed and caught in a drainage bottle. This prevents odors and keeps the patient dry but must be inspected frequently by the nurse. In many cases, when this appliance is not available, a very satisfactory dressing may be made from a large square of rubber tissue with a small opening cut in the center (Fig. 162). Liquid adhesive is applied to the abdomen about the cystostomy opening, and the rubber tissue is sealed to the skin. One sterile dressing and two sterile pads of absorbent cotton are placed over the opening, and the rubber is folded over them. The whole dressing is secured by several Montgomery straps. These dressings should be changed every half hour for the first 48 hours, then hourly, and after that p.r.n., depending upon the fluid intake. It is very important to prevent the dressings from becoming saturated.

Complications. Bedsores are not infrequently seen after cystostomy, but usually they can be averted by maintaining a clean, dry bed and by attention to the skin over the sacrum. Pulmonary complications, bronchopneumonia and hypostatic congestion may become manifest after several days in bed in one position. In their prophylaxis, deep respiration and frequent change of position should be remembered. As soon as it is advisable these patients are allowed to get out of bed and to walk about.

Convalescence. A cystostomy may be temporary or permanent, depending upon the original purpose of the operation. The patient is often sensitive about his "bottle and tube" which he carries with him. If he is with other similar patients, the inconvenience and the awkwardness do not seem so great. However, if he is by himself or on a floor where he is the only one with such a device, diversional activity should be sought which will meet his particular interests.

Odors will not be a problem if drainage tubing and the bottle are changed daily. They must be cleaned thoroughly with soap and water.

For the patient who is going home with a cystostomy, the use of a rubber urinal is effective. This is an oval-shaped rubber bladder. To one end of the bag a rubber tubing is attached which can be connected to the drainage tube in the patient. The other end has a screw cap. The bag can be strapped to the inner aspect of the thigh or calf in male patients or to the thigh in female patients. When it fills, it is quite easy to empty into the toilet by unscrewing the cap. The patient should be instructed regarding adequate cleaning of the bag with soap and water to prevent odors. At night, he may use the drainage bottle at the side of the bed as the collecting unit; during this time, the rubber bag can be exposed to fresh air.

MALE GENITO-UROLOGY

In the male, several organs serve both as parts of the urinary tract and of the reproductive system. Disease of these organs may produce functional abnormalities of either or both systems. For this reason diseases of the entire reproductive system in the male usually are treated by the urologist.

Prostate Gland

The prostate is a pyramidal-shaped walnut-sized gland situated just below the bladder in the male. It is pierced by the urethra, and from it arises a mucous secretion which enters the urethra with the secretion from the seminal vesicles. Infection

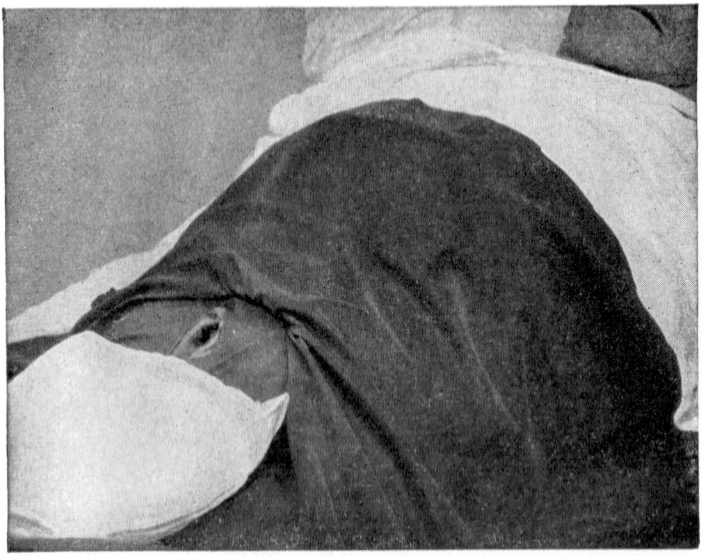

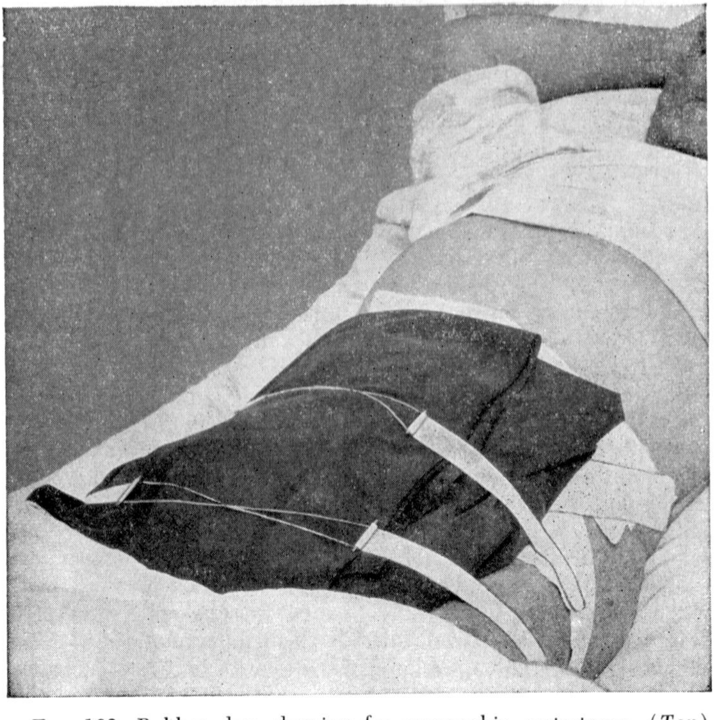

FIG. 162. Rubber dam dressing for suprapubic cystostomy. (*Top*) Rubber dam applied to the abdomen about the opening into the bladder. (*Bottom*) Dam folded over a pad and held with tapes.

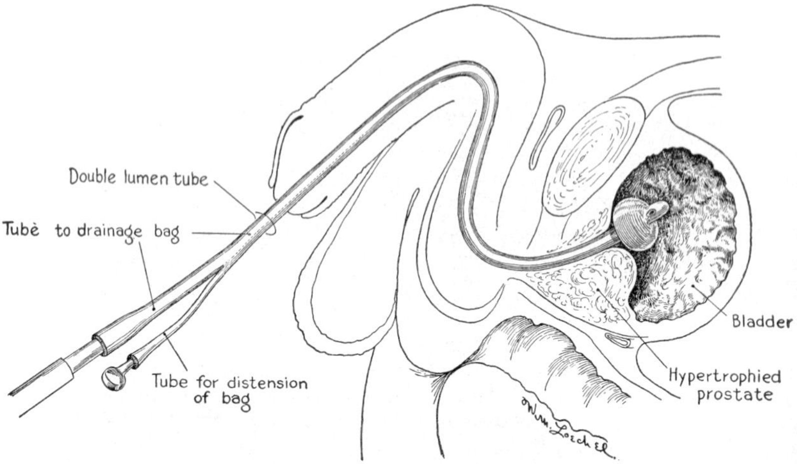

FIG. 163. Diagrammatic drawing to show Foley catheter in place. This is a two-way catheter: One part leads to the drainage bottle; the other part, shown plugged with a peg, is used to inflate the rubber balloon at the end of the catheter. After a known amount of air or water is injected into the balloon, the tube is plugged with a peg or folded upon itself and held with a rubber band in order to prevent the escape of the medium from distending the bag. Only when the catheter is withdrawn is this tube opened.

extending from the urethra often produces acute and chronic inflammations in the gland.

Benign Prostatic Hypertrophy. In patients past 50 years of age, the gland often enlarges, extending upward into the bladder and producing obstruction to the outflow of urine by encroaching upon the vesical orifice. This condition is known as enlargement of the prostate, or prostatic hypertrophy. Since this produces an obstruction to the flow of urine, a gradual dilation of the ureters (hydro-ureter) and kidneys (hydronephrosis) results. The hypertrophied lobe extends upward into the bladder and forms a pouch which retains urine. This pouch is not emptied when voiding takes place, and the remaining urine (called residual urine) decomposes and may produce calculi or a cystitis. Considerable difficulty and frequency in urination develop gradually and finally the patient is unable to void at all.

Carcinoma of the Prostate

Cancer of the prostate occurs in patients in the older age group. The symptoms may or may not be marked. If neoplasm is large enough to encroach on the bladder neck or cause obstruction of urine, then the patient has the same signs as noted in benign prostatic hypertrophy. However, many prostatic carcinomas are extremely malignant with few local symptoms and yet are widely disseminated. Metastases occur in bone, brain and lungs. On rectal examination, the prostate usually is found to be "stony hard" and fixed. Symptoms due to metastases are backache, loss of weight, loss of appetite, and anemia. These can be alleviated and improved by castration and estrogen administration or by both.

Treatment. If a patient is admitted as an emergency because he is unable to void, the physician immediately tries to catheterize him. If this is unsuccessful, suprapubic cystostomy is performed (Fig. 161). This relieves the urinary obstruction. Treatment depends on the extent of disease. If the cancer has not invaded the capsule, then total radical prostatectomy by perineal method is the procedure of choice. If metastases are present or the process has invaded beyond the capsule and the patient is having symptoms of urinary obstruction, then transurethral resection to allow an adequate channel for the passage of urine is indicated.

Preoperative Nursing Care

Estimation of kidney function, the administration of fluids in large quantities, and constant drainage of the bladder by an inlying catheter are important parts of this regimen. During this time, the nurse is able to help her elderly patient adjust to his environment. By conversation and observation, she will note his idiosyncrasies, physical incapacities and mental attitude. The nurse should attempt to make his adjustment to surgery and its implications as smooth as possible. Any complications such as cardiac and pulmonary must be investigated before the patient has surgery. If the urinary obstruction has been nearly complete for a considerable period, a marked distention of the bladder occurs.

The Foley catheter is preferred when an indwelling catheter is desired. This catheter has an inflatable rubber bag near its tip. After it is inserted into the bladder, the bag is inflated with water or air. The inflated bag is too large to pass through the vesical orifice, and the catheter will remain in the bladder without other fixation until the rubber bag is deflated. The nurse will note that one outlet of the catheter leads to the bag. Before these catheters are sterilized for use, she must check the bags to see that they do not leak. The bag is inflated to the desired amount (usually 5 cc.) by the physician after he inserts the catheter. A clamp, a cork or a rubber band is used to keep the fluid from running out of the bag. This never should be removed by the nurse.

The Foley catheter may be "2-way" or "3-way" (Fig. 163). The "2-way" catheter allows for drainage from one channel. The other outlet is for the purpose of inflating the bag. The "3-way" catheter allows saline to flow into the bladder by one route and to return to the drainage bottle by the other channel. The larger of these two pathways is for drainage. The third opening is to permit water or air to inflate the bag near the tip of the catheter. The "3-way" Foley catheter can allow for constant bladder irrigation. The flow of saline is regulated so that the number of drops per minute can be seen in the glass Murphy drip. Usually from 30 to 60 drops are sufficient per minute.

Catheterization is often a difficult operation in these cases. The ordinary rubber catheter frequently will

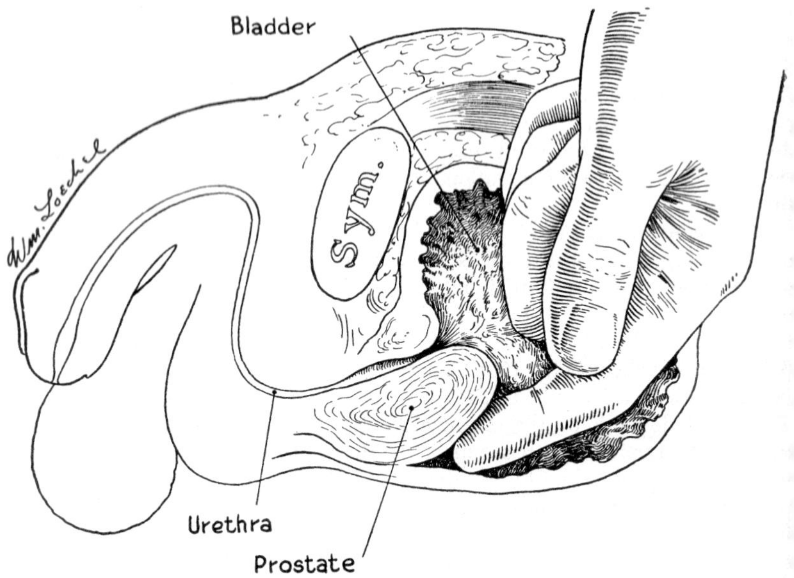

FIG. 164. Diagrammatic drawing to show how the prostate is shelled out of its bed with the finger in suprapubic prostatectomy.

be too soft and pliable to pass through the urethra into the bladder. A thin wire, called a stylet, can then be introduced into the catheter which will prevent the catheter from collapsing when the resistance is met. The surgeon often employs a catheter of woven silk coated with wax whose end is upturned to form a slight angle (called a coudé-woven catheter).*

In obstinate cases metal catheters must be employed. These have a curve more marked than the ordinary, called the prostatic curve. Often a suprapubic cystostomy is necessary to give adequate drainage.

In addition to any one of the three temporary measures (suprapubic cystostomy, indwelling cath-

* The sterilization of the woven catheters is best performed by wrapping them separately in gauze and boiling them in a catheter tray. In removing them from the sterilizer the catheters are often damaged. Being waxed, the heat will soften them, and picking them up by forceps will break off large pieces of the coating, making them useless. Therefore, they should be allowed to cool in the air without removing them from the catheter tray. When cooled they may be picked up without damage, because the wax is hardened. Other surgeons prefer to have woven catheters sterilized by immersing them in a solution of 5 per cent formalin for 20 minutes. If this method is used, the nurse should have at hand a flask of sterile cold water for rinsing them before their insertion into the urethra.

eter, or repeated catheterization) to make the patient comfortable prior to major surgery, he is encouraged to eat a high-caloric diet. Eggnogs can be given between meals. Attention must be given to his own personal preferences and habits if he is to accept surgery favorably.

Prostatectomy

When the tests of the kidney show that the function has returned more nearly to the normal, the patient is considered ready for operation. The gland may be removed through an abdominal wound, a *suprapubic prostatectomy*. An opening is made into the bladder, and the gland is removed from above (Fig. 164). The gland may also be removed through an incision in the perineum—*perineal prostatectomy*. Instruments have been devised with an ocular and operating system which can be introduced through the urethra to the prostate. Under vision, small pieces of obstructing gland tissue can be removed with an electrical wire. This is called *transurethral resection* of the prostate (Fig. 165). A fourth technic is to make a low abdominal incision and approach the prostate gland between the pubic arch and the bladder (without entering the bladder). This is called *retropubic prostatectomy*.

There are advantages and disad-

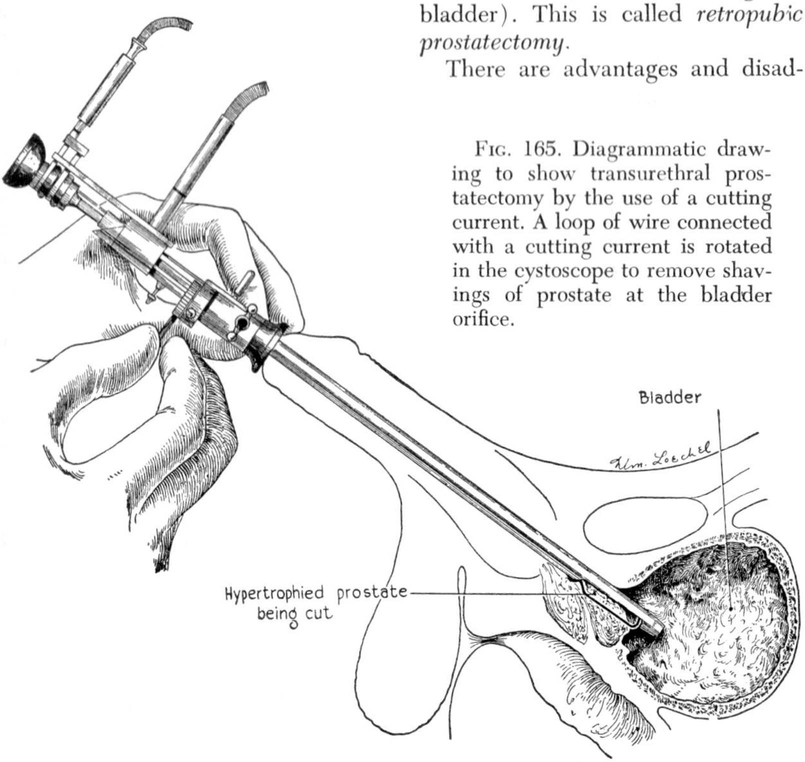

Fig. 165. Diagrammatic drawing to show transurethral prostatectomy by the use of a cutting current. A loop of wire connected with a cutting current is rotated in the cystoscope to remove shavings of prostate at the bladder orifice.

vantages to most of these methods. The suprapubic prostatectomy requires an abdominal incision. It is the easiest to perform; however, it carries with it all the hazards of abdominal surgery, primarily shock. Perineal prostatectomy requires skill on the part of the surgeon so that the rectum and other organs are not injured. This area is very vascular, and hemorrhage is often likely. Postoperatively, the wound is contaminated easily by virtue of the position of the incision. Transurethral resection also must be performed by a skilled operator. Hemorrhage is a common complication. The real advantage of this method, however, is that there is no incision. The retropubic approach is less traumatic than the suprapubic prostatectomy; however, occasionally, there are evidences of prolonged drainage, pelvic cellulitis or osteitis pubis.

Postoperative Nursing Care

As soon as the patient returns from the operating room, the nurse should check his pulse and blood pressure, because the immediate dangers following prostatectomy are shock and hemorrhage.

Hemorrhage may occur from the bed of the prostate so that before completion of the operation many surgeons pack the cavity or produce pressure on the walls by distending a small rubber bag attached to a tube which leads out through the urethra. The packing or bag is removed later through the suprapubic wound. In spite of these precautions, the nurse must watch the patient carefully for signs of hemorrhage.

An intake and output chart is also very important in these cases. Any complaints of pain can usually be relieved by a sedative. Frequent changing of position is comforting and will prevent pulmonary complications.

Following perineal prostatectomy, the surgeon will change the dressing the first day postoperatively; often after that it may become a nurse's dressing. Aseptic technic must be practiced in changing such a dressing, for the possibilities of infection are great. Dressings can be held in place by a double-tailed T-binder. The tails can cross over the incision which will give double thickness, then each tail is drawn up on either side of the scrotum to the waist line and fastened. Rectal temperature should not be taken, and a rectal tube should be used only on specific order by the physician. Any signs of oozing, infection, tenderness or pain should be reported. The nurse must be tactful and professional in working with male patients to avoid embarrassment for each.

As the days pass and drainage tubes are removed, the patient often shows signs of discouragement and depression because he is not able to gain control of his bladder immediately. It is important for him to know that it is a gradual process and that even though he may be discharged with "dribbling" it should gradually diminish. His wife or some other responsible member of the family should be told of his condition. It is well for them to realize that he should be made to do as much for himself as possible. He needs mental stimulus to prevent boredom, despondency and physical lassitude.

When a cystostomy has been performed the nursing care discussed on page 379 should be carefully given.

Management of Neurogenic Bladder

Under this heading we are concerned primarily with the acute urinary retention secondary to the paralysis of the bladder in cases of spinal-cord injury and disease. These patients die, not from the cord injury but from infection introduced into the bladder by catheterization, finally reaching the kidney, causing death by sepsis. These injuries to the cord usually result in retention, then incontinence of overflow (dribbling), and finally "automatic" micturition. This is best obviated by adhering to the following regulations:

Do not catheterize but rather manually express the urine by massaging the bladder every few hours. The massage should be from above downward toward the symphysis with the patient lying on his side. The patient should be instructed to try to urinate during this time. This manual treatment is contraindicated only if the urine becomes infected (cystitis). Daily specimens should be collected and examined. Should the above not suffice, a suprapubic cystostomy is the best recourse. Munro's apparatus for tidal drainage has also been used in the treatment of neurogenic bladder. (See p. 521.)

Urethral Strictures

Strictures result from inflammation or trauma of the urethra. They produce symptoms of obstruction and retention of urine. One of the most common causes of inflammation is that produced by the gonococcus organism. It is important for the nurse to know if the disease is in its infectious stage, and if so, to take the necessary precautions.

Treatment. The treatment may be palliative (gradual dilatation of the narrowed area with metal sounds), or operative (incision of the stricture—urethrotomy). If the stricture has become so small as to prevent the passage of a catheter, several small filiform whalebone bougies are used in search of the opening. When one bougie passes beyond the stricture into the bladder, it is fixed in place, and urine will drain from the bladder beside it. The stricture can then be dilated to larger size by the passage of a larger sound (Gouley follower) over the filiform as a guide. Sometimes a suprapubic cystostomy must be performed. The postoperative treatment of these cases is similar to that described for cystostomy, page 379.

ANATOMY AND PHYSIOLOGY OF THE MALE REPRODUCTIVE SYSTEM

The structures included in the male reproductive system are the testes, the vas deferens and the seminal vesicles, the penis, and certain accessory glands, such as the prostate gland and Cowper's gland. The testes are formed in embryonal life within the abdominal cavity near the kidney. During the last month of fetal life, they descend posterior to the peritoneum, to pierce the abdominal wall in the groin and to progress along the inguinal canal into the scrotum. In this descent, they are accompanied by blood vessels, lymphatics, nerves and ducts, which, along with supporting and investing tissue, make up the spermatic cord. This cord extends from the internal

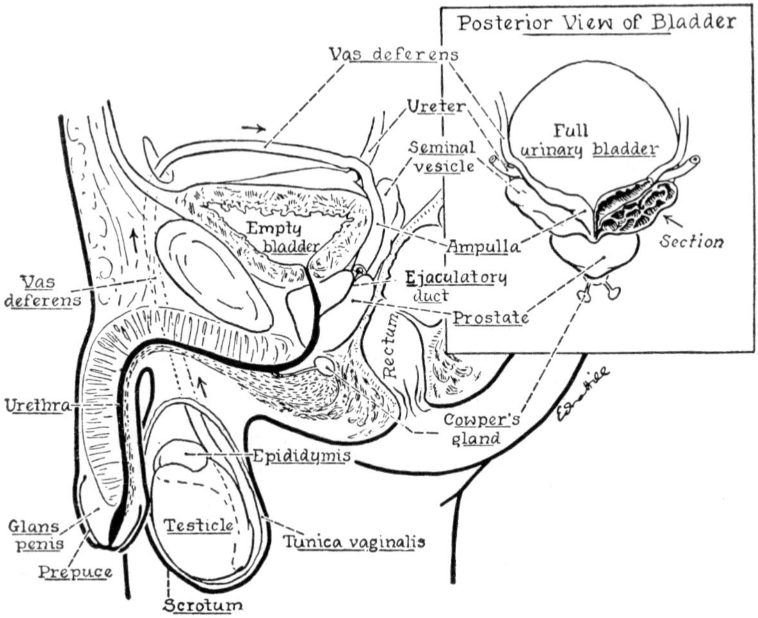

FIG. 166. Semidiagrammatic drawing showing anatomy of male reproductive system.

inguinal ring through the abdominal wall and the inguinal canal to the scrotum. As the testes descend into the scrotum, a tubular process of peritoneum accompanies them. This normally is obliterated, the only remaining portion being that which covers the testes, the tunica vaginalis. (When this peritoneal process does not obliterate but remains open into the abdominal cavity, a potential sac remains into which abdominal contents may enter to form an indirect inguinal hernia.)

The testes proper consist of numerous seminiferous tubules in which are formed the male reproductive elements, the spermatozoa. These are transmitted by a system of collecting tubules into the epididymis, which is a hoodlike structure lying on the testes and containing tortuous ducts that lead into the vas deferens. This firm tubular structure passes upward through the inguinal canal to enter the abdominal cavity behind the peritoneum, thence extending downward toward the base of the bladder. An outpouching from this structure is the seminal vesicle, which acts as a reservoir for the secretion of the testes. The tract is continued as the ejaculatory duct, which then passes through the prostate gland to enter the urethra. The secretion of the testes is carried by this pathway to the end of the penis in reproduction.

The testes have a dual function. The primary function is reproduction, the formation of spermatozoa from the germinal cells of the seminiferous tubules. The testes, however, are also important glands of internal secretion. This secretion is produced by the so-called interstitial cells and is called male sex hormone. It has to do with the preservation of the male sex qualities.

The prostate gland lies just below the neck of the bladder. It surrounds the urethra posteriorly and laterally and is traversed by the ejaculatory duct, the continuation of the vas deferens. This gland produces a secretion which is chemically and physiologically suitable to the needs of the spermatozoa in their passage from the genital glands.

The penis has a dual function of being the organ of copulation and of urination. Anatomically it consists of a glans penis, a body and root. The glans penis is a soft rounded portion at the end which retains its soft structure even when erect. The urethra opens at the extremity of the glans. The glans is normally covered or protected by an elongation of skin of the penis known as the foreskin, which may be reflected to expose the glans. The body of the penis is composed of erectile tissues, numerous vessels which may become distended during sexual excitement. Through it passes the urethra, which extends from the bladder through the prostate to the end of the penis.

Congenital Malformations

Many disturbances of normal growth may occur in the formation of the genital organs of the male. The most common is a failure of the testes to descend into the scrotum. This condition is called *cryptorchism*. The testes may remain within the abdomen, may pass through the abdominal wall but be arrested in the inguinal canal, or may pass through the external abdominal ring but not descend into the scrotum. In almost all cases of undescended testicle, there is a potential if not a concomitant indirect inguinal hernia. In addition, the testicle not in the normal position may atrophy, and there is a considerable tendency for such an organ to undergo malignant degeneration. In many boys, the testicle may descend spontaneously shortly after puberty and, in other instances, the descent may be brought about by hormonal therapy. In cases in which the testicle does not descend normally, often an operation is performed to place it in the scrotum.

Failure of the urethra to form normally in the penis is known as *hypospadias* when the urethral opening is on the lower wall of the penis; when it is a groove on its upper surface the condition is called *epispadias*. These anatomic abnormalities may be repaired by various types of plastic operations. Unfortunately, all too frequently two or more attempts at repair are necessary with only indifferent ultimate results.

DISEASES OF EXTERNAL GENITALIA

Gonorrhea

This disease occurs as a result of an infection with the gonococcus, which penetrates the tissues of the urethra as a result of sexual exposure. The time elapsing from the moment of infection until the development of disease may be from two to seven days, sometimes longer. The infection produces a marked purulent, usually painful, urethral discharge. At first the anterior portion of the urethra is invaded, but not infrequently the infection extends posteriorly to involve the prostate and to extend along the vas deferens to produce infection in the seminal vesicles and in the epididymis. A systemic infection may occur to produce a disabling arthritis. The disease is diagnosed by the examination of a stained smear of the pus from the urethra. The gonococcus appears as a bean-shaped organism in pairs lying within the pus cells and staining in a characteristic manner (see p. 634).

Early treatment of the infection is most likely to prevent development of the complications of gonorrhea. It must not be forgotten that the transmission of the infection from the urethra to the eyes may produce a very marked ophthalmia (see p. 449). Penicillin prophylaxis and therapy have given excellent results.

Penile Ulceration

Ulcerations occurring on the penis may be of several types, but because of the danger of chancre (syphilis), all lesions are considered syphilitic until proved otherwise. The method by which diagnosis is made is by a combination of history of the disease, a microscopic examination of a darkfield specimen removed from the lesion, and a Wassermann examination. The treatment of penile ulceration varies greatly, depending upon the cause of the ulceration. It is not started until the diagnosis is made.

A chancre is a firm ulceration which is the primary lesion of syphilis (see p. 636). It occurs as a result of sexual exposure; the method of diagnosis has been described. Local treatment is usually unnecessary other than a mild antiseptic and a protective dressing, the main portion of the treatment being confined to systemic measures which usually result in a rapid healing of the local lesion. Penicillin produces a rapid cure.

The chancroid is an ulceration produced by a mixed infection, usually associated with marked lymphadenopathy in the groin. Treatment often necessitates circumcision and cauterization of the ulceration.

Balanitis

Balanitis is an ulceration produced by a spirochete and a fusiform bacillus commonly found in the oral cavities. These organisms are largely anaerobic; therefore, the infection always occurs under the foreskin. Circumcision, cauterizing or oxidizing antiseptics are frequently used in the therapy.

Herpes

Herpes of the glans penis begins as a small blister which produces secondary ulceration. This is not a venereal disease, and the ulcerations heal rapidly under protective dressing or with a mild antiseptic treatment.

Phimosis

Phimosis is a condition in which the foreskin is narrowed so that it cannot be retracted over the glans. It may be corrected by circumcision. The operation consists in the removal of the foreskin so that the glans penis is not covered. It is frequently performed in infancy and in adults as a hygienic or therapeutic measure.

Carcinoma of Penis

Carcinoma of the penis occurs in the skin of the penis and rarely, if ever, occurs in circumcised individuals. It represents about 3 per cent of all skin cancer. Local treatment or complete amputation of the penis may be necessary.

DISEASES OF TESTES AND ADJACENT STRUCTURES

Epididymitis

Infection of the epididymis is produced most often as a complication of gonorrhea. The infection passes upward through the urethra and the ejaculatory duct, thence along the vas deferens to the epididymis. The infection may occur at any time during the course of the disease, but most often in its early stages. The patient complains of pain and soreness in the inguinal canal along the course of the vas deferens and then develops pain and swelling in the scrotum and the groin. The epididymis becomes swollen and extremely painful; the temperature is elevated.

Treatment. The treatment of the disease is the treatment of the gonorrheal infection (p. 635). In addition, the patient should be put to bed and the scrotum elevated. Only on rare occasions is surgery necessary.

Orchitis

An inflammation of the testes may occur as a result of some systemic infection, such as pneumonia, influenza, smallpox, typhoid, syphilis, tuberculosis. In addition, torsion of the spermatic cord or severe trauma may be factors in the production of an orchitis. The symptoms are characteristic. The testicle becomes swollen, tense and painful, often accompanied by a high temperature, nausea and other systemic symptoms. The marked swelling inside the dense capsule of the testes may be sufficient to shut off the blood supply to the organ so that gangrene of the testes is not infrequent. The sudden cessation of pain is a symptom of this complication.

Treatment. Rest, elevation and the application of hot or cold compresses are the usual local measures. The general systemic infection causing the local lesion should be cared for. If suppuration occurs, incision and drainage are often necessary.

Tumors of Testicle

Tumors of the testicle usually occur in the adult during the years of greatest sexual activity. They are almost always malignant and most frequently arise as the result of congenital abnormalities in the testis itself. The tumors tend to metastasize early to distant areas. The symptoms appear very gradually, a gradual swelling of the testicle followed by backache, pain in the abdomen, loss of weight, and general weakness. The metastatic growth may be more marked than the local testicular one. The enlargement of the testicle without pain is a significant diagnostic finding.

Treatment. Irradiation followed by removal of the testicle, orchiectomy and further irradiation is the accepted method of therapy.

Hydrocele

Hydrocele is a collection of fluid in the tunica vaginalis. It may be acute or chronic. The acute type occurs in association with acute infectious diseases of the epididymis or as a result of local trauma or of a systemic infectious disease, such as mumps, diphtheria, typhoid. This type of hydrocele usually disappears spontaneously with the improvement in the causative disease, and no local treatment is necessary. Chronic hydrocele is that which occurs as a result of a low-grade infection of the testes or the epididymis. It may occur also without any evident infection of these structures. The tunica vaginalis becomes widely distended with fluid, and this lesion is differentiated from a hernia by the fact that it transmits light when transilluminated.

Treatment. Treatment of the chronic type of hydrocele is sought because of the inconvenience of the large scrotal mass. Palliative therapy may consist of simple aspiration of the fluid; this usually results in a reaccumulation of the fluid so that frequent tappings are necessary. Some patients with hydrocele may be treated by aspiration of the fluid and injection of some irritating or sclerosing fluid. This irritating solution sets up an inflammation in the wall of the hydrocele which results in its contraction and eventual obliteration.

In the surgical treatment of hydrocele, an incision is made through the wall of the scrotum down to the distended tunica vaginalis. The sac is opened and excised or everted around the testicle. In the postoperative care of these patients, a suspensory bandage is usually worn for a period of time. Such a support usually is made commercially and obtainable in the pharmacy. However, gauze, muslin or adhesive suspensories can be made.

Varicocele

Varicocele is a dilatation, elongation and tortuosity of the veins of the spermatic cord. This occurs most frequently in the veins on the left side in young adults. Very few if any subjective symptoms may be produced by the enlargement of the spermatic vein, and as a rule no treatment is required. When pain, tenderness and discomfort in the inguinal region are symptoms, therapy may be instituted. This usually consists in excision of the enlarged veins. In the postoperative care of these patients, a suspensory bandage is worn for a time.

REFERENCES AND SUGGESTED READING

Unit Five: Nursing in Conditions of the Urinary Tract—Male Urology

General

(See also those for Unit One, p. 205.)

Cawker, A.: Nursing care of urologic patients, Canad. Nurse **43**:514-522, 1947.

Daut, R. V.: Urological conditions in women, Am. J. Nursing **50**:479 482, 1950.

Emerson, C. P., and Bragdon, J. S.: Essentials of Medicine, ed. 17, pp. 397-438, Philadelphia, Lippincott, 1955.
Lowsley, O. S., and Kirwin, T. J.: Urology for Nurses, ed. 2, Philadelphia, Lippincott, 1948.
Newton, Kathleen: Urologic nursing, Am. J. Nursing **50**:167-170, 1950.

KIDNEY AND URETER

Emerson, C. P., and Bragdon, J. S.: Essentials of Medicine, ed. 17, pp. 411-432; pp. 413-424 (nephrosis and nephritis); pp. 806-807 (tuberculosis), Philadelphia, Lippincott, 1955.
MacLean, J. T.: The use of the artificial kidney, Canad. Nurse **45**:95-99, 1949.
Schweishimer, Waldemar: Kidney stones, Trained Nurse & Hosp. Rev. **120**:40-43, 1948.

BLADDER AND PROSTATE

Buchtel, H. A., and Pace, J. R.: Transurethral prostatic resection—nursing care, Am. J. Nursing **42**: 1136-1141, 1942.
Cordonnier, J. J.: Ureterosigmoid anastomosis, Surg., Gynec. & Obst. **88**:441-446, 1949.
Emerson, C. P., and Bragdon, J. S.: Essentials of Medicine, ed. 17, pp. 433-435 (bladder); p. 435 (urethra), Philadelphia, Lippincott, 1955.
Hayes, B. A., and Millsap, J. G.: Retropubic prostatectomy and nursing care, Am. J. Nursing **50**: 435-438, 1950.
Kuehn, C. A., and Simon, M.: The colon as an artificial bladder, Am. J. Nursing **53**:688-691, 1953.
Seidel, E. S.: Tidal drainage, its present status, Am. J. Nursing **50**: 702-705, 1950.
Van Schoick, M. R., and Higgins, Charles: Carcinoma of the prostate, Am. J. Nursing **48**:427-429, 1948.
Wilhelm, O. J.: Exstrophy of the bladder, J. Urol. **59**:1108-1120, 1948.

MALE REPRODUCTIVE SYSTEM

Emerson, C. P., and Bragdon, J. S.: Essentials of Medicine, ed. 17, pp. 719-725; pp. 681-682; pp. 781-782 and pp. 844-850, Philadelphia, Lippincott, 1955.
Rosenthal, Theodore: The modern treatment of venereal disease, Am. J. Nursing **49**:93-94, 1949.
Wright, L., and Prince, C. L.: Hypospadias, Am. J. Nursing **46**:686-689, 1946.

CLINICAL SITUATIONS

NEPHRECTOMY

Katie Matz noticed that a pain in her left loin was becoming worse but attributed her difficulty to the fact that, as a clerk, she was on her feet a great deal. One day the pain became very acute. She was nauseated and vomited. After a series of tests, it was determined that her difficulties were caused by hydronephrosis and renal calculi; a nephrectomy was performed.

1. During an acute attack of renal colic, the physician prescribed morphine sulfate 0.03 Gm. This was given to

——(1) constrict renal blood vessels
——(2) relieve spasm
——(3) dilate kidney cortex
——(4) lower the blood pressure

2. All urine passed by Miss Matz was collected in a glass urinal and strained. This was in order to

_____(1) detect and save for analysis any malignant tissue
_____(2) detect and save for analysis any calculi
_____(3) prevent the spread of infection
_____(4) ensure an accurate intake and output record

3. Miss Matz was concerned about losing a kidney for fear she would be an invalid. The nurse can reassurer her by saying
_____(1) "By restricting your fluid intake to half the usual amount, you will have adequate kidney function."
_____(2) "The remaining kidney is normal and can assume the work of two."
_____(3) "Allowing your mind to accept the fact that you will be an invalid is three quarters of the battle."
_____(4) "Perhaps at a later time you will have a kidney transplant. This is a new operation which can be done."

4. A serious postoperative problem for which the nurse must be alert is evidence of
_____(1) clear fluid drainage, suggesting urine leakage
_____(2) hemorrhage, usually indicated by bloody drainage under the back
_____(3) postural changes indicating overprotection of operated side

Suprapubic Prostatectomy

Mr. Flanders, a bank teller nearing the retirement age, had been uncomfortable because of frequency of urination. He put off seeing his physician until one day he was unable to void. After 12 hours, he became acutely uncomfortable and visited his physician. The physician attempted catheterization but was unsuccessful and admitted Mr. Flanders to the hospital, where a suprapubic cystostomy was performed.

1. For a cystostomy, the skin area to be shaved is
_____(1) the entire abdomen and the upper pubic area
_____(2) the complete perineal area
_____(3) the abdomen and the perineum
_____(4) none; adequate cleaning of the genitalia is sufficient

2. Following a suprapubic cystostomy, fluids are
_____(1) encouraged
_____(2) restricted
_____(3) limited
_____(4) taken in normal amounts

3. The reason for the response to Question 2 is that this procedure
_____(1) reduces nonprotein nitrogen
_____(2) decreases bladder drainage
_____(3) decreases danger of ascites

4. When a suprapubic drainage tube is removed from the bladder, the usual procedure is to
_____(1) suture the skin and the bladder under local anesthesia
_____(2) insert a smaller tube
_____(3) place a dressing over wound
_____(4) insert a gauze pack and cover with petrolatum gauze

5. This procedure is selected because

_____(1) it is important to facilitate prompt, rapid healing
_____(2) it is important to permit gradual healing
_____(3) the bladder edges will approximate without interference

6. The surgeon eventually performed a suprapubic prostatectomy. The most common complication following this operation is
_____(1) shock
_____(2) distention
_____(3) incontinence
_____(4) paralytic ileus

7. A satisfactory method of controlling odors from urine drainage is to
_____(1) leave bottle uncapped so that air can circulate through the receptacle
_____(2) deposit a chlorophyll tablet in the bottle once every 24 hours
_____(3) use a 2-holed stopper for the bottle—one hole to serve as an air vent, the the other for the drainage tube

8. When Mr. Flanders prepared to go home following his suprapubic prostatectomy, he complained to the nurse of some "dribbling." In reply, the nurse should say
_____(1) "I shall tell the surgeon about it and have him talk to you before you leave."
_____(2) "You may think you have 'dribbling' but you do not. This is a natural feeling which will become less as time goes on."
_____(3) "This is a common symptom. By wearing pads or a rubber urinal, you will be more comfortable. In a week or two, this difficulty should disappear."

UNIT SIX

Nursing in Conditions of the Integumentary System (Including the Subcutaneous and the Areolar Tissue and the Breasts)

CHAPTER NINETEEN

Surgery of the Skin

GENERAL CONSIDERATIONS

The skin, or its appendages, covers and protects our entire body and has many functions. It conserves body heat and helps to cool us by sweat evaporation; it protects against invasion by organisms, and a break in its continuity may be the portal of entry for pathogenic bacteria. It has great healing properties and can be transplanted from one part of the body to another. The skin is the natural habitat of many organisms; therefore, it is necessary to use antiseptics in its preparation for surgery.

STAPHYLOCOCCIC INFECTIONS

Furuncles (Boils)

The staphylococcus is a common inhabitant of the skin surface and of the circulating air. Frequently it causes surface infections by invading a hair follicle or the duct of a gland. The infection may be a very slight one, characterized by a small, red, raised, painful "pimple" that may subside very rapidly with the drainage of a tiny drop of pus. Frequently, however, the infection may progress and involve the skin and the subcutaneous fatty tissue in a tense, raised, reddened mound. The hardened area of induration is the body's effort to localize the infection. The bacteria produce a necrosis of the invaded tissues, and in a few days the characteristic pointing appears and the boil is said by the laity to "come to a head."

Treatment and Nursing Care

If treated conservatively, the body

may control the infection by eventual evacuation of the central necrotic core and of the pus contained in this necrotic center. Hot moist applications will hasten this process. These may be applied in the form of hot compresses or poultices. In the conservative treatment of staphylococcic infections it is important not to rupture or destroy the protective wall of induration that has localized the infection. Therefore, the boil or pimple should never be squeezed, and it is well, when possible, to apply a splint to immobilize the part and thus protect the wall from being destroyed by movement. This procedure relieves the pain, as movement of the part produces tension on the infected area.

In staphylococcic infections, penicillin is most effective, but in some cases the organisms may develop a resistance to penicillin, in which case other antibiotics may be used. It is important that the sensitivity of the organism be tested against commonly used antibiotics. The antibiotic is chosen to which the organism is most susceptible. Those which can be employed other than penicillin are chlortetracycline, Terramycin and neomycin.

Sometimes the pain is so intense that it is wise not to wait for localization and spontaneous evacuation

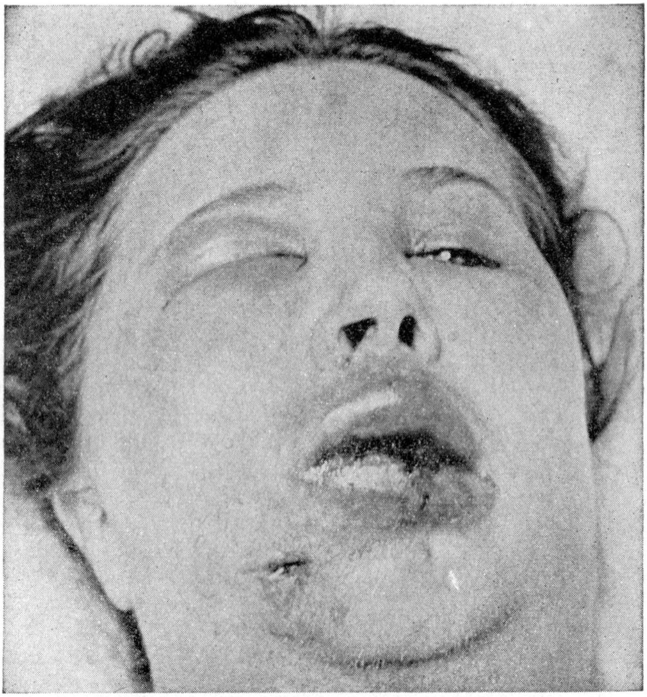

Fig. 167. Carbuncle of upper lip with marked edema of eyelids.

of the necrotic material. In such cases a crucial incision may be made through the area of infection to permit relief of tension and more direct evacuation of the pus and slough.

CARBUNCLES

A carbuncle is a staphylococcic infection similar to a boil, except that the infection spreads widely in the subcutaneous fatty tissues, producing numerous sites of pointing and, therefore, a much more extensive area of acute inflammation. Carbuncles appear most commonly in areas in which the skin is thick and the subcutaneous tissues are more fibrous; therefore, they are seen most frequently on the back of the neck and less frequently on the back and other parts of the body. They are more apt to occur in older and debilitated people, and they are especially frequent in diabetics. So frequent is this latter association that every patient past middle age with a carbuncle should be suspected of diabetes until it is disproved. In carbuncles, the extensive inflammation frequently is not associated with a complete walling-off of the infection, so that absorption with production of high fever, leukocytosis and even the extension of the infection to the blood stream may occur.

Treatment and Nursing Care

In many cases a carbuncle may subside very rapidly by the administration of the antibiotic to which the infecting organism is sensitive. The antibiotic must be continued until the infective process is controlled. If the process already has gone on to form pus, incision and drainage may be necessary.

In caring for patients with carbuncles, the nurse must consider not only the surgical lesion but also the general care of an extremely toxic patient. Furthermore, as many of these patients are diabetic, the question of diet, the administration of insulin and intravenous glucose and the complications of diabetes, such as acidosis, must be borne in mind.

Carbuncle of Upper Lip

Infection of the upper lip, especially carbuncle, is an unusually serious disease because of the danger of thrombosis and embolism of the veins of the face and of the nose. Some of these vessels drain into the cavernous sinus, a large venous channel in the skull, and an extension of the process in that direction is attended with grave consequences. Some surgeons recommend early incision in the treatment of such patients but, since the advent of penicillin, incision rarely is necessary and by the use of this drug in large doses at regular intervals the danger of spreading infection usually is controlled. The nurse never should attempt to squeeze the lesion because of the danger of breaking the protective wall and thus producing an extension of the process. Rapid death may result from an intracranial extension causing septicemia or meningitis. Therefore, this apparently minor condition must be regarded as a most serious disease with a very high mortality.

INFECTIONS OF HAND AND FINGERS

Infections of the fingers and the hand are of extreme importance to the nurse, not only because she must know how to take care of these lesions but also because there are frequent accidents in nursing that may lead to a development of these infections in the nurse herself. Therefore, it is important that she know the cause, and especially the prophylactic treatment, of these infections, because they may lead to serious disability, if not to fatal consequences.

Since almost all of these hand and finger inflammations are due to infection, it is important to identify the organism and to determine its sensitivity to the antibiotics. In the treatment of these infections, the appropriate antibiotic properly administered will permit rapid subsidence of the inflammatory process; it may abort the infection in some cases, and in other well-established infections it will hasten its resolution.

PARONYCHIA (RUNAROUND)

Paronychia is a common infection, especially in females. It results most often from an infection of a hangnail and is seen frequently after manicuring. The infection extends between the soft tissues and the nail on the dorsum of the fingertip and forms a tense, painful, throbbing area of inflammation at the side of the nail. If the infection is allowed to go untreated, it may progress underneath the eponychium (cuticle) and then invade the space underneath the base of the nail. This gives this infection its common name.

Cleanliness of the hands and careful care of the nails are the best prophylaxis against paronychia. If the

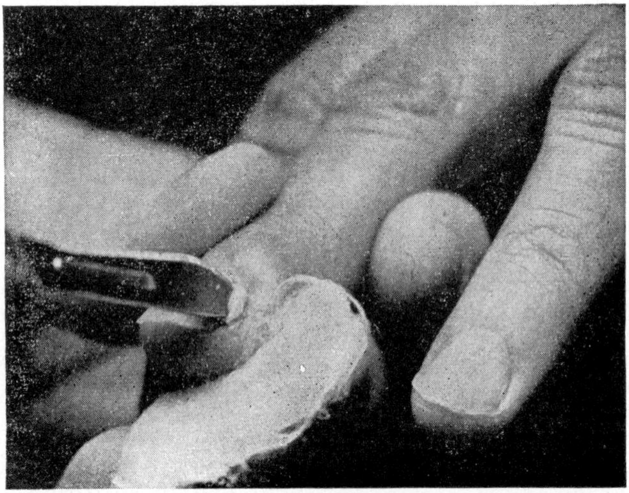

FIG. 168. Paronychia or runaround. The infection lies between the soft tissues and the side of the nail. Drainage by inserting the tip of a scalpel along the edge of the nail is customary surgery.

infection does occur, it can be drained easily by lifting up the soft tissues from the edge of the nail with the tip of a scalpel. Once the pus is evacuated, the inflammation usually will subside with the use of hot moist applications.

Infections of Fingertip

Infections of the pulp of the fingertip usually are the result of a puncture wound, the stick of a pin or a needle, when bacteria are carried into the layers of the skin or into the fatty tissues underlying it. When the infection lies between the layers of the skin, the abscess which is formed is spoken of as an *epidermal abscess*. This lesion is diagnosed easily because it forms a small, tender, blisterlike mound at the site of the pinprick. Puncture and removal of the overlying skin may be performed without anesthesia, exposing the true skin below. In workmen and in others, in whom the surface skin is thick, the infection may not progress to the surface so readily and, instead, it may perforate through the true skin and invade the subcutaneous fatty tissues. This process is known as a *collar-button abscess*, one abscess cavity lying between layers of the skin connected by a narrow tract and a second abscess lying below the skin. In the treatmean of such abscesses it is important naturally to drain both the superficial and the deep collection by incision.

Felon (*Distal Closed Space Infection*)

The most common and serious type of infection of the fingertip is that due to the streptococcus in the pulp of the finger. There usually is a history of needleprick or pinprick or some other form of puncture, followed several days later by throbbing pain, which may be of such intensity as to prevent sleep. The swelling and the edema produced by the infection may be sufficient to impair or shut off completely the arterial supply to the soft tissues, so that rapid necrosis and even invasion of the bone may occur. The resulting disability often is great because of the extreme importance of the fingertips in the use of the hand and the fingers.

Treatment. Early incision and drainage will prevent the progress of the necrosis; therefore, wide incision often is practiced for what may appear to be a relatively small area of infection. It is surprising to note that radical incision is conservative therapy when dealing with infections of the pulp of the finger.

After incision, the wound is held open by rubber dam or gauze drainage and immobilized by an appropriate splint. Warm moist dressings are used until the area of slough has separated entirely, after which time healing may be permitted to take place.

Prophylaxis. In the prophylaxis of fingertip infections, the nurse who has pricked her finger with a needle or a pin should report it to her head nurse at once. Frequently, a slight enlargement of the incision or cauterization of the needle puncture with phenol may abort a serious infection. If throbbing pain becomes a prominent symptom, no time should be wasted in consulting a surgeon. Because the infecting organisms are usually those effectively controlled by penicillin, this antibiotic is used in full doses both as a prophylactic and therapeutic measure.

Infections of Tendon Sheaths of Hand—Tenosynovitis (Whitlow)

Infections of the tendon sheaths on the palmar surface of the hand occur most frequently from puncture wounds. Most often they are caused by the streptococcus. They are serious because they may lead to a rapid destruction of the tendon itself and, therefore, to a marked finger and hand disability. An infection may involve the sheaths of the tendons in the fingers and the thumb; it may invade the fascial spaces of the hand, or it may advance along the tendon sheaths of the thumb and the fifth finger and invade the bursal space through which the tendons pass at the wrist. It produces a tense swelling of the involved finger with extreme pain when motion is attempted.

Treatment. Early incision and drainage are necessary to prevent necrosis of the tendon. Petrolatum gauze usually is laid in the wound to provide drainage.

Often penicillin is of value. In the early phases of the infection it may prevent necrosis and the necessity for incision. After incision, it is used to prevent extension of the infection and to hasten healing.

Postoperative Nursing Care

In the postoperative care of these patients, the nurse usually finds the part bandaged and on a splint, and for a time hot moist applications are applied through the dressings directly or through tubes fastened in them. The nurse must be extremely careful to carry out a sterile technic in moistening the dressings because of the danger of producing a mixed infection which usually is associated with the extension of the inflammatory process. Elevation of the part must be enforced to reduce the inflammatory edema and to give comfort to the patient. This usually is accomplished by means of pillows, which should be protected with a plastic cover. (See p. 27, Hot Wet Dressings.)

After the acute inflammatory process has been controlled, the infected hand often may be treated in a warm saline bath two or three times daily. The basin and the solution should be sterilized and the solution placed in the basin at a temperature as warm as the patient can stand comfortably. This temperature is maintained as well as possible by adding more solution at intervals. The bath usually is continued for at least 30 minutes. Its purpose is to apply heat to aid in the discharge of the necrotic materials from the wound. After removal from the bath the hand is placed in a sterile towel and dry heat may be continued by the use of an electric light in a bed cradle. The nurse must be careful to avoid scalding or burning.

BURNS

Burns are injuries to the skin, usually caused by heat but occasionally caused by irradiation, electricity and so forth. The prevention and the care of burns is an outstanding health problem with which a nurse must be familiar. Burns are among the commonest of household injuries, and in disaster and war burns take a tremendous toll.

Heat, either moist, such as steam or boiling water, or dry, such as a flame, a hot-water bottle, hot metals.

Chemicals, strong acids, such as sulfuric or nitric; strong alkalies—for example, caustic soda (lye), and other strong chemicals. (In most cases, dilution by flushing the part with water is the best treatment.)

Electricity, the effects of which vary widely, depending on the type, the voltage and the amperage of the current. Accidental burns usually are noted where the current enters and leaves the body. In addition to these local effects, systemic changes that produce respiratory, circulatory and central nervous system disturbances may be noted.

Irradiation, which may be by ultraviolet rays, x-rays and radium. Sunburn and burns from ultraviolet lamps usually are superficial and produce short-lived effects. Those from x-ray and radium are slow to appear, and the most marked effects, such as ulceration, may not occur for years.

Friction. This is caused by a prolonged rubbing of the skin.

Classification and First Aid Treatment

First-degree burns produce only redness (erythema) of the skin. Treat by occluding air with any soothing application such as oil, baking-soda paste and so forth.

Second-degree burns produce blisters (vesicles). Treat the same as first-degree burns. Do not disturb blisters until later.

Third-degree burns produce sloughing and destruction of the skin and the deeper tissues. Apply sterile protective dressings or any clean white linen available. Two body surfaces should not be wrapped together. Do not remove clothing if matted in burn and never apply ointments, grease or oil. Such application would have to be removed later, which is traumatizing and time-consuming. Treat the patient for shock by keeping him quiet, administering a sedative and fluids. Have him see a physician or be transported to a hospital immediately.

Treatment and Nursing Care

The nurse will give intelligent care to her patient with burns if she recognizes that the indications for treatment in the order of their importance are (1) to prevent shock and pain, (2) to prevent fluid loss and to replace lost fluid (plasma), (3) to prevent infection, (4) to promote early healing, (5) to prevent emotional upset, (6) to prevent contracture formation and (7) to achieve normal function, if possible.

Burns produce systemic as well as local effects, and the combined result may lead to shock and, often, death. The shock is the result of two factors—the pain of the burned area that produces a nervous or psychological shock and the dilatation of the capillaries produced by the burn that causes a loss of circulating fluid by allowing the plasma to escape into the tissues. These factors account for the early deaths in most extensive burns.

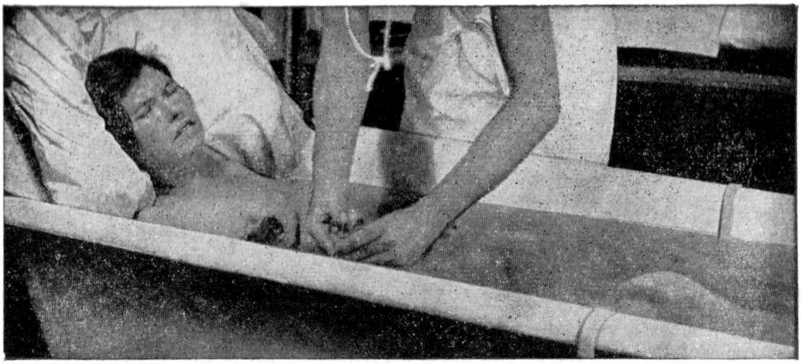

FIG. 169. Débridement and cleansing of burn with patient in saline bath.

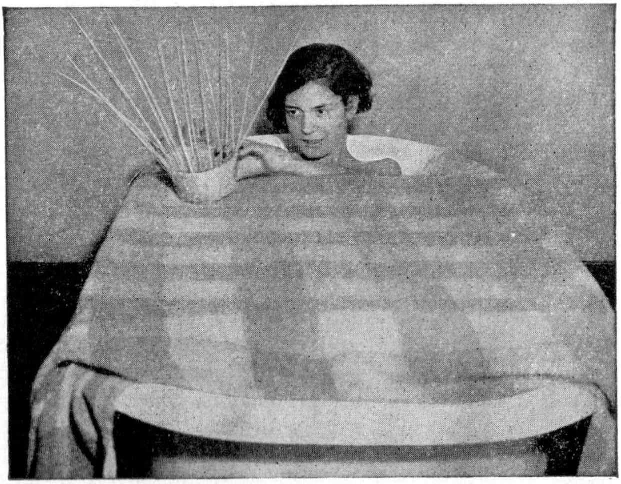

FIG. 170. Patient with severe burn of leg who has started occupational therapy for burned contracted fingers even before operation. (Brown, J. B., and McDowell, F.: Skin Grafting of Burns, Philadelphia, Lippincott)

Pain is relieved best by adequate doses of narcotics. The kind and the amount of medication used will depend upon the condition of the patient and the desires of the physician.

Any kind of burn is painful. A patient so afflicted is entitled to every consideration as regards both his physical and his mental comfort. The nurse must be gentle when she cares for his needs. Sudden jarring or careless handling is inexcusable. During a dressing of the burned area, the

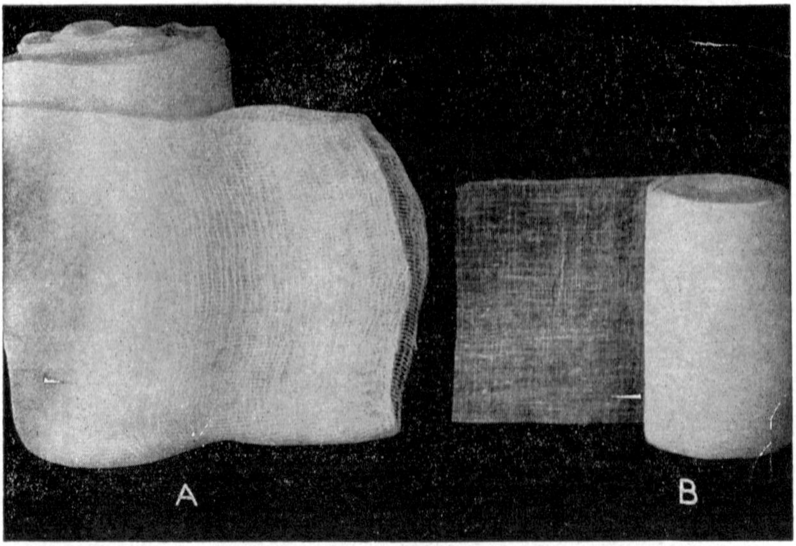

FIG. 171. (A) Gauze rolls used for application of pressure in large dressings. (B) Fine-mesh (No. 44) bandage gauze used next to all open wounds and grafts, either wet or with ointments. Granulations do not grow up through meshes of this gauze, which can be removed with nearly no pain or bleeding. (Brown, J. B., and McDowell, F.: Skin Grafting of Burns, Philadelphia, Lippincott)

physician and the nurse must take time and care when removing dressings that adhere to the tissues. Often the saturating of a dressing with saline will help.

To prevent infection, everyone attending the severely burned patient should wear a mask and sterile gown and gloves.

With warm water, soap and soft wash material the burned area is cleansed and the shreds of burned epidermis and loose tissue are removed with sterile instruments. At the same time the blebs are punctured. All finger rings should be removed.

Patients who can tolerate fluids orally should be given electrolytes by mouth.

During these procedures intravenous plasma, whole blood, or saline and glucose (5 per cent solution or other substitutes) is given. Hematocrit readings offer a good index of the patient's condition.

Local dressings are important adjuncts to good treatment. Several layers of fine-meshed gauze (bandage) saturated with petrolatum should be applied snugly and smoothly. This should be covered with a voluminous gauze dressing plus sterilized waste or oakum, all held firmly with an elastic bandage, tricot hose or stockinet. The chief

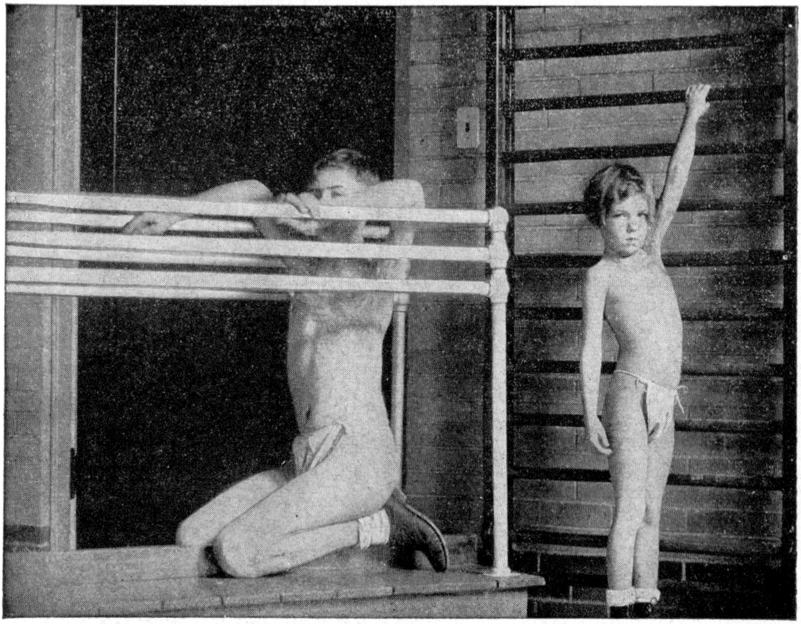

FIG. 172. Simple equipment useful in working out postoperative stiffness or even secondary contractures. Even a trapeze hung in a transom of the hospital or at home may suffice. The instillation in the patient of a will to help himself may be more important than the type of equipment. Massage, baking and baths seldom are necessary if restoration has been adequate and the patient is able to exercise. (Brown, J. B., and McDowell, F.: Skin Grafting of Burns, Philadelphia, Lippincott)

advantages of such a pressure dressing are: (1) further fluid loss is prevented, (2) swelling and further injury are prevented, and (3) healing is promoted with least loss of function.

Additional splinting is very desirable, and often necessary, for tranquillity of the part as well as of the patient. This dressing is left on for from 10 to 12 days.

There are many other methods of local treatment advocated by excellent authorities.

In severe burns, the marked disturbance of fluid balance may last for several days. Frequent estimates of hemoglobin or hematocrit are necessary, and blood and/or plasma often is given in large (from 3,000 to 5,000 cc.) amounts. As fluid balance is extremely important, an accurate recording of intake and output is essential. Frequent specimens of urine are sent to the laboratory to determine the fluid status of the patient and to reveal any kidney damage.

After the danger from shock is past, the care of the patient is a

PLATE 2

AGES IN PROGRESSIVE HEALING OF SECOND- AND THIRD-DEGREE BURNS

(From "Management of the Cocoanut Grove Burns at the Massachusetts General Hospital.")

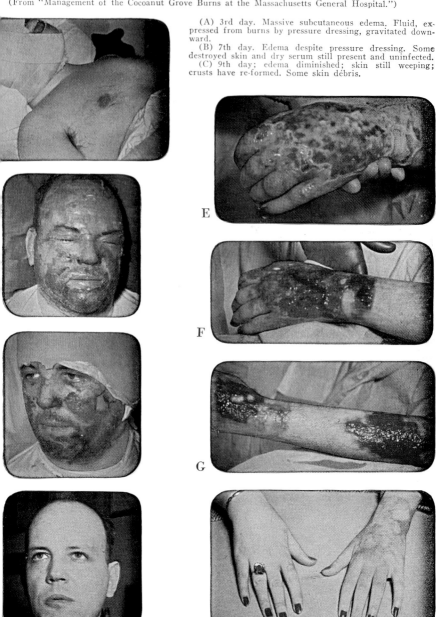

(A) 3rd day. Massive subcutaneous edema. Fluid, expressed from burns by pressure dressing, gravitated downward.
(B) 7th day. Edema despite pressure dressing. Some destroyed skin and dry serum still present and uninfected.
(C) 9th day; edema diminished; skin still weeping; crusts have re-formed. Some skin débris.

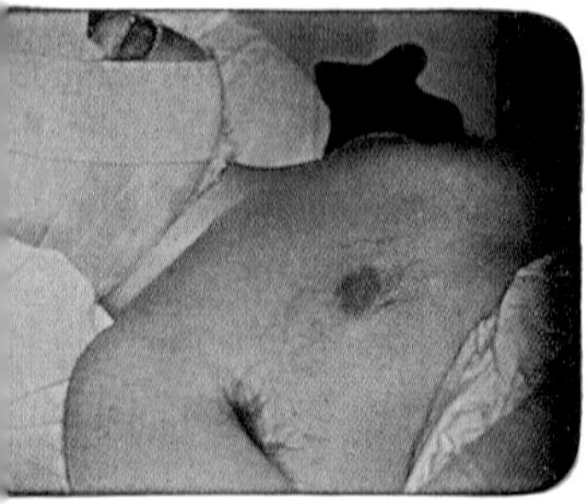

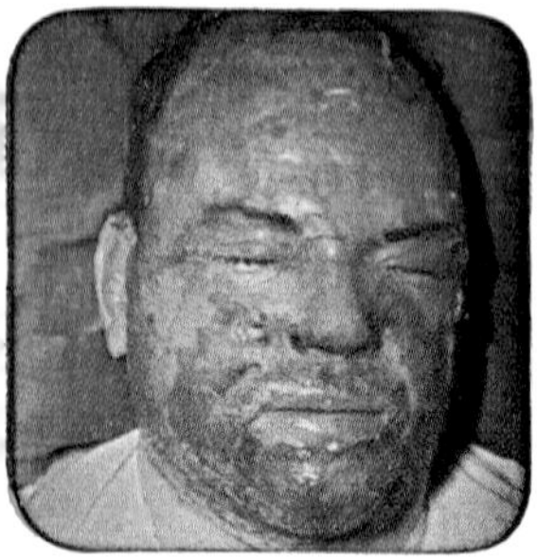

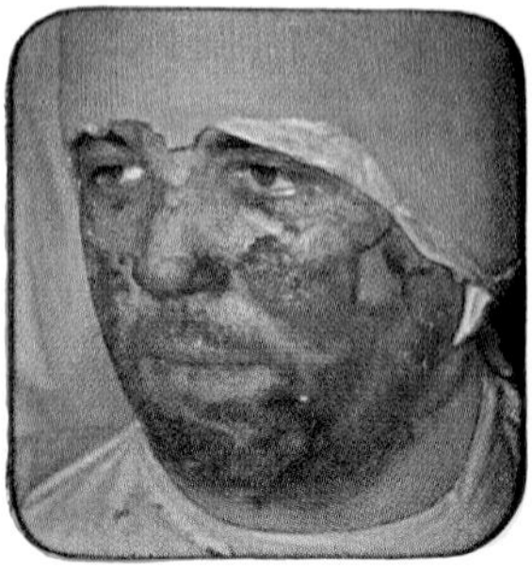

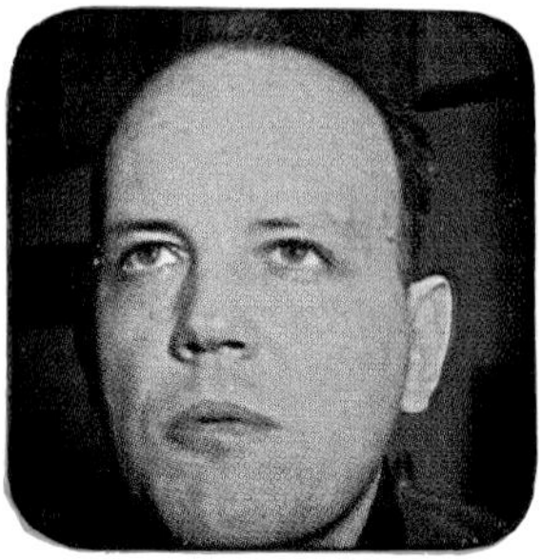

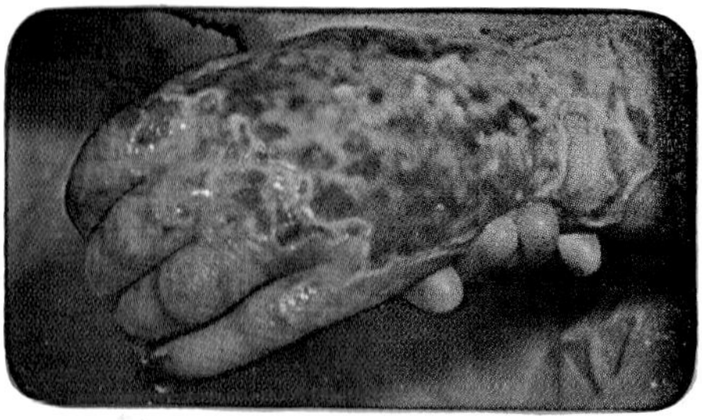

E

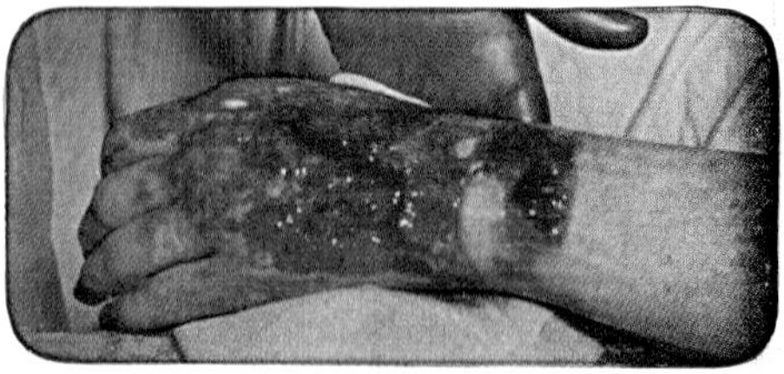

F

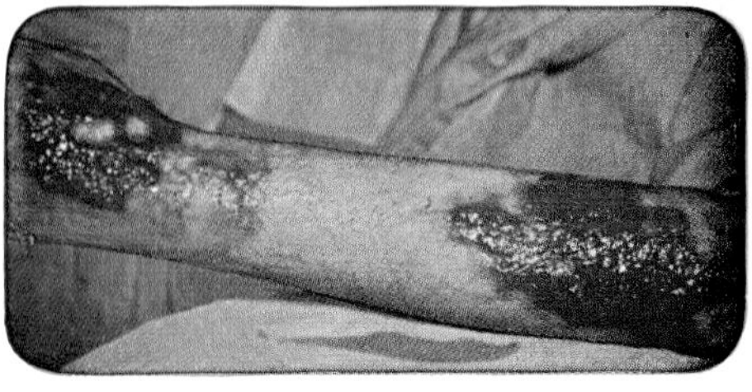

G

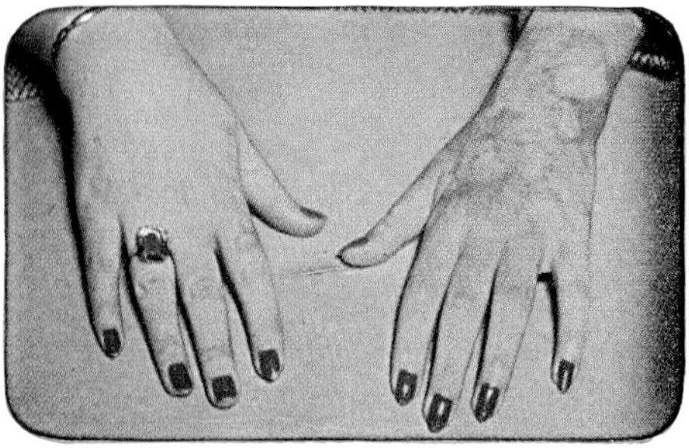

H

(D) 55th day. Absence of scarring; return to rmal contours. Scalp healed without grafting.
(E) 19th day. Slough still in place. Skin immetely adjacent normal; no evidence of infection.
(F) 30th day. Most of the slough has separated. Granulations are edematous; infection is minimal.
(G) 51st day, the day of grafting. Note healthy appearance of granulations and islands of viable skin in center of raw surface on back of hand.
(H) Final view of hands at 3½ months.

matter of the care of the burned area. As the eschar loosens it is cut away, so that eventually a few granulating surfaces are formed. In many situations new skin may have covered the burned area. When all the necrotic tissue has disappeared, skin grafts may be used to hasten healing. Early skin-grafting has shortened the recovery period of many patients.

It is in the stage of granulation formation that serious deformities may develop, due to contractures. The nurse must attempt to keep the part in the position that will give the best functional result. Often this may be accomplished by the application of splints.

As soon as permissible, exercises of each part should be instituted under the direction of the physician, first by the physical therapist and the nurse and then by the patient himself. Occupational and diversional therapy also play a helpful role in rehabilitation (Figs. 170 and 172).

Throughout the patient's illness, a high caloric and high protein diet should be maintained. Many times, the patient is nauseated or not interested in food, and it is up to the nurse to tempt him with smaller feedings offered more frequently. They should be served attractively and with an appreciation of his likes and dislikes. An inadequate protein intake will lead to poor wound healing, anemia and ultimate death.

A nursing problem is the disturbing odor that arises when tissue becomes necrotic. This can be combated by the frequent changing of dressings and the liberal use of deodorants.

Such a patient will need diversion to keep him from thinking of himself. Time weighs heavily and worry about possible disfigurement is great. By finding out what the patient's interests and hobbies are, she may be able to help him in this regard.

ULCERATIONS

The superficial loss of surface tissue due to death of the cells is called an *ulceration*. A simple or a healthy ulcer, such as is found in a small superficial second-degree burn, tends to heal by granulation if kept clean and protected from injury. If exposed to the air, the serum that escapes from it will dry and form a scab, under which the epithelial cells will grow and cover the surface completely.

Special diseases cause characteristic ulcers—thus, there are tuberculous ulcers of the skin and syphilitic punched-out ulcers of the leg.

Ulcers of the Skin. These arise usually either from infection or from an interference with the blood supply. Infectious ulcers are not uncommon. They develop usually from an infection with an anaerobic streptococcus or from a combination of infections in which a hemolytic anaerobic streptococcus lives in symbiosis with a staphylococcus. Ulcers of this type tend to progress peripherally and are seen often in the lower extremity or on the abdomen or the chest after operation. They are characterized by an overhanging edge, and culture from them usually shows the type of organism causing the infection. These ulcers tend to resist ordinary forms of treatment, but the application of zinc peroxide,

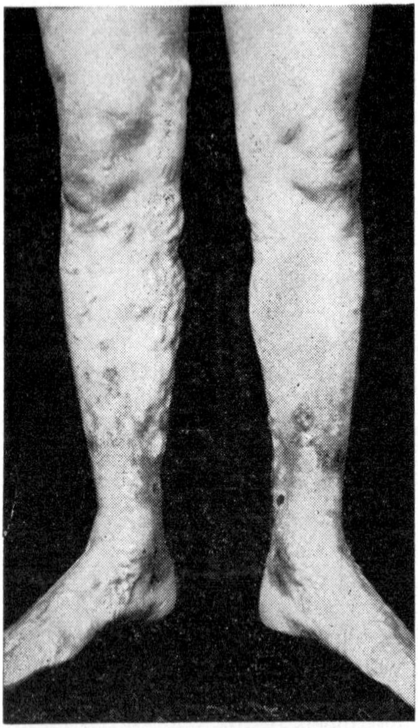

Fig. 173. Varicose ulcers at usual locations.

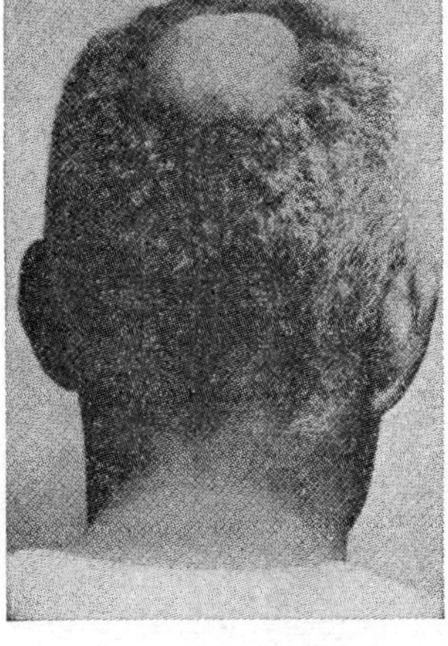

Fig. 174. Large sebaceous cyst of the scalp.

which liberates oxygen over a long period of time, converts the anaerobic portions of the wound into an aerobic area. Penicillin locally or intramuscularly also is highly effective. Healing occurs rapidly due to the inability of the anaerobic streptococci to live in an unfavorable environment.

Ulcers Due to a Deficient Arterial Circulation. These are seen in patients with peripheral vascular disease, arteriosclerosis, Raynaud's disease and frostbite. In these patients the treatment of the ulceration must be carried out in conjunction with the treatment of the arterial disease. The danger is from secondary infection. Frequently, amputation of the part is the only curative therapy.

Varicose Ulcers

The prolonged venous stasis and edema seen in patients with varicose veins (see Varicose Veins, p. 273) result in a gradual replacement of subcutaneous fatty tissue by fibrous tissue. The skin becomes discolored and, on pressure, is firm and brawny. These tissues have a poor resistance to infection, so that minor trauma and abrasions result in ulcerations that tend not only to remain but to enlarge and progress. The ulcers are surrounded by an area of hard edema and frequently are characterized by a burning pain. In advanced cases, the ulcers may progress to involve the entire circumference of the leg. They are seen most often in patients who have had a previous phlebitis.

In most instances, the ulcers will heal if the venous stasis and the associated edema can be relieved. This may be accomplished by rest in bed with elevation, but frequently patients are unable to carry out this method of therapy. Another method of treatment is to supply external support to prevent edema and to compress the superficial veins so as to relieve the venous stasis. This is produced by applying firm bandages and often incorporating in them a warmed gelatin mixture that cools and forms a rubberlike supporting casing to the part (Unna's boot). Elastic bandages and stockings often are used instead of gelatin boots, but as a rule they do not provide the firm support obtained by the gelatin boot.

The thin epithelium that eventually heals the ulcer is traumatized easily, and recurrence of ulceration is not infrequent. In many cases, a better and more permanent healing may be obtained by excision of the fibrous subcutaneous tissue and the application of skin grafts.

CYSTS AND TUMORS

Sebaceous Cysts

Cysts of the sebaceous glands are seen very frequently on the hairy parts, especially on the scalp. These result from a blockage of the drainage duct, the continued secretion of the gland being dammed up within the dilated duct. The cysts cause relatively few symptoms, except disfigurement, but occasionally they become infected and, in older people, may undergo a malignant degeneration. They may be removed easily under local anesthesia without the necessity of hospitalization.

Verrucae (Warts)

Verrucae are benign skin tumors that appear more commonly in children, but that are seen also in older people. Occasionally they are painful, and they may become infected. Usually they can be cured by irradiation therapy or by destruction by electrocoagulation.

Nevi (Birthmarks)

Nevi are vascular tumors of benign nature affecting the skin and, often, the subcutaneous tissues. They may be simple dilatations of cutaneous vessels, and these are spoken of as *portwine birthmarks*. They may disappear with age, but usually they are treated with irradiation or carbon dioxide snow. The *strawberry birthmark* is a true benign tumor of the capillaries. It is raised very slightly above the surface of the skin, and it occurs most often in the upper part of the body or on the face or the neck. Nevi respond very well to irradiation therapy as a rule.

Moles

Moles are of various types: flat or raised, smooth or lobulated, always pigmented, some of them containing hair. Generally they are benign, but those deeply pigmented and raised above the surface of the skin may take on a malignant change suddenly and become melanotic tumors. As a rule, no treatment is necessary unless the mole is disfiguring, but in cases in which the mole is lobulated, raised above the surface and in a position in which frequent irritation may induce malignant change (as, for instance, under the arm or on the back of the neck), excision is indicated as a prophylactic measure against the development of malignancy.

Keloids

A keloid is an overgrowth of

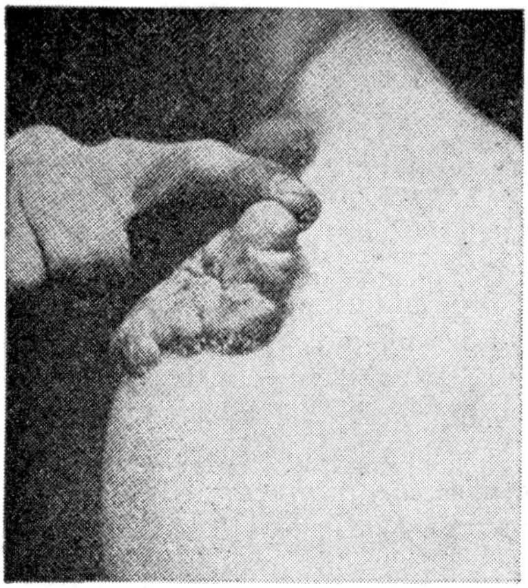

FIG. 175. Keloid of shoulder after minor injury.

fibrous tissue at the site of a scar. It may occur without warning and is especially prone to develop in scars in the Negro. It causes no particular difficulty, except disfigurement, and frequently responds to irradiation therapy. Excision is advisable occasionally (Fig. 175).

Malignant Tumors of Skin

A nurse can be most helpful to an individual with a noninvading skin lesion by urging him to see a physician. If the sore or the lump is a cancer, it is the most curable of all cancers if treated early; in spite of this, these lesions are responsible for 6 per cent of all cancer deaths.

Carcinoma of the skin or epithelioma may occur from either the superficial cells of the skin (the so-called prickle-cell epithelioma) or from the deeper cells of the skin (the so-called rodent ulcer or basal-cell carcinoma). The former type occurs at any site on the body, most often on the hands and round the various orifices of the body. The basal-cell carcinoma or rodent ulcer appears on the face, especially on the temples. Of the two, the prickle-cell epithelioma is the more malignant. Both respond very well to local therapy, either irradiation with radium or destruction of the tumor by electrocoagulation.

Basal-cell Carcinoma

The face, especially the cheeks about the nose and the eyes and in front of the ears, is a common site for the development of cancer in patients past middle age. The growth may spring from an old warty or papillomatous tumor, or frequently from areas of hornified skin, a condition spoken of as senile keratosis. Such lesions, therefore, should be regarded as predisposing to cancer and the patient should be referred to a physician for competent treatment. These cancers are of the slow-growing type, called rodent ulcers, and are characterized by invasion and erosion of contiguous tissues but by very late and infrequent metastatic growths.

Treatment and Nursing Care

Treatment may be by one of several methods: the excision of the growth (curative only if done early), the application of radium or a combination of both. This cancer is one that is benefited and often cured by radiation therapy.

The nursing care consists of the application of sterile dressings to the lesion and careful observation for any signs of hemorrhage. Hemorrhage often occurs after operation, but it may result simply from the erosion of a large vessel without any reference to operation.

The nurse can explain the nature of radiotherapy to the patient receiving this treatment for the first time.

Being alone in a small room with a huge machine will be less frightening when the patient has some understanding of it. Reassure the individual who fears that this treatment will cause sterilization, for it will not. Explain to him that he may experience some reddening and perhaps blistering of the treated skin. Lanolin or any soothing lubricant will keep the skin soft after radiation therapy is completed. The patient should know that he always will have delicate skin; therefore, he must protect it from excess exposure to the sun, cold and so forth. The importance of follow-up care must be stressed, for there is always the possibility of recurrence or of a new primary lesion.

PLASTIC OR RECONSTRUCTIVE SURGERY

By this term is meant that type of surgery which takes care of the repair of defects and malformations, both congenital and acquired. This type of surgery is applicable to many parts of the body and to numerous structures, including bone, cartilage, muscle, nerve and cutaneous structure, bone inlays and transplants for deformities and nonunion, muscle transference, and reconstruction and the splicing of nerves, cartilage replacement and, lastly, but as important as any, the reconstruction of the cutaneous tissues round the neck and the face, to which also is added the term cosmetic surgery.

Precautions. Before making any attempt at such surgery anywhere in the body, it is important that the tissues concerned be free of infection as well as the causative factors, such as syphilis, tuberculosis, diabetes and neoplasm, and that the general condition of the patient be good with regard to nutrition, age and morale. As has been stated aptly, the surgeon must treat what is behind the deformed face as well as the deformity itself. The surgeon should explain to the patient in minute detail the hazards of the job and that absolute perfection is not to be expected. The nurse can be of great help here in building up the proper psychological state and in overcoming any inferiority complex by suggestion, hopefulness and assurance.

General Considerations. In all reconstructive work, tissue must be obtained from a distance or near by to fill the defect. This is accomplished by flap or graft. A *flap* is a piece of tissue used to cover or fill a defect. It has been lifted from its bed but still has a partial attachment by a pedicle, from which it receives its blood supply until healed in its new location. A *graft* is a piece of tissue separated completely from its normal and original position and transferred by one or more stages to correct a distant defect. Transfers or transplants from the same person are termed *autografts*; from a different person *homografts*. The former type is much the better, being safer and more likely to be successful.

For plastic surgery of the nose, see also page 213; for cleft palate and harelip, see page 282.

Skin Grafting

As this type of reconstructive or plastic surgery most often is found necessary to correct unsightly and embarrassing deformity around the

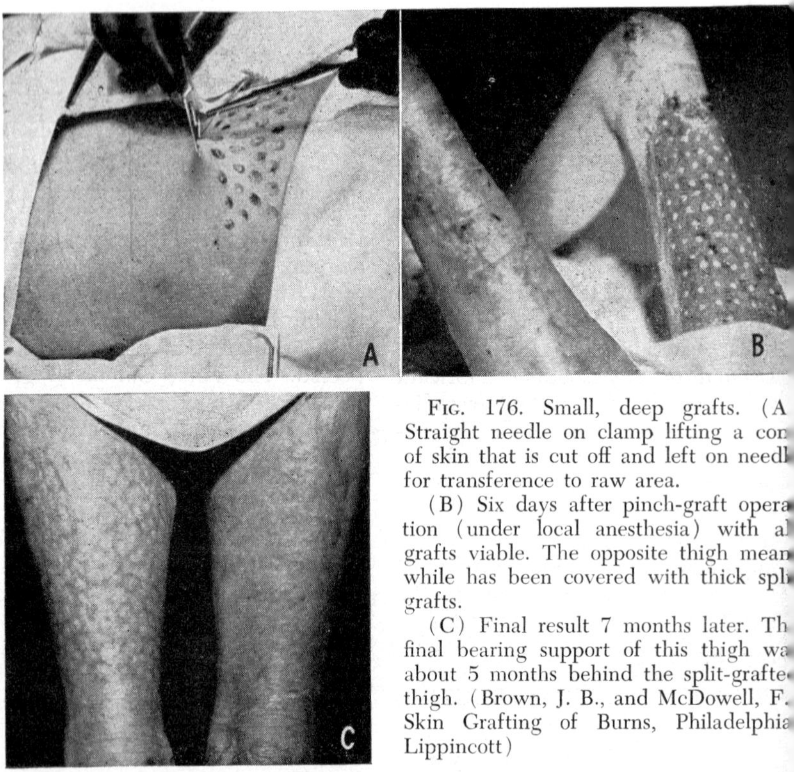

FIG. 176. Small, deep grafts. (A) Straight needle on clamp lifting a con[e] of skin that is cut off and left on needl[e] for transference to raw area.

(B) Six days after pinch-graft operation (under local anesthesia) with al[l] grafts viable. The opposite thigh meanwhile has been covered with thick spli[t] grafts.

(C) Final result 7 months later. Th[e] final bearing support of this thigh wa[s] about 5 months behind the split-grafted thigh. (Brown, J. B., and McDowell, F.: Skin Grafting of Burns, Philadelphia, Lippincott)

face, mouth and neck, attention will be given especially to the maxillofacial technic and nursing care.

So that the operation may be a success, the area to be covered with grafts must be free of infection and sloughs, because grafts "take" or grow only on a clean "granulating" surface. Therefore, a period of preparation of the wound usually is necessary before the operation can be undertaken. Warm saline or penicillin dressings often are used, and penicillin usually is given systemically. The donor area most often is the anterior thigh but, because the nurse cannot tell where it is to be, she should ask for specific instructions. The preparation of the donor area consists of a shave and a thorough cleansing by soap and water.

Several types of grafts are in common usage. To cover small surfaces, the *Reverdin* or *pinch graft* often is used. Bits of skin are picked up on the point of a needle or with forceps, cut off with the scissors and applied to the area to be grafted. This operation may be performed easily under local anesthesia.

The *Thiersch graft* is used to cover larger surfaces. Strips of superficial

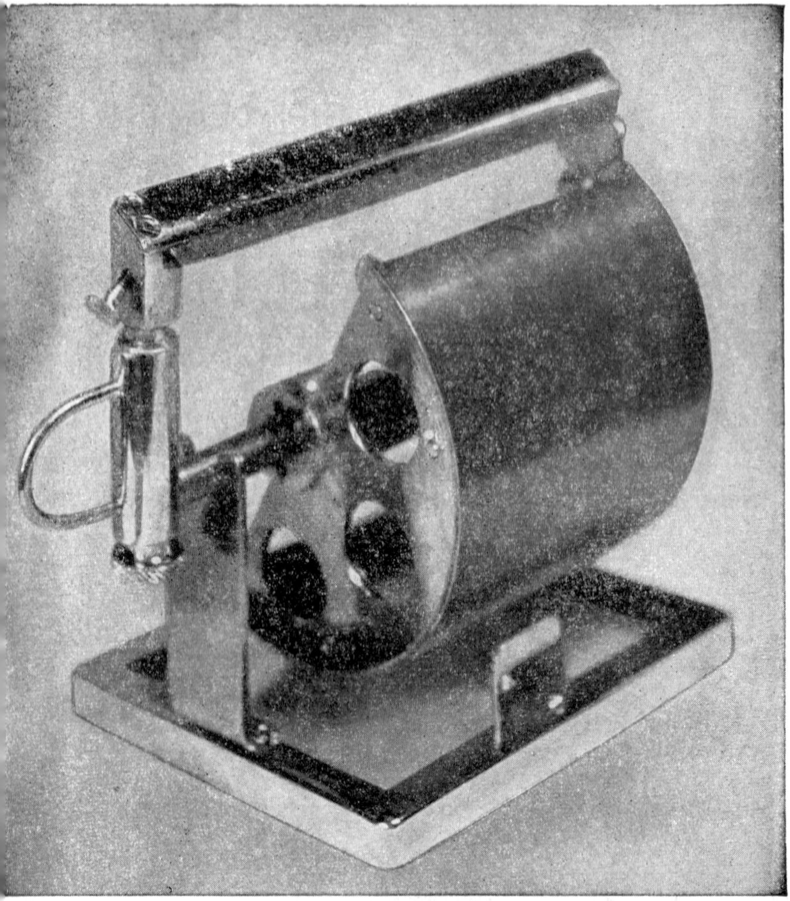

Fig. 177. The dermatome. The knife blade is set so that it is very close to the drum. Rubber cement is applied to the drum and to the skin, and the drum is applied firmly to the skin. Then the drum is rotated slowly and picks up the skin to form a diaphragm as the knife is pushed back and forth. (Brown, J. B., and McDowell, F.: Skin Grafting of Burns, Philadelphia, Lippincott)

skin are shaved off with a razor and applied to the granulating wound.

Split-thickness grafts are grafts of approximately one half the thickness of the skin, removed by a knife or a dermatome.

Wolfe-Krause grafts differ from the previous types in that they consist of the full thickness of the skin.

In the treatment of contractures from scars of old burns or injuries, especially those of neck and chin, it

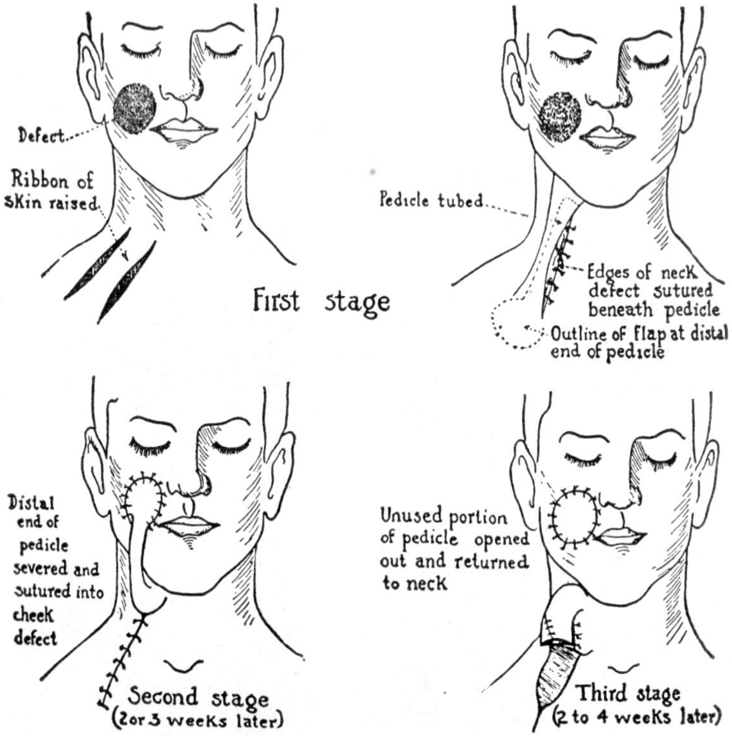

FIG. 178. Diagram showing preparation of tube pedicle flap, after Gillies. (Ivy, R. H.: Plastic and reconstructive surgery of the face, mouth, and jaws in Nelson's Loose Leaf Surgery, vol. II, p. 682)

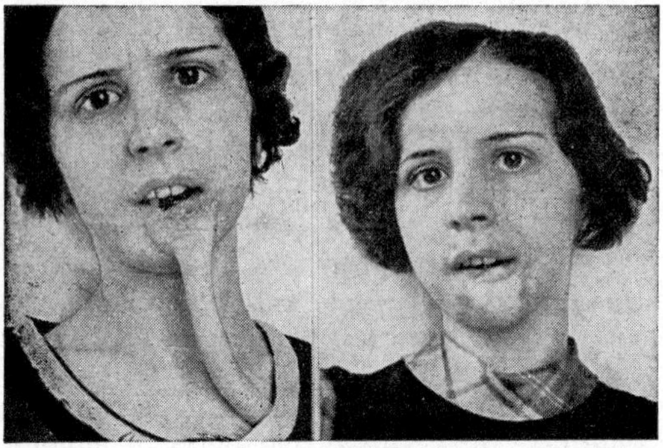

FIG. 179. (*Left*) Showing tube pedicle flap from chest, used for repair of chin defect. (*Right*) After pedicle had been severed. (Robert H. Ivy, M.D.)

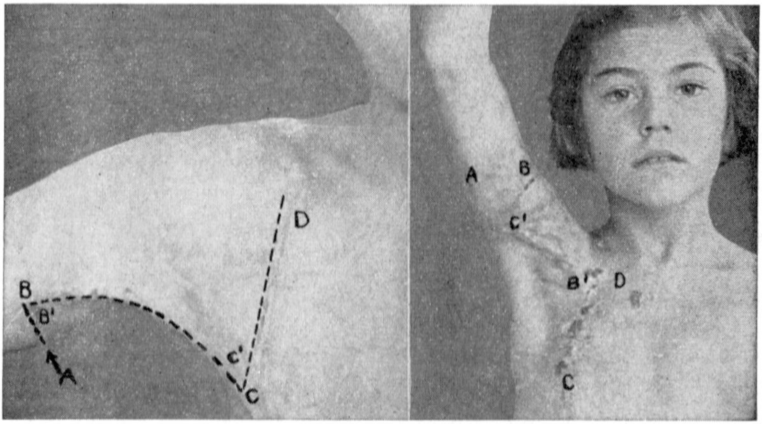

FIG. 180. (*Left*) Scar contracture of axilla, causing restricted elevation of arm, suitable for correction by Z-plasty. Incisions indicated by dotted lines. (*Right*) After operation, showing free elevation of arm. Lettering indicates relocation of flaps. (Robert H. Ivy, M.D.)

is necessary often to excise a large amount of contracted (scar) tissue. The area thus denuded most often is covered with a *pedicle* or *Gillies tube flap*. This flap is so cut that a tube or pedicle may be left attached through which the graft may obtain its blood supply. The flap is applied to the surface to be covered with the pedicle still attached. After the flap is well united to its new location, blood vessels grow into it and the pedicle can be removed (p. 414).

Other areas of the body may require plastic work of greater surface magnitude, the result of extensive burns, mutilated limbs and crippling scar contractures. Here will arise the problem of donor areas for Reverdin, Ollier-Thiersch or sliding grafts. The Thiersch type may be made with a sharp razor blade or by the Padgett dermatome for the larger sheets of skin split of a definite thickness. When a cavity such as the orbit, the mouth or the nostril is to be relined, the graft may be sutured round a previously fashioned mold of dental rubber or plastic material.

In some circumstances, instead of free grafts or pedicle flaps, "sliding" flaps of skin and subcutaneous tissue from the surrounding area can be used. One application of the sliding flap method is the Z-plastic, very useful for relieving comparatively narrow scar contractures about the neck or about joints such as the axilla, the elbow, the knee or the wrist. The application of the Z-plastic to a scar contracture of the axilla is shown in Figure 180.

Fascial transplants have numerous uses. They are obtained generally from the fascia lata of the thigh and are adaptable for use as suture material, for repair of hernia defects and for replacement of tendon loss.

Cartilage transplantation may be immediate and direct, taken from the costal cartilages and transferred to the nose.

Bone grafts demand meticulous aseptic technic and rigid fixation in their new site. They may be taken from the crest of the tibia, the upper border of the iliac bone or a rib.

All donor areas should receive the same careful treatment given any other surgical wound. If possible to close safely by suture, such is done. For the raw, wide area left from the Thiersch method, paraffin mesh, albolene or petrolatum gauze permits a painless dressing within 8 to 10 days.

The area from which the free graft is to be taken, usually the anterior surface of the thigh or the abdomen, is designated by the surgeon for preparation. The hair should be shaved from it, but generally no antiseptics are used until the patient is taken to the operating room.

After the application of the grafts, the area is covered with paraffin mesh and a dressing is applied to hold the grafts firmly in place. Frequently, more adequate pressure is maintained by incorporating in the dressings sponge rubber, moist sea sponge or cotton waste. No redressing is necessary for from 3 to 5 days, at which time only the gauze is removed, the paraffin mesh being left in place. Care must be exercised in removing the dressings so as not to disturb the grafts.

Nursing Care of Maxillofacial Patients

While these patients require the same general care as all other surgical patients, there are a few special points to which the nurse's attention should be called.

Preoperative Attention. In maxillofacial patients a mild laxative the night before and a simple enema the morning of operation are sufficient. Starvation is unnecessary. The patient may have a good meal the evening before, and no breakfast or fluid for 4 hours before the operation. For the comfort of the patient, operation is done best in the morning. If it is necessary to postpone the operation until afternoon, there is no reason why a very light breakfast should not be allowed. Fluids may be included.

The mouth should be made as clean as possible to lessen the danger both of lung complications after general anesthesia and of infection in the wound. If special dental care is unavailable, the nurse can accomplish much by swabbing the gums with hydrogen dioxide.

A hypodermic injection of morphine sulfate, 0.016 Gm. (gr. ¼) or 0.011 Gm. (gr. ⅙), and atropine sulfate, 0.4 mg. (gr. 1/150), three-quarters of an hour before starting the anesthesia always is advisable in maxillofacial patients, who often are more difficult to anesthetize because the field of operation is so near the anesthesia inhaler. The atropine also helps to reduce the secretion of saliva and mucus.

Preparation of the Part. If the patient is a man, the skin of the face should be shaved closely and, of course, well cleansed with soap and water. If the operative field extends up toward the scalp, this should also be shaved as far as is necessary. It is not necessary to apply dressings o the skin before operation, unless here already is a wound.

If the operation is to be done under local anesthesia, no laxative or enema need be given and food need not be withheld. The preliminary hypodermic of morphine and atropine should be given just as for general anesthesia.

Postoperative Management. The nurse watching the patient recover from general anesthesia should keep the patient's head turned away from the operated side, so that the wound and dressings will not be soiled by vomited material.

Occasionally, after operation within the mouth, the nurse may be alarmed by undue bleeding from the gums. All ordinary hemorrhage of this nature can be controlled by inserting a gauze pad in the mouth against the bleeding part of the jaw and bringing pressure of the opposing teeth to bear against it. If the patient is conscious, he can be made to bite on the pad. This pressure of the jaw often can be applied even when no teeth are present. In case of difficulty, the nurse should make pressure with the pad until the doctor arrives. The gauze pad can be changed as it becomes soaked with blood or saliva. After plastic operations on the face, frequently no dressings are used. If the incisions have been closed accurately with sutures, no dressings are necessary unless it is desired to control oozing of blood by pressure. Particularly near the mouth, dressings tend to become soaked with saliva and food, which may lead to infection of an otherwise clean wound. Slight oozing of blood from the incisions generally occurs for a short time after operation. If this blood is allowed to clot on the wound, infection may occur under the clot and spoil the cosmetic result. For the first hour or so after operation the nurse should wipe the blood that oozes from the incision with an alcohol sponge, so that it will not clot on the surface.

In plastic operations the flaps sometimes become blue and congested, due to partial obstruction of the venous circulation. The surgeon sometimes scarifies the surface of the flap, making numerous small openings to relieve the blood congestion and avoid gangrene of the flap. The blood flow from these small incisions then can be kept up by the continuous application for several hours of hot fomentations of 1 per cent sodium citrate. These must be applied in an aseptic manner in order not to infect the flap. Probably the most convenient way is for the nurse to drop some of the warm sodium citrate solution on the dressings from time to time with a syringe.

Pain is more likely to follow operations involving the jaw bones than the soft tissues alone. For postoperative pain, either a hot-water bag or an ice bag may give relief. Whichever works best in the individual case is employed. Sedatives ranging from aspirin to morphine may be required.

In maxillofacial patients there is no reason to withhold fluids for any length of time after operation, as may be the case after abdominal operations. The patient may have cracked ice or water as soon as postanesthetic vomiting is over, and liquid diet may be started as soon as the patient has a desire for food. Very often soft diet is started the day after operation.

When there is a wound of the

mouth, the mouth should be cleansed after each feeding. It is not sufficient always for the patient to use a mouthwash. Frequent swabbing of the gums and the teeth with cotton on applicators soaked in hydrogen dioxide will accomplish a great deal in keeping the mouth clean. The mouth, and especially the wounded or diseased part, should be irrigated three or four times a day with some antiseptic fluid—it makes little difference what the fluid is. Boric acid, liquor antisepticus, or even normal saline, will do. The syringe should require only one hand to operate it, leaving the other hand free to retract the cheek or hold a light. A very convenient syringe is the one used for irrigating eyes. This consists of a fairly large rubber bulb and a small glass nozzle of the medicine dropper type. An all-rubber ear-and-ulcer syringe or a power spray also may be used. When very frequent irrigation is required, a reservoir (rubber bag or douche can) may be suspended over the head of the bed, not more than 2 feet above the patient's head, and the fluid carried to the mouth through a glass nozzle. Sometimes the patient himself can use this.

Gauze packing frequently is placed in mouth wounds. This should not be allowed to remain longer than 48 hours without change. If no packing is used in the mouth, no treatment other than frequent irrigation is required.

Suppurating superficial wounds can be cleansed with hydrogen dioxide. Granulating surfaces are treated by application of penicillin solution and covered with boric acid or petrolatum gauze.

Bandage. All nurses should know how to apply a good bandage to the head—a bandage that will stay in place. The head bandage commonly taught is the Barton, but this has the disadvantage of pulling backward on the chin—a very serious objection, particularly in cases of fracture of the lower jaw. A bandage that is universally useful in cases of fracture or for holding dressings on any part of the head, the face or the neck is a modified Barton or figure-of-eight that does not pull back on the chin. A 2 or 2½ inch gauze or muslin bandage is used.

Diet. The diet for maxillofacial patients is very important. Many of them, particularly those with fractures of the jaws, have to have the upper and the lower teeth fastened together for weeks and, therefore, can take only liquid food. Others are able to take soft food, but are unable to masticate. These patients are not to be classed with the ordinary postoperative patient on liquid diet, to whom the liquid is given in small amounts because he is in no condition to assimilate more, and to whom a soft and, finally, a full diet is given after a short time.

In patients obliged to remain for a long time on liquid diet because of an injury to the jaw, sufficient quantity and quality should be given to maintain them in a state of good nutrition. Under this regimen a loss of weight will be noted at first, but if properly carried out it is possible to obtain a gain in weight. As a basis for the diet of the average patient for 24 hours, the following is suggested: Milk, 4 pints; soup, 2 pints; eggs, 4. This diet should be prepared and varied as far as possible to avoid monotony. Ingenuity must be exercised in this respect. Much can be accomplished with the liberal use of stewed fruits and fruit juices, soft cereals, malted milk, cocoa, coffee, tea and so forth. A proper vitamin content must not be overlooked. The soft diet for patients able to manage it also demands careful preparation. The usual routine soft diet in hospitals is not suitable always for patients unable to masticate. All meat, vegetables and cooked fruits should be divided finely or mashed. The patient must be fed often in order to obtain the equivalent of a full diet.

Psychological Aspects. The nurse is in a unique position to help these patients to accept their many experiences more easily. Many times, the ultimate objective requires a number of operations separated by long intervals of time. Patience is a real factor. Recreational, occupational and spiritual therapies need to be explored fully with the interests of the individual patient kept intact.

Often, the kinds of dressings that have to be worn, the unusual positions that have to be maintained and the temporary incapacities that must be experienced can be very upsetting to the best of patients. The nurse must be able to offer hope and encouragement and to combine this with a wholesome sense of humor. Tact and patience, attention to small details will make the nurse an invaluable colleague as the patient regains his self-assurance and more normal usefulness and appearance.

CLINICAL SITUATION: THIRD-DEGREE BURN

In attempting to save his 4-year-old son from the flames of a rapidly progressing fire in their one-story home, Mr. Valice was burned severely. A helpful neighbor stripped the remains of the shirt from the victim's back and applied heavy automobile grease (the most accessible lubricant) to his burns. Then he was rushed to the hospital, where it was estimated that he had sustained a third-degree burn of 50 per cent of his body.

1. A third-degree burn means that

____(1) the skin and the deeper tissues have been destroyed

____(2) the deepest third of dermal tissue has been destroyed

____(3) a burn less severe than a first-degree burn has been received

2. The use of any type of grease or oil on a third-degree burn is

____(1) desirable, for it prevents air from contacting raw tissues and lessens the possibility of infection

____(2) undesirable, since it has to be removed later when the wounded area is cleansed

____(3) questionable; some cases are helped, while others are not

3. Because Mr. Valice had been unable to save his son, he did not care whether he lived or died. Such an attitude

____(1) cannot be changed

_____(2) will not affect the regeneration of tissues
_____(3) will definitely hinder his recovery

4. If Mr. Valice were conscious, the best kind of fluid to give him as emergency treatment and thereafter would be
_____(1) hot tea or coffee
_____(2) whiskey or brandy
_____(3) salt and soda bicarbonate solution

5. Pressure dressings are applied to a burned area after it has been cleaned and débrided because they
_____(1) are the most comfortable type of dressing
_____(2) help to prevent fluid loss
_____(3) can absorb large quantities of fluid

6. The best emergency measure would have been to
_____(1) leave charred clothing in place; cover patient with blanket
_____(2) leave charred clothing in place; cover burned area with clean cloth
_____(3) strip charred clothing from burned area

CHAPTER TWENTY

Surgery of the Breast

INTRODUCTION

Up to the time of puberty it is impossible to find microscopically any difference in the breasts of the two sexes. At puberty, some slight swelling appears in the male breast. At the same time, a pronounced increase in size occurs in the female organ. This begins about the tenth year and increases rapidly up to between the fourteenth and the sixteenth years. The development of the mammary gland is a result of hormone action that begins with puberty in the female. At this time, the nipple takes on its natural protruding form. In the male, contrary to some statements, breast tissue always exists and may take on growth.

The breast is a glandular organ with many lobules; its secretion passes via collecting ducts to the nipple. In some women, there is a cyclic engorgement of the breasts, associated with tingling and tenderness. This is due to a hormonal disturbance. The symptoms begin usually in the latter part of the menstrual cycle and disappear when menstruation occurs. About eight weeks after conception, the breasts enlarge greatly, the nipples become more prominent and sensitive, and the breast is prepared to nourish the infant to come. When pregnancy is over and lactation has ceased, the breast shrinks, loses its excessive fat and often becomes flabby and flattened. Surgical conditions may arise from inflammations and tumors developing in it.

FISSURE OF NIPPLE

Fissure of the nipple is a longitudinal ulcer that develops frequently in any woman who is nursing a baby. The ulcer is irritated constantly by the act of suckling and causes the mother considerable pain, often associated with bleeding of the nipple. Prophylactic treatment, cleanliness and washing and drying of the nipple after each nursing usually will prevent the occurrence of this condition. If a fissure develops, it should be washed at frequent in-

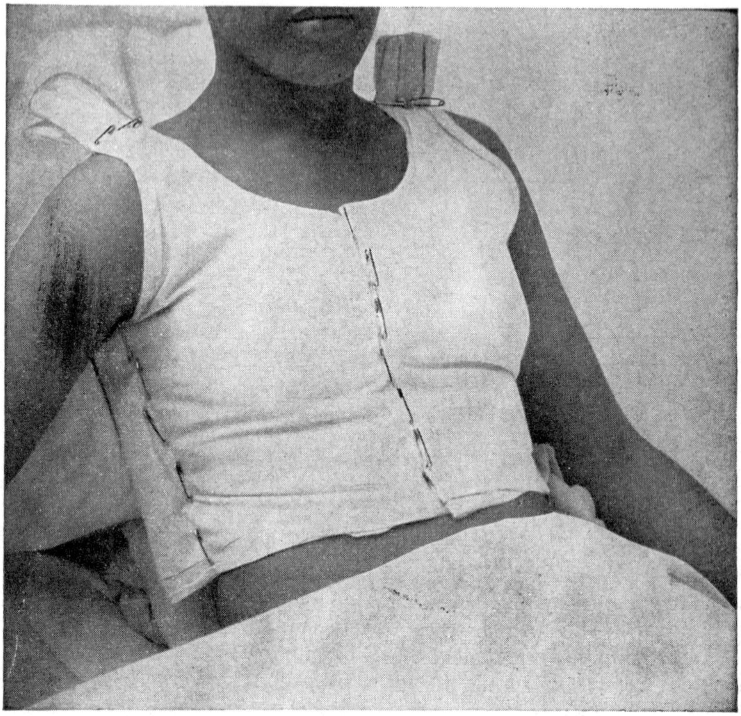

Fig. 181. Breast binder. Safety pins are used to make a snug fit.

tervals with saline solution, and nursing should be permitted only with an artificial nipple. If healing does not occur promptly, or if the case is severe and painful, nursing should be stopped and a breast pump substituted for it. Ulceration that persists suggests carcinoma or a primary luetic lesion.

INFLAMMATIONS

Acute Mastitis

Acute mastitis usually occurs at the beginning or the end of lactation. It results from insufficient care of the nipple. An infection of the ducts results, with stagnation of milk in one or more lobules. The breast becomes tough and doughy, and the patient complains of dull pain in the region affected. A nipple that is discharging pus, serum or blood demands investigation.

Treatment and Nursing Care

Treatment consists of care of the nipples, the application of icebags, and, twice daily, massage of the engorged lobules. Massage should be toward the nipple, holding the rest of the breast with the other hand.

The milk gradually is expressed from the affected lobules, and the breast then should be supported with a tight binder. Nursing from the affected side should be prohibited, but the breast should be evacuated at regular intervals with a breast pump.

Mammary Abscess

Breast abscess usually develops as a sequela of an acute mastitis, although it may occur independent of lactation. The area affected becomes very tender and dusky red, and pus may be expressed from the nipple. Chemotherapy and antibiotic therapy are being used with success; however, incision and drainage may be indicated. Dressings soaked in hot solution increase the drainage and hasten resolution. The use of the suction cup has proved to be valuable in the treatment of such abscesses.

Chronic Cystic Mastitis

Chronic cystic mastitis is a disease of the breast in which many small cysts are produced, due to an overgrowth of fibrous tissue about the ducts. The disease occurs most commonly between the ages of 30 and 50 and is characterized by an uncomfortable feeling in the breast, the presence of small nodules that feel like tiny lead shot, and, occasionally, by shooting pains.

Any mass in the breast should raise a suspicion of malignancy, and for that reason surgical advice should be obtained. If the disease occurs before the age of 38, when it is important to preserve the function of the breast, the lesion may be kept under close observation for a time, or the larger cysts may be removed for pathologic examination. At times, aspiration of a solitary cyst is justified.

In older women, or in younger women, when any doubt exists as to the diagnosis, it is safer to amputate the entire breast.

TUMORS OF THE BREAST

Paget's Disease

Paget's disease of the nipple is seen most frequently in women over forty, and usually it is unilateral. Most often it begins as a mild eczematoid condition of the nipple that may spread over the areola and even part of the breast; later, it may become ulcerated or eroded. In the more advanced stages, there may be retraction of the nipple. This is a true carcinoma of the ducts of the breast that converge at the nipple.

When any lesion of the nipple is not healed in a few weeks under treatment by simple cleansing and protective measures, a suspicion of Paget's disease should be confirmed by biopsy examination. It demands the same treatment; that is, early and total removal of the mammary gland, as does carcinoma of the mammary gland itself.

Carcinoma

The breast is a most frequent site of development of carcinoma in the female. It is so common that one author states that most tumors of the breast in women over 40 years of age are carcinomatous. Every tumor of the breast should be viewed with suspicion and should be removed unless there is a contraindication.

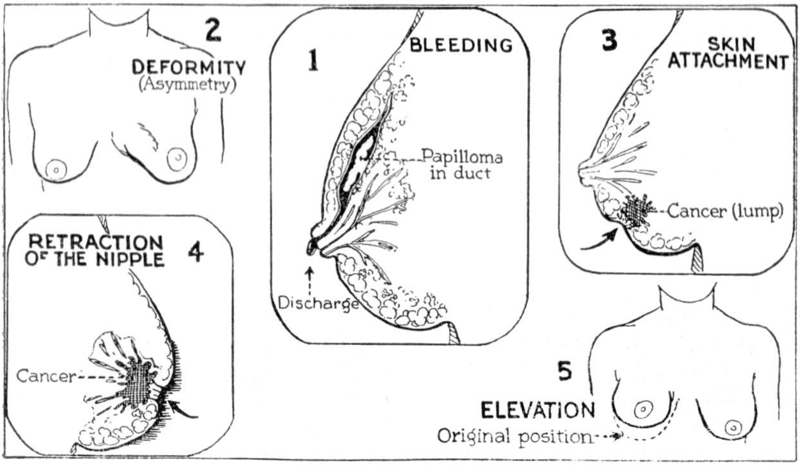

FIG. 182. Signs of cancer of the breast. (1) Bleeding from the nipple arising from a papilloma in the duct. This may be a benign lesion at first but it is definitely considered to be a premalignant lesion. (2) Deformity or asymmetry of the breast. (3) Skin attachment at the site of a malignant mass. (4) Retraction of the nipple when cancer appears at the center of the breast. (5) Elevation of the breast involved due to contraction and shortening of the fibrous tissue trabeculations brought about by the malignant tumor. (American Cancer Society, New York)

Of tumors diagnosed as benign before operation, 10 per cent are found after removal to be cancerous.

Symptoms. The symptoms of the disease, unfortunately, are insidious. The patient finds a non-tender lump in the breast, usually the upper outer quadrant. However, it may be movable. As it grows it becomes attached to the chest wall or to the overlying skin. Pain usually is absent, except in the very late stages. Eventually, a dimpling or "orange peel" skin may be observed. Upon examination in the mirror, the patient may note asymmetry and an elevation of the affected breast. Bleeding from the nipple may be evident, as well as nipple retraction. If no treatment is given, the tumor invades the surrounding tissues and extends to the lymph glands of the adjacent axilla, producing more or less fixation of the breast on the chest wall and nodules in the axilla. Finally, ulceration occurs and cachexia becomes prominent. Metastases may be to lungs, bone, brain or liver. In untreated cases death usually results in two or three years.

Diagnosis and Treatment. Women now are educated to regard any lump appearing in the breast with suspicion. There are numerous benign masses, adenofibroma and cysts, that have no serious implication, but a painless mass appearing in a woman past thirty-five should be looked upon as a carcinoma until this is disproved. In many instances the physician is able to make a positive diagnosis by palpation and inspection, but many times a diagnosis cannot be made with certainty. The only safe method is removal of the mass and microscopic examination. In many cases the examination is made immediately by a technic known as a "frozen section." If a positive diagnosis of cancer is received, a radical removal of the breast is performed while the patient still is under anesthesia. If the tumor is benign, the small wound is sutured and only a small scar results.

The treatment of carcinoma of the breast is removal or destruction of the whole tumor. It is evident that complete removal of the tumor can be accomplished more surely when the cancer still is confined to the breast. This is borne out by clinical experience, which shows a rate of cure of better than 70 per cent if the tumor is confined to the breast. When it has spread to the nodes of the axilla, the cure rate falls to 40 per cent.

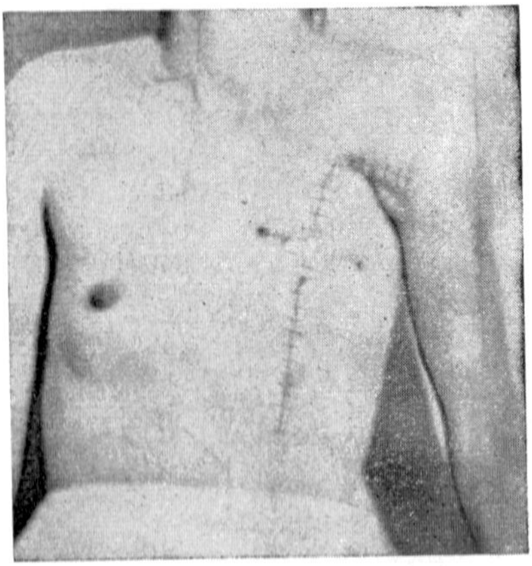

Fig. 183. End result following radical resection for carcinoma of the breast. Note that the breast and the muscles of the chest wall have been removed, so that the skin lies directly upon the chest cage. (Geschickter, C. F.: Diseases of the Breast, Philadelphia, Lippincott)

Surgical removal of the breast and the muscles of the chest wall beneath it, as well as of the lymphatic pathways if the cancer has spread to the axilla, is looked upon as the best method of treatment in operable cases. In a few cases, in which the tumor is inoperable so far as cure is concerned, the surgeon may remove the breast to free the patient from a foul, ulcerating lesion. There are other methods of treatment, however, that are used in addition to surgery or by themselves. X-rays may be used before and after operation. Radium needles may be introduced into the tumor mass in inoperable cases. There is evidence to support the belief that ovarian hormones influence the growth of breast carcinoma. In some instances, surgical or x-ray castration may be performed, especially in menstruating women. Male sex hormone, testosterone, has been found helpful especially in the treatment of bone metastasis. In some cases removal of the adrenal glands has produced regression of the recurrent growth. There is no reason to believe that any of these measures will produce a cure of breast carcinoma, but they may have a palliative effect for a time.

The situation of the patient with

an inoperable cancer of the breast is a most distressing one. It is distressing also to the surgeon, who realizes that there was a time when the tumor was curable, but that the patient through ignorance, neglect or fear appeared for treatment when it was too late. The situation of the inoperable patient also is distressing because the tumor spreads to such areas as the brain, the lungs, the liver and to bone and causes symptoms that are hard to relieve. Pain, cough, ascites, paralyses and fractures are a combination of terminal symptoms for which little can be done. Sedation in increasing doses and sympathetic nursing offer some relief.

The nurse can help greatly. In her contacts she can point out the importance of frequent self-examination of the breasts and of obtaining early medical advice if a mass is found. She can help in the psychological preparation of the patient for breast surgery. She can point out that the breast usually is functionless in most patients with cancer and that loss of the breast as against loss of life is a small price to pay. She may be able to allay the patient's fear of disfigurement by describing artificial appliances that can be used.

The Male Breast

The male breast may be the site of inflammatory or malignant changes, although this is much less common. The same treatment as for corresponding lesions of the female breast is indicated.

Plastic Surgery of the Breast

Hypertrophy, with the production of unilateral or bilateral pendulous breast, not infrequently is the cause of pain and of psychological trauma that bring the patient to the surgeon. Plastic operations have been devised by which much of the hypertrophic tissue is excised and a breast of normal size is produced.

Nursing Care for Breast Operations

Before Operation. One of the responsibilities of every nurse is to know and disseminate information regarding the earliest signs of cancer. Carcinoma of the breast is one type of malignancy that can be detected early because it is accessible to palpation and observation. Every woman should palpate her breasts frequently and examine them carefully before a mirror. Any untoward sign or noticeable change should be sufficient reason for her to seek medical advice. Upon admission to a hospital for a questionable tumor of the breast, most women have a real fear of cancer. Unfortunately, many times this fear has made them delay seeking treatment until the tumor has metastasized. Fear also stems from the emotional trauma of knowing that the breast may be removed. The only delay before operation should be that necessary to check the physical and the nutritional needs of the patient. If radical surgery is anticipated, there may be fluid and blood loss—therefore, blood replacement must be available. The patient is told by the surgeon that there is a possibility of radical surgery if it is indicated. No patient should go to the operating room anticipating a half-inch incision for a tumor excision and return having had a radical mastectomy. Because the emotional factor is a significant one, encouragement and reassurance must be given. A hypnotic is given, and the usual physical preoperative preparation is carried out. Skin preparation should be extensive enough to meet the maximum possible surgery (see p. 58). If it is known that radical surgery, including a skin graft, is to be done, the donor skin area also must be shaved and cleaned. This usually is the anterior aspect of the thigh.

Operation. The dorsal position is used on the operating table, the arm of the affected side being carried upward to expose the axilla. A radical mastectomy comprises removal of the breast and the underlying muscles down to the chest wall after removal of the nodules and the lymphatics of the axilla. Such a radical operation is necessary to remove the tumor and the area of lymphatic spread. Bleeding points are ligated and the skin is closed as well as possible over the chest wall. A drainage tube usually is placed in the axilla. A blood transfusion often is given during the operation to compensate for blood loss.

After Operation. The anesthetic of choice usually is general for a radical mastectomy. Postoperative care is given with special attention to pulse and blood pressure, as they are valuable indices in detecting shock and hemorrhage. Dressings must be inspected for bleeding, especially under the axilla and the area on which the patient is lying.

After the patient has recovered from the anesthesia, sedatives are given for the relief of pain and the patient is encouraged to turn and take deep breaths to avert pulmonary complications. The dressing usually is fairly snug; however, it should not be so tight that lung expansion is restricted. Some surgeons prefer to include the arm (flexed at the elbow) in the dressing to give added pressure. In other instances, gauze fluffs, mechanics' waste or foam rubber sponge may be added to the dressing within the binder to provide pressure. Positioning of the patient depends upon the dressing; semi-Fowler usually is desirable. The arm, if free, may be propped on a pillow. Whether the arm is flexed or extended depends on the orders of the physician. Such elevation, however, helps to prevent lymphedema, which is a common postoperative occurrence due to interference with the circulatory and the lymphatic systems. After 24 hours, the arm on the affected side should have passive exercise. This can be increased each day with the patient doing more herself. By the tenth day she should be able to reach the top of her head and comb her hair. Failure to encourage exercises, such as "climbing the wall with the fingers," may prolong the disuse of the arm and promote the development of a contracture. Exercise should not be accompanied by pain; if the patient has plastic reconstruction or the incision was closed with considerable tension, such exercises will be limited greatly and done very gradually.

The patient usually is allowed out of bed on the second or the third day after operation; often the arm on the affected side is held in a sling for a time to prevent tension on the wound. A normal diet may be given unless nausea is a symptom. If a drainage tube has been inserted, it is

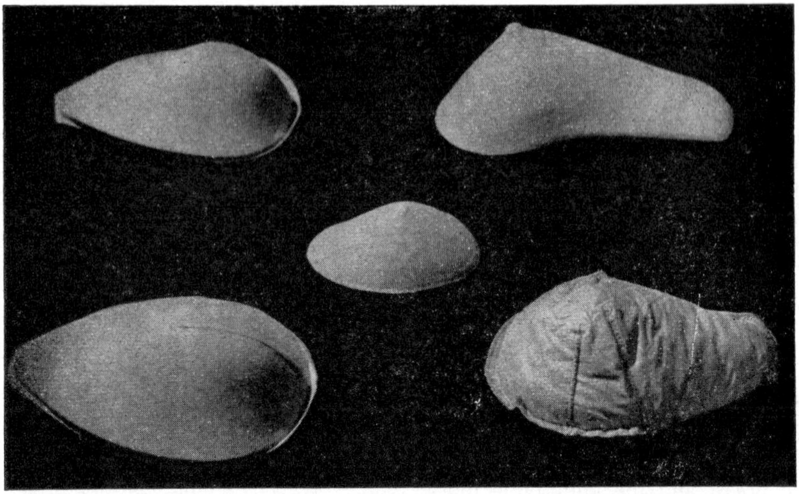

FIG. 184. Various types of prostheses for use after breast amputations. By the use of these appliances, held in place with a suitable brassière, deformity is minimal.

removed usually on the second day. She may be advised to have x-ray treatment after operation to lessen the possibility of recurrence. Anorexia, nausea and vomiting are not infrequent symptoms after irradiation; to abstain from eating and drinking three hours before and after these treatments often helps.

Follow-up care is important in an effort to detect possible recurrences or metastases. When the wound has healed sufficiently the surgeon will give instructions regarding the use of a prosthetic. Easily washed plastic material with a cotton filler can be worn effectively in a comfortable uplift brassière. Plastic air-foam replicas can be made to match the size and the shape of the breast removed. They are inexpensive and easy to clean with soap and water. Another product that is available is a prosthetic made of a plastic film cover and filled partially with a slow-flowing thick fluid. The principle which is followed is that the breasts readily follow the law of gravity and change their contour and position with every body motion. Often, when a patient knows that such appliances are available, her fear of disfigurement is eliminated. No prosthetic should be worn until the physician has authorized it.

The patient who is admitted to the hospital with an inoperable carcinoma of the breast calls for the utmost in sympathy and understanding: her physical and mental comfort is the primary goal. Details of care follow the regimen used in terminal carcinoma of any part of the body.

Psychological Aspects. The woman who has undergone a radical mastectomy cannot help but have innumerable questions. The nurse should convey to her patient that she has time to discuss any problems that may be troubling her. Frequent questions are these: Is it normal to drain so much? Will the swelling of my arm go down? How will my husband react to my deformity? Will I be able to wear a regular bathing suit? Will people be aware that I am a cripple? Will I be able to swim, play tennis or golf, drive a car?

After studying this chapter, the nurse should be able to answer these questions intelligently. Her attitude should not be impersonal; this patient needs someone with whom she can share her troubling thoughts.

A point that should not be overlooked is the preparation of the husband. An example of this need is illustrated by the husband who thought that he was being kind by not looking at his wife, whereas she interpreted his reaction as one of rejection and repulsion. If time had been taken to tell the husband how he might help his wife in making her adjustment, such an experience would have been avoided.

REFERENCES AND SUGGESTED READING

Unit Six: Nursing in Conditions of the Integumentary System (Including the Subcutaneous and Areolar Tissue and the Breasts)

GENERAL

(See also those for Unit One, p. 205)

Emerson, C. P., and Bragdon, J. S.: Essentials of Medicine, ed. 17, pp. 443-504, Philadelphia, Lippincott, 1955.

BREAST

Emerson, C. P., and Bragdon, J. S.: Essentials of Medicine, ed. 17, pp. 498-502, Philadelphia, Lippincott, 1955.

Haagensen, C. D.: Carcinoma of breast, J.A.M.A. **138**:195-205, 1948.

Self-examination of the breasts, Am. J. Nursing **52**:441, 1952.

Seligmann, W.: New breast form for mastectomy patients, Am. J. Surg. **86**:466-467, 1953.

Sugarbaker and Wilfley: Cancer of the breast, Am. J. Nursing **50**:332-335, 1950.

Smith, G. W.: When a breast must be removed, Am. J. Nursing **50**: 335-339. 1950

BURNS

Armistead, N. B.: Preventing deformities following severe burns, Am. J. Nursing **50**:162-163, 1950.

Hirshfeld, J. W.: The treatment of thermal burns, Am. J. Nursing **46**: 158-162, 1946.

Peterson, G. G.: A method of treating burns, Am. J. Nursing **50**:785-786, 1950.

Schwartz, D. R.: Pyruvic acid paste for burns, Am. J. Nursing **48**:283-284, 1948.

CANCER

Clark, R. L., and Maisel, C. J.: Cancer of the skin, Am. J. Nursing **51**: 334-335, 1951.

Emerson, C. P., and Bragdon, J. S.: Essentials of Medicine, ed. 17, pp. 488-495, Philadelphia, Lippincott, 1955.

INFECTIONS AND HAND INJURIES

Hirshfeld, J. W., and Pilling, M. A.: Injuries of the hand, Am. J. Nursing **44**:967-973, 1944.

Wilson, J. D., and Sister Mary: Open injuries of the hand, Am. J. Nursing **52**:1104-1107, 1952.

PLASTIC SURGERY

Hamm, W. G., and Hyde, A. C.: The care of massive injuries to the face, Am. J. Nursing **45**:439-443, 1945.
Ivy, R. H.: Plastic and reconstructive surgery of the face, mouth, and jaws, *in* Nelson's Loose Leaf Surgery, vol. 2, pp. 679-722A.
Pearlman, L. M.: Plastic surgery, Am. J. Nursing **51**:618-620, 1951.

CLINICAL SITUATION: RADICAL MASTECTOMY

Annette Lawrence fidgeted as she sat with several other women at the club meeting watching the movie, "Breast Self-examination." As soon as she got home, she went to her bedroom and carefully examined her breasts. The results prompted her to see her physician, who recommended a biopsy. An early carcinoma was noted, and Annette gave permission for a radical mastectomy.

1. In the self-examination of the right breast done in the dorsal position, a flat pillow or a folded towel should be placed under the
_____(1) head
_____(2) left shoulder
_____(3) right shoulder

2. Annette was worried about the possibility of losing the complete function of her right arm postoperatively. The nurse can reassure her by saying
_____(1) "Function can be regained by a series of graduated exercises."
_____(2) "It is useless to worry, for loss of function is inevitable."
_____(3) "Use of the arm will come back of its own accord."

3. The area of skin to be prepared for a breast biopsy on Annette is
_____(1) the front and the back upper trunk past the mid-line
_____(2) the entire right breast
_____(3) the right breast, the neck to the umbilicus, the right axilla to the left nipple

4. In a radical mastectomy
_____(1) only the involved tumor is removed
_____(2) the breast, the underlying muscles and the axillary lymphatics are removed
_____(3) all the tissue identified as breast tissue is removed

5. Dressings must be inspected for bleeding, especially
_____(1) near the nipple site
_____(2) under the axilla
_____(3) at the anterior mid-line cleft

6. Follow-up care for Annette is
_____(1) unnecessary, since radical surgery has been performed
_____(2) optional, depending upon Annette's emotional make-up and her reaction to treatment thus far
_____(3) imperative, for metastasis is possible

UNIT SEVEN

Nursing in Conditions of the Eye and the Ear

CHAPTER TWENTY-ONE

Surgery of the Eye

INTRODUCTION

The eye is such an important organ that its care and protection are a major consideration. Care begins at birth and is continued throughout life because, with advancing age and conditions of life, changes occur in the eye, and these can be corrected in various ways. The recognition of the importance of eye care is extending to industry. Protective devices now are a necessity in industrial procedures in which there is danger of injury from foreign bodies, dust and so forth. The importance of adequate and well-placed light in preventing eyestrain is essentially no longer a medical problem but one of general and social interest.

The National Society for the Prevention of Blindness and other medical groups have been responsible for the dissemination of invaluable pamphlets on eye care. It is important for the nurse to become familiar with them so that she may offer sound advice when confronted with such questions by the patient as the following: Will watching television damage my eyes? Are tinted glasses helpful for night driving? What kind of sun glasses are safe to wear? The nurse needs to practice the principles of good eye health in her care of all patients, not only of those with eye disorders.

The care of the eye is undertaken by three groups of specialists:

1. The *optician* usually not a physician, whose concern it is to

grind, mount and dispense lenses.

2. The *optometrist,* who is licensed to examine for refractive errors in the eye by mechanical means and to provide appropriate corrective lenses. He may not be a physician, and he does not use drugs in the examination of the eyes.

3. The *oculist,* the *ophthalmologist* or the *ophthalmic physician,* who is skilled in the treatment of all diseases of the eye. Because of training and experience, he is able to make a more thorough and complete examination of the eye for refractive errors and other changes.

ANATOMY AND PHYSIOLOGY

Anatomy

The eyeball is a spherical organ situated in a bony cavity called the *orbit.* It is rotated easily in all the necessary directions by six muscles attached to its outer surface. For the purpose of study, the eyeball may be divided into 3 coats or tunics.

The dense white fibrous outer coat is called the *sclera.* Anteriorly it becomes continuous with the *cornea,* the translucent structure that bulges forward slightly from the general contour of the eye. Posteriorly, there is an opening through which the optic nerve passes into the eyeball. The nerve spreads out over the posterior two-thirds of the inner surface of the globe in a thin layer called the *retina.* In it are situated the tiny nerve endings. These, when properly stimulated, transmit visual impulses to the brain which are interpreted as sight.

Between the sclera and the retina is the pigmented middle coat known as the *uveal tract.* This tract is composed of three parts. The posterior part, the *choroid,* contains most of the blood vessels that nourish the eye. The anterior part is a pigmented muscular organ, the *iris.* It gives the characteristic color to the eye (blue, brown and so forth). The circular opening at its center, the *pupil,* is made smaller or larger, according to the intensity of the light, by its two sets of muscle fibers. The circular fibers by their contraction constrict the pupil; the radial fibers enlarge it. Between the iris and the choroid is the third portion of the uveal tract, a muscular body known as the *ciliary body.* It is composed of radial processes, the ciliary processes arising from a triangular-shaped muscle (ciliary muscle). Between these processes and to them are attached delicate ligaments that pass centrally and become inserted in the capsule of the crystalline lens.

The *lens* is a semisolid body enclosed in a transparent elastic capsule. It is capable of being modified to varying degrees of convexity by the contraction and the relaxation of the ciliary muscle, thus changing the focus of the eye as it looks from one object to another.

The cavity within the eye is divided by the lens into two parts. The posterior part contains a jelly-like translucent substance called the *vitreous humor,* which is the chief factor in maintaining the form of the eyeball. The anterior part contains a clear, watery fluid, the *aqueous humor,* which is secreted by the ciliary processes. It bathes the anterior surface of the lens, escapes at the pupil and enters the space between the iris and the cornea known as the *anterior chamber.* Finally it is

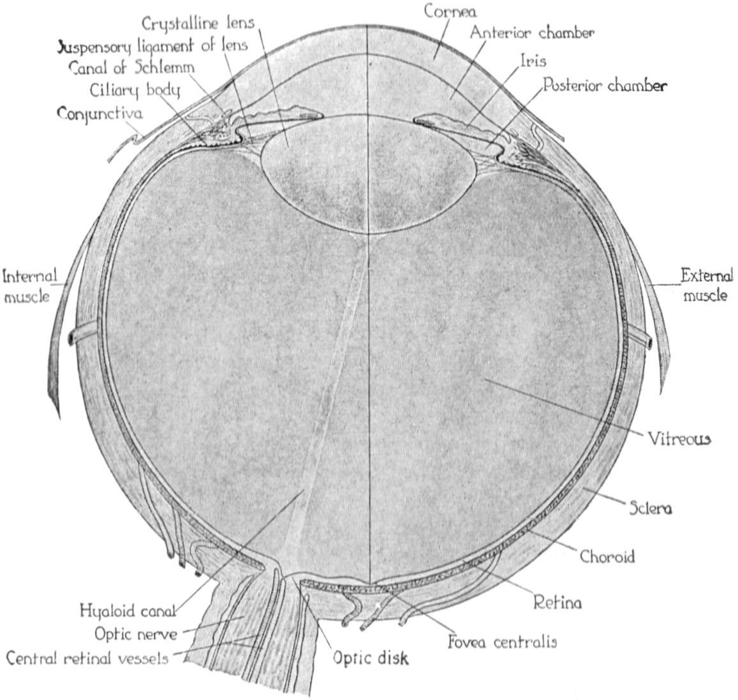

FIG. 185. Diagrammatic horizontal section of right eye (× 3½). (Piersol, G.: Human Anatomy, Philadelphia, Lippincott)

drained from the eye through lymph channels (the canal of Schlemm) located at the junction of the iris and the sclera.

Appendages. The eyelids are the protective coverings of the eye. Lining the lids and entirely covering the anterior part of the eye is a highly sensitive membrane, the *conjunctiva,* the surface of which is kept moist by a constant flow of lacrimal fluid (tears). This fluid is excreted from the lacrimal gland, which is located in the upper and outer part of the orbit. It flows downward and inward across the eye and drains into tiny channels (lacrimal punctae). By these channels it is conducted to the lacrimal sac and duct, which pass downward, backward and outward and open into the nasal cavity beneath the inferior turbinate bone.

Physiology

Vision is made possible by the passage of rays of light from an object through the cornea, the aqueous humor, the lens and the vitreous humor to the retina. In the normal eye, rays coming from an object 6 meters distant will be brought to a focus on the retina by the lens while perfectly at rest. If, under the same conditions, the rays of light are brought to a focus in front of the retina, the condition is spoken of as *myopia*, or nearsightedness, and *hyperopia* (farsightedness) is the condition in which the rays are focused behind the retina. In such conditions glass lenses are prescribed. These, in association with the lenses of the eye, will correct the fault and restore a normal focus at the retina.

Rays from objects situated at shorter distances (less than 6 meters) require a "stronger" lens to focus them on the retina. This is brought about by a contraction of the ciliary muscle that relaxes the lens capsule and causes the lens to become more convex. This function is called *accommodation*, and by its means objects at different distances from the eye can be seen distinctly. As age approaches, the elasticity of the lens decreases, and accommodation for near vision is not complete. It is common to see older people reading with the paper held at arm's length, an example of this condition, which is called *presbyopia*. Lenses may be given these patients that enable them to focus rays from near objects on the retina—"reading glasses."

Astigmatism results from uneven curvature of the cornea so that, instead of the curve being equal in all directions, it is shaped somewhat like the bowl of a spoon. Two foci thus are given the eye instead of one and, as a consequence, the patient is unable to focus horizontal and vertical rays on the retina at the same time. These defects also may be corrected with appropriate lenses.

The drug atropine paralyzes the nerve endings that function in accommodation, and for this reason "drops" of this drug or homatropine, a short-acting derivative, are placed in the eye before an examination for "glasses." The ophthalmologist thus is able to ascertain the function of the eye with the lens completely at rest.

EXAMINATIONS AND DIAGNOSTIC PROCEDURES

The eye is an organ that can be examined with relative ease both as to its function and its structure. In its functional examinations are included its ability to move in its orbit and the reaction of the pupil to light and accommodation.

The usual function of the eye is tested in several ways. The patient may be asked to identify illuminated letters or objects of varying sizes on what is known as the Snellen chart. Usually each eye is tested alone. Letters or objects are of the size that can be seen by the normal eye at a distance of 20 feet from the chart. Rows of letters of larger sizes are designated as 30, 40 and so on. These really are letters of a size that should be seen by the normal eye at distances of 30 feet, 40 feet and so on. When an eye can identify letters of size 20 at 20 feet, the eye is said to have 20/20 vision. If it can identify only the letters of the number 40 line, it is said to have 20/40 vision. The visual fields are spot tested by a perimeter, an instrument that tests the lateral vision with the eye fixed at a central point. Tests for color vision are made by having the patient identify various colors of wool yarn or figures or letters that can be seen only if the patient can identify colors in a color plate.

Examination of the structural part of the eye may be made in several ways. Tension within the eyeball is measured by a tonometer. In certain diseases, especially glaucoma, the tension in the eyeball is increased markedly. (Normal tension is 14 to 28/mm.) The surface of the eyeball and the conjunctiva may be more closely inspected by the magnifying loupe. This also is used in the search for the removal of foreign bodies. The slit-lamp is an instrument that projects a beam of light through the pupil for the purpose of detecting opacities in the various media of the eye. With the ophthalmoscope, a small beam of light is reflected through the pupil and, through a small opening in the mirror, the examiner may view the interior of the eye. The instrument is fitted with a series of lenses that permit measurements of structural changes. Thus, in certain diseases of the brain, the optic nerve may be pushed forward into the eyeball. This is spoken of as *choking of the disk* and, by means of the lenses in the ophthalmoscope, the amount of choking may be estimated and described in diopters; for example, choked disk of 3 diopters. In addition, the blood vessels of the interior of the eye may be visualized and, since this is the only area in the body in which blood vessels can be observed by direct vision, it is an important source of information, not only in diseases of the eye, but also in many systemic conditions; for example, hypertension.

A more recently devised type of diagnostic examination is the *gonioscopy*. By means of a contact glass and a magnifying device, the angle of the anterior chamber may be seen. Such visualization is desirable in congestion, inflammation, tumors, cysts, trauma, glaucoma and congenital anomalies.

Refraction

The normal eye, by reason of its lens apparatus and the cornea, is able to refract parallel rays of light so that they focus on the retina. By this mechanism, we are able to see. Due to abnormalities in the eye structure or in the lens structure, defective vision may occur because objects are not focused correctly on the retina.

By various examinations and tests with trial lenses, the ophthalmologist can determine the strength and the type of lens that will overcome the refractive error. In the case of presbyopia, two different types of lenses may be used—bifocals—one for far distance and one for near vision and reading. Most lenses are prescribed for use in "glasses," but in some cases this may be avoided by the application of a lens directly to the surface of the eye (contact lens).

DRUGS USED FREQUENTLY IN EYE DISEASES

In caring for ophthalmic patients nurses are advised to wash their hands before and after the instillation of drops. To carry any of the solutions to their own eyes would cause serious inconvenience.

Adrenalin Chloride. This drug is used in solutions of 1:1,000 as an astringent and hemostatic. It is of use in preventing hemorrhage during slight operations on the eye, in contracting the blood vessels in inflammatory conditions of the eye and in increasing the rapidity of action of certain other drugs; for example, atropine in iritis.

Adrenalin chloride should be kept in dark bottles, as it undergoes changes when exposed to the light.

Dionin, 1 to 5 per cent solution, is a drug used in the treatment of diseases of the cornea and the ciliary body and in glaucoma. The instillation of the drug causes at first a smarting sensation and redness of the conjunctiva. This "Dionin reaction" lasts for only a short time and is followed by relief of pain. If the drug is given over a long period of time, an immunity develops and stronger solutions must be used or the drug must be discontinued for a time.

Fluorescein Solution. This is a yellowish-green fluid that is used to detect corneal abrasions and ulcers. One drop of the solution is placed in the eye and is followed by an irrigation with normal saline solution. The corneal injury then appears stained a bright green. The surgeon thus is enabled to locate the site of the injury and estimate its exact extent. It is used most often as a 2 per cent solution in a 3 per cent solution of sodium bicarbonate.

Sulfonamides. The various sulfa derivatives may be used in inflammatory diseases of the eye orally, parenterally and locally. Applied locally they may be used in powder form, in a solution of the sodium salts or in an ointment base. The indication for their use is the establishment of the presence of organisms against which the sulfonamides are effective.

Antibiotics. Penicillin is an antibacterial agent that is effective both locally and parenterally. It has been used in eyes and found to be dramatically effective for both superficial and intra-ocular infections, particularly those caused by gram-positive cocci. It has been found to be promising in the treatment of interstitial keratitis, as well as other forms of syphilis. The eye tolerates easily a solution containing from 1,000 to 2,000 units per cubic centimeter.

Bacitracin ointment and neomycin ointment have been found effective in specific infections of the eye.

Drugs Used for Antiseptic Action

Argyrol. Argyrol (silver proteinate), a combination of albumin and silver, often is used in solutions of from 5 to 10 per cent as a soothing antiseptic in all forms of conjunctivitis.

Protargol. Protargol, a combination of silver with alum, combines the antiseptic action of the silver with the astringent action of alum. It is used in all forms of discharging conjunctivitis in from 5 to 10 per cent solutions.

Silver Nitrate. Silver nitrate, in from 1 to 3 per cent solutions, is used as an astringent and antiseptic in acute contagious diseases of the eye, especially those due to the gonococcus. As a rule, it is brushed directly on the everted lids after irrigation. A second irrigation of physiologic saline should follow this application to lessen the pain and the irritation caused by the drug. Silver nitrate solutions must be kept in dark bottles because of the rapid decomposition caused by the access of light.

Boric Acid. Boric acid is used in a

per cent solution as a mildly anti-ptic, nonirritating lotion. For irri-ıting the eyes, the solution should ɜ warmed. The use of boric acid ash is being viewed with suspicion y some writers, who report ill fects.

Bichloride of Mercury. Bichloride mercury in 1:10,000 solution is ften used as an irrigating fluid.

Yellow Oxide of Mercury. This rug, from 1 to 2 per cent, long has een used in the form of an oint-ıent in the treatment of eye affec-ons, especially affections of the lid argins (blepharitis).

Penicillin G Potassium Ointment. ach gram of this ointment contains om 200 to 2,500 units of penicillin. Iany physicians believe that peni-illin should be used only for serious ıfections because of the possibility f developing sensitivity to it.

Drugs That Dilate the Pupil (Mydriatics) and Paralyze Accommodation (Cycloplegics)

Atropine Sulfate. Atropine sulfate, n from 0.5 to 2 per cent solutions, robably is used more commonly han any other drug in ophthalmol-gy. It is used in the treatment of nflammatory diseases of the uveal ract (iritis and cyclitis) and the ornea, to rest the iris and the ciliary ody, and to prevent adhesions of he iris to the lens (posterior syne-hia). In refraction of the eyes it ets the lens at rest by causing pa-alysis of accommodation. Its effects ısually are complete in half an hour nd last from 7 to 10 days. During his time the pupil is unable to con-ract; therefore, the eyes should be protected from bright lights by the vearing of dark glasses, and no attempt should be made to use the eyes because accommodation for near vision cannot take place.

Toxic symptoms sometimes appear after the use of atropine in the eyes. Swelling of the lids, dryness of the mouth and the throat with difficulty in swallowing, dizziness, flushed skin with pallor round the mouth, rapid full pulse, restlessness and, at times, delirium are symptoms that should warn the nurse of atropine poisoning. The administration of the drug must be discontinued until the surgeon can be notified. The use of atropine is contraindicated absolutely in cases of primary glaucoma and in most cases of conjunctival affections.

Homatropine Hydrobromide. This drug, in solutions of from 1 to 2 per cent, acts as a weak atropine. It dilates the pupil and paralyzes accommodation more quickly, but its effects disappear within 24 to 48 hours. Its short-lived action makes it useful for examination of the eye for glasses or of the retina with the ophthalmoscope.

Euphthalmine Hydrochloride. This drug, in 5 per cent solution, is used in examinations of the eye. Its action is short-lived and it has the advantage of dilating the pupil without affecting accommodation.

Drugs Used to Contract Pupil (Myotics)

Eserine Sulfate. Eserine sulfate, in solutions of from 0.25 to 1 per cent, is much used in diseases of the eye caused by increased tension within the eyeball (glaucoma). By the contraction of the pupil caused by the drug, the aqueous humor is permitted to escape more easily into the lymph channels, which drain it from the eye. Eserine also is used in preventing prolapse of the iris after wounds of the cornea. Its action is rapid and lasts from five to eight hours. This drug must be kept in dark bottles. Exposure to light causes it to turn pink or red and, although in this form it retains its original properties, it is much more irritating than a clear, fresh solution would be.

Pilocarpine Hydrobromate. This drug, in from 0.5 to 1 per cent solutions, acts in the same manner as eserine, but its action is less powerful.

Drugs Used to Produce Anesthesia

Cocaine. Cocaine is employed in 2 and 4 per cent solutions to produce anesthesia of the conjunctiva for short operations on the eye. It may be instilled with a sterile pipet—one drop every 3 minutes to a total of 4 drops in the eye to be operated upon. Besides producing a loss of sensation, it causes a contraction of the capillaries and dilates the pupils. When instilled into the eye the patient often experiences a smarting sensation, but this may be avoided in large measure by dropping the solution on the everted lower lid while the patient is looking upward. Both eyes should be kept closed after the instillation of each drop. For deeper anesthesia, from 1 to 2 cc. is injected into the conjunctiva with a 2-cc. syringe and a 23-gauge needle.

Holocaine. This drug is used in from 1 to 2 per cent solutions. Its anesthetic action is rapid and without any effect on the pupil. It is especially useful in operations for glaucoma and in the removal of foreign bodies from the cornea.

Procaine. Procaine, in 1 and 2 per cent solutions, also is used by injection for lid anesthesia, as well as for the O'Brien facial nerve block and the Van Lint block.

Pontocaine. This drug, a brand of tetracaine hydrochloride, in 0.5 and 1 per cent solutions, is at present one of the most popular drugs used for surface anesthesia. The aqueous solution is unaffected by prolonged boiling and can be sterilized easily this way. It exhibits a higher efficiency than cocaine solutions of corresponding strength, usually it is unattended by irritation or tissue injury, and it does not exert any effect upon the blood vessels. It is less likely than cocaine to affect the corneal epithelium, and it does not dilate the pupil, disturb accommodation or increase intra-ocular pressure. The stronger concentrations may produce a sensation of burning. This, however, is transient. It is valuable not only for operations but as an anesthetic for removing sutures and relieving tension and other painful procedures, such as the discomfort after the removal of a foreign body from the eye.

Nursing Care of Ophthalmic Patients

The mental anxiety frequently experienced by the ophthalmic patient requires as much consideration as does his physical condition. When permissible, the nurse should use such means as the radio and occupational therapy to keep the patient's mind occupied. She should not be oversolicitous, but she should show interest, sympathy and understanding. Because of differences of personality, her tactics to overcome mental anxiety will vary. When per-

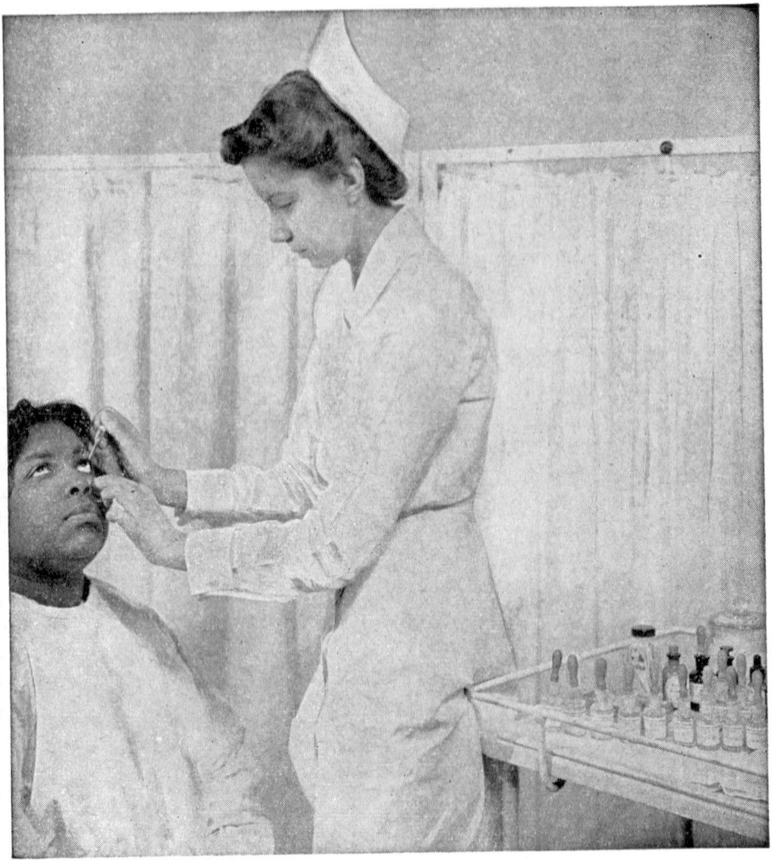

FIG. 186. Instilling drug into the eye. Note that the nurse, in using the dropper, rests her right hand against the patient's forehead and with her left hand depresses the lower lid. The eyedropper is held directly above the sulcus, between the lower lid and the eyeball. Note eye tray with solutions marked plainly and an individual dropper for each bottle.

manent blindness is apparent, reeducation may be done by others so afflicted or by people specially trained for this. In this way the process of development of a well-adjusted individual will be hastened.

The daily care of ophthalmic patients should be the same as for other bed or ambulatory patients. The patient should be assisted as much as possible; at the same time, he should be encouraged to help himself so that he will not feel that he is a burden. A patient who cannot see should be fed; or, if he is accustomed to feeding himself, he should be supervised. Proper elimination should be promoted by cathartics or enemas, as ordered. Ambulatory patients should have a daily rest period in the afternoon.

Ophthalmic patients should not read, smoke or shave unless given permission by the surgeon. They must be cautioned against rubbing their eyes or wiping them with a soiled handkerchief. All patients receiving atropine should wear dark glasses.

Light. As light causes pain in many cases of disease of the eye, and as the eyes should be rested as much as possible before and after undergoing operation, it is well to treat the ophthalmic patient in a darkened room. Dimmed artificial lights may be used by the nurse for her own needs.

Eyedrops. Solutions of various drugs are employed in the treatment of nearly every kind of eye disease. The administration of these drops often is the duty of the nurse. Therefore, it is important that she familiarize herself with the proper method of procedure.

Before instilling drops the nurse must be absolutely sure that she has the prescribed solution of the proper drug. Some drugs (for example, atropine and eserine) act in exactly opposite ways (see above). Therefore, if one of these drugs is indicated in the treatment of a certain eye disease, the other is contraindicated. It may seem needless to emphasize this warning, but experience has taught how easy it is in a dimly lighted room to pick up the wrong bottle from a tray containing similar vials.

After making sure that she has the prescribed drug, the nurse should inspect the solution for changes in color or sedimentation. These sigr are evidences of decomposition, anc if present, the solution should be di carded and a fresh one ordered an sterilized for use.

An eyedropper usually is en ployed for the instillation of drop This instrument is composed of glass pipet fitted with a small rul ber bulb. The glass part is washe and sterilized easily, but the rubbe undergoes gradual deterioration, an for this reason only a small amour of solution should be drawn into th pipet. The dropper never should b inverted or filled too full, as the is risk of contaminating the solutio by contact with the rubber bulb. A excess of solution remaining after in stilling the drops should be discarde because of the risk of contaminatio if it is returned to the bottle.

Procedure for Instilling Eye drops. When instilling drops int eye, the head of the patient shoul be tilted backward and incline slightly to the side so that the solu tion will run away from the tea duct. This latter precaution is es pecially necessary when poisonou solutions such as atropine are em ployed, because absorption of th excess drug via the nose and th pharynx may lead to toxic symp toms. In most cases it is well to pres the inner angle of the eye after in stilling the drops to prevent th excess of the solution from enterin the nose. The lower lid is depresse with the fingers of the left hand, th patient is told to look upward, an the solution is dropped on th everted lower lid. Care must b taken that the pipet does not touc any part of the eye or the lids t guard against contamination of th

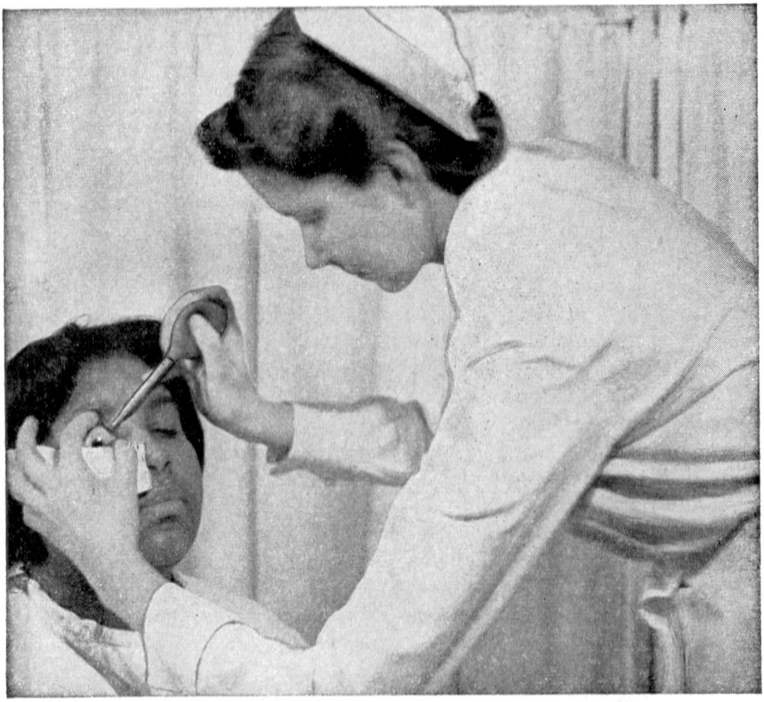

FIG. 187. Eye irrigation with rubber syringe and glass tip. This technic now is used more often than the older undine method.

dropper and injury to the parts. After placing the drops (1 or 2 at most) in the eye, the lid is released and any excess of fluid is sponged gently from the lids and the cheeks with sterile cotton.

After using the dropper, if contamination has been avoided, it may be replaced in the bottle, but in no circumstances should it be used for other solutions until after it has been cleansed thoroughly.

To instill drops in the eyes of children often is a difficult procedure. Two methods are employed commonly. If there is no discharge, the child may be placed flat on his back in bed and, while the eyes are closed, the prescribed drop may be placed at the inner corner of the eye. As soon as the lids are opened, the fluid enters the eye. The second method requires two persons, who sit facing each other. The child is placed across their laps so that the head can be held between the knees. The lids can be opened easily, forcibly if necessary, and the drops are instilled.

In the older patient, it will help the nurse to remember that he is often likely to jump or grab the nurse's hand; therefore, precautions are necessary. After the medication is instilled, the nurse can tell her patient to close his eyes gently; this patient often has a tendency to "squeeze" his eyes closed, thereby expelling the medication.

Ocular Irrigations. Ocular irrigations are indicated in various forms of inflammation of the conjunctiva, in the preparation of the eye for operation and in the removal of inflammatory secretions. Also, they are used for their antiseptic effect. The fluid to be employed depends upon the condition present, but the solutions in most common use are: boric acid from 2 to 4 per cent, physiologic sodium chloride solution, bichloride of mercury 1:10,000, Mercurophen 1:8,000, and occasionally, in purulent cases, potassium permanganate 1:5,000. They should be warmed before using.

The irrigating apparatus is simple, consisting of a sterile eyedropper, an irrigating syringe or an undine, a bottle of warmed fluid and a small curved basin and cotton for catching the fluid and the secretions.

The patient should be flat on his back or sitting with the head tilted backward and inclined slightly toward the side to be treated. The basin may be held by the patient, if sitting, or so placed that when he is lying down it will catch the fluid as it runs from the eye. The nurse stands in front of the patient, in order that she may see exactly what she is doing.

After carefully cleansing the lids of dust, secretions and crusts, she holds them open with the thumb and the fingers of one hand, and with the other hand she flushes the eye gently, directing the stream away from the nose. The fluid never should be directed toward the nose because of the danger of spilling over into the other eye. The procedure should be continued until the eye is entirely free of secretions. It must be remembered that very little force should be used because of the danger of injury. For the same reason and to prevent contamination, no part of the irrigator should touch the eye, the lids or the lashes. When the irrigation has been completed, the eye and the cheek should be dried gently with cotton.

Hot Compresses. Heat relieves pain and increases the circulation, thereby promoting absorption and reducing tension in the eye. It is especially valuable for the deep-seated inflammations of the eyeball, iritis, acute glaucoma and so forth, as well as for such superficial ones as keratitis and conjunctivitis. It is best applied in the form of compresses of 7 or 8 thicknesses of gauze or cotton, just large enough to cover the eye.

The patient is moved to the side of the bed and a towel is used to cover the chest. The skin of the lids and the adjacent cheek may be anointed with cold cream or petrolatum. The compresses then are moistened in a basin of water or any other prescribed solution that has been heated by an electric hot plate placed on a table beside the bed. The fluid, which should be kept at a temperature of between 115° and 120° F., should be expressed from the pad and, after being tested for temperature on the back of the hand, the compress is placed gently over the closed lids. The pads should be changed every 30 to 60 seconds for 10 or 15 minutes, and the application should be repeated every 2 or 3 hours. At the completion of the period of application, the lids should be dried gently with cotton. New pads should be used for each application and, if the eyes have a purulent secretion, the compresses should be applied to one eye at a time, the solution and the basin being changed between applications in order not to carry infection from one eye to the other.

Cold Compresses. Cold causes a capillary constriction that tends to reduce the amount of secretion and relieve pain during the early stages of acute inflammatory conditions of the conjunctiva. It is indicated also in the treatment of injuries or after operations on the eye, as it tends to reduce swelling and to retard bacterial growth.

The patient is prepared in the same manner as for the application of hot compresses. The pads are moistened in boric acid solution and placed in rows on a block of ice suspended by a gauze sling over a basin. They are applied to the closed lids and are changed every 15 to 30 seconds. The duration of the application usually is from 5 to 15 minutes each hour. Cold compresses never are used in the treatment of deep-seated inflammations of the eye (iritis, keratitis) because cold, by constricting the capillaries, interferes with the nutrition of the cornea.

Leeching. Leeches have been used for centuries to remove blood from congested parts. Practically their only use in present-day surgery is the treatment of inflammations of the iris and the ciliary body. Then the tension in the congested vessels and irritation of the nerves may be relieved largely by local bloodletting.

The artificial leech, consisting of a scarifying instrument and a piston suction syringe, has replaced largely the live leech. A local injection of procaine is given, the skin is disinfected again, and dried carefully and the skin surface is scarified so as to draw blood about an inch from the angle of the orbit. The leech is applied, suction being made by carefully keeping out all air. The thumbscrew is tightened as the piston is withdrawn slowly. The barrel is filled almost full of blood if possible. The thumbscrew is released and the leech is removed. The skin is scrubbed with alcohol and a sterile dressing is applied to the area. The leech should be cleaned in cold water, sterilized in 70 per cent alcohol and, when not in use, kept dry in a sterile towel with the barrel and the plunger separate.

Ointments. Ointments of various kinds are used frequently in the treatment of inflammatory diseases of the lids, the conjunctiva and the cornea. Those ordered most commonly are boric acid, penicillin, sulfonamides, bacitracin, neomycin, zinc oxide, bichloride of mercury, yellow oxide of mercury and pontocaine ointments. These are applied best with a bit of cotton wound around a toothpick. The lower lid should be everted and a small amount of the ointment transferred from the applicator to the conjunctiva of the lower lid. The lid then is massaged gently in such a way as to distribute the drug over the eyeball.

Preoperative Nursing Care. The

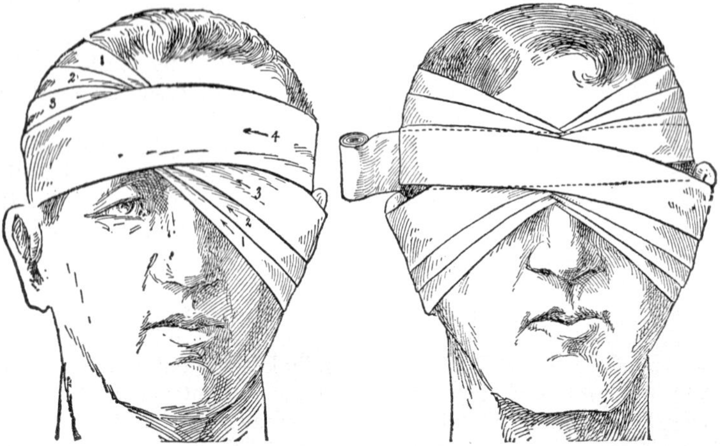

FIG. 188. Crossed bandages of (*left*) one eye and (*right*) both eyes.

preparation of the patient for ophthalmic operation must be carried out with the most scrupulous care. The lower bowel is evacuated in the morning of the day of operation, and only liquid diet is given after that.

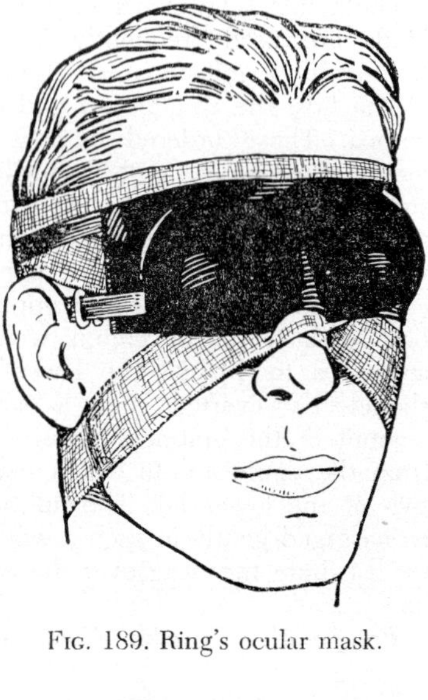

FIG. 189. Ring's ocular mask.

The hair of female patients shoul be so arranged that it will remain i place for several days, and band ages may be applied over it. Usuall it is recommended that long hair b plaited into two braids that may b pinned up over the head. Befor preparing the eyes for operation, th heads of all patients should be cov ered with a stockinet cap. The mal patient should have his face shaved The eyebrow above the eye to b operated upon is shaved only in spe cial cases ordered by the surgeon The eyelashes of the eye to underg operation are cut with blunt scissor covered with petrolatum in order t catch the lashes. Both eyelids, th nose, the forehead and the cheek are scrubbed thoroughly with gree soap and then are rinsed with salin solution; sterile cotton sponges an forceps are used. After this proce dure both eyes are irrigated with per cent saline solution, followed b drops of an antiseptic or antibioti solution into the eye to be operate

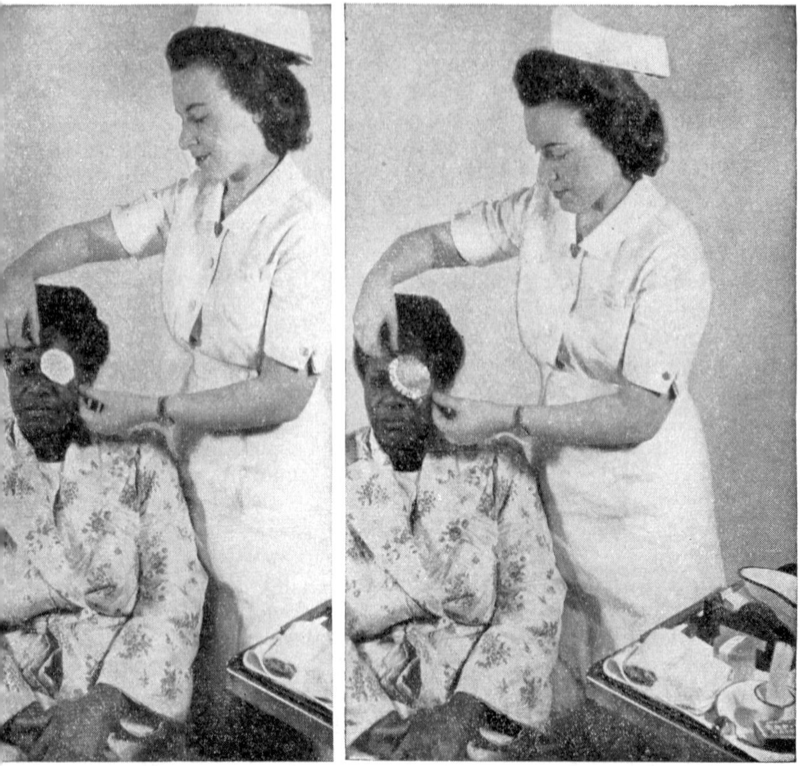

FIG. 190. (*Left*) Application of eye dressing, using Scotch tape. (*Right*) Application of metal eye shield.

pon. This varies in different clinics. small cross mark then is made with colored solution on the forehead ver the eye to be operated upon. oth closed eyes then are covered ith eye patches wet with boric acid olution, and the eyes and the forehead are protected with sterile gauze ressings bound in place with a 2-ich bandage. In the preparation of atients for operations on the eye, o adhesive should be used on the kin.

Before the patient is taken to the perating room, precautions as to the removal of glass eyes, false teeth and so forth must be taken. These are the same as those described for any other surgical operation. If the patient is to have local anesthesia, he should be instructed to hold his head still and to look up or down as directed by the surgeon. He should be cautioned not to "squeeze" the eye during or after operation.

Postoperative Nursing Care

After operation the patient is returned to bed to lie in the supine position with a small pillow under the head. Sandbags may be used under the pillow on each side of the head to keep the head quiet. Where possible, the patient should have a call bell and should be instructed to ring when necessary rather than to move or strain in an attempt to be self-sufficient. Inasmuch as the patient often has both eyes covered, it is well for any personnel who enter his unit to announce himself. The application of bed sides to the bed of a patient with bandaged eyes frequently gives him a sense of security.

The surgeon should be notified immediately if the patient is restless, if he coughs, turns, develops a rhinitis, has excessive pains or disturbs the dressing.

The mouth should be swabbed twice daily, but the teeth should not be brushed until permission is given by the surgeon. Female patients should not have their hair combed until they are allowed out of bed. When the patient complains of abdominal discomfort due to gas, a hot-water bottle to the abdomen and the insertion of a rectal tube often give relief. Catheterization may be necessary when there is difficulty in voiding. Morphine never should be given to ophthalmic patients unless it is certain that vomiting will not injure the eye.

The eye dressing tray should contain:

Sterile cotton squares in sterile container
Sterile saline in jar with irrigator and cover
Sterile applicators
Small crescent basin
Atropine solution 1 per cent } sterile, with medicine droppers
Pontocaine solution 1 per cent } sterile, with medicine droppers
Sulfonamides and/or penicillin i solution or ointment as desired b the physician
Sterile eye patches
Bichloride of mercury ointment
Scotch cellulose tape—½ in. wide, wit dispenser
Bandage scissors
Hand lens

As indicated in the preoperativ care of these patients, diversional o recreational therapy is importan This should be of such a nature tha the eyes are not fatigued in any way Even the environment of this patien is an important consideration. Th walls and the ceiling should b painted in soft pastel shades. Ligh should be regulated so that it is no bright and does not produce a glare

Before the patient leaves the hos pital, he must be informed thor oughly by the physician regardin medications, eye aids ("glasses") the type of work he can do and hi follow-up visits.

TRAUMA TO THE EYE

Foreign Bodies. Foreign bodie (dust, cinders and so forth) fre quently cause considerable discom fort, due to irritation of the sensitiv conjunctiva. If the body has been i the eye only a short time, it ma often be removed by a nurse. Th lower lid should be everted, the pa tient instructed to look up and th lower half of the conjunctival sa examined. If the body is not found he upper eye should be examined y everting the upper lid.

In examining the upper eye, the urse stands in front of the patient nd instructs him to look down at is feet. She then takes the lashes etween thumb and fingers of one and and with the other places a natchstick, an applicator or a toothick across the upper part of the id. The lashes are pulled downward nd forward away from the eye as he applicator is pressed downward ently. The foreign body may be emoved by touching it gently with small applicator wound with cotton nd moistened in saline solution.

If removal by this method is unuccessful, or if the offending particle as been in the eye for a considerble period of time, the nurse should ot attempt to remove it. It may ave become embedded in the corea and there is considerable danger f serious injury if removal is atempted by unskilled hands. The urgeon usually requires Holocaine, hand lens, fluorescein, an eye spud, ormal saline for irrigating the eye nd penicillin solution to instill after emoval of the offending particle as prophylaxis against infection. If the ffending foreign body is known to e a metal, the doctor may use a nagnet to remove it.

Hematoma ("Black Eye"). Hemrrhage into the orbit from trauma a frequent occurrence. The bleedng that takes place into the loose issues of the orbit spreads rapidly nd produces a discoloration of lids nd surrounding skin. In itself the njury is not too serious, but frequently it is frightening to patients ecause of discoloration and marked swelling in such a prominent site. The bleeding usually stops spontaneously, but it may be reduced in amount and the swelling made less by the application of cold compresses (see p. 443). Absorption of the blood may be hastened after the first 24 hours by the use of hot compresses applied fifteen minutes at a time at intervals throughout the day.

Lacerations. Lacerations of the eyelids are not serious unless they are accompanied by an injury to the eyeball. Injuries to the lids are treated in the same way as any other wound but, because of his special training, the ophthalmologist usually is requested to care for them. Lacerations of the eyeball are more serious because of the danger of the production of visual defects, and more extensive injuries may even endanger the entire eye. These are referred invariably to the ophthalmologist for appropriate care. They may entail transplantation of conjunctival flaps to prevent leakage of ocular fluids, excision of prolapsed iris and, in severe injuries, even removal of the eye.

Retinal detachment is a separation of the retina from the choroid. This may appear as tears or holes as a result of trauma or arise from degeneration, frequently in myopia. Flashes of light, blurred vision, a sensation of a veil coming across the eye and, finally, loss of vision are the usual symptoms. The patient may be treated with absolute bed rest in the supine position, both eyes bandaged, in the hope that the retina will regain its normal position. Usually, however, surgery is required. With a diathermy needle, holes are made in the retina to allow the subretinal collection of fluids to escape. The retina falls back into place and becomes adherent to the choroid, due to the reaction caused by the diathermy current.

NURSING CARE. When the patient returns from the operating room, he must be reminded of the position that he is to maintain. This will depend on the nature of the repair and the specific orders of the surgeon. Small pillows and sandbags are useful. Side rails also will remind him that he must remain in bed. The patient should not brush his teeth or comb his hair until the surgeon gives permission. All comfort measures are instituted which will allow the patient to relax while maintaining a restricted position. He is cautioned about sudden motion, sneezing or coughing; such activity may redetach the retina. After 10 days, peep-hole glasses are worn, which allow central vision but limit the movement of the eyes. He is allowed out of bed, and physical activity is increased gradually.

The psychological nursing care of this patient is of major importance. Diversion that is relaxing is desirable, such as conversation, listening to music, having someone read a favorite book and so forth. These individuals become depressed easily; therefore, every attempt should be made to prevent this reaction. The nurse should be sure that the patient understands all instructions for posthospital care and follow-up visits.

Enucleation. Removal of the eyeball is called *enucleation.* It is necessitated by such trauma that the contents of the globe escape, by infections and by other injuries in which there is a fear of sympathetic oph thalmia. This is a condition in whic the uninjured eye may develop a inflammatory reaction after an injur to one eye. During the removal o the eye, muscles are cut as close t the globe as possible. By using tan talum sutures, these muscles are ap proximated to the plastic prosthesi thereby providing the means for co ordinated motion with the patient real eye. After the healing proce is well under way, a plastic shell inserted into an opening of the im plant. This shell is colored to matc the patient's eye. In successful case it is difficult to distinguish the pros thesis from the normal eye.

DISEASES OF THE EYE

STYE (HORDEOLUM)

A *stye* is an infection of the tin glands that empty at the free edg of the eyelid. The area become swollen, red, tender and painful. A eyelash will be found in the cent of the yellow point that appear Hot compresses, applied in the ear stage, will hasten the pointing of th abscess. Removal of the central las often is followed by drainage of pu but incision sometimes is necessar

CHALAZIA

A *chalazion* is a cyst of the me bomian glands. It is noted as a sma lump, hard and painless, in the li Occasionally, such a cyst may b come infected. When this occur hot compresses are used; it may b necessary to do an incision and drainage. For the uninfected cys massage may help it to be rea sorbed; however, the usual trea nent is to make a small incision and xpress the cyst. The incision is made fter the cosmetic effect has been onsidered.

Conjunctivitis

Simple conjunctivitis, caused by rauma or organisms of low viruence, is characterized by redness of he eyes, some photophobia (dread f light), moderate lacrimation and arying degrees of purulent disharge. Frequent saline irrigations re required to remove the discharge, nd the instillation of Argyrol, from 5 to 10 per cent solution, twice daily usually suffices to cure the ordinary ase. Dark glasses should be given o the patient for photophobia.

Gonorrheal Ophthalmia

This is an acute purulent conjunctivitis that occurs in newborn babies and is due usually to the gonococcus. The infection occurs at the time of birth from the infected birth canal of the mother. It is such a serious disease, often causing blindness, that every child should be given prophylactic treatment. As soon as the baby s born, the lids should be cleansed and 2 drops of a 1 per cent solution of silver nitrate dropped into the outer angle of each eye. Penicillin solution eventually may replace silver nitrate as the prophylactic measure of choice, but this is still in the experimental phase.

The acute stage of the disease begins on the third day after birth, with gradually increasing swelling of the lids and severe pain. The discharge, at first only turbid, becomes yellowish and profuse. If untreated, he disease causes ulceration of the cornea and the whole eye may become involved. Recovery from the advanced stages of the disease is accompanied by varying degrees of blindness. Both eyes usually are affected.

Nursing Care

After the disease has developed, the treatment falls largely into the hands of the nurse. The patient must be isolated. The nurse should wear a gown and rubber gloves to protect herself from infection. Some surgeons ask nurses to wear goggles, because of the danger of accidental infection of the eyes. If this should occur, the conjunctival sac should be irrigated thoroughly with penicillin solution (1,000 units per cc.) and repeated every half hour for several applications. After treating these cases, the nurse should thoroughly disinfect the gloves and her own hands.

Treatment in the early stages consists of the application of cold compresses 15 minutes out of every hour to help control chemosis. The eye involved is irrigated with normal saline solution at room temperature and followed by a medicine dropper full of penicillin solution (1,000 units per cc.). This routine is carried out every 15 minutes for the first 12 hours; after that time, it may be extended to every half hour for the next 12 hours. Less frequent irrigations may be necessary on the second day if the eye smear is negative for gonococcus organisms and if pus is no longer present. Penicillin also is administered intramuscularly as an adjunct to the local treatment. Infants up to two years of age are given from 50,000 to 100,000 units daily. The adult dosage of 300,000 units daily may be given beyond this age.

In making these applications, the nurse should wrap the child in a sheet or a small blanket to hold its arms and legs. After the irrigation, the lids should be anointed with liquid petrolatum or boric acid ointment to prevent them from sticking together. If only one eye is infected, the other should be protected with a dressing saturated with penicillin solution (1,000 units per cc.) and bandaged in place. The infectious nature of the pus always must be borne in mind by the nurse. All bits of cotton, gauze compresses and so forth which might be infected should be wrapped in paper to be burned. The utensils used must be sterilized frequently.

Gonorrheal Conjunctivitis in Adults. The infection is carried to the eyes by contact with soiled fingers or linen. The symptoms are similar to those described for ophthalmia neonatorum, except that very often only one eye is infected. The pain is very severe, necessitating morphine for relief. The treatment is the same as that recommended for infants. If corneal ulcerations appear, atropine drops are used.

Extreme care must be taken not to infect the other eye when only one eye is involved. The patient should lie so that the discharges drain away from the nose. The uninfected eye should be protected by dressings saturated with penicillin solution (1,000 units per cc.), or by the application of a Buller's shield. This consists of a watch glass fitted in a square piece of adhesive plaster applied carefully to the brow, the temple, the lower margin of the orbit and the nose. Reinforcements of adhesive strips often are used, and the area over the bridge of the nose always should be sealed with collodion.

Corneal Ulcers

Inflammation of the cornea is called *keratitis* and, if this process is associated with a loss of substance, a corneal ulcer results. The inflammatory reaction often spreads deeper to the iris (iritis), with the result that pus is formed and collects as a white or yellow deposit behind the cornea (hypopyon). If the ulceration perforates, the iris may prolapse through the cornea, or other serious complications may follow. Because of the importance of the cornea to vision, any ulceration must be considered as a most serious condition. The healing of any but the very superficial ulcers is attended with some degree of opacity of the cornea and, therefore, with some diminution of vision.

Symptoms. The symptoms of corneal ulceration are pain, marked photophobia and increased lacrimation. The eye usually appears somewhat injected or "bloodshot" (lay term).

Treatment. In the treatment of corneal ulcers, dark glasses should be provided to relieve the photophobia. Atropine and dionin drops usually are given at frequent intervals. Holocaine may be used to relieve pain. Penicillin 1:1,000 is employed in irrigations of the eye several times daily. Hot compresses go far in relieving the pain in this condition. If the ulcers show no tendency to heal, the surgeon often applies some strong antiseptic locally: silver nitrate 2 per cent, phenol followed by alcohol and so forth. Fluorescein generally is used to outline the ulcers before the application of the healing solutions.

Fever Therapy. Other methods of treatment of corneal ulcers are small doses of x-ray and fever therapy, a bacterial antigen of typhoid bacilli, consisting of 20 million per cubic centimeter, being used. In this treatment the nurse must have available a tray containing alcohol sponges, tourniquet, sterile medicine glass, sterile 5-cc. syringe, tuberculin syringe and 23- and 22-gauge needles. Sterile physiologic salt solution is used for diluting the antigen.

Nursing Care in Fever Therapy

After the injection of the antigen, the patient's temperature, pulse, respiration and blood pressure are taken every hour until the temperature reaches 100° F. At this time the readings are made at 15-minute intervals so long as the temperature is elevated. The patient should be placed in bed after the temperature reaches 99° F. If a chill occurs, hot-water bottles should be placed round him and blankets should be added immediately. Hot liquids should be encouraged and other food given as the patient desires it. Codeine often is prescribed for the patient's comfort.

After the fever subsides, an alcohol rub should be given and the patient placed in dry clothing and a clean bed. Wet clothing should be changed p.r.n. during and after the temperature rise.

Fever therapy is used frequently in many inflammatory diseases of the eye. The temperature should not exceed 104° F.

Corneal Transplantation (Keratoplasty)

All too frequently, the sight in the eyes of patients with corneal ulcers is badly impaired, even to complete loss of vision following extensive scars due to trauma or infection. Here the plastic procedure of corneal transplantation is employed, with marvelous success in many cases. Transplants may be taken from the same person or from a donor, or from the eye of a recently deceased person.

Treatment and Nursing Care

The patient's general condition is checked and attempts are made to attain optimum health. The day before surgery, cultures usually are taken of the conjunctiva, and the flora of organisms is reduced by antibiotic eyedrops. The psychological factor cannot be dismissed; therefore, these patients must be reassured.

The care after operation is the same as that after operation for cataract, except that the time of lying in bed without moving the head is longer; this is about a week. The first dressing then is done and pressure dressings are retained from two to four weeks. Skin care, mouth care and adequate semisoft diet are given during the first week; a mild cathartic followed by an oil retention enema will eliminate undue straining on defecation. Every precaution is taken to prevent infection. Home care is directed primarily at avoiding straining of the eyes. Gradually strength and vision in the eye are regained.

Glaucoma

Glaucoma is the name given to the disease characterized by increased tension or pressure within the eye. This disease ordinarily occurs in individuals past 40 and may be classified as primary or secondary, acute or chronic. The cause of primary glaucoma is unknown, although it often is associated with emotional disturbances, endocrine imbalance, allergy or vasomotor disturbance. Secondary glaucoma results as a complication of some other disturbance within the eye. This increased intra-ocular tension may be noted with the fingers, but more accurately by means of a *tonometer*. Normally, fluids which enter the eye globe are balanced by those which leave the eye. In glaucoma, more fluid is secreted than is absorbed, which results in an increased intraocular tension. When this imbalance occurs gradually, symptoms are slight; however, when it occurs rapidly, pain results because of the pressure on the optic nerve. Peripheral vision is impaired long before there is any effect on central vision. Artificial lights appear to have a rainbow around them. Vision becomes cloudy or smoky. These symptoms are aggravated after the patient has been in dim light (e.g., watching movies or television) or following an emotional upset. If untreated, glaucoma leads to blindness.

Treatment and Nursing Care

Early detection of glaucoma means that the patient may have the condition controlled by myotic drugs. (See Drugs Used to Contract Pupil, p. 437.) By their use the pupil is contracted and the iris is drawn away from the cornea, thus allowing the aqueous humor to drain through the lymph spaces into the canal of Schlemm. Pilocarpine, eserine or Carcholin are the drugs employed.

There are many types of surgery. In acute cases, an incision is made through the cornea so that a portion of the iris may be drawn out and excised (*iridectomy*). This permits drainage of lymph from the anterior chamber and reduction of intraocular tension. Other operations on the iris (*iridencleisis* and *iridotasis*) are modifications having the same objective, that is, to permit fluid to escape.

Chronic glaucoma often is treated by making a small opening with a circular knife at the junction of the cornea and the sclera. This operation, called *corneoscleral trephining*, leaves a permanent opening through which aqueous humor may drain. Usually it is covered by a flap of conjunctiva. In the preoperative treatment of these cases, irrigations of both eyes are often prescribed and weaker solutions of eserine are instilled in the unaffected eye.

After operation, the patient is kept flat and relatively quiet for 24 hours and liquid diet is permitted. Narcotics or sedatives may be given if necessary. After the first dressing is changed, the patient is allowed more freedom. Usually, he is discharged on the fifth day. He is expected to visit the ophthalmologist regularly since surgery is only palliative and recurrences are likely.

Teaching Suggestions. Remind the patient of the importance of avoiding worry, fear, anger and excitement. Tight clothing such as a tight belt, collar or corset should not be worn. Perform exercises in moderation to keep the blood circulation active. Alcoholic beverages are to be avoided, and coffee as well as tea should be limited to a cup a day. Bowel habits should be regular. Keep the teeth clean and healthy. Take care of acute or chronic colds. Avoid dark rooms as much as possible; go to movies only if the ophthalmologist permits. Use eye drops or eye washes only with the consent of the eye physician. Be conscientious about keeping appointments for eye examinations.

Cataract

Cataract is the term applied to an opacity of the crystalline lens or of its capsule. The most common type occurs in adults past middle age, but it may occur in younger individuals as a result of trauma or disease. Occasionally it occurs at birth (congenital cataract). As the rays of light entering the eye must pass through the pupil and the lens to reach the retina, any opacity in the lens behind the pupil will produce alteration in vision. Very often the opacity is not complete at first, so that vision may be improved by an iridectomy (removal of a piece of iris), which allows light to pass through the part of the lens uncovered by the operation. As time goes on, the degenerative processes separate the lens from its capsule, opacity becomes complete and the cataract is said to be ripe or mature. The ripe or mature cataract can be cured only by operation.

The preparation for operation has been described (see p. 444). The nurse should explain to the patient some of the restrictions he will face immediately postoperatively. He will accept these limitations more gracefully at that time. At the operation, an incision is made through the sclera barely outside of the cornea, the lens capsule is excised and the lens is expressed by pressure on the eye from below with a metal spoon. This is called an *extracapsular extraction.*

Another type of cataract operation is known as an *intracapsular extraction.* In the operation, the lens is removed within its capsule. The incision is closed with very fine black silk sutures.

After the extraction of the cataract, both eyes are covered with sterile eye patches held in place with two pieces of Scotch cellulose tape, and additional protection is supplied by a metal eye shield. Often an ocular mask of black buckram is applied to cover the entire dressing.

At present, some eye surgeons are trying plastic lens as a substitute for the real lens when it is removed. If successful, such a procedure will minimize greatly the postoperative discomforts and complications.

Postoperative Nursing Care

The patient is permitted a low firm pillow immediately after operation and may have the head of the bed slightly raised within the first 24 to 48 hours after operation. Any strain felt by the patient may be relieved somewhat by placing pillows under the knees or the small of the back. Liquid diet is supplemented with custards, junkets, gelatin and so forth. Iced water, fruit juices, milk and other gas-producing foods are avoided. Soft diet usually is resumed on the second day. An enema is ordered after 48 hours. During this procedure the patient must be cautioned against straining.

Most patients wear a face mask which covers both eyes. It helps the patient if anyone who comes near his bed speaks to him. He wonders what is going on about him and is apt to be less apprehensive if he knows. Crib sides often give the patient a feeling of security, and they should be used especially at night.

Sneezing and vomiting should be prevented as much as possible.

Splints often are applied to the elbows of patients who persist in interfering with the bandages.

During the first 24 to 48 hours many patients become anxious and worried over the results of the operation. This is not to be wondered at if it is remembered that the patient's mind may be active, even though both eyes are closed. The efficient nurse can do much to reassure her charge and direct his thoughts away from himself toward other and more diverting subjects.

Many of these patients are in the older age group. Psychoses as well as pulmonary and circulatory complications have occurred postoperatively in cataract patients as a result of covering both eyes and restricting their physical activities. Consequently, there is a trend to increase their activities earlier. Some eye surgeons do not cover the unoperated eye. The rule which usually is followed is that the older the patient, the fewer the restrictions.

Pain usually is slight after cataract extraction but, should it become severe, the surgeon should be notified at once, as this may be the symptom of a serious complication, such as hemorrhage.

The surgeon usually will dress the eye 24 hours after operation, and once daily thereafter until the seventh or the eighth day.

For the contents of the dressing tray, see p. 446.

If the surgeon finds that the corneal wound is sealed at the first dressing and examination, the patient is permitted to be turned on the unaffected side. If, however, the anterior chamber has not re-formed, it indicates that there is still some leak of aqueous humor through the wound and turning must not be allowed for 48 hours or longer.

Under normal conditions the unoperated eye may be uncovered on the third or the fourth day, and at the end of a week the patient needs only the protection afforded by dark glasses. When the sutures are removed, the eye is anesthetized with 1 per cent pontocaine, and sterile eye speculum, forceps and scissors are required. The patient is discharged when his eyes have become accustomed to ordinary daylight.

Six or 8 weeks after the removal of the cataract the patient may be fitted with glasses, which in a measure take the place of the crystalline lens. In 6 months' time the eyes will have made their adjustment and permanent glasses may be ordered. However, the power of accommodation is lost, so that two glasses must be used, one for distant and one for near vision.

Strabismus (Squint)

Strabismus or *squint* is a condition in which one eye deviates from the object at which the person is looking (lay term "cross-eyed"). It may result from paralysis of the nerves supplying the extra-ocular muscles, due to injury or disease. Double vision or diplopia results. In children, a strabismus due to ocular defects often develops. It is characterized by single vision usually because the image seen by the divergent eye is suppressed involuntarily.

The strabismus in children often may be corrected by the wearing of properly fitted glasses. Orthopedic training for muscle disturbances, such as strabismus, is successful in many instances without operation. It consists of a series of muscle exercises carried out by means of various instruments, cards and test objects. Patients who have a marked degree of squint usually are operated upon after having had some training; then, after the eyes are straightened, the exercises are employed again. Early detection and immediate medical consultation are to be encouraged if the defect is to be corrected satisfactorily.

The Nurse and the Newly Blind

When an individual has marked visual impairment or is newly blind, he needs a great deal of help in making the adjustment so that he emerges as a confident, happy and useful person. For the most part this care is entrusted to those skilled in this work. However, there are certain practices which a nurse can follow as she cares for such a person.

A blind person always should be treated as a normal human being. Avoid expressions of pity and sympathy. Keep him from becoming discouraged by seeing that he has someone with whom he can talk or some other form of diversion such as a radio. Help him to overcome his feeling of awkwardness as he performs simple activities. If he is allowed out of bed, the blind person should survey his room by walking around and touching the furniture. Thereafter, the nurse should be sure that the furniture remains in the same position. Never leave a door half open; it should be either open or shut. When walking with a blind person, allow him to follow you by lightly touching your elbow. Do not push him ahead of you. When he walks alone, a lightweight walking stick can be used as an extended hand to warn him of obstacles. It should not be used for tapping the sidewalk or the floor.

Personal appearance is a significant part of the patient's care. He should be allowed to dress by himself; a woman even can learn to fix her hair and use cosmetics. Table etiquette, smoking, writing and so forth all are activities that can be acquired with practice. The nurse should be familiar with the programs offered by such groups as The Seeing Eye, Inc., Morristown, N. J., where blind persons can learn the value of a dog guide.

CLINICAL SITUATION: SURGERY FOR GLAUCOMA

Jake Kayko, now 62 and slowly facing blindness due to a chronic glaucoma, was admitted to the hospital for more eye surgery. He was a mason but is no longer able to work; he also has a small chicken farm.

1. Normal eye tension as measured by a tonometer is
_____(1) 15 to 29 mm.
_____(2) 25 to 35 mm.
_____(3) 35 to 55 mm.

2. Mr. Kayko has minimal vision of the affected eye. He probably has no vision
_____(1) when looking straight ahead
_____(2) from the "corner of his eye" as he crosses the street
_____(3) for colored objects

3. Pilocarpine is used to
_____(1) contract the pupil, draw the iris away from the cornea and allow aqueous humor to drain into the canal of Schlemm
_____(2) contract the pupil, allow the iris to move toward the cornea and prevent aqueous humor from draining into the canal of Schlemm
_____(3) dilate the pupil, draw the iris away from the cornea and prevent aqueous humor from draining into the canal of Schlemm

4. Mr. Kayko was somewhat confused during his first postoperative night and tried to get out of bed to go to the bathroom. The nurse should
_____(1) have told him preoperatively that it is imperative for him to remain in bed
_____(2) apply restraints; only in this way can he be reminded that he must remain in bed
_____(3) explain why he must not get out of bed; attach sideboards to the bed if this has not been done already

5. On previous occasions, Mr. Kayko never was too concerned about keeping his clinic appointments. The result probably was that
_____(1) the time of doctors and nurses as well as supplies were not wasted; eventually, such a patient must have surgery anyway
_____(2) his eyesight continued to get progressively worse, and the possibility of total blindness is greater
_____(3) he saved a good bit of money, which will help to take care of his surgery now

6. The worry that was uppermost in the mind of Mr. Kayko was, "How will I take care of my chickens if I can't see?" The best reply by the nurse is
_____(1) "You can learn how to do this, so don't worry about it."
_____(2) "Maybe you should consider selling them and develop another hobby."
_____(3) "Think of getting well yourself and don't worry about the chickens."

7. The purpose of surgery for glaucoma is to
_____(1) remove the causative factor in order to prevent malignancy
_____(2) restore sight to within normal limits
_____(3) prevent blindness, if possible, and relieve tension

CHAPTER TWENTY-TWO

Surgery of the Ear and the Mastoid

INTRODUCTION

The ear is one of the most important sense organs of the body. It is the seat of the sense of hearing, and upon its normal function depends reception of all sound. Defects in this function result in defective hearing which may arise from various causes and may even be present to a greater or lesser degree without the notice of the patient. Many of the causes of defective hearing may be remedied very easily, such as a collection of wax in the external ear so the sounds are not transmitted to the eardrum. By simple irrigation of the ear, such collections can be removed with restoration of normal hearing. Defects due to diseases of the ear itself are less easily remedied. These may arise as the result of disease of the transmitting apparatus of the ear, or due to disease of the auditory nerve itself. Various diagnostic tests are available to demonstrate the site of the difficulty in defective hearing.

The *audiometer* is an instrument by which the intensity and the pitch of pure tones can be varied. This is used to test the acuity of hearing. *Tuning forks* of various sizes with variations of vibrations are used to test the tones which the patient can hear. These tuning forks may be held a distance from the ear or may be placed directly upon the skull, on the forehead or over the temporal bone, thus testing the acuity of hearing when it is transmitted by the air as compared with that transmitted by bone. When the acuity of the sound is greater when transmitted by bone than it is when transmitted by air, the inference is that the difficulty in the ear is in the conduction apparatus within the ear, rather than due to a nerve disease.

In addition to the hearing function, the ear also has a function in maintaining equilibrium of the body. This function is carried on by the semicircular canals and it is disturbed in various sorts of brain tumors which involve the eighth nerve. Tests for this vestibular function are performed by syringing the ear with hot or cold water, or by rotation of

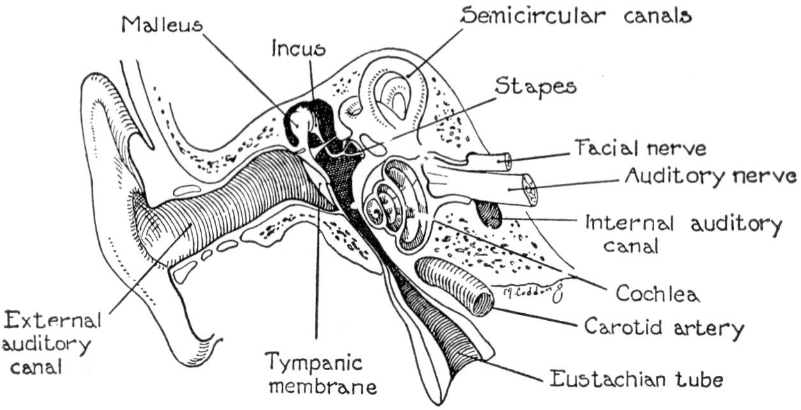

FIG. 191. Semidiagrammatic drawing of the ear to show the relations of the structures of the external and the internal ear. (Wolf, G. D.: Ear, Nose and Throat, Philadelphia, Lippincott)

the patient with the head held in position, which stimulates certain of the semicircular canals. These tests of ear function are more commonly employed in suspected neurosurgical disease.

ANATOMY

To understand the diseases of the ear, it may be necessary for the nurse to review its anatomy briefly. The ear consists of three principal parts. The *external ear* is composed of a narrow canal leading to the tympanic membrane, a drumlike structure stretched across the canal, which transmits sound waves to the bones of the middle ear. The *middle ear* is located within the temporal bone and is separated from the covering of the brain by only a thin osseous plate. It contains three tiny bones which transmit the sound vibrations to the organ of hearing located in the internal ear. Extending anteriorly from the middle ear into the nasopharynx is a narrow canal called the eustachian or auditory tube. (See Fig. 197, p. 482.) Posteriorly, there is an opening into a honey-comblike group of air cells, located in the bony prominence back of the ear called the mastoid process. The *internal ear* contains the organs of hearing and equilibration.

EXTERNAL EAR

The external ear is subject to various congenital deformities which, for cosmetic reasons, may require surgery. Undue prominence of the auricle, supernumerary or loosely attached auricles and tiny fistulae on the helix may need attention. Then, too, many deformities due to injuries, such as the cauliflower or prizefighter ear, the complete avulsion of the member, human bites and infections, require surgery.

Foreign bodies are found frequently in the external auditory canal. They may be anything from

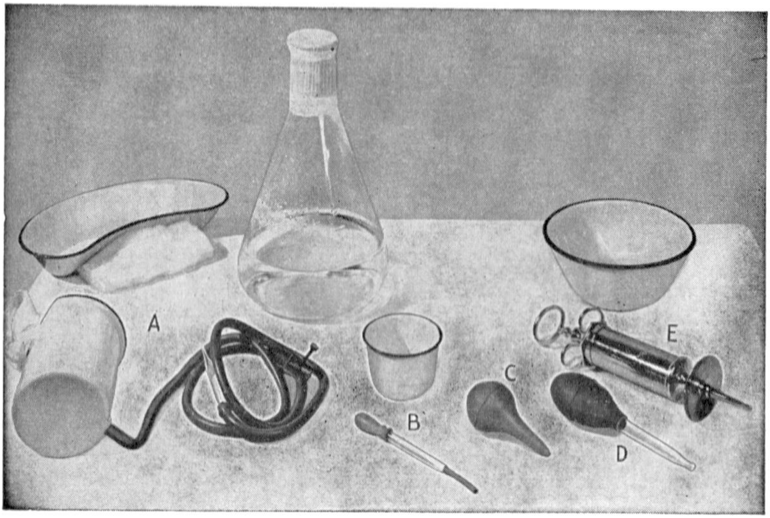

FIG. 192. Five types of equipment used for irrigation of the ear. (A) Irrigating jar, tubing with pipet tip. (B) Medicine dropper with rubber tube protecting glass tip. (C) All-rubber pointed syringe. (D) Glass-tipped syringe. (E) Metal syringe with shield.

seeds, beads or buttons to insects (fleas, ants). As long as the foreign body is present, it occasions considerable discomfort to the patient. After an examination with a head mirror and an ear speculum, usually the body can be removed by irrigating with warm sterile boric-acid solution. Seeds (beans, peas) which swell with moisture may be removed by a hook or forceps. Extreme care must be taken in doing this so that the body may not be pushed farther in toward the ear drum.

The sebaceous glands of the canal secrete an oily brownish material known as *cerumen*. Not infrequently there is an accumulation of this material, forming a mass which cannot be removed easily. This impacted cerumen may cause deafness on the affected side and sometimes aching. Usually it may be removed by irrigating with warm solutions. The instillation of a drop or two of warm olive oil softens the mass and makes its subsequent removal easier.

The solutions for irrigating the ear should be used at a temperature of about 105° to 110° F. Solutions which are too hot or too cold or are used with too much force may result in pain or dizziness to the patient.

MIDDLE EAR

OTITIS MEDIA

The middle ear is the most important from the point of view of surgery, because it is involved most frequently in infections, and from these may arise very serious complications. The infections usually originate in the nasopharynx, extending thence along the eustachian tube to the middle ear. If the infection is acute, there is intense pain, headache, fever and impairment of hearing. The ear drum may appear red and bulging if viewed through an aural speculum. This inflammation of the middle ear is spoken of as *otitis media* and is a very common complication in children following infections of the nose and the throat, especially after measles, scarlet fever, diphtheria and "sore throat." As the infection progresses, swelling closes the orifice of the eustachian tube, and the distention may cause a perforation of the ear drum with a discharge of pus. In many cases of purulent otitis media, there is an extension of the inflammation into the mastoid cells, causing an acute mastoiditis.

Treatment. The treatment of an early inflammation may be conservative for 24 hours, consisting of nasal irrigations and gargles, with instillation of mild antiseptics, such as Argyrol 10 per cent solution, into the nasopharynx. The sulfonamides and/or penicillin are indicated. In addition to this, warm aural irrigations of boric-acid solution should be given. This treatment may suffice in mild inflammations of the catarrhal type. If the symptoms continue, and the ear drum is found to bulge, it should be incised (*myringotomy*), allowing free drainage of pus to take place. This operation is very painful; therefore, it is best performed with general anesthesia. Myringtomy is indicated in many cases even though perforation of the ear drum has occurred. The membrane usually heals well, and hearing is impaired only slightly, if at all.

Nursing Care

After incision of the drum fo purulent otitis media, the nurse i called upon to irrigate the ear wit warm antiseptic solutions every tw or three hours. The irrigation is bes performed by the use of a steril soft rubber ear syringe or of an ordi nary dressing syringe to the end o which is attached a small rubbe tube. The solution is received in small curved basin held snugly be low the auricle. To be effective th fluids must reach the ear drum, an to this end the nurse is advised t pull the auricle upward and back ward in order to straighten the ex ternal auditory canal. In childre this canal may be straightened b pulling the auricle down and back Extreme gentleness should be used and care must be taken that the flui has free exit so that it will not b driven into the middle ear. Afte each irrigation the external meatu should be plugged lightly with ster ile cotton, which is changed whe necessary.

Heat applied to the mastoid are may give considerable relief to th patient, but sedative drugs may b required also. The best drainage i secured by having the patient lie o the affected side. Treatment of th nasopharynx should be carried ou simultaneously.

Mastoiditis

Mastoiditis is the most commo complication of middle-ear diseas Fortunately, the use of the sulfona mides and the antibiotics has re duced the incidence of this condition tremendously. The infection involves the numerous tiny air cells in the mastoid process and produces what is, in effect, an acute osteomyelitis. It is a serious disease because only a thin plate of bone separates these cells from the membranes covering the brain. Extensions to these structures may result in a meningitis, brain abscess, or more frequently a thrombosis of the lateral sinus, a large venous channel which lies between the layers of the dura on the cerebral side of the mastoid. Since the thrombosis is infectious in origin, the infecting organisms are carried all over the body, producing septicemia.

Symptoms. The symptoms of acute mastoiditis are those of an acute infection, fever is usually quite high, and there is swelling behind the ear with extreme tenderness, redness, edema and pain.

Treatment. Conservative treatment is begun at once. This includes bed rest, adequate diet and fluids, chemotherapy and sedatives for discomfort. Most cases will subside within a day or two. When the infection is more persistent, surgery is indicated because of the dangers of intracranial extension. A simple or radical mastoidectomy may be performed. Under certain indications the endaural approach is chosen in place of the retro-auricular route. If this is done, the shaving of the hair is not necessary. The auricle must be cleaned thoroughly, because the incisional approach is made through this structure.

Nursing Care

If not contraindicated, the hair should have a shampoo the day before the operation. In preparing the patient for a mastoidectomy, the nurse should shave the head for a distance of about two inches around the auricle. In female patients, the preparation should be done carefully with due regard to cosmetic results. This area can be shaved in such a way that longer hair from above and in front of the scar can later be drawn over the operative site. On female patients, a single layer of gauze can be fastened to the periphery of the shaved area with collodion; this dressing can then be drawn back to cover the hair and keep it out of the way.

In the operating room, the patient is placed on the operating table with the head turned to the unaffected side and supported by a firm pillow. A curved incision is made posterior to the ear down to the bone. The mastoid cells are opened with a chisel and a mallet. All mastoid cells should be removed with a curet. Packing is inserted, and the upper part of the incision may be sutured.

After the patient has recovered consciousness following the anesthesia, he may have discomfort which can be relieved with sedatives. Diet may be increased as tolerated, and the patient usually is allowed out of bed the day of surgery if he so desires. The nurse must be on the alert for signs suggestive of a facial nerve injury. This may affect the entire side of the face, shown by the inability to close the eye completely or to move that side of the mouth, to whistle or to drink without the fluid's escaping. The corner of the mouth droops or the face is expressionless when the patient smiles.

INNER EAR

The Labyrinth Fenestration Operation for Otosclerosis

The surgical treatment of the chronic progressive deafness condition called otosclerosis has been under development for about 75 years and only within the last 15 years has it progressed into the practical modern surgical technic of the labyrinth fenestration operation.

In otosclerosis the deafness is the result of the blocking of sound vibrations from reaching the auditory nerve elements in the inner ear mechanism by a deposit of bone around the footplate of the stapes—a part of the sound-conducting apparatus. The fenestration operation restores a conduction channel around the obstruction and permits sound impulses again to reach the perceptive mechanism in the inner ear. This is accomplished by (1) a partial mastoidectomy, (2) a reconstruction of the outer and the middle parts of the ear whereby a new drum or skin flap is fashioned and (3) by the creation of a new window (the fenestration) into the internal ear mechanism which is covered and sealed by the newly established drum or skin flap. The new conduction mechanism thus established restores the hearing to a practical serviceable hearing level in from 75 to 80 per cent of properly selected otosclerosis patients.

Nursing Care

These operated patients require skillful nursing care because they are heavily narcotized from the preoperative sedation and prolonged anesthesia and because they are very nauseated and dizzy for from 1 to 3 days after operation. The sickness is similar to severe seasickness and is due to the irritation of the equilibrium apparatus in the internal ear as the result of the creation of the new window at that area.

The most comfortable position for the patient is the supine one or on the side of the operated ear. Usually nothing can be tolerated by mouth for at least 6 or 8 hours. Dramamine is given for the first 2 or 3 days after operation. This drug has been very effective in reducing the postoperative nausea, vomiting and vertigo. Some surgeons prescribe dramamine preoperatively as well. Liquids by mouth can be tolerated 6 or 8 hours after operation, but the patient often is given intravenous fluids by slow drip over a period of 10 hours. Vitamin K often is a part of the pre- and postoperative regimen.

The nurse must watch the breathing rate carefully, as in some of the patients the respirations are reduced to 5 or 6 per minute. Penicillin is given routinely, starting before operation or immediately after operation, either by injection every three hours or the one injection per day method.

On the day following operation the patient is permitted to take any position desired, even sitting up or out of bed, and is encouraged to move around as much as possible, short of losing any ingested fluids or food by vomiting. This requires judgment and skill on the nurse's part. During the first 24 hours and sometimes during the second day the patient is apt to have difficulty in voiding. Frequently, catheterization is necessary, but the patient may be

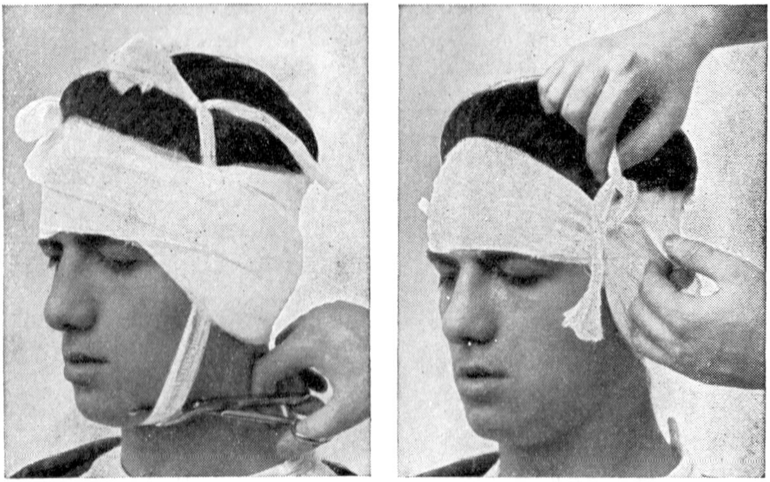

FIG. 193. Improved ear bandage. (*Left*) Extra piece of bandage tied loosely around the head and the chin before bandage is applied. (*Right*) Extra bandage cut in two pieces and tied over each temporal region, the end of the bandage being tied in a knot on one side.

held in a sitting position or even a standing position if the vertigo and the vomiting are not too severe.

During the second day after operation the patient is usually able to take care of himself; he is encouraged to walk as much as possible and is placed on a full diet as rapidly as his condition permits. Usually no bowel movement is expected or desired for at least three days after operation, and then often some help, such as mild laxatives or enemas, is required. As soon as the patient can walk sufficiently well to be able to take care of himself with no danger of falling he can be discharged from the hospital. This is usually on the sixth or the seventh day after operation.

The dressings on the operated ear are changed approximately every second day. The only sterile instruments necessary are a pair of scissors, a thumb forceps and a straight hemostat. The dressings consist of sterile gauze squares and a 2- or 3-inch bandage. Frequently, a skin graft is taken from the arm at the time of operation for placement in the ear. When this is done the arm requires a change of dressing (petrolatum gauze and gauze squares) from 3 to 5 days after operation.

In his posthospital instructions, for several months after surgery this patient should be told not to dive or swim, because moisture in the cavity will make it susceptible to infection. He should be reminded of the importance of follow-up visits to his physician so that the cavity is kept clean during the healing process.

There is much gratification in finding that a patient's hearing has improved as a result of the operation. On the other hand, the nurse must use great tact and understanding with a patient who has not been helped.

Talking with the Person Who Is Hard of Hearing. Remember which is the person's better ear and speak quietly and distinctly on that side. In drawing his attention, raise your arm. Place yourself in a position where light is on your face and lips. Speak in sentences and avoid word-by-word utterances. If the person does not understand what you have said, repeat the thought, using other words.

When a person wears a hearing aid, do not get too close to it; instead, experiment to see how close you should stand for his effective hearing.

REFERENCES AND SUGGESTED READING

Unit Seven: Nursing in Conditions of the Eye and the Ear

General

(See also those for Unit One, p. 205)

Manhattan Hospital: Nursing in Diseases of the Eye, Ear, Nose and Throat, ed. 9, Philadelphia, Saunders, 1953.

Parkinson, R. M.: Eye, Ear, Nose and Throat Manual for Nurses, ed. 7, St. Louis, Mosby, 1953.

Wolf, G. D.: Ear, Nose and Throat, ed. 1, Philadelphia, Lippincott, 1947.

Eye

Blake, E. M.: Glaucoma, Am. J. Nursing **52**:451-452, 1952.

Blodi, F. C.: Retrolental fibroplasia, Am. J. Nursing **53**:718-720, 1953.

Brinkley, D.: Focus on vision, Am. J. Nursing **53**:1224-1226, 1953.

Calhoun, F. P., Kilgo, A. P., and Mills, E.: Detachment of the retina, Am. J. Nursing **53**:1316-1320, 1953.

Castroviejo, R.: Corneal transplantation, Am. J. Nursing **46**:31-34, 1946.

Deming, D.: Fearless eyes, Am. J. Nursing **44**:765-768, 1944.

Giuner, I., and Klimek, A.: Surgical treatment of patients with cataract and glaucoma, Am. J. Nursing **54**:292-294, 1954.

Kirby, D. B.: The Surgery of Cataract, Philadelphia, Lippincott, 1950.

Kuhn, H. S.: Emergency nursing care of the eyes in industry, Am. J. Nursing **47**:24-26, 1947.

Lancaster, W. B.: Crossed eyes in children, Am. J. Nursing **50**:535-537, 1950.

Lovejoy, M. A.: The blind use inner vision, Trained Nurse & Hosp. Rev. **115**:420-421, 1945.

Miller, R. V.: I had a detached retina, Am. J. Nursing **54**:608-609, 1954.

The Newly Blinded, Morristown, N. J., The Seeing Eye, Inc., 1948.

Parfitt, R. E.: Dropper instillation of eye medications, Am. J. Nursing **49**:91-92, 1949.

Romes, B.: The eyes and vitamins, Am. J. Nursing **52**:728-730, 1952.

Siniscal, A. A.: Trachoma, Am. J. Nursing **52**:1508-1510, 1952.

Weaver, H. E.: Glaucoma: a problem for the public health nurse,

Pub. Health Nursing **41**:93-95, 1949.

Weiss, M. O.: Psychological aspects of nursing care for eye patients, Am. J. Nursing **50**:218-220, 1950.

Wright, H. B.: Corneal transplantation and nursing care, Am. J. Nursing **46**:35-36, 1946.

EAR

Cutler, H.: Otitis media, Am. J. Nursing **53**:573-574, 1953.

Jaros, J. F.: Surgical applications of electrocoagulation, Am. J. Nursing **48**:36-37, 1948.

Lewis, D. K.: Deafness, Am. J. Nursing **52**:575-578, 1952.

Neuschutz, L.: The hard of hearing patient, Am. J. Nursing **44**:134-135, 1944.

Nichols, R. E.: The newly deafened patient, Am. J. Nursing **46**:223-224, 1946.

Pedersen, T. E.: The fenestration operation for otosclerosis, Am. J. Nursing **45**:726-727, 1945.

Rosenberger, H. C., and Bukdvina, E.: Fenestration, Am. J. Nursing **47**:730-731, 1947.

CLINICAL SITUATION: FENESTRATION OPERATION

Was Mrs. Janeway intentionally neglecting her 3-month-old baby when he cried so pitifully? The reason for her inattention was a progressive loss of hearing. After several tests she was scheduled for a fenestration operation. Her convalescent discomforts soon were minimized when the joys of hearing were experienced.

1. The diagnosis of otosclerosis can be established by the use of

______(1) an audiometer
______(2) a tuning fork
______(3) an otoscope

2. The nurse should offer psychological support to Mrs. Janeway by saying (after checking with the physician)

______(1) "It must be wonderful to know that you will soon be able to hear again."
______(2) "There are as many failures as successes in this operation, so try not to get your hopes too high."
______(3) "About three fourths of patients having this operation have improved hearing; let us hope you are one of the fortunate ones."

3. The fenestration operation is essentially

______(1) the removal of one of the middle ear ossicles
______(2) the cureting of fibrous adhesions of the inner ear
______(3) the creation of an opening in the internal ear mechanism

4. It is to be expected that Mrs. Janeway may experience the following annoying symptoms:

______(1) vestibular imbalance
______(2) auricular headache
______(3) tinnitus

5. In addressing Mrs. Janeway, the nurse should remember to

______(1) speak quietly and normally, facing Mrs. Janeway's good ear

_____(2) exaggerate the movements of her lips

_____(3) speak loudly when standing close to the affected ear

6. Dramamine is given to Mrs. Janeway pre- and postoperatively to

_____(1) accelerate the process of auditory nerve activity

_____(2) dull the pain experienced when the semicircular canals are disturbed

_____(3) minimize the sensation of equilibrium irritation and imbalance

7. Mrs. Janeway should be told not to

_____(1) wear her hair over the operated ear

_____(2) go swimming or diving for the first year

_____(3) participate in gymnastic exercises

_____(4) wear wool headgear

UNIT EIGHT

Nursing Conditions of the Endocrine Glands

CHAPTER TWENTY-THREE

Surgery of the Thyroid and Other Endocrine Glands

INTRODUCTION

The ductless or endocrine glands have a very important influence on the bodily metabolism, beginning early in life (in utero) and continuing with varying degrees of activity until death. They give their secretion directly to the blood as it passes through them without the use of ducts. By the production of hormones, these glands exert their function on various portions of the body. Some of the glands have no other function, as for instance the thyroid, the parathyroid, the pituitary and the adrenal glands. Others are located in organs which have definite other functions, such as the ovary, the testis and the islet cells of the pancreas. All of these glands have important interrelationships with each other; at the same time each has its own definite function. They become important surgically due to abnormalities in the gland which produces hormones in abnormal amounts, or of abnormal nature, or due to inflammations or tumors.

THE THYROID GLAND

Physiology. The thyroid is located in the anterior part of the neck, being composed of two lobes which lie on either side of the trachea, joined anteriorly by a narrow band called the isthmus. The thyroid secretion called *thyroxin*, of which iodine is an element, has the function of speeding up the metabolic processes. It is one of the hormones whose chemical structure is known, and it is high in iodine content. During puberty, pregnancy, and often at the menstrual periods, the gland may seem

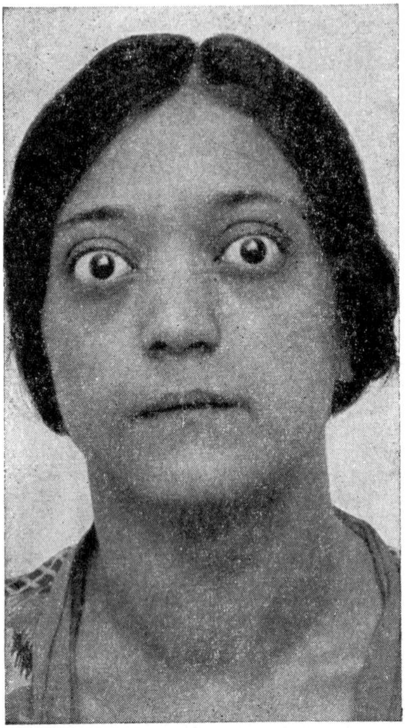

FIG. 194. Exophthalmic or toxic goiter.

to enlarge slightly, because of increased function demanded by the growth of youth or of the fetus.

CRETINISM AND MYXEDEMA

In childhood when the thyroid secretion is deficient the child is fat, has coarse sparse hair, subnormal temperature and practically no mental development. This condition is called *cretinism*. If the secretion becomes insufficient in adult life, either from disease or because too much of the gland has been removed at operation, the patients are sluggish mentally, their faces become expressionless, their motions slow, and the tissues are boggy. The condition is called *myxedema*.

Treatment. In these conditions of hypothyroidism (deficient thyroid secretion) the administration of thyroid extract by mouth brings about a marked improvement.

GOITER

Any abnormal enlargement of the thyroid gland is called a goiter, of which there are several kinds.

Simple colloid goiter (diffuse nontoxic goiter) is an enlargement of the thyroid which is found very commonly in certain parts of the world (around the Great Lakes, Switzerland, etc.) and is thought to be due to a deficiency of iodine in the drinking water. Since iodine is one of the constituents of the secretion of the thyroid, an abnormal secretion results, the gland enlarges, forming a prominent swelling in the neck, and causes symptoms due to pressure on the trachea (shortness of breath), or on the esophagus (difficulty in swallowing). Often these case can be benefited markedly by medical treatment, but if the pressure symptoms are prominent, the excess of the gland must be removed surgically.

Adenomatous goiter (nodular nontoxic goiter) is caused by a benign tumor of the thyroid. It usually occurs in older adults, mostly women, and is characterized by a nodular enlargement of the gland. At times the adenomatous goiter may take on toxic symptoms (nodular toxic goiter, see toxic goiter below). The benign adenomas may undergo malignant changes. The best treatment is surgical removal of the greater part of the gland with the tumor.

Exophthalmic goiter (Graves's disease, diffuse toxic or hyperplastic goiter) is really a state of hyperthyroidism, that is, increased activity of the thyroid gland. Due to an increased or perverted secretion, all the metabolic processes of the body are stimulated to abnormal activity. The pulse rate is rapid, often from 100 to 120 when the patient is at rest. There are frequent hot flushes, and sweating is observed, even of the hands. The eyes are prominent and pushed forward, a condition known as *exophthalmos*. The patient becomes highly nervous, marked tremors appearing in the outstretched fingers, frequently he is subject to emotional states of laughter, crying and depression. Often the patient is driven to activity, yet is apprehensive and overly affected by minor irritations. Palpitation is often evident when the patient lies down. Indigestion and diarrhea are common, and after a short time the patient becomes emaciated. The thyroid is usually enlarged, although in most cases the enlargement is less marked than in the colloid type.

As the disease progresses the patient grows weaker, totally incapable of doing any sort of work. The slightest excitement aggravates symptoms.

Toxic goiter occurs in both sexes but more frequently in the female.

Preoperative Treatment and Nursing Care

Patients suffering with exophthalmic goiter cannot be operated on without requisite preoperative preparation. These extremely nervous individuals must have some considerable period of rest in bed in the most quiet atmosphere possible. They must be protected from disturbing sights and should be placed so that they will not come in contact with very ill patients. In the care of these patients it may be well to place them beside a patient who has made a satisfactory recovery from operation. The nurse should see that they have an abundance of fresh air and an ample amount of carbohydrate and protein foods. Usually this patient is embarrassed about his unusually large appetite and may hesitate to ask for another helping. The nurse should recognize this dietary need because of the increased metabolic activity. A daily caloric intake of from 4,000 to 5,000 calories is not only desirable but essential. Tea or coffee is not given without the permission of the physician.

The nurse should gain the complete confidence of her patient and by every method attempt to keep the patient free from worry and anxiety. Some forms of occupational therapy are quieting and are given at the direction of the surgeon.

The patient with a hyperthyroidism often comes to the hospital from a home made tense and unhappy by restlessness, nervousness and loss of efficiency, which are the symptoms of the disease. It is necessary to protect the patient from a continuance of such unpleasantness and unhappiness. Therefore, the nurse should watch carefully the effect of visitors upon the patient. If there is any evidence of nervous upsets by their visits, it may be advisable to limit the visiting privileges during the preoperative period.

Sedatives (bromides) are frequently administered, and because many older patients with hyperthyroidism have associated cardiac disease, digitalis may also be given.

Three methods of treatment may be used in the treatment of hyperthyroidism. Certain drugs, thiouracil, propylthiouracil and methylthiouracil in appropriate dosages, prevent the thyroid from utilizing iodine to make thyroxin. Since an excess or abnormal formation of thyroxin produces hyperthyroidism, this action reduces the toxic symptoms and brings the basal metabolic rate back to normal. In mild cases, lengthy remissions of hyperthyroidism may be produced, and the patients may need no other treatment. Experience has shown that severe cases of toxic adenomas cannot be cured by this method alone, but the drugs are used to prepare these patients for thyroidectomy. They are not without danger, in that they may produce toxic symptoms, one of which is a depression of the white blood count (agranulocytosis). For this reason blood counts are taken at frequent intervals.

Subtotal thyroidectomy is the treatment for hyperthyroidism which has been employed for many years. But operation upon a patient in the "toxic" state is so dangerous that efforts to reduce the toxicity and bring the basal metabolism back to normal are employed regularly before operation is considered. The administration of iodine as Lugol's solution or potassium iodide is known to reduce the glandular hyperplasia and the metabolic rate. The thiouracil drugs are so much more effective in reducing the basal metabolism that usually they are employed first; iodine is given in addition in the last week before thyroidectomy. With this method of preparation, operation can be performed with a mortality that is almost nil.

Radioactive iodine as a therapeutic drug in hyperthyroidism is a development of the atomic age. The thyroid is known to absorb and utilize iodine in the formation of thyroxin. Radioactive iodine given by mouth is absorbed and produces an effect on the thyroid by giving off rays which destroy the glandular cells. The radioactivity is short-lived, so that repeated doses may be given, depending upon the course of the disease. This method of treatment usually is reserved for the older patient and for malignancy of the thyroid.

Basal Metabolism. That the doctors may estimate the rapidity with which the metabolic processes are working, the basal metabolic rate is determined at frequent intervals. In order to carry out the test properly, it is necessary that the patient be as quiet as possible and without food or water for at least 12 hours previously. Therefore, this estimation usually is made in the morning, the nurse having been instructed to withhold the breakfast until after the test. The basal metabolism estimation, although painless, is often looked upon with considerable apprehension by the patient. This may be overcome easily if the nurse will take the trouble to explain briefly to the patient what is done during this procedure. The slightest amount of exertion increases the metabolic rate and will give an inaccurate reading; therefore, the patient always is transferred to the metabolic department in bed when possible or certainly on a stretcher or a wheel chair.

Many different conditions and factors have to be considered in the interpretation of a basal metabolic rate. The person taking it must have the entire confidence and co-operation of the patient. There should be no disturbing elements. If the patient has had a stormy night or has been upset in any manner whatever previous to the time set for the test, too much importance should not be attached to the reading. These patients should be sent back with a request for a future reading as a checkup. A non-co-operative patient will frequently produce a high metabolic rate. Furthermore, the type of machine, as well as the ability of the person conducting the examination, must be considered in the final decision.

Operation. The immediate preparation of thyroid patients for surgery includes a good night's rest the preceding night, adequate shaving of the neck (see p. 58), nothing by mouth after midnight and a preanesthetic hypodermic about 20 or 30 minutes before surgery. The operation is performed with the patient in the dorsal position, with a sandbag or air pillow under the shoulders and the head low to make the neck more prominent (see p. 91). The patient's hair should be tightly enclosed in a cap. Through a transverse incision in the lower part of the neck, the thyroid is exposed and excised, leaving only a small amount of glandular tissue on the posterior capsule of the gland on each side. This small amount of thyroid tissue is all that is necessary for normal function, and an inadequate removal of the gland predisposes to a recurrence of hyperthyroidism. The wound is usually closed with clips and is often drained for a day or two.

Nursing Care of Patients After Thyroidectomy

The patient should be moved carefully, care being taken to support the head so that no tension be placed on the sutures. The most comfortable position is the semi-Fowler with the head elevated and supported by pillows. The utmost quiet is observed, and morphine is given hypodermically to relieve the painful effects of the operation. Occasionally the patient is placed in an oxygen tent for the first few hours to facilitate breathing. The nurse should anticipate any apprehension on the part of her patient and inform him that by being in the tent his breathing will be easier and he will be less tired. Fluid may be given by vein, but water may be given by mouth as soon as nausea ceases. The nurse should inspect and reinforce the dressings when necessary, remembering that when the patient is in the dorsal position, evidences of bleeding should be looked for at the sides and the back of the neck as well as anteriorly. In addition to checking the pulse and the blood pressure, it is also important to be on the alert for complaints from the patient of sensation of pressure or fullness at the incision site. These may be indicative of hemorrhage and should be reported. Ice caps applied over the dressing are routine in many hospitals to help in bleeding control. Usually, there is a little difficulty in swallowing, and in this condition experience has taught that cold fluids, or ice, may be taken better than others. Often a soft diet is preferred by many patients rather than a liquid diet. Occasionally, difficulty in respiration is observed with the development of cyanosis and noisy breathing, due to an edema of the glottis or to an injury to the recurrent laryngeal nerves. Since this complication demands the insertion of a tracheotomy tube, the surgeon in charge should be summoned at once.

Little talking should be permitted, but when the patient does speak, the nurse should watch for voice changes which might indicate injury to the recurrent laryngeal nerves which lie just behind the thyroid next to the trachea.

When the nurse is not in constant attendance an overbed table is a great comfort to the patient. On it may be placed the materials which are needed frequently, such as paper wipes, water pitcher and glass, small emesis basin, etc. These are kept within easy reach so that the patient is not required to turn the head in search of them. It is also convenient to use this table when inhalations are given for the relief of excessive mucous secretions.

The patient is usually permitted out of bed on the first postoperative day and has a diet of choice. A well-balanced high-caloric diet is to be preferred to regain any weight loss. Stitches or skin clips are usually removed on the second day. By the fifth day, the average patient is ready for discharge from the hospital.

Complications. Hemorrhage, edema of glottis and injury to the recurrent laryngeal nerve are complications which have been reviewed in the preceding section. Other noteworthy complications are tetany and acute thyrotoxicosis.

Tetany. Occasionally, in operations upon the thyroid, the parathyroid glandules may be injured or removed. This produces a disturbance of the calcium metabolism of the body. As the blood calcium falls, there appears a hyperirritability of the nerves, with spasms of the hands and the feet and muscular twitchings. This group of symptoms is termed tetany, and its appearance should be called to the attention of the surgeon at once. Tetany of this type is usually relieved by the administration of parathyroid extract or calcium in some form.

Acute Thyrotoxicosis. The most serious postoperative complication after thyroidectomy for toxic goiter is a condition called acute thyrotoxicosis. The symptoms usually appear soon after operation, with a marked rise in temperature, often 105° to 106° F., rapid thready pulse, profuse perspiration and extreme restlessness. Delirium and death may follow in rapid order. At the appearance of any of these symptoms the surgeon should be notified.

In the treatment of thyrotoxicosis, the application of cold has been most effective. Icebags may be used—8 or 10 for temperatures of 102° to 103° F., but if the temperature reaches 104° F., a complete ice pack may be used. Rubber sheets are placed under and over the patient, protected of course by a cotton sheet. Several pounds of cracked ice are placed on the upper sheet, and an electric fan is put at the foot of the bed and directed toward the patient's face. The ice pack is maintained as long as the

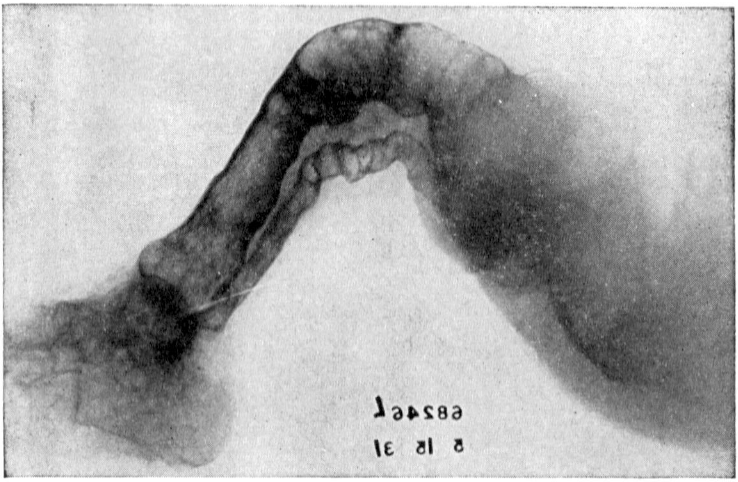

FIG. 195. Roentgenogram of the lower limb of a male patient who had a large adenoma of a parathyroid gland that caused decalcification, multiple fractures, cystic degeneration and skeleton deformities and resulted in a loss of stature. Removal of tumor stopped the loss of calcium and recurrent fractures.

marked elevation of temperature continues. In addition to the external cold, cold fluids may be given by mouth, along with sedative drugs, sodium bromide 1 Gm. (gr. 15), third hour, or luminal .06 Gm. (gr. 1), b.i.d. It has been shown that the preoperative and postoperative administration of 10 per cent glucose solution intravenously will prevent the severe toxic reaction after operation. This form of treatment is especially valuable when dealing with the very toxic patient in whom thyrotoxicosis is most likely to develop. Vitamin B_1 is a valuable adjunct.

Convalescence. After recovery from operation for toxic goiter, the convalescence should be long, to give the patient adequate time to regain his strength before resuming active life. It is often possible to arrange for these patients to spend some time after operation in a convalescent home if their own home surroundings are not convenient or suitable.

Carcinoma of the Thyroid

The thyroid may develop tumors, both benign and malignant. The benign tumors, adenomas, develop malignant changes in a fair percentage of cases; this is one of the indications for operation in nodular goiter. Carcinoma of the thyroid usually is diagnosed preoperatively if far advanced, but often the malignancy is discovered only in microscopic section or at operation in less-advanced cases. The treatment consists of total removal of the thyroid gland, or of the involved lobe, and the removal of the lymph nodes

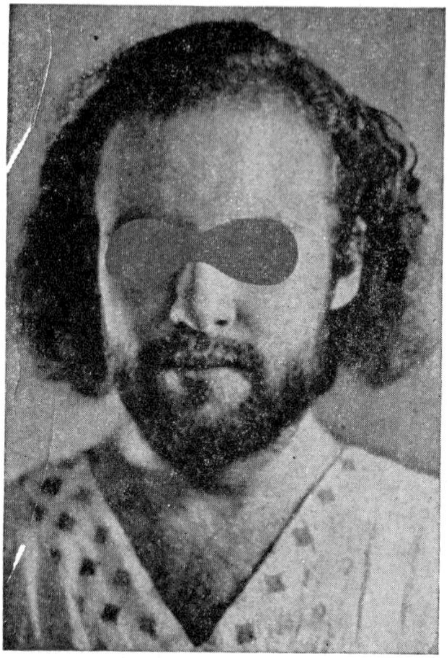

FIG. 196. A 16-year-old girl with developed hirsutism, masculinity and a heavy beard that grew with great strength in childhood. She menstruated 1 day only when she was 16 years old. A large adrenal shadow was demonstrated by roentgenogram after perirenal injection. At operation a large cortical adrenal adenoma was removed.

draining the involved area. X-ray therapy is a valuable adjunct. Radioactive iodine is also used in repeated doses instead of or in addition to surgery.

THE PARATHYROID GLANDS

Hyperparathyroidism. The small parathyroid glands, four in number, regulate the metabolism of calcium in the body. Occasionally, they are the seat of benign tumors, and their abnormal secretion causes a decalcification of bones, resulting in pathologic fractures and calcium deposits elsewhere in the body (tendons, kidney, pelvis, etc.). In such cases, improvement or cure may be obtained by removal of the parathyroid tumor.

THE ADRENAL GLANDS

The adrenal glands are small triangular organs which lie in the retroperitoneal fatty tissue above the kidneys. (Fig. 156.) They are important parts of the ductless glands, and the hormones which they secrete have to do with the development and growth of the sexual characteristics of the individual and with the regulation of the blood pressure by the well-known hormone adrenalin. These glands become of surgical importance when tumors develop in them. The tumors which arise in the cortical or outside portion of the gland give rise to changes in the sexual characteristics of the patient, virilism in women and feminism in men. They occur most often in young women and produce symptoms depending upon the age and the sex of the patient.

Virilism is characterized by the appearance of masculine and the recession of feminine physical and mental traits. There is an excessive growth of hair on the face (hirsutism), the breasts atrophy, the menses cease, the clitoris enlarges, and the patient's voice and habits approach the masculine. Arrhenoblastoma of the ovary will simulate the above symptom complex. When the disease occurs in children a precocious puberty results. If these changes occur in utero, a true hermaphrodite may be the result. If the change begins in early childhood, pseudohermaphrodism will result.

Diagnosis of Tumors. This is often somewhat difficult because many similar symptoms may be produced by certain tumors of the pituitary gland and by some ovarian tumors.

The tumors which arise from the medulla or central part of the adrenal are less frequent. They give symptoms of paroxysmal hypertension accompanied by pallor, tachycardia, headache and sweating.

Because these glands are so small their tumors cannot usually be palpated and, in an effort to make a diagnosis, sometimes air is injected into the fatty tissue around them to make them visible on an x-ray plate.

Operation. When the tumors are diagnosed or their presence is suspected, remarkable recovery may take place if they can be removed. The operation is performed through an incision in the loin or through an abdominal incision. In the treatment of these cases sodium chloride and sodium citrate are given in large amounts both preoperatively and postoperatively. Frequently, there is a very marked and rapidly developing insufficiency of the adrenal gland after operation, the signs of which are anorexia, hiccough, nausea, vomiting, sleeplessness, weakness, restlessness or apathy, an increase of pulse rate and a fall in blood pressure. To avoid these complications, extracts of adrenal cortex are given both before and after operation. The blood pressure must be estimated at intervals of four hours. A diet low in potassium is usually given.

SURGERY IN DIABETES

It is generally conceded that a patient with diabetes is a poor operative risk. This is due, in part, to the fact that the majority of such patients are old in years and are already in a state of general decline or are prematurely "old" because of early arteriosclerosis. The resistance to infection is low, healing is usually delayed, and serious diabetic complications, such as coma, often follow minor infections and even minor operative procedures.

With the advent of insulin and the facilities for chemical analysis of the blood, the prognosis for the diabetic has improved materially. The metabolic problems which previously complicated nearly every surgical operation now can be solved rapidly and often surely by proper pre- and postoperative treatment. Insulin and the administration of glucose, either by mouth (orange juice) or intravenously, are the usual preoperative measures. Fluids should be supplied in abundance. The operation should take place not more than two hours after the last prescribed food given in liquid form.

The anesthetics which experience has shown to be best fitted for the diabetic are the gasses (nitrous oxide or ethylene) or spinal anesthesia. Postoperatively, food and fluids are given as soon as possible, with sufficient insulin to prevent acidosis. Because postoperative vomiting may often occur, it is the practice in some clinics to pass a nasal tube before or immediately after operation (Fig. 272, p. 631). Fluids and liquid foods may be given slowly by this method almost immediately after operation. The operations most commonly performed are amputations for gangrene. The utmost care must be employed in dressing the wounds of diabetics to prevent infection. (See Chap. 6, p. 115.)

Gangrene of the toes and the foot is the most frequent surgical complication of the diabetic. It occurs due to an early development of arteriosclerosis. Many prophylactic measures have been suggested, the chief of which is cleanliness of the feet. A second is a warning against the promiscuous cutting of corns and calluses. A frequently obtained history is one of the onset of gangrene immediately after cutting a corn on unclean feet. The cold and painful extremities which are the premonitory signs of gangrene are often carelessly treated by heat. Burns which too often occur may mark the onset of gangrene. The treatment of early gangrene has been described elsewhere (p. 270).

Diet for Surgical Diabetics

The preoperative treatment is to store sufficient glycogen in the liver to protect the patient against the anesthetic. This carbohydrate may be given in the form of tea and toast, orange juice, oatmeal, or oatmeal gruel. Insulin must be given in order to burn sufficient of it. After operation, as well as before, hyperglycemia and its threatening acidosis or hypoglycemia due to starvation caused by insufficient food or excess of insulin to burn the food eaten must be guarded against. For the first 24 hours after nausea ceases oatmeal gruel or orange juice, plain or with glucose added, is given. If not tolerated by mouth, glucose is given intravenously. The carbohydrate feedings should be stopped 3 hours prior to the operation and resumed 3 hours after the operation. Insulin should be given before each feeding to ensure the utilization of the food.

When liquid diet may be replaced by soft and light diet, the patient will gradually be put back on his former diet or one that is found to be more suitable.

Nursing Care of Surgical Patients with Diabetes

Any infection is a source of potential danger because organisms thrive and spread more rapidly when blood sugar content is above normal. Whether the patient with diabetes has had surgery or is to have surgery, the principles of care remain the same. Essentially, trauma to tissues must be minimized if not eliminated, and the metabolic balance must be maintained. If not, the patient risks the hazards of spreading infection with necrosis and experiences the metabolic imbalances of diabetic coma or insulin shock.

A furuncle or corn never should be squeezed or cut; scratches and burns must be prevented. Once a local infection is present, it is difficult to control. The nurse has an opportunity to teach ways of preventing skin breaks. Pressure points, such as corns, calluses, blisters and ingrown toenails, can be eliminated if properly fitting shoes and stockings are worn. The feet should be washed daily and patted dry with a soft towel. No friction should be exerted. Lanolin spread thinly is effective in keeping the skin soft, and the placing of lamb's wool between the toes will help to prevent friction. Nails may be cut straight across.

The patient must be made aware of the dangers of bruises resulting from accidentally bumping into carelessly placed footstools and other furniture. Proper lighting and well-fitting eyeglasses are necessities to these individuals.

When a wound is present, aseptic technic must be followed in an attempt to prevent infection from spreading.

The nurse is responsible for serving an attractive diet, noting what has not been eaten and reporting it so that a proper substitute may be made to maintain metabolic balance. She is also responsible for the collection of urine and blood specimens and their proper disposition to the laboratory. These two functions are as important as the giving of medications.

The surgical patient may face any one or all three of the following disturbances which interfere with a properly balanced metabolism: (1) Vomiting. This should be inspected for food loss and reported so that essential food value may be replaced intravenously. (2) Starvation. Prior to surgery, a patient is placed on nothing by mouth. Infusions of glucose and injections of insulin are used to maintain balance. (3) Febrile reactions are sufficient to upset carbohydrate metabolism, and appropriate steps must be taken to maintain metabolic balance by increasing insulin. In addition to the above, an adequate protein reserve must be established prior to operation and the salt and water balance must be maintained.

Diabetes with the threat of coma or insulin shock requires close attention and observation on the part of the nurse. She should have insulin and intravenous glucose solution on hand for immediate use in any possible emergency.

REFERENCES AND SUGGESTED READING

Unit Eight: Nursing in Conditions of the Endocrine Glands

General

Emerson, C. P., and Bragdon, J. S.: Essentials of Medicine, ed. 17, pp. 523-578, Philadelphia, Lippincott, 1955.

(See also those for Unit One, p. 205)

Grollman, A.: Essentials of Endocrinology, ed. 2, Philadelphia, Lippincott, 1947.

Thyroid

Bartels, E. C.: Thiouracil and allied drugs in hyperthyroidism, New England J. Med. **238**:6, 1948.

Corrigan, K. E.: Use of radioactive isotopes, Am. J. Nursing **48**:309-311, 1948.

Emerson, C. P., and Bragdon, J. S.: Essentials of Medicine, ed. 17, pp. 526-541, pp. 527-529 (B.M.R.), Philadelphia, Lippincott, 1955.

Evans, F. A.: The basal metabolic rate determination, Am. J. Nursing **53**:1322-1323, 1953.

King, B. T., Felton, V., and Stoleson, H.: Nursing care in hyperthyroidism, Am. J. Nursing **46**: 773-775, 1946.

Lidz, Theodore: Emotional factors in the etiology of hyperthyroidism, Psychosom. Med. 11:2-8, 1949.

Means, J. H.: The Thyroid and Its Diseases, ed. 2, Philadelphia, Lippincott, 1948.

DIABETES

Beardwood, J. T., and Kelly, H. T.: Simplified Diabetic Management, ed. 6, Philadelphia, Lippincott, 1954.

Emerson, C. P., and Bragdon, J. S.: Essentials of Medicine, ed. 17, pp. 542-566, Philadelphia, Lippincott, 1955.

Maureen, Sister M., and Beland, Irene: The nurse and the diabetic patient, Am. J. Nursing **46**:606-609, 1946.

Rosenthal, Helen, Stern, Frances, and Rosenthal, Joseph: Diabetic Care in Pictures, ed. 2, Philadelphia, Lippincott, 1953.

CLINICAL SITUATION: THYROIDECTOMY

Cynthia Swann, a young newspaper reporter, announced to her roommate that she "simply could not take it anymore." She was irritable, losing weight and easily upset. Her friend insisted that she see a physician and offered to go with her. Shortly thereafter, Cynthia was hospitalized with a presumptive diagnosis of exophthalmic goiter.

1. Thiouracil was given to Miss Swann in order to

____(1) produce atrophy of the gland
____(2) lower the blood calcium and increase the blood phosphorus
____(3) reduce the hyperplasia of the gland
____(4) give off rays that destroy the glandular cells

2. A suitable form of relaxation which the nurse might suggest to Miss Swann preoperatively is to

____(1) listen to a college football game on the radio
____(2) watch an absorbing mystery play on television
____(3) join another patient in learning how to tat (make fine lace)
____(4) play cards with other patients

3. A basal metabolic test is done to determine

____(1) the vital capacity of the pulmonary system
____(2) the rapidity with which the metabolic processes are working
____(3) the extent of growth of the thyroid gland and the pressure exerted upon the trachea
____(4) the degree to which a highly nervous patient can relax when conditions are favorable

4. On recovery from anesthesia after a subtotal thyroidectomy, Miss Swann's most desirable position will be

____(1) prone
____(2) high Fowler's
____(3) supine
____(4) Trendelenburg

5. Hemorrhage may be detected by noticing the following symptoms:

____(1) complaint of a sensation of fullness at the incision site
____(2) a fall in pulse, shallow respirations, increase in blood pressure
____(3) apathy, drowsiness, a forward nodding of the head
____(4) apprehension, thirst and a flush of the face

6. Upon discharge, Miss Swann

will be instructed to return for follow-up visits because

_____(1) radiation therapy must be instituted

_____(2) a series of radioactive iodine treatments is necessary

_____(3) a general check-up including a basal metabolic test should be done

_____(4) the skin clips have to be removed

7. Before leaving the hospital, Miss Swann asked the nurse if she had any suggestions to offer about making her incision less conspicuous. The best reply would be:

_____(1) "Wear your usual clothes. The only person to whom such an incision would appear conspicuous is yourself."

_____(2) "The best thing to do is wear high-necked dresses. Use lace insertions in the dresses you now have."

_____(3) "Colorful scarves and costume jewelry will help to hide the scar."

_____(4) "Don't cover the incision line with anything, for it may irritate scar tissue and produce an infection."

UNIT NINE

Nursing in Conditions of the Nervous System

CHAPTER TWENTY-FOUR

Surgery of Brain and Spinal Cord

HISTORY

Neurosurgery is a division of general surgery that has made most of its advances since the beginning of the twentieth century. Paul Broca (1824-1880), a French surgeon, was the founder of modern surgery of the brain.* Sir Victor Horsley (1857-1916), an English neurologist and surgeon, is credited with the recognition of neurosurgery as a special field.† In the United States, training of personnel for this specialty preceded that of European countries. Dr. Harvey Cushing (1869-1939), of Johns Hopkins, Harvard and Yale Universities, and Dr. Charles H. Frazier (1870-1936), of the University of Pennsylvania, were two of the pioneer neurosurgeons.

* Garrison, F. H.: History of Medicine, p. 492, ed. 4, Philadelphia, Saunders.

† Frazier, C. H.: A review, clinical and pathological, of parahypophyseal lesions, Surg., Gynec. & Obst. **62**:1.

In England, in 1888, Sir Victor Horsley and William Richard Gowers (1845-1915) were the first to remove a tumor from the spinal cord;* soon such operations were performed in the United States.

It was not until 1918 that Dr.

* Garrison, F. H.: History of Medicine, p. 643, ed. 4, Philadelphia, Saunders.

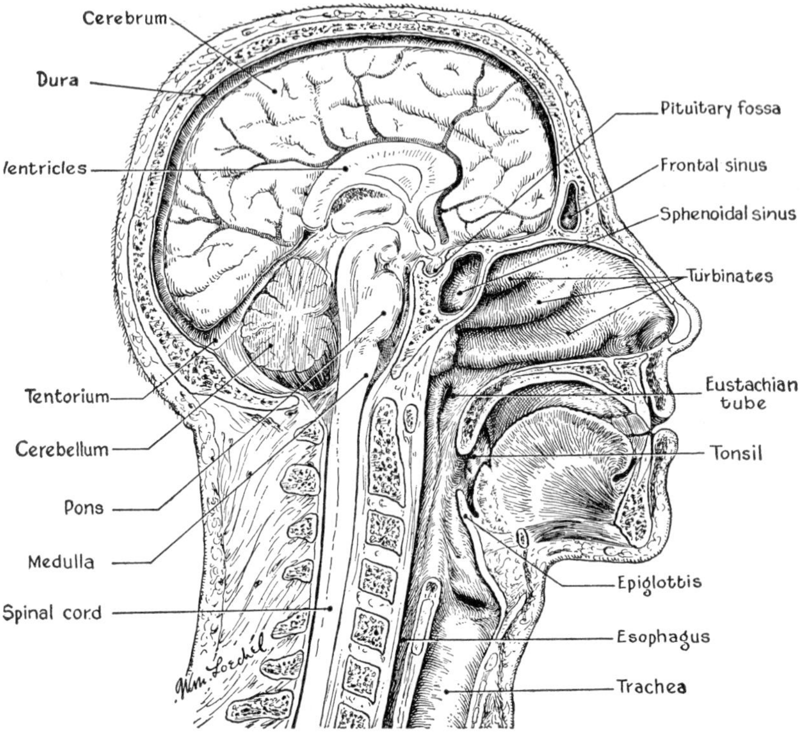

FIG. 197. Cross-sectional view, showing the anatomic position and relation of structures of the head and the neck.

Walter E. Dandy, of Baltimore, injected air into the ventricles for the diagnosis of brain tumors by x-rays (ventriculography). In 1919 he extended this method of air injection by using the lumbar route (encephalography). Other significant contributions have been the x-ray visualizations of the blood vessels of the brain (arteriography) and the recording of the minute electrical currents of the brain (electroencephalography).*

* Davidoff, L. M., and Dyke, C. G.: The Normal Encephalogram, p. 11, Philadelphia, Lea.

Due to the work of these men and many others in the field of research, surgery of the nervous system has developed into the highly specialized branch of surgery which it is today.

Neurosurgical Nursing

The field of neurosurgical nursing is a fascinating one. Within its scope the nurse has an opportunity to utilize all her powers of observation. By her careful charting, she is a vital source of information for the surgeon as he makes a diagnosis and in the postoperative care of her patient.

By her optimism, nursing ability

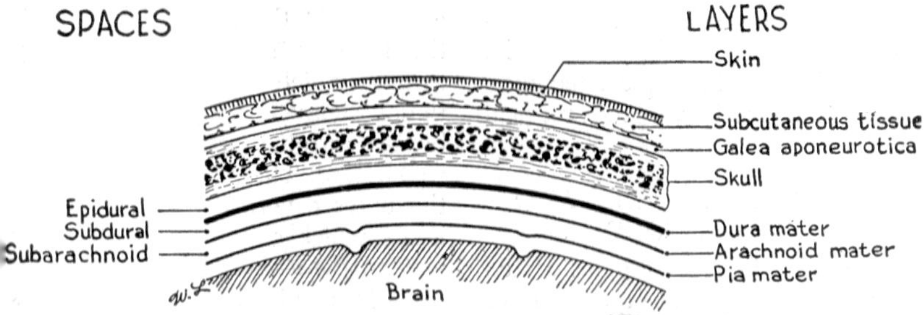

FIG. 198. Diagrammatic drawing showing the various layers from skin to brain. (*Left*) The intracranial spaces are indicated. (*Right*) The various layers of tissue structure.

and concern for the patient as a person, the nurse can help to ease many of the difficult experiences of her patient and his family. When one realizes that the behavior and the personality of a person can be affected markedly by organic lesions of the brain, she is less inclined to think of an individual as an un-co-operative patient with a foul disposition but rather as one who needs help and understanding. His reactions may be beyond his control; the nurse must realize this.

The many interesting diagnostic tests in which the nurse participates are much like solving a puzzle. But more interesting, the diagnosis is not the end; it is merely a steppingstone to the removal of the cause. Surgery must be done accurately for otherwise the penalty may be the death of the patient or the reduction of his mental and/or physical abilities to that of mere existence. Although surgery has its numbers of successful cases, there are instances in which the injury is too great to repair, or the tumor too extensive to remove, and the patient's prognosis is hopeless. It is important that even in these instances the nurse must exercise as much concern for the comfort and the feelings of her patient as she does in situations where the prognosis is more encouraging. This is significant, not only from the point of view of the individual patient, but also from that of his family.

The neurosurgical nurse has an opportunity to use many procedures in giving sound conscientious bedside care. It is important to apply the principles of good body mechanics, since the position of the patient must be changed frequently. From the moment the patient shows response after his operation, the nurse is on the alert to help him in his rehabilitation. Often every activity may have to be relearned, such as using his fingers to hold a spoon, learning to say words and sentences, acquiring the ability to write, etc. In addition he needs psychological assistance in the form of encouragement. The nurse is a key person in that she is with him day and night and therefore is responsible for much of his future progress.

Neurosurgery is becoming increasingly more common because of the many advances in surgical technics. There is a need for good surgical nurses.

ANATOMY OF BRAIN AND SPINAL CORD

The brain is a soft organ, located in a rigid, bony box—the skull or cranium. At the base of this box is the foramen magnum, an opening through which the spinal cord is continuous with the brain. Three membranes surround the brain and the spinal cord. These are (1) the dura, the outer covering of dense fibrous tissue which closely hugs the inner wall of the skull, (2) the arachnoid and (3) the pia mater, which adheres

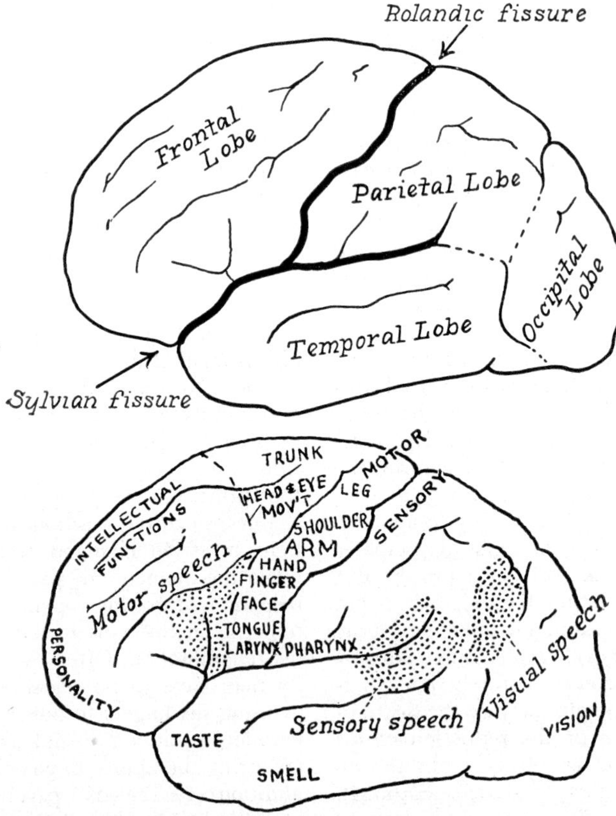

FIG. 199. (*Top*) Diagrammatic representation of the cerebrum, showing relative locations of various lobes of the brain and the principal fissures. (*Bottom*) Diagrammatic representation of cerebral localization for motor movements of various portions of the body.

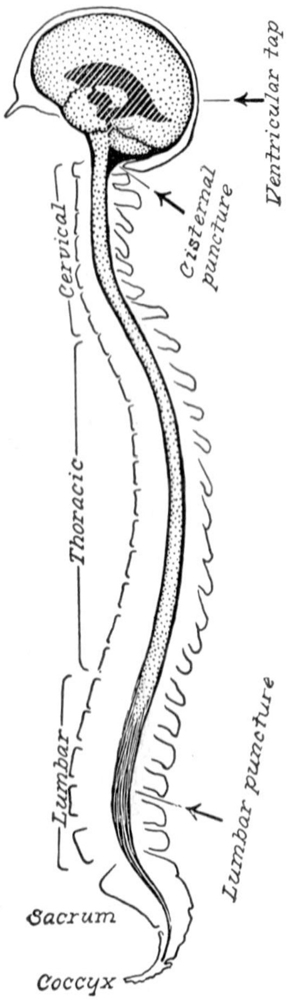

FIG. 200. Diagrammatic representation of the cerebrospinal system, showing the brain, the cord and the spaces occupied by cerebrospinal fluid, ventricles and dural sac. The sites for the introduction of needles for ventricular tap, cisternal puncture and lumbar puncture are indicated.

closely to the brain and spinal-cord surfaces (meninges).

Divisions of Brain. The brain is divided into cerebrum, midbrain, cerebellum, pons varolii and medulla oblongata or brain stem.

The *cerebrum* is divided into 2 hemispheres and consists of 5 lobes: frontal, parietal, temporal, occipital and insular. The cerebrum is the largest part of the brain, and on its surface or cortex are located the "centers" from which motor impulses are carried to the muscles and to which sensory impulses come from the various sensory nerves.

The *midbrain* connects the pons and the cerebellum with the hemispheres of the cerebrum.

The *cerebellum* or "little brain" is located below and behind the cerebrum. Its function is the control or co-ordination of muscles and equilibration.

The *pons varolii* is situated in front of the cerebellum between the midbrain and the medulla and is a bridge of union between the two halves of the cerebellum as well as between the medulla and the cerebrum.

The *medulla oblongata* transmits the fibers from the brain to the spinal cord, motor fibers crossing at this point. It also contains important centers controlling the heart, respiration and blood pressure and gives origin to a number of cranial nerves. The 12 cranial nerves find exit from the brain at the base of the skull.

There are two glands present in the brain: the pituitary and the pineal. The pituitary gland is frequently approached surgically. It lies at the base of the brain in a bony fossa termed the sella turcica, just posterior to the optic chiasm, upon which it may press when the gland is enlarged.

Spinal Cord. The spinal cord, surrounded by the vertebral column, extends from the foramen magnum of the skull, where it is continuous with the medulla oblongata, to the first lumbar vertebra, where it tapers off into a fine thread of tissue. The spinal cord is an important center of reflex action for the body and contains the conducting pathways to and from the higher centers in the cord and brain.

Nervous System. The nervous system has two main divisions: the voluntary (that portion over which the being has control) and the autonomic (that portion over which control is not possible). The latter is divided into (1) the parasympathetic system, of which the vagus nerve mainly determines the function, and (2) the sympathetic nervous system, a separate set of nerve fibers from the spinal cord which supply the vital organs, the blood vessels, the sweat glands and the pupils of the eye.

CEREBROSPINAL FLUID

The soft structure of the brain is protected not only by its three coverings, but it is also bathed and, in a manner, cushioned by cerebrospinal fluid. This fluid is secreted by the choroid plexuses in the cavities of the brain called ventricles. It circulates by well-defined channels from the lateral ventricles through narrow tubular openings to the third and the fourth ventricles. From this narrow cavity it escapes to the subarachnoid space to bathe the entire surface of the brain and the spinal cord. The cerebrospinal fluid is normally absorbed by the large venous channels of the skull and along the spinal and cranial nerves.

The spinal fluid is clear and colorless, having a specific gravity of 1.007. The average patient's ventricular and subarachnoid systems contain about 150 cc. of this fluid. Inasmuch as the fluid is considered to be a dialysate from the choroid plexuses, its composition includes those substances also present in blood plasma, which is its source. Disease produces changes in the composition of this fluid. Determinations of the protein content and the quantity of glucose and chloride present constitute the chief chemical examinations. In a state of health there are a minimal number of white cells and no red cells in the spinal fluid, thus the examination for cells is important. Other diagnostic examinations include the Wassermann reaction for syphilis and the colloidal-gold reaction, which is a colloidal precipitation test based upon the protein content in the spinal fluid.

The ventricular system is important to the neurosurgeon for another reason. By means of air replacing cerebrospinal fluid, he is able to visualize with x-rays (encephalogram and ventriculogram discussed later) the size, the shape and the position of these structures. Any interference or distortion may be suggestive of a space occupying lesion. (See Fig. 204.)

PHYSICAL AND NEUROLOGIC EXAMINATION

In addition to the usual complete physical examination, the neurosurgical patient has a neurologic examination. (See below.) The nurse and the physician can help the patient to assist in this vital diagnostic procedure by explaining what he is expected to do. All equipment should be available in one place.

An examination of the motor and the sensory systems is also done. Motor tests include observation of posture and gait, reflex tests, coordination observations, etc. Sensory tests determine skin sensation and deeper tissue sensation as well as ability to recognize objects by sense of touch.

NEUROLOGIC EXAMINATION FOR TESTING CRANIAL NERVES

Nerve	*Equipment*	*Procedure*
I. Olfactory	Four small bottles of volatile oils, such as: (1) turpentine, (2) oil of cloves, (3) oil of wintergreen, (4) vanilla	Instruct patient to sniff and identify the odors. Each nostril used separately.
II. Optic	Ophthalmoscope	In darkened room, patient is examined with this instrument. More detailed examination with special equipment is used for accurate visual fields determination.
III. Oculomotor IV. Trochlear VI. Abducens	Flashlight	Because of close association these nerves are examined collectively. They innervate pupil and upper eyelid and are responsible for extraocular muscle movements.
V. Trigeminal	Test tube of hot water Test tube of ice water Cotton wisp from cotton applicator stick Pin	*Sensory* branch – Vertex to chin tested for sensations of pain, touch and temperature. This includes reflex reaction of cornea to wisp of cotton. *Motor* branch—Ability to bite is tested.
VII. Facial	Four small bottles with solutions which are salty, sweet, sour and bitter (Four clean medicine droppers)	Observe symmetry of face and ability to contract facial muscles. Instruct patient to taste and identify substance used. He should rinse his mouth well between each drop of solution. This is a test for the anterior ⅔ of tongue.
VIII. Acoustic	Tuning fork	Tests for hearing, air and bone conduction.

Nerve	Equipment	Procedure
IX. Glosso-pharyngeal	Cotton applicator stick	Test for taste of posterior ⅓ of tongue and gag reflex.
X. Vagus	Tongue depressor	Checking voice sounds, observing symmetry of soft palate will give suggestion of function of vagus.
XI. Spinal Accessory		Since this innervates the sternocleidomastoid and the trapezius muscles, the patient will be instructed to turn and move his head and elevate shoulders with and without resistance.
XII. Hypoglossal		Tongue movements observed.

The nurse should know the results of the findings of the neurologic and physical examination because only then is she able to observe intelligently any diversion in symptoms or reactions of her patient. These deviations must be charted accurately if they are to be meaningful to the neurosurgeon.

LUMBAR AND CISTERNAL PUNCTURES

Inasmuch as the quality of the cerebrospinal fluid, as well as its pressure, may be a diagnostic aid to the surgeon, punctures to obtain such fluid may be done. The pressure in the cerebrospinal system may be estimated and a specimen of the fluid readily obtained by inserting a needle into the subarachnoid space between the third and the fourth lumbar vertebrae or at the base of the skull. Normal pressure averages 125 mm. of water. Values from 75 to 200 mm. are considered within physiologic limits. The puncture in the lumbar region is called a *lumbar* or *spinal puncture;* the insertion of the needle into the cisterna magna at the base of the brain is called a *cisternal puncture.*

The tray prepared by the nurse for these punctures should contain:

1. Local anesthesia syringe, needle, and procaine 0.5 per cent solution.
2. Covers—sterile.
3. Skin antiseptics and sterile cotton.
4. Spinal-puncture needle with stilets to fit. (It is important that before setting up the spinal-puncture tray, the nurse inspect the spinal needles, being particularly careful that the stilet and the needle fit exactly, especially at the tip. Frequently, the stilet fits perfectly at the handle end, but the bevel of the needle and the stilet do not coincide. Such a needle is difficult to introduce and may cause an unnecessarily large hole in the dura. The difficulty usually lies in the fact that the stilet and the needles have been interchanged.)
5. Water manometer and rubber tube attachment. (All of these parts must be tested beforehand by the nurse to insure patency of the tubes and accurate fitting

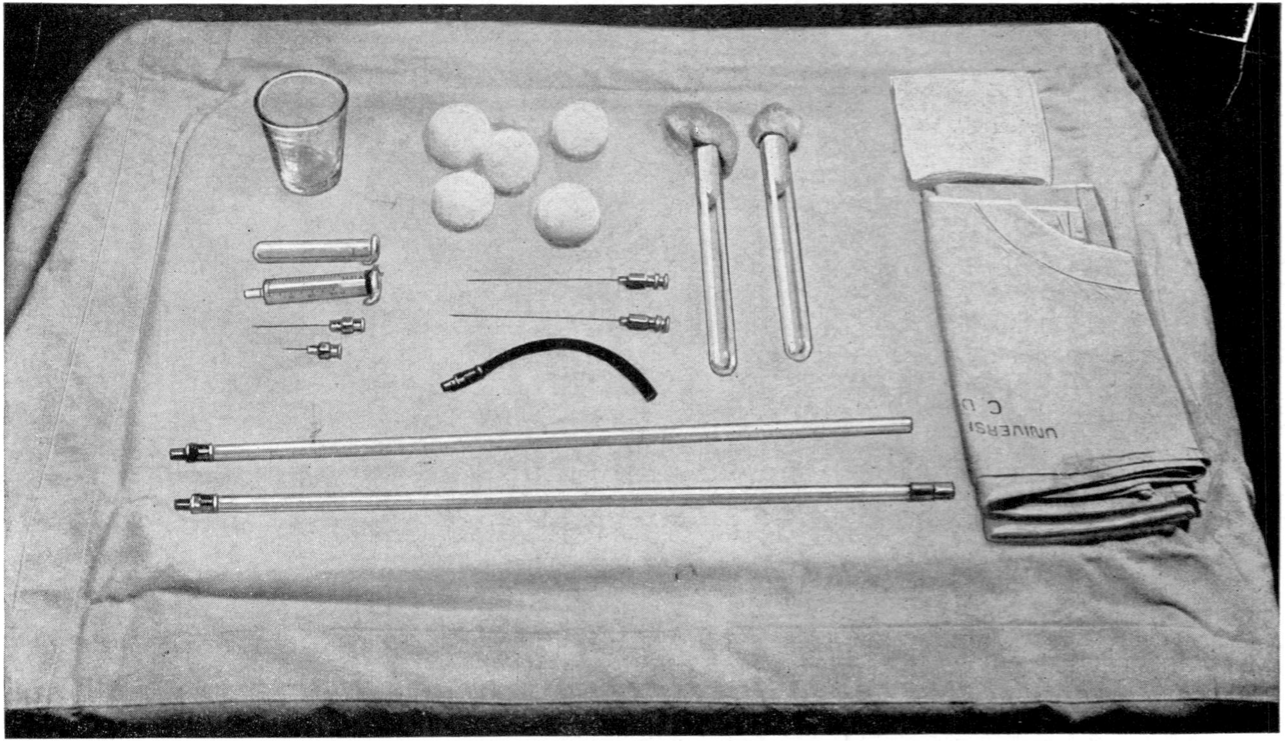

Fig. 201. Sterile lumbar-puncture tray. The tray is set up as pictured and sterilized in an autoclave. The medicine glass is for procaine solution. Note water (glass) manometer and attachments, tubes for spinal fluid and drapes. A 3-way stopcock may be used instead of a metal adapter and rubber tubing.

of the parts to the manometer and the needles.)

6. Sterile test tubes—2, with non-absorbent cotton plugs or corks.

The nurse should have a pair of sterile rubber gloves ready for the physician. During the procedure the patient is placed upon his side with his back to the operator at the edge of the bed. The thighs and the head are flexed, and the body is bent forward as much as possible to increase the space between the vertebrae. It may be necessary for the nurse to hold the patient in this position, especially in the case of children and nervous adults (see Fig. 202).

Queckenstedt Test. A test to determine the presence of an obstruction between the cranial cavity and the lumbar-puncture needle is called the *Queckenstedt test.* Pressure is made firmly upon the jugular veins in the neck for 10 seconds, then released. The increase in intracranial pressure caused by the compression should be noted, and if the pressure does not return to its original position in 10 seconds, the pressure is noted at 10-second intervals until it has returned to its original level. If there is any obstruction in the spinal subarachnoid space, the rise and the fall of the pressure will be slow and gradual or none at all. A blood-pressure cuff may be used to apply compression about the neck at 20, 30, 40 and 50 mm. of pressure and respective cerebrospinal-fluid pressure measurements made.

Nursing Care

To prepare a patient for a cisternal puncture, the neck is shaved to the external occipital protuberance in the midline. The patient is placed on his side with the head flexed upon the chest. The tray is the same as that for a lumbar puncture.

After either puncture, the patient may complain of headache. All patients complaining of headache and dizziness when the head is elevated should be kept in bed until these complaints have disappeared.

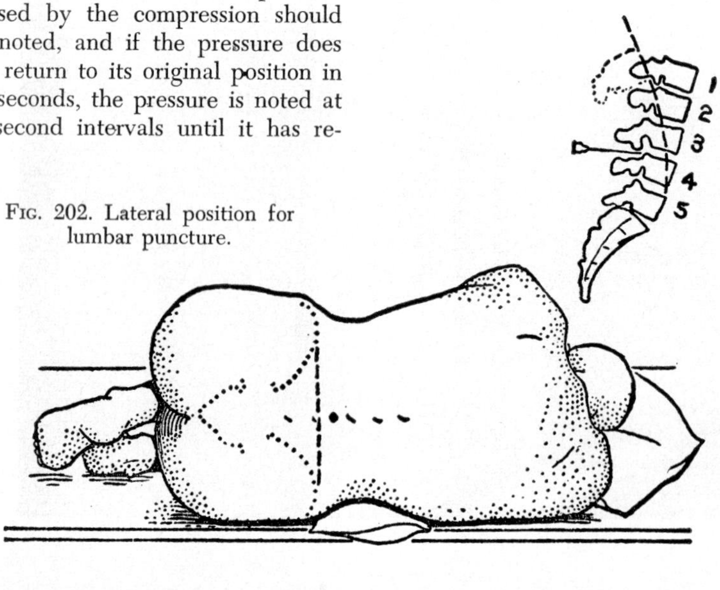

FIG. 202. Lateral position for lumbar puncture.

When a specimen of spinal fluid is removed for examination, it should be sent to the laboratory immediately. Changes which would alter the result of the examination may take place if the fluid is allowed to stand.

Nursing Care of the Unconscious Patient

Unconsciousness is a condition in which there is a depression of cerebral function. This may range from stupor to coma. In stupor, the patient will elicit symptoms of annoyance when stimulated by something unpleasant such as a pin prick, loud clapping of hands, etc., by drawing back, facial grimaces and making unintelligible sounds. In coma there is no response.

Nursing care of this type of patient is more important than with a conscious patient. His every need should be attended to, and conversation about him must not take place in his room. Detailed nurses' notes are to be kept, and the physician should be notified of any change in activity, reflex action, vital signs, pupillary variations, etc.

Temperature of his environment will be determined by his condition. If he has a temperature elevation, he should have a sheet or perhaps only a loin cloth covering him. The room may be cooled to 65° F. However, if the patient is older and does not have an elevation, he needs a warmer atmosphere. Regardless of the temperature, the air should be fresh and free from odors. Body temperature is never taken by mouth on these patients. Rectal temperature is preferred to the less-accurate axillary temperature.

Special attention is given to these patients because they are insensitive to external stimuli. He must be turned frequently and positioned properly (see Fig. 203). Attention should be given to those areas where pressure is greatest to prevent decubiti. Sheets must be free of wrinkles, crumbs and moisture. Lanolin may be used where the skin is unusually dry. In the unconscious patient, the mouth is an area which also needs conscientious care. The mouth should be swabbed carefully and rinsed thoroughly. The tongue as well as the space underneath must be included. A soothing lubricant within the mouth and on the lips will prevent drying and the formation of encrustations.

There are occasions when the corneal reflex is absent. Because of this, the cornea is likely to become irritated or scratched. It may be necessary to irrigate the eyes with a weak germicidal solution and lubricate them with mineral oil. A patient following head surgery will often have periocular edema. Cold compresses may be used, and care must be exerted to avoid contact with the cornea.

If there is ear or nasal bleeding, or oozing of cerebrospinal fluid, the physician should be notified immediately. A small cotton pledget may be placed loosely in the nostril, but no attempt to clean the nose should be done until the physician sees the patient.

The accumulation of secretions in the pharynx presents a serious problem which demands energetic and conscientious treatment. Since the unconscious patient is unable to swallow and has absent pharyngeal reflexes, these secretions must be re-

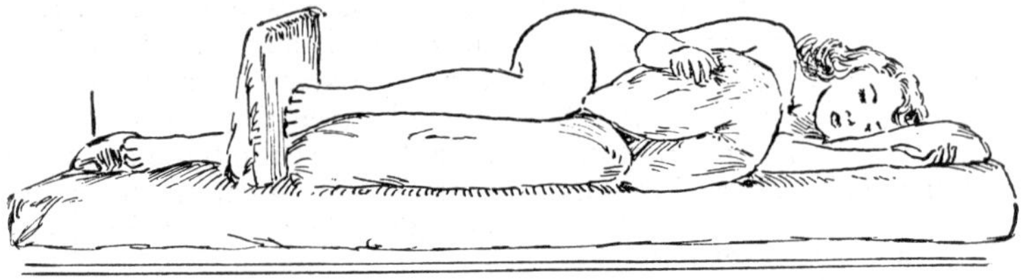

FIG. 203. Posture for nursing an unconscious patient. Note pillows placed at the feet and underneath the upper leg and arm and the head to maintain the patient in correct posture. (Redrawn from Gutiérrez-Mahoney and Carini: Neurological and Neurosurgical Nursing, St. Louis, Mosby)

moved in order to eliminate the danger of aspiration. Portable electric suction or wall suction with a No. 16 multiholed, soft rubber catheter can be used. Oral and nasal routes may both be tried; by the latter method accumulations deep in the pharynx can be reached more easily. Petrolatum used sparingly is the most acceptable lubricant. The force of the suction should not exceed 5 lb./sq. in.; the catheter should be closed while it is being passed through the vestibule of the nose. Gently gliding the catheter back and forth in the hypopharynx is most effective and occasionally withdrawing the tube completely so that it can be flushed with water will prevent its becoming clogged. The frequency of suctioning is determined by the needs of the patient.

The nutritional needs of this patient are met by giving the required fluids intravenously. Intravenous solutions and blood transfusions must run in slowly on patients with intracranial conditions. If given too rapidly, they may increase the intracranial pressure. Sixty drops per minute is the average rate of flow. In addition, a nasal tube may be passed, and the patient can be fed by gastric feedings. The procedure is much the same as for gastrostomy feedings (see p. 307). One way of testing to see whether the patient is able to swallow without choking is to give him a swab wet with water to suck. *Never give fluids by mouth to the patient who cannot swallow.*

Urinary incontinence can be taken care of by inserting a retention catheter such as the Foley. A full bladder, on the other hand, may be the overlooked cause of retention. Some neurosurgeons recommend colonic irrigations every second or third day to eliminate frequent involuntary stools.

Maintaining good body position is important; equally important is passive exercise to the extremities so that contractures are prevented. The use of a foot board will aid in the prevention of footdrop and eliminate pressure of bedding on the toes. A trochanter roll supporting the thigh will keep the leg in good position. The arm should be in abduction, and a folded pad can serve as a comfortable hand support.

If the patient is restless, crib sides should be provided. If it is possible for him to sustain injury against the side attachments, they should be padded satisfactorily. Every conceivable method of keeping a patient quiet should be attempted before restraints are used. The reasons are several: Any form of restraint antagonizes a person, whether he is conscious or not, and as a result he may injure himself by rebelling physically and mentally. Finally, any strain may hasten the development of an increased intracranial pressure.

CONVULSIONS (SEIZURES)

A very important aspect of observation on the part of the nurse is that of a convulsion or seizure. Convulsive seizures are a common symptom of a neurologic lesion. They may be major or minor in their intensity. A major seizure may be preceded by a warning (an aura). Respirations often cease, the patient is cyanotic and has tonic spasm alternating with clonic movements. There may be much jerking of the muscles, the face and the extremities. As the seizure continues he may froth at the mouth, clench his teeth and breathe noisily and heavily. This may continue for a while, and the patient may then go into a more quiet unconsciousness. There often is bladder incontinence. A minor seizure is less severe and does not exhibit the violent movements, frothing at mouth and incontinence. Following such an episode, the individual may or may not have any recollection of the attack.

A focal convulsion or jacksonian seizure is limited at first to a muscle or group of muscles but may spread to involve the entire body. In neurosurgery watching an attack is very important as it is a means of locating the cause. As the physician in charge frequently is unable to reach the patient at the time of an attack, it devolves upon the nurse to note and describe as many of its important features as possible.

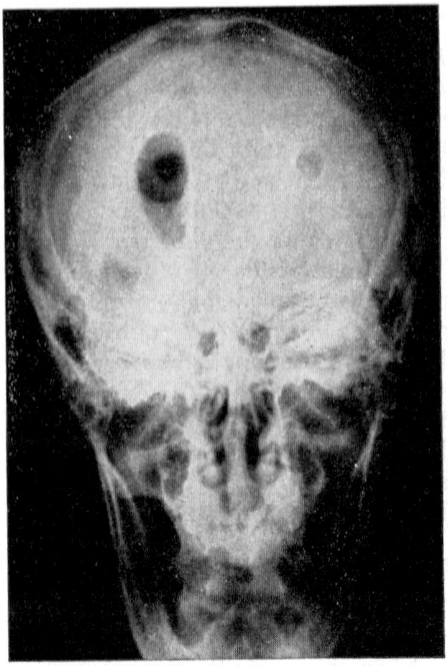

FIG. 204. Ventriculogram. Note the lateral ventricles displaced toward the right; the left lateral ventricle is deformed markedly and filled poorly with air due to a large tumor on the left side.

The nurse has several responsibilities in caring for such a patient. By her understanding she will make it easier for the patient to adjust to the hospital environment. She must prevent psychological trauma to other patients who happen to be near by protecting and screening him. The nurse is aware of the fact that she cannot stop a convulsion, therefore, her objective is twofold: (1) *Protection of the patient from injury.* A padded tongue depressor should be placed between the molar teeth to prevent the tongue from being bitten and the front teeth broken. If the patient is subject to seizures this tongue depressor should be at the bedside. If a tongue depressor is not available any soft firm object will serve the purpose. If he is in bed, padded side boards should be available. When an ambulatory patient has a seizure, it is best to lay him on the floor, place a soft pillow, or any soft article, under his head and loosen all tight clothing. (2) *Observing and recording the march of symptoms.* The most important part of the attack is the beginning. Note should be made of:

1. The first thing the patient does in an attack, where the movements or stiffness starts and the position of the eyeballs and the head at the beginning. (In recording, always state whether or not the beginning of the attack was observed.)
2. The type of movements of the part involved.
3. The parts involved. (Turn back bed covers and expose patient.)
4. The size of both pupils.
5. Incontinence of urine or feces.
6. Duration of each phase of the attack.
7. Unconsciousness, if present, and its duration.
8. Any obvious paralyses or weakness of arms or legs after the attack.
9. Inability to speak after the attack.
10. Whether or not the patient sleeps afterward.

Immediately following the attack the nurse should make a brief but clear record of her observations, stressing those noted when the attack started.

DIAGNOSTIC TESTS

Encephalography-Ventriculography

The cerebrospinal-fluid spaces in and around the brain can be seen in x-ray examination when the contained fluid is replaced with air or oxygen. The injection of these directly into the ventricles through openings in the back of the skull is called *ventriculography.* A similar injection made by the spinal subarachnoid route is called *pneumoencephalography.*

These procedures are of great diagnostic value to the neurosurgeon. Encephalography is not performed when there is increased intracranial pressure because of respiratory collapse which may result from the herniation or dislocation of the medulla into the foramen magnum following the removal of spinal fluid. Pressure of bone upon the medulla compresses vital centers.

Preparation of Patient. The night before encephalography or ventriculography the patient should have a good rest. If rectal anesthesia is to be administered the rectum should be evacuated. On the morning of operation the breakfast is withheld to avoid vomiting. The back of the head should be shaved previous to ventriculography, the whole head if it is to precede a craniotomy. Prior to making an encephalogram, all hairpins should be removed; long hair should not be braided, since braids cast a shadow on the x-ray plate. As with other surgical patients, dentures are removed.

Operative Procedure. In pneumoencephalography, the patient is placed in an open-back chair with wheels. The procedure is much the same as for a lumbar puncture. When air is injected to replace spinal fluid removed, the surgeon usually desires a record of these amounts. This can be kept by the nurse. After air replacement is complete, the patient is wheeled in this chair to the x-ray department where pictures are taken.

The patient for ventriculography is placed on the operating table, and the posterior half of the head is scrubbed and draped with sterile towels. Small scalp incisions are made, and trephine holes are made in the skull, exposing the dura. The dura is opened and a blunt ventricular needle having a stilet is inserted into the ventricle on each side. After a sufficient amount of air has replaced the fluid, the patient is taken to the x-ray room.

Postoperative Nursing Care

The patient is frequently in a state of shock after either of these procedures. Hot-water bottles and blankets may be necessary to bring the temperature to normal. The most favorable postoperative position is flat in bed.

The pulse, respirations and blood pressure should be taken every 15 minutes for the first hour, every 30 minutes for the second and the third hours, and then every hour for the fourth, the fifth and the sixth hours. If at this time the patient's condition seems to be satisfactory the notations may be made at less frequent intervals, but constant observation should be made for stupor and other signs of increased intracranial pressure. When these appear the physician should be notified immediately. If nauseated, the patient should be turned on his side to prevent aspiration of vomitus.

Medication can be given for the headaches, and an ice cap applied to the head. As these headaches will persist until the gas is absorbed usually they will be troublesome for 1 or 2 days. When all headaches have disappeared the patient may be allowed out of bed.

Liquid diet is usually given the first day, and the fluid intake should be adequate. Soft diet is often given the second day, and light diet the third.

Electro-encephalogram. This is a visual record of the electrical activity of the brain. Inasmuch as there are definite rhythms of brain electric potentials, any abnormality such as tumor, hemorrhage and infection will show as an abnormal record.

Arteriogram. By the injection of a radiopaque substance into the internal carotid artery or the vertebral artery, it is possible to visualize by means of x-rays the cerebral arterial system. This is significant in detecting aneurysms, abscesses, tumors and other lesions. The procedure may be done by the "open" or "closed" methods. In the "closed" arteriogram, a needle with syringe containing the dye is inserted into the desired artery in the neck. In the "open" method, full aseptic technic is carried out, and a small incision is made in the neck, exposing the artery. Dye is injected in this artery in the x-ray department. Following the taking of roentgenograms, the incision is sutured; this area is observed for swelling or hematoma and the pulse is checked frequently.

In a small percentage of cases, un-

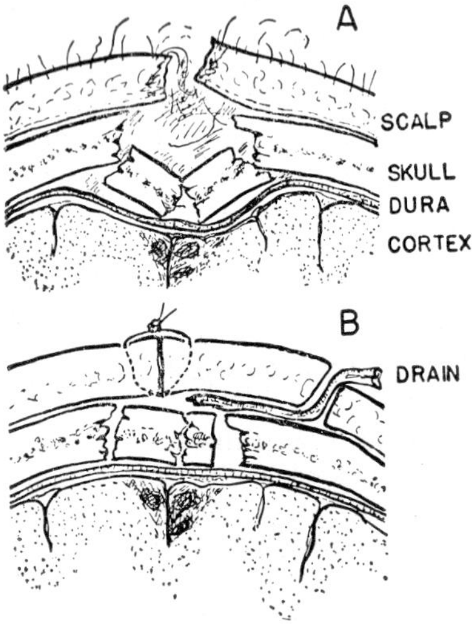

FIG. 205. Diagrammatic drawing showing a depressed fracture of the skull. (A) The fracture has not punctured the dura but it has caused contusion of the underlying cerebral cortex. (B) Shows the relation of the structures after operation and elevation of the depressed fragment. (Penfield: Canadian Army Manual of Military Neurosurgery, Ottawa, Government Distribution Office)

toward effects result from the irritant effect of the dye on the blood vessel lining. These include alteration in the state of consciousness, weakness on one side, tingling in the extremities, and perhaps disturbance of speech. These may appear very shortly after the injection or may be delayed several hours. It is necessary for the nurse to observe the patient for such symptoms following this procedure and to report them. Treatment may be a stellate ganglion block which counteracts the effect of vasospasm and/or thrombosis.

Radioactive Technic to Locate Brain Tumors. The location of cerebral tumors recently has been rendered even more precise by the use of a "radioactive mapping technic." An intravenous injection of radioactive phosphorus or potassium is given either before or during surgery. Cerebral tumors absorb greater amounts of these substances than normal brain tissue absorbs. A type of Geiger counter is used to locate the tumor.

SCALP, SKULL AND CRANIAL INJURIES

Parts of the head which may be injured are the scalp, the skull and the periosteum, the meninges and the blood vessels and the brain itself.

Scalp Injury. Because of the many blood vessels, the scalp bleeds readily when injured. Trauma may be an abrasion ("brush wound"), contusion, laceration or avulsion. Before such a wound can be cared for properly, an area of about two inches should be shaved around the wound. The injection of procaine makes it easier for the surgeon to clean the wound thoroughly and to treat it. If the patient is unconscious, showing evidence of shock, this type of wound is the last to receive attention except for the application of a sterile dressing.

Skull Injury. If there is a depression of cranial bones, the likelihood of increased intracranial pressure is great and must be watched for. When the fracture is compound, the area must be cleansed, débrided and closed as early as possible because there is the added danger of infection.

Fracture of the skull is treated as a neurosurgical condition because the fracture in itself is of less importance than the injury to the brain which may be produced. For this reason, every case of head injury, even though it appears to be slight, should be under the constant observation of a surgeon for several days.

Symptoms. The symptoms, besides those of the local injury, depend upon the amount and the distribution of brain injury. Fractures of the vault produce swelling in the region of the fracture, and for this reason an accurate diagnosis cannot be made without an x-ray picture. Fractures of the base of the skull frequently produce hemorrhage from the nose, the pharynx, or the ears, and blood may appear under the conjunctiva. The escape of cerebrospinal fluid from the ears and the nose is a diagnostic sign of importance. Bloody spinal fluid, if present, suggests brain laceration or contusion.

BRAIN INJURY

Serious brain injury may occur following blows or injuries to the head, with or without fracture of the skull. When the lesions produced are microscopic and the immediate symptoms are mild and not of long duration, the condition is spoken of as a *concussion*. The jar of the brain may be so slight as to cause only dizziness and spots before the eyes (spoken of as "seeing stars"), or there may be complete loss of consciousness for a time.

In more marked cerebral injuries, with bruising of the brain or hemorrhage on its surface, unconsciousness is present for a considerable period. These are spoken of as cerebral contusions, and the symptoms, as would be expected, are more marked. The patient lies motionless with feeble pulse, shallow respiration and pale, cold skin. There is often involuntary evacuation of the bowels and the bladder. He may be aroused with effort but soon slips back into unconsciousness. The blood pressure and the temperature are subnormal, and the picture is somewhat similar to that of shock. The patient may never recover from this primary state. On the other hand, however, he may recover completely and perhaps pass into a second stage of cerebral irritability. Vomiting is commonly the first symptom indicative of recovery from the stage of primary shock.

In the stage of cerebral irritability the patient is no longer unconscious. On the contrary, he is easily disturbed by any form of stimulation, noises, light and voices, and he may even become maniacal at times. Gradually the pulse, respiration, temperature and other body functions return to normal. However, recovery is not complete at once. There are commonly residual headache and vertigo and often impaired mentality or epilepsy as a result of irreparable cerebral damage.

Extradural Hemorrhage. In cases of injury to the head, with or without fracture of the skull, rupture of the middle meningeal artery may occur. This artery runs between the dura and the skull, and hemorrhage from it causes pressure on the brain as a clot is formed in this location.

The symptoms are characteristic.

There is usually a momentary loss of consciousness at the time of injury, followed by an interval of apparent recovery. Then, often suddenly, signs of compression appear, usually with muscular twitchings or convulsions because the clot presses upon the region of the cortex which sends impulses to the muscles (the motor cortex).

Treatment. The treatment consists in making an opening through the skull, removing the clot and controlling the bleeding artery.

Subdural Hematoma. Not infrequently, either with or without injury, hemorrhage may take place over the surface of the brain underneath the dura. This hemorrhage may give few symptoms at the time it occurs, but as time goes on, a thick-walled pseudocyst may be formed which causes pressure on the brain surface and may produce very alarming symptoms. This lesion is one which is most amenable to treatment. A simple trephine opening through the skull will permit a puncture of the cystic mass and relief of the pressure which it produces. When this condition occurs in infants, it is possible to do a subdural tap through the coronal suture. The presence of old blood aspirated from this space is diagnostic of hematoma. Subdural hemorrhage may occur at birth due to injury attendant upon delivery.

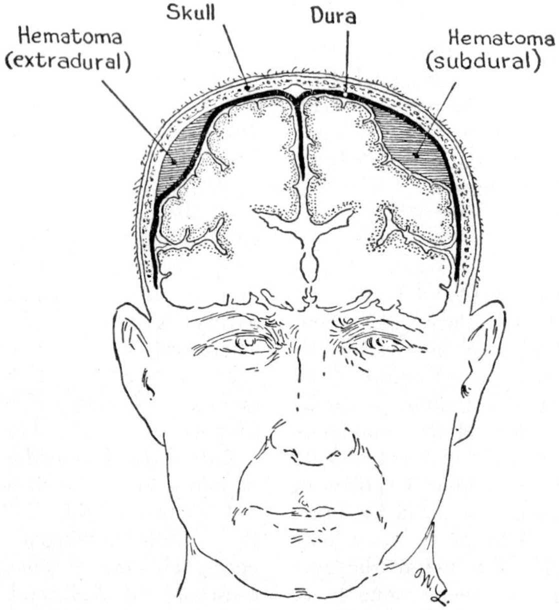

FIG. 206. Diagrammatic views showing the difference in the relations of an extradural hematoma (*left*) and a subdural hematoma (*right*).

Treatment and Nursing Care

In fractures of the vault, an operation is always necessary if the fracture is compound or if fragments are so depressed as to press upon or be driven into the brain. After shaving the scalp, the wound is cleaned by cutting away the infected and devitalized tissue. Bone fragments are removed or elevated. A metal or polyethylene plate can be shaped to fit the opening.

Fractures of the base are much more serious because of the danger of grave cranial complications and meningitis. The nasopharynx and the external ear should be kept clean, and usually a plug of sterile cotton is placed in the latter channel to absorb discharges. At times repeated lumbar punctures are performed to remove the bloody fluid in an attempt to lessen adhesion formation between the spinal cord and its membranes, which would otherwise occur.

All fractures of the skull should be suspected of brain injury until proved to be otherwise. The successful treatment of this condition falls largely to the nurse. The patient should be placed in bed, often with the head slightly elevated. Treatment of the initial shock should include the application of warm blankets, and hot-water bottles if ordered by the neurosurgeon. Close observation of the patient's temperature, pulse, respirations and blood pressure should be made.

The general treatment consists in absolute mental and physical rest in a cool, darkened room. Absolute quiet should be preserved, including the exclusion of all visitors. During the stage of recovery the patient should be watched very closely for the development of neurologic signs, convulsive movements, spasms, or stupor. These symptoms of increased intracranial pressure, including a rise in blood pressure and fall in respiration and pulse, or increasing drowsiness may appear rapidly (see p. 500) and should be reported to the neurosurgeon at once.

An icebag may be applied to the head, and sedative drugs administered. Every form of stimulation is to be avoided at first, and mental as well as physical rest should be enforced. Reading and even conversation should be resumed very gradually.

Liquid diet should be continued until the danger of complications is past. A limited fluid intake is necessary when signs of increased intracranial pressure are noted. Glucose or sucrose, 25 or 50 per cent, is usually administered intravenously to relieve the pressure, as well as magnesium sulfate by mouth or by enemas.

If the patient is irrational he should be restrained by physical means only when there is danger that he may injure himself. It is imperative that he be kept quiet, and medications such as chloral hydrate, bromides and barbiturates are given. The nurse should note the urine output; a distended bladder may be the cause for the restlessness.

Following cranial trauma, the patient must be kept constantly in bed for a minimum of 14 days. The greater the period of rest following the injury the less likely the occurrence of the so-called post-traumatic syndrome of periodic headache.

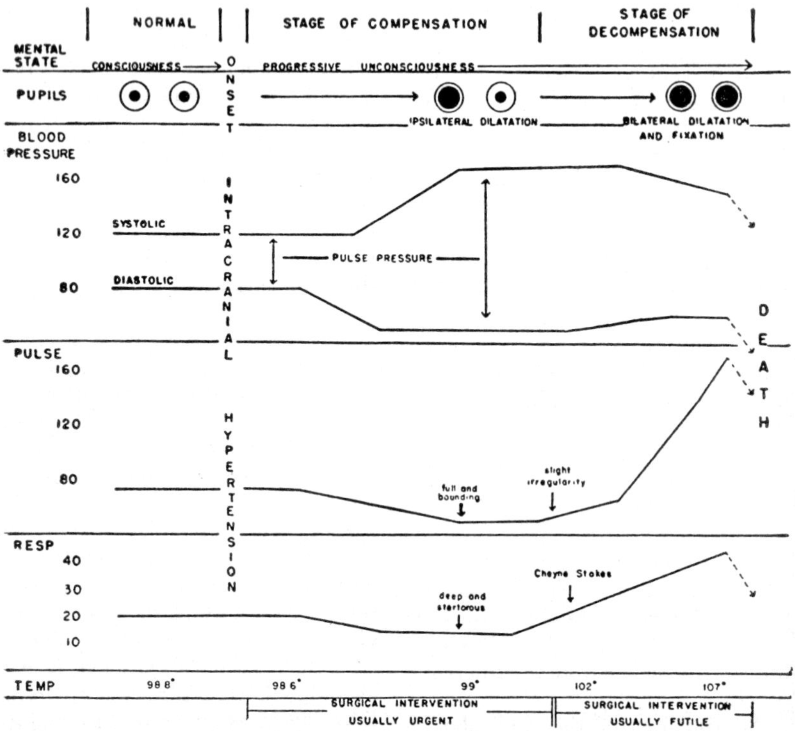

FIG. 207. Chart showing changes in mental state, pupils, blood pressure, pulse rate, respiration rate and temperature before and after the onset of fatal increase of intracranial pressure. (Penfield: Canadian Army Manual of Military Neurosurgery, Ottawa, Government Distribution Office)

INCREASED INTRACRANIAL PRESSURE

Compression of Brain. The brain, although a soft structure, is incompressible, and the bony box surrounding it is firm and unyielding. Therefore, any abnormal intracranial content, depressed fracture, blood clot, edema of the brain substance, inflammatory swellings or tumors, must cause pressure upon the brain. The fluids, blood and cerebrospinal, are the first materials to be extruded from the skull. A cerebral anemia and an increase in the pressure of the cerebrospinal fluid result. At times in fetal life and infancy, the fluid is not absorbed as rapidly as it is formed, or there is an obstruction to its circulation. This results in a distention of the ventricles with a progressive enlargement of the head, as the cranium is not ossified at that early age. This condition is called *hydrocephalus*, and the child usually dies in early life.

Increased intracranial pressure is expressed in many cases by its effect upon the optic nerve. Pressure in the subarachnoid space surrounding the nerve compresses it and produces the "choked disk" or "papilledema" seen by examination of the fundus of the eye with an ophthalmoscope.

EFFECTS. The important centers controlling respiration, blood pressure and the heart rate are early affected by lack of proper blood supply, with a resulting increase in blood pressure, slowing respiration, and a full, slower pulse. Headache, dizziness, vomiting and restlessness are the result of compression of the cerebrum. If the cause of the increased intracranial pressure continues, the patient becomes stuporous, the pupils become dilated, and respiration becomes more and more labored, often being of the Cheyne-Stokes type (respirations gradually increasing in depth, then decreasing until they apparently cease altogether, only to begin again the same cycle). Blood pressure continues to rise, and the pulse tends to become slower. The temperature also often increases rapidly. Finally, the increase in intracranial pressure may become sufficient to paralyze the vasomotor and respiratory centers; blood pressure falls, respiration fails, and death ensues.

The rapidly rising temperature alone may be a fatal complication if not controlled. Such a complication is recognized under the term "hyperthermia." Excessive temperature of this character is recognized by its rapid ascension, usually occurring immediately following operation with or without increased intracranial pressure. Characteristically, the extremities are cold, while the trunk is excessively warm. Every effort must be made to control the mechanism producing the condition.

TREATMENT. Compression of the brain may be treated by the removal of the compressing factor, by reducing the amount of normal fluids in the skull, or by removing portions of the skull to allow the brain room to expand.

Removal of the compressing factor such as a depressed fracture or blood clot may be possible by operation. Removal of the fluids from the skull cannot be accomplished safely by lumbar puncture, because of the danger of removing the support of the brain from below, forcing the medulla downward into the opening in the base of the skull, the foramen magnum, and causing instant death. A ventricular tap, removing cerebrospinal fluid directly from the ventricles through openings in the back of the skull, will prevent this catastrophe. However, hypertonic solutions of glucose or sucrose (50 to 100 cc. of 50 per cent or 250 cc. of 20 per cent solution) may be given intravenously for its effect in this direction. By injecting this hypertonic solution, fluid is drawn into the blood in order to reduce the sugar solution to the concentration normally found in the blood. Therefore, a hydremia is produced with a resultant increase in urine secretion. The fluid which enters the blood is drawn in part from the brain and, in so doing, intracranial pressure is reduced. The same end is accomplished by a somewhat slower method when a concentrated solution of magnesium sulfate is injected into the rectum. Fluid is drawn into the rectum from the blood, which, theoretically, takes up fluid from the brain and other tissues.

The operation whereby compression of the brain is reduced by removal of some of the overlying cranium is called a *decompression*. It is usually done in the temporal region by removing the bone and allowing the brain to herniate outward underneath the temporal muscle (subtemporal decompression).

Nursing Care

In cranial trauma, increased intracranial pressure may occur suddenly due to edema or hemorrhage in the brain. To detect these changes, the pulse, respiration and blood pressure should be taken every 15 minutes. Warning signs are: evidence of stupor, notable decrease in pulse or respiration, and increasing blood pressure and pulse pressure. (See Fig. 207.) These alarming symptoms should be reported immediately, and the nurse should be prepared for such treatments as intravenous injection of 50 per cent glucose.

Brain Tumor. The signs of increased intracranial pressure develop more slowly when caused by a brain tumor unless the tumor is rapidly growing and obstructs the circulation of the cerebrospinal fluid. Warning signs as stated above should be watched for and reported. Since straining increases intracranial pressure, these patients should not be allowed to expel enemas. Hyperthermia should be treated at once by cold or alcohol sponges, ice-water enemas, or ice packs.

BRAIN ABSCESS

Abscess of the brain may occur following intracranial injuries and fracture of the skull, and in septicemia. The most common etiologic factor, however, is middle-ear disease and mastoiditis (see p. 459). The symptoms (persistent headache, vomiting, slow pulse, subnormal temperature and drowsiness) usually become manifest after the acute stage of the middle-ear disease has passed. Localizing signs—neurologic symptoms—aid in the diagnosis.

Treatment. Multiple brain abscesses are usually fatal; however, a single abscess may be cured by incision and drainage. Here again, the use of the antibiotics has resulted in dramatic cures.

Nursing Care

After operation copious dressings should be applied, and the patient should lie with the opening downward to promote drainage. The nurse should watch these patients carefully for retraction of the head, stiffness of the neck, headache, chills, sweats, etc.—symptoms suggestive of a postoperative meningitis.

It is important that this type of patient be maintained on a high caloric diet. Palatable forms of carbohydrates and proteins should be administered at 3-hour intervals in addition to the usual diet.

INTRACRANIAL TUMORS

Brain tumors may be classified into three groups: (1) Those arising from the coverings of the brain, such as the dural meningioma; (2) those developing in or on the cranial nerves, best exemplified by the acoustic neurinoma and the optic-nerve spongioblastoma polare; and (3) those originating in the brain tissue, as the various gliomas, sarcoma, tuberculoma, gumma and metastatic lesions. Tumors may be benign or malignant. However, because it may be in a vital area, a benign tumor may have malignant effects.

Cerebellar Tumors. These are the most common brain tumors found in children. The vomiting, the staggering gait and the headaches gradually become very severe unless operation is performed. As tumors in the cerebellum lie very near the medulla oblongata, death may occur very suddenly.

Pituitary-Gland Tumors. The pituitary gland is a small olive-shaped body located in a small pocket just below the optic nerves. The functions of this gland (which among other things has to do with the growth and the development of secondary sexual characteristics) may be increased or decreased by the presence of a tumor in it. Increased function (hyperpituitarism) accelerates growth, which in children results in gigantism. In adults the face becomes coarse and the hands large, a condition called *acromegaly*.

A decrease in function leads to hypopituitarism, characterized by marked adiposity and loss of sexual characteristics. In addition to these disturbances of function, the tumor, by pressure on the optic nerves, causes increasing loss of vision resulting in blindness. X-rays are an important aid in the diagnosis, showing an enlargement or deformity of the bony shell surrounding the pituitary gland.

Symptoms

The symptoms of brain and meningeal tumors may be divided into general and local.

General Symptoms. These are caused by a gradual compression of the brain due to the tumor growth. The pressure of the cerebrospinal fluid is usually increased when estimated by lumbar puncture. The most common symptoms produced by this increased intracranial pressure are headache, vomiting, choked disk and stupor. Headache is most common in the early morning and increases in severity and frequency. Vomiting occurs often without preceding nausea and without relation to meals. It is of the forceful type described as "projectile" vomiting. Papilledema or choking of the disk is present in 70 to 75 per cent of the cases.

Localizing Symptoms. These are the neurologic signs produced by the tumor. Because the surgeon knows the functions of the different parts of the brain, he is able to diagnose the location of the tumor from disturbances of function brought about by its presence. For example, a tumor of the motor cortex manifests itself by causing convulsive movements localized to one side of the body, spoken of as "jacksonian epilepsy"; tumors of the occipital lobe cause blindness of half of each eye, by involving the centers or tracts for vision of one side of the brain; tumors of the cerebellum cause dizziness and a lack of muscular coordination of one side of the body; tumors of the frontal lobe cause a disinterested mental attitude, and the patient often becomes extremely untidy and careless and uses obscene speech. Many tumors are not so easily localized, because they lie in the so-called silent areas of the brain (i.e., areas the functions of which are not definitely determined).

Since definite localization of the tumor must be ascertained before an operation for its removal can be attempted, the surgeon frequently resorts to encephalography or ventriculography. (See Fig. 204.)

Treatment. "An untreated brain tumor uniformly leads to death." If the increase in intracranial pressure continues without relief, headache and increasing blindness become the most distressing symptoms. If the tumor cannot be localized, or if the condition of the patient does not warrant an attempt at a curative operation, a decompression may be performed (see p. 502). This may restore sight and relieve all symptoms for a time. Often the tumor may be removed later.

If the tumor is of the cerebrum, an attempt to remove it may be made by an operation called a *craniotomy*. A large flap of scalp and bone is turned down, the dura is incised, and the tumor is removed. After bleeding is controlled, the bone flap is replaced, and the muscle and the scalp are sutured.

Tumors in and about the cerebellum are removed by an operation called a *suboccipital craniectomy*. The scalp and the muscles are dissected away from the base of the skull, and the bone is removed by rongeur forceps. After removal of the tumor, the dura is sutured, and the soft tissues are closed over it, leaving a defect in the bone.

Nursing Care

Preoperative Care. The nurse should become familiar with the symptoms of the patient so that she can make comparisons postoperatively. These should include observations on paralysis, vision, personality, speech and incontinence. Paralysis of the hand can be tested by the hand grip. Observations of leg movement should be specially noted if the patient is not ambulatory. Patients with leg paralysis should have protection of these parts, especially the feet, with bed cradles or other supports to relieve the pressure of bedding.

The mental preparation of the patient is important. Many times he does not realize that he is about to undergo surgery. Even so, encouragement and attention to his needs will usually make him amenable to any form of treatment. Some surgeons prefer that the patient not read. The environment should be conducive to rest. Loud-playing radios and too many or noisy visitors must be eliminated. Reassurance and consideration for the family is extremely important, for they recognize the seriousness of a brain operation.

Preparation for Operation. The preparation for an operation on the brain or the skull consists first in shaving the entire scalp. Usually a shampoo of the scalp on the day before operation is advisable. Any infection found on the scalp should be reported to the surgeon before the operation. The patient's weight must usually be determined for the calculation of rectal anesthesia. All evacuations of the rectum should be made without causing straining by the patient, as death may occur due to the increased intracranial pressure.

Morphine sulfate is usually not given to neurosurgical patients because of its action as a respiratory depressant and because it masks pupillary signs.

Postoperative Treatment. This is almost as important as the operation itself. While the patient is in the operating room, the postoperative bed is made as usual for any surgical patient except that in head cases, the foot end of the bed will be the head end. This will make for easy access to the head when changing a head dressing. A sponge rubber mattress or an air mattress (not filled to its fullest) are preferred, inasmuch as they help in the prevention of decubiti. Equipment which should be available in the room includes the following:

Suction set with catheter for aspiration of mouth secretions.

Padded tongue depressor to be used during seizures.

Ventricular tap set to be used if there is evidence of increasing intracranial pressure.

Emergency drugs such as stimulants and hypertonic solutions with syringes and needles.

Lumbar puncture set.

Sphygmomanometer, stethoscope and vital sign sheet.

It is preferable that a nurse be in attendance for at least the first 24 hours. When the patient is unconscious, the care outlined on page 491 is followed.

In order to follow the case accurately, the surgeon requires that the blood pressure, pulse and respiration be taken and recorded every 15 minutes for 3 hours, then every half hour for 3 hours, then every hour for the remaining 24 hours. The temperature should be taken every half hour for 6 hours and every hour for the remaining 24 hours. Any marked changes should be reported to the neurosurgeon at once.

Shock. The operations are usually long, and shock is the earliest postoperative complication. The nurse should see that the bed is warm and that heat is available. If shock develops, the usual treatment is carried out, blood transfusion being particularly effective in these cases. The patient is placed in Trendelenburg position only upon the order of the physician, for this head-low position may increase intracranial pressure, which is undesirable.

Respiratory Failure. This is more apt to occur in the patient operated upon for cerebellar tumor. Removal of the cerebrospinal fluid is usually the treatment which the neurosurgeon carries out at once. This procedure is called a *ventricular tap*. For convenience, a sterile brain cannula is attached to the head of the bed at all times. The treatment for increased intracranial pressure also includes giving intravenous injections of 50 per cent glucose or sucrose (see Treatment, p. 501).

State of Consciousness. The nurse should be particularly observant of the state of consciousness after a local anesthetic or after a reasonable period of time following a general anesthetic. This can be determined by first addressing the patient by his name. If he does not respond, command him to do something such as showing his tongue or moving his leg. If still no response, observe his reaction to painful stimuli, such as a pin prick.

The nurse must remember that the patient may display signs of mental disturbance and confusion following head surgery, particularly if the frontal lobe was involved. Therefore, it does not help to scold the patient if he wets the bed. Tolerance and a patient attitude must be assumed by all who care for him. Prolonged unconsciousness, cyanosis, or abnormal color changes in the skin should be noted and reported promptly.

ELEVATED TEMPERATURE. This must be treated immediately. Every effort should be made to keep the room cool. Some neurosurgeons order the following treatment: if the temperature reaches 102° F., the patient is covered with only a sheet; at 103° F., a loin cloth is applied, the sheet is removed, and an alcohol sponge is given every half hour; at 104° F., ice-water enemas are injected and siphoned off every half hour until the temperature drops. An ice-water enema consists of a glass of finely cracked ice shaken with a glass of cold water. After quickly injecting the solution, the rectal tube is clamped and left in place until it is siphoned off. At least 20 minutes should elapse before a rectal temperature is taken after an ice-water enema. Another popular enema for temperature reduction is the aspirin enema. The ordered amount of aspirin is dissolved first in about 75 cc. of hot water. To this is added 75 cc. of cold water. Temperature should be that of the room. It is given slowly through a small rectal tube.

TURNING AND MOVING PATIENTS. The patient is kept quiet immediately after operation; later, turning is ordered at frequent intervals to prevent pneumonia and pressure sores. These should be prevented on the scalp and the ears as well as the sacrum, the hips, etc.

In the uncomplicated case, the head may be raised slightly when recovery from anesthesia occurs, and the general care is given as for any postoperative case.

Paralysis of the legs or the arms, the hand or hands, or of the swallowing function, and incontinence or aphasia should be watched for and reported. The extent of these abnormalities should be compared with preoperative observations.

Dressings. The dressing is often stained with blood shortly following operation. It is important that sterile pads be placed immediately about the dressing by the attending nurse.

The wound is usually dressed on the third to the fifth day. At times, especially in wounds following suboccipital craniectomy, there may be a leak of cerebrospinal fluid through the wound. This complication is dangerous, because of the possibility of meningitis. Any sudden discharge of fluid from a cranial or spinal wound should be called to the surgeon's attention at once.

When the dressings are removed, the nurse may notice a piece of silver foil directly over the incision line. This is frequently used to prevent dressings from adhering to the wound. A convenient head rest for a patient receiving a dressing is a piece of sponge rubber (3 in. x 8 in. x 8 in.) which is covered with a towel. Some surgeons prefer to use gauze dressings to clean the incision rather than cotton balls because wisps of cotton may cling to short hairs and stitches. Head dressings can be held in place by a gauze roll, ace bandage, gauze bandage or by a stockinet cap.

On healing of the wound, the scalp should be cleaned thoroughly. Often crusts are removed more easily after the application of warm oil dressings for a few hours.

Suboccipital Craniectomy. Patients with suboccipital craniectomy are dressed with firm adhesive strappings to prevent movement of the head and the neck. These patients must be turned from side to side at frequent intervals to prevent the development of pressure sores at the back of the head. In turning the patient, it is important to turn the body and the head as one piece to prevent any strain on the wound with resultant tearing of sutures.

Water must not be given to a patient who has had a suboccipital craniectomy until ordered by the physician. Due to the operation, the patient temporarily may not be able to swallow. Aspiration of fluids or mucus may cause pneumonia, a complication avoidable by good nursing care.

Rehabilitation and Convalescence. The convalescence of a neurosurgical patient is dependent upon the extent of trauma and the success with which treatment was carried out. When a tumor is benign and is removed successfully, it is most gratifying to help the patient make his recovery. Good nursing will eliminate untoward complications. As a result, the emphasis can be placed on regaining function. Gradual exercises to extremities, getting out of bed, learning to feed himself, are all ways in which the nurse can help the patient to help himself. Doing everything for the patient is a hindrance to his successful rehabilitation. Close co-operation between the nurse and the physical therapist will help the patient to achieve good muscle function. He should be accompanied when walking, for sudden attacks of dizziness or unconsciousness may occur. In cases of aphasia, the patient may have to be taught to talk. This can be a painstaking process to the patient and deserves patience and encouragement by the nurse. With regard to appearance of the head, following surgery, men usually have no problem because of short hair. In women where there is still very short hair, attractive turbans, scarfs, etc., can be worn. The family must be aware of the limitations of the patient but should be informed of his progress and how they can help to continue his recovery.

When tumor, injury, or disease is of such a nature that the prognosis is poor, convalescence is geared to making the patient comfortable and as happy as is possible. Perhaps he is left with a paralysis, is blind, or suffers from seizures. The family is kept informed of the progress of the patient by the surgeon; however, many times the real expression of their emotions takes place after the physician leaves. It is then that the nurse must help them to accept their responsibility. Often the care of this patient is transferred to some member of the family. Whoever is responsible must have proper instruction regarding the physical and mental care of the patient. If some member is not able to do this, perhaps some adjustment can be made with a visiting nurse to assume part care as needed. The medical social worker may be called in to assist in making

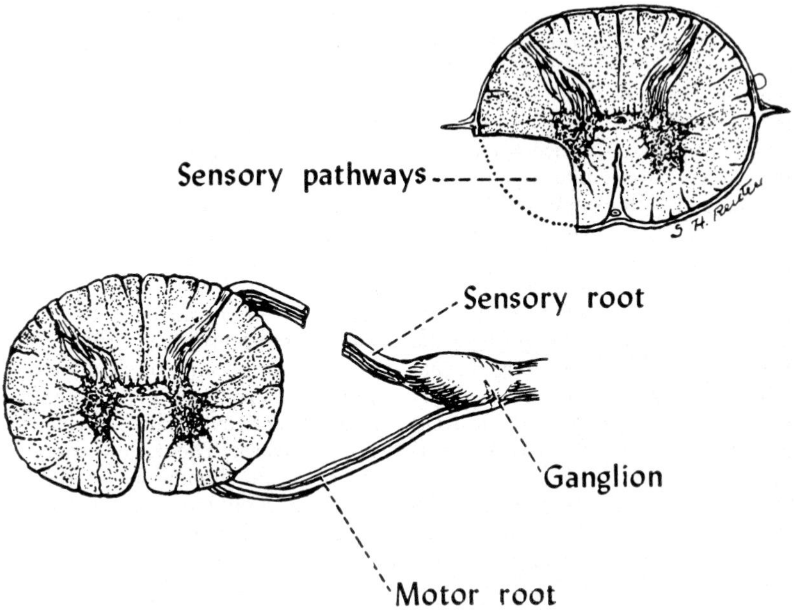

FIG. 208. Cordotomy and rhizotomy. (*Top, right*) In the cordotomy, incision is made through that portion of the cord carrying pain and temperature pathways. (*Bottom, left*) In the rhizotomy a section of the sensory root is removed. (Newton, Kathleen: Geriatric Nursing, St. Louis, Mosby)

financial arrangements or to help in placing this individual in good hands.

LOBOTOMY

In certain psychoses and in painful states which cannot be relieved otherwise (inoperable carcinoma), neurosurgeons have helped by an operation which is called prefrontal lobotomy (leukotomy). The principle of the operation is to cut the association tracts leading from the prefrontal lobes.

Nursing Care

Mental preoperative preparation may be unsuccessful, for often the patient is not in a condition to understand. However, the nurse is able to care for his nutritional and physical needs, and to observe his personality reactions as well as his behavior.

Postoperatively, he is cared for in the same way as any other patient after operation. When he has responded, the nurse must realize that the patient will not remember much that has passed and will have to make his reorientation to time and place. This may or may not be possible. The chief nursing problem is attention to skin, mouth and elimination, but he should be encouraged to do as much as he can for himself. This will demand supervision, for his behavior may be childlike. When eating, he may literally play with his food. In taking a bath, he may splash water around. He may tear his dressings off. Patience is required to guide him in the right direction. Encouraging him to void at frequent intervals may curb incontinence of urine. Every attempt should be made to get him interested in some form of diversional therapy. The nurse will have to be firm and encourage him to "hurry up," for he is likely to dawdle with any activity. He should be praised when he does something well. By stepping up his activities so that he continues to progress, one is able to get such a patient to care for himself and not be a burden to his family. The need for this type of care to continue after he leaves the hospital is a real one. If no one is interested in helping him, he will regress rapidly. Therefore, the physician and the nurse have a challenge to meet in passing on their interest and motivation to those who care for this patient after he leaves the hospital.

RHIZOTOMY AND CORDOTOMY

Rhizotomy and cordotomy are done in most instances to relieve intractable pain. The approach for both procedures is the same as for a laminectomy. The cordotomy is the more complicated procedure; the sensory pathway portion of the cord is severed (Fig. 208). In the rhizotomy, the sensory roots of the spinal nerves are cut before they join with the motor root.

Nursing Care

It is important for the patient to know what changes in sensation will take place as a result of surgery. The length of the incision for rhizotomy varies directly with the number of nerves to be cut; the incision for cordotomy is relatively small. After operation, the nurse will be on the alert for signs of shock, respiratory distress, bladder disturbances, paralyses and constipation. Since sensations will be limited, the patient may lie in an uncomfortable position and develop pressure sores without realizing it. Those responsible for his care at home must recognize that his sensations are limited. However, this seems a small price to pay when compared with his being free of pain.

TRIGEMINAL NEURALGIA (TIC DOULOUREUX)

Tic douloureux, or trifacial or trigeminal neuralgia, is a neuralgia of the cranial nerve which carries sensory impulses from the face, the forehead, and the jaws. It occurs in adults, usually past midlife, and is characterized by attacks of terrific neuralgic pain along the distribution of the nerve. The attacks may be brought on by insignificant stimuli, such as a draught of cold air, talking, laughing, or eating, and the pain is so severe that even morphine may not entirely relieve it.

Treatment. Two forms of treatment have been used. The injection treatment, injecting alcohol into the nerves, may bring about relief for from 6 to 18 months. The operative treatment consists in dividing the nerve paths which carry the painful impulses to the brain. The operation is performed in the sitting position. An opening is made into the skull in the temporal region, and after elevating the dura the nerve is cut as it enters the brain stem. The wound is sutured.

After the operation, the patient has a complete loss of sensation in the area supplied by the divided nerves. This "woodeny" feeling may alarm the patient, but the nurse should reassure him. Herpes labialis (fever blister) frequently appears but soon disappears without treatment.

An operation for this affection is that directed toward the tract of the fifth nerve in the brain stem. This requires a suboccipital approach, similar to that used for tumors of the cerebellum. This operation is termed *tractotomy.* Its advantage lies in the preservation of the sense of touch in the face and the eye.

Nursing Care

Preoperative care of a patient with trigeminal neuralgia includes a recognition on the part of the nurse that certain factors may aggravate excruciating facial pain. Food which is too hot or too cold may initiate this pain; careless handling, such as jarring a bed, may also precipitate discomfort. Even washing the face, combing the hair or brushing the teeth may produce acute discomfort. The nurse can lessen these discomforts by using cotton pads to wash the face, substituting a blunt-tooth comb to comb the hair and so forth. When the nurse realizes that he may be irritable and nervous, she is able to give more considerate care.

The most dangerous symptom after these operations is the development of an infection of the cornea (keratitis). The sensation of the eyes is supplied by a part of the trigeminal nerve, so that destruction of the nerve may make the cornea insensitive to injury and foreign bodies, with the result that frequently infection may occur. To protect the eyes from this danger, they are irrigated 3 times daily with warm saline solution and sometimes kept covered with an eye shield. The patients are later provided with a special form of protective glasses for a time. If sensation of the eye has not been destroyed, these precautions are unnecessary.

As the patient with trigeminal neuralgia is usually an older individual, every precaution should be taken to prevent pulmonary complications. Turning, deep breathing and early ambulation are the usual preventive measures.

An uncommon complication following this operation is the occurrence of epidural hemorrhage. The signs and symptoms are similar to those occurring in traumatic middle meningeal hemorrhage (see p. 497). The stay of this patient in the hospital is usually less than a week. His chief adjustment is to become accustomed to the lack of sensation in the area involved and to recognize and avoid anything which might irritate his face or eyes without his feeling it. A specific point to remember is that he should visit his dentist regularly, since he may not have a toothache in the presence of dental caries.

SURGERY OF SPINAL CORD

Fractures and Dislocation of Spinal Column

Fractures and dislocations of the spine are serious injuries because of the danger of injury to the spinal cord. They appear most commonly in the neck (cervical region) and the lower back (lumbar region).

The first-aid and later handling of these patients is extremely important because much damage can be done to the spinal cord by inexpert care. The patient should lie where he is injured until he is moved correctly by 2 or 3 people. Careful moving of the patient as though he were one piece is imperative. This means that there should be no flexion, extension or torsion of the spine, and that lying on the back is desirable. He should not be moved from the stretcher until he has been transported to the operating table, a hospital bed or a bakelite x-ray table. Particular attention must be paid to injuries of the cervical vertebrae. The head should be immobilized with sand bags, covered bricks or whatever is available. Movement may cause such damage to the spinal cord that the patient may have permanent paralysis of his 4 extremities (quadriplegia). The other risk is that of causing acute respiratory failure because of intercostal nerve involvement. Shock also is a concomitant symptom and must be treated promptly and adequately.

Symptoms. The symptoms of fracture—deformity, tenderness, swelling, etc.—may be present, but the most striking symptoms are those due to the crushing of the cord, caused by the displacement of the vertebrae. If the injury has been severe, there are loss of sensation and complete paralysis of all the muscles supplied by nerves arising from the cord at the level of the lesion and below. The paralysis at first is flaccid but later becomes of the spastic type with rigid spasms of the muscles in the paralyzed limbs.

Fractures of the Cervical Vertebrae

In fractures of the cervical vertebrae, usually the body is crushed due to hyperflexion of the neck. Such injuries occur in diving accidents, auto accidents and from being struck on the head by a heavy object. During the war gunshot injuries were not uncommon. The danger from cervical vertebral fractures is injury to the spinal cord, which in this area is relatively large, and its injury may produce paralysis of the entire lower body. The injury usually results from crushing the cord by acute hyperflexion of the neck. For this reason the neck must be extended and the head held well back even in the first-aid care of these patients.

In the treatment of fractures lower down in the spine, hyperextension can be obtained by the use of a Bradford frame or other appliances. In cervical fractures, however, this is not so easy, and some form of weight extension is often used. Leather-covered slings under the chin and the occiput have been used, but they are uncomfortable. More positive traction can be obtained by the use of a Crutchfield or Barton tongs apparatus. Through small incisions, the short pins of the tongs are inserted through the outer table of the skull. Traction can then be provided by weight and pulleys. With the chest slightly elevated on pillows and the head low, hyperextension can be maintained easily. About 25 lbs. weight may be applied. Extension of the neck is more effective if the head of the bed is raised (Fig. 209). After a period of 6 to 8 weeks, the patient may be fitted with a leather-covered steel collar to hold the neck in extension.

When there is evidence of spinal cord injury, a laminectomy may be performed to free (decompress) the cord from pressure that may arise from deformity or swelling in the cord.

Nursing Care of a Patient with a Cervical Vertebral Fracture

In a compression fracture, an attempt is made to restore the normal contour of the spine by producing hyperextension. This can be accomplished by a head halter or tongs to which traction is applied. The head halter is made of heavy canvas or leather and can cause considerable pressure on the skin. Thin, soft padding inside the halter may make it more comfortable for the chin and the ears. For the male patient, it is sometimes possible to obtain the consent of the physician to remove the halter long enough to permit the barber to shave him. (Traction can be maintained by exerting manual pull on the same parts as the halter, e.g., chin and occiput.) Care to the back is achieved by pressing down on the mattress with one hand and washing or massaging with the other. Other pressure areas which especially need attention are shoulders, sacrum and heels. More leeway is permitted in the turning of the patient who has Crutchfield tongs. During this process, the patient must be observed carefully for signs of respiratory impairment.

Usually the patient is placed with

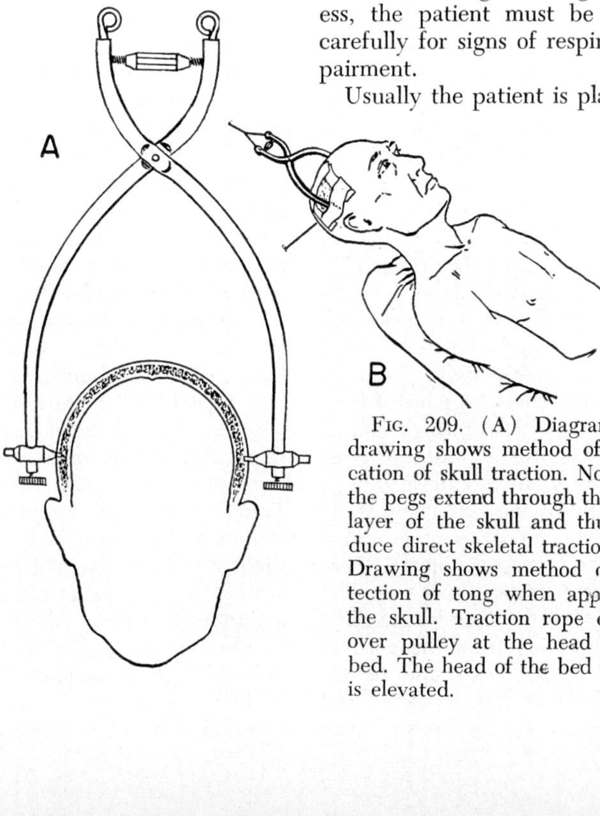

Fig. 209. (A) Diagrammatic drawing shows method of application of skull traction. Note that the pegs extend through the outer layer of the skull and thus produce direct skeletal traction (B) Drawing shows method of protection of tong when applied to the skull. Traction rope extends over pulley at the head of the bed. The head of the bed usually is elevated.

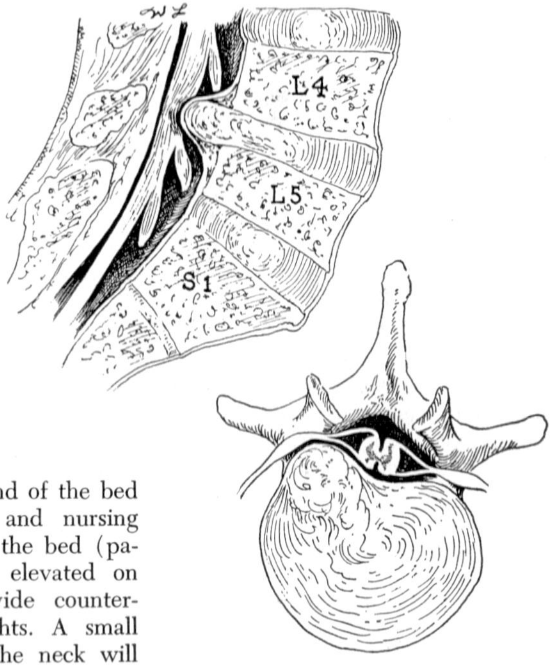

FIG. 210. Diagrammatic drawing shows herniation of the nucleus polyposis. The upper drawing shows how such herniation presses upon the structures of the spinal cord. The lower drawing shows how such herniation may press upon the exit of the spinal nerve and produce pain and other symptoms.

the head at the foot end of the bed to facilitate medical and nursing care. The foot end of the bed (patient's head) can be elevated on shock blocks to provide countertraction for the weights. A small pillow placed under the neck will help to maintain the normal contour of the cervical vertebrae. The back of the head must be checked periodically for signs of pressure; massage will help. All extremities should be put through the normal range of motion at least once daily.

The use of the Stryker frame for this patient is an added advantage, inasmuch as the nurse can turn him more easily and administer care more satisfactorily (Fig. 215).

Diversional activity such as the radio, visitors, etc., may be helpful. A frame can be made to hold a book conveniently for this kind of patient. Reassurance and patience are essential. The period of time an individual is thus incapacitated varies with the nature of the problem. Often a plaster collar or a Thomas collar is used to replace traction, and greater freedom is permissible.

RUPTURED INTERVERTEBRAL DISK

(Herniation of the Nucleus Pulposa)

One very distressing complaint is pain in the back. This may arise from various muscular strains or ligamentous sprains, but these usually improve rapidly. Lumbar back pain which persists, is severe and radiates into the groin and down the leg is often due to pressure on a spinal nerve from a ruptured intervertebral disk.

The intervertebral disk is a cartilaginous plate which forms a cushion between the vertebral bodies. This tough gristlelike material is incorporated in a capsule. A ball-like condensation in the disk is called the *nucleus pulposa*. Incidental to back injury, falls, automobile accidents, lifting strains, etc., the cartilage may be injured. In most cases the immediate symptoms of trauma are short-lived, and those resulting from the injury to the disk do not appear for months or years. Then with degeneration in the disk, the capsule pushes back into the spinal canal or it may rupture and allow the nucleus pulposa to be pushed back against the dural sac or against a spinal nerve as it emerges from the spinal column. This produces pain due to pressure in the area of distribution of the involved nerve. The pain is intensified when the pressure is increased by coughing, sneezing, bending or lifting. Continued pressure may produce degenerative changes in the involved nerve, such as changes in sensation and reflex action. X-ray examinations and air or radiopaque oil injected into the dural sac (*myelogram*) may demonstrate the area of pressure.

The treatment of this injury may be by conservative means, rest in bed with extension, heat and massage, fitted back braces, etc. This often does not give permanent or complete relief, and in such cases a more direct attack is decided upon removing the offending pressure by excision of the fragments of the disk which protrude into the spinal canal. Frequently, an additional stabilizing procedure is added, in which a bone graft from the tibia or the fibula is used to fuse the spinous processes. The spinal fusion has the purpose of bridging over the defective disk to ensure against a recurrence of pain or deformity.

Nursing Care

Preoperative preparation is a shave and a soap-and-water scrub of the back, from mid-thorax to the middle of the buttocks. In addition, a leg should be prepared if spinal fusion is to be done also. Most patients possess a fear of surgery of any part of the spine and therefore need assurance and explanations all along the way. The usual preanesthetic drugs are given as ordered.

Postoperatively, the patient's bed is kept flat. There need be no restriction of diet. Frequent turning from side to side relieves pressure, and the change of position is welcomed by the patient. He must be reassured that no injury will result from such turning. Sometimes immediately after operation or more often after removal of the sutures, a body cast is applied from armpits to groin. This must be inspected for areas of pressure. The patient wears the cast from 6 to 8 weeks and is then fitted for a brace to be worn for an additional 3 to 6 months. Some surgeons keep patients in bed from 6 to 8 weeks in the cast, others allow them to be up and about, their activities limited only by the cast.

Spinal fusion adds the additional danger of a longer and more shocking procedure. The patient has an additional wound and cast of the leg, and it may be several days before he is alert and relatively pain-free. Postoperative care also includes attention in moving the operated leg, pillows must be adjusted for support and comfort, and care must be taken to avoid sudden flexion and extension at the knee, which causes pain. The recovery period is somewhat slower than in those with simple removal of the ruptured portion of the disk, because bony union must take place, which takes 6 to 8 weeks.

Other details of nursing care are similar to those mentioned in the care of patients with spinal cord injuries and tumors.

SPINAL-CORD TUMORS

Tumors within or pressing on the spinal cord cause symptoms which are, in effect, the same as those caused by fracture of the spine, except that they are slower in development. There is usually sharp pain in the distribution of the spinal roots arising from the cord in the region of the tumor, associated with increasing paralysis below the level of the lesion. The level of the tumor may usually be detemined by a neurologic examination. An important diagnostic measure in the exact localization of the lesion is the use of Lipiodol, introduced in 1921. This is an iodized oil, opaque to x-rays. By injection of the oil, either into the lumbar subarachnoid space or into the cisterna magna, the medium may be brought in contact with the suspected tumor. Defects in the oil shadow will then appear by contrast in the x-ray plate if a lesion is present. This diagnostic procedure is called a *myelogram.*

Operation. The treatment consists in a laminectomy with the removal of the tumor. This operation, for the exposure of the spinal cord, is performed with the patient in the prone position. A median incision is made over the spinous processes, and the soft tissues are separated on each side. These bony projections are removed with large bone-cutting forceps, and the posterior part of the vertebral arch is removed in order to expose the dura. After obtaining a bloodless field, the dura is incised, and the tumor or clot is removed. The dura is then closed, the soft tissues are sutured over it, and an adhesive dressing is applied.

Nursing Care of Patients with Spinal-Cord Injuries and Tumors

Nursing care of a patient with spinal-cord damage is more effective if the nurse knows what has been found by the physician in his physical and neurologic examinations. The nurse is called upon to help the physician and the patient as he has blood tests, roentgenograms, lumbar puncture, spinal dynamics such as Queckenstedt's test, and myelography. These individuals are usually quite concerned if they have loss of function of one or more extremities. Often any treatment or procedure which might help is tried willingly.

A patient having a fracture of the cervical vertebra with possible cord damage presents a difficult nursing problem. In addition to the care outlined for spinal-cord patients, it is necessary for traction to be maintained by means of Crutchfield tongs (see p. 512) or some other device. Nothing is given by mouth until specifically ordered by the physician. Oxygen is usually administered because of respiratory impairment. The chief emphasis in nursing care of all cord patients is placed on posture of the patient, skin care, adequate nutritional and fluid intake, and psy-

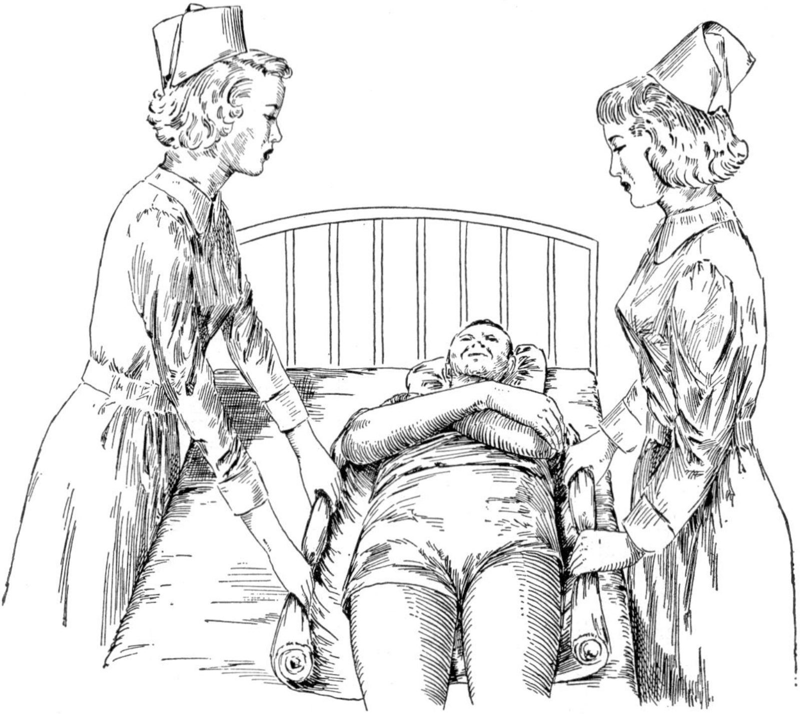

FIG. 211. Method of turning the patient after a spinal injury or a spinal-cord tumor or operation. It is important for the nurse to remember that the patient should be turned as a whole. Two nurses are required to do this. The turning or the draw sheet has been placed upon the bed before the patient is put in the bed. Then the patient is positioned in the middle of the turning sheet, with arms folded across his chest. He should be instructed not to take any part in the turning maneuver. The turning sheet is rolled toward the center from each side by the nurses, and with tension exerted by the nurses' hands on the rolls, the patient is pulled toward the side of the bed. (Redrawn from Gutiérrez-Mahoney and Carini: Neurological and Neurosurgical Nursing, St. Louis, Mosby)

chological and rehabilitative encouragement.

Posture. If acutely ill or too disabled, he is confined to bed where specific attention is given to proper posturing. A fracture board is placed under the mattress to prevent its sagging. An air or sponge-rubber mattress is recommended because there is more equal distribution of body weight. An air mattress should not be filled to its maximum nor should it be so relaxed that the patient's body touches the bottom of

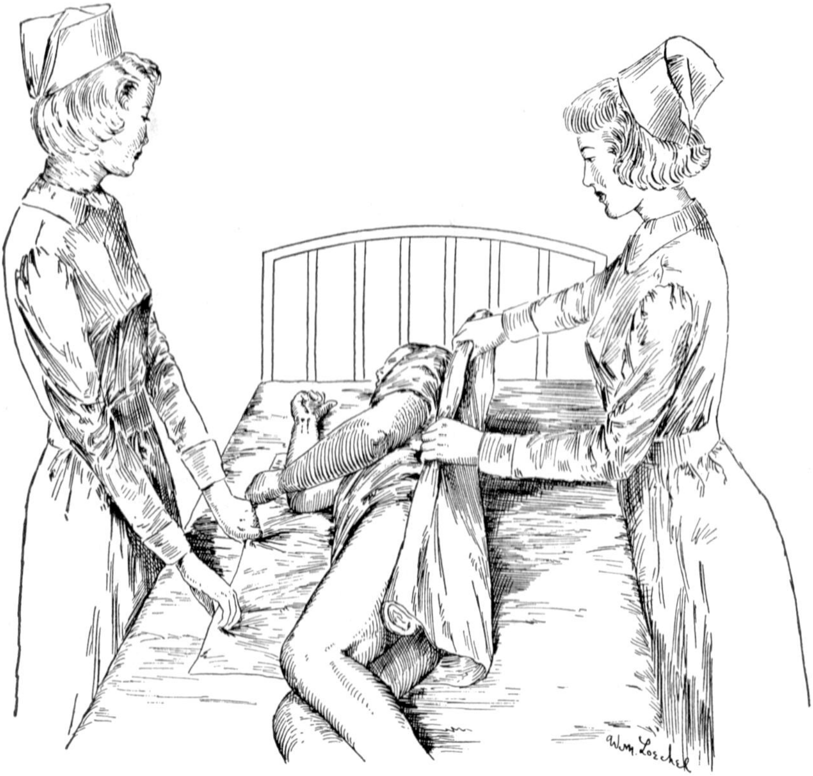

FIG. 212. The patient is rolled on to his right side by the nurse on his left. This is done by pulling upward on the rolled sheet, rolling the patient over like a log. (Redrawn from Gutiérrez-Mahoney and Carini: Neurological and Neurosurgical Nursing, St. Louis, Mosby)

the bed. Caution must be observed in handling a patient on this mattress. If weight other than that of the patient is placed against the mattress it may be sufficient to displace the air and cause the patient to be thrown to the floor. Sponge-rubber mattresses should be covered with a water-repellent material to facilitate cleaning. To prevent footdrop, a foot board must be used when the patient is on his side or back. When placed in the prone position, a small blanket rolled and placed under the dorsum of the ankle will be comfortable. Since the weight of bedclothes often causes pressure, the use of a cradle may help.

Extreme care must be exercised in turning a patient with a spinal-cord injury lest additional trauma be given to the cord. He should be

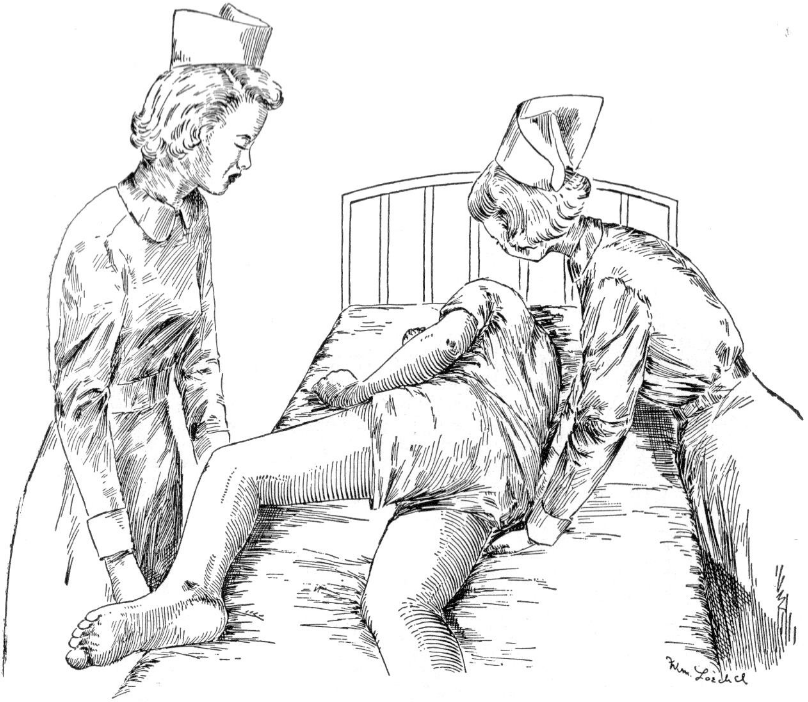

FIG. 213. The patient has been rolled on to his right side, and the nurses are making ready to position him properly in bed. (Redrawn from Gutiérrez-Mahoney and Carini: Neurological and Neurosurgical Nursing. St. Louis, Mosby)

turned as one piece; often this is accomplished best by having the patient lie on a folded draw sheet so that it comes above the shoulders and below the hips. Three people are usually needed to turn such a patient. When he is on his side, a pillow should be placed between his legs to prevent pressure. The Stryker frame (Fig. 215) is effective for several reasons: (1) one nurse can turn the patient; (2) the nurse has easy access to her patient because the frame is narrow; and (3) when in the prone position, the patient is able to read, eat, play solitare, etc., in a comfortable position.

Physical therapy may be given before and after operation. Close co-operation between the physical therapist and the nurse is necessary if the patient is to use his muscles to their fullest capabilities. This is not a function which can show much improvement if the patient does his exercises during a half-hour visit with the therapist and then forgets to do them the rest of the day.

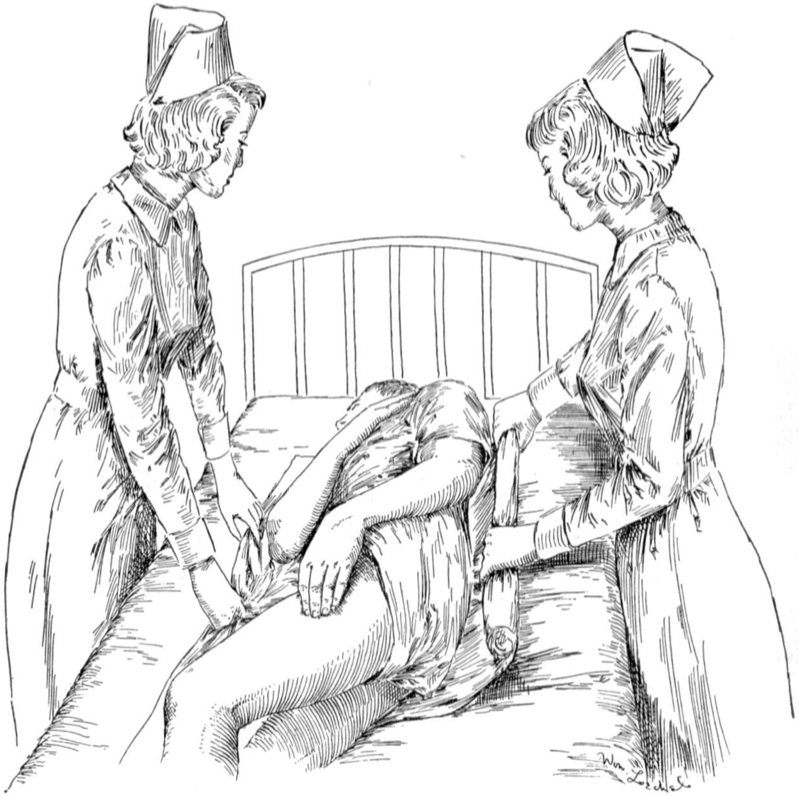

FIG. 214. When it is desired to turn the patient or place him on his back, the nurse at the patient's back rolls the sheet again and holds it taut while the nurse on the patient's right pulls the sheet so that the patient is rolled again on to his back. (Redrawn from Gutiérrez-Mahoney and Carini: Neurological and Neurosurgical Nursing, St. Louis, Mosby)

Skin Care. Simple cleanliness can prevent many problems, the chief of which is decubitus ulcer. The stimulation of a bath, as well as good care to vulnerable areas, is essential; these are sacrum, trochanters, heels, elbows, scapula and back of the head. Proper posturing and turning will help to prevent prolonged pressure. Alternating pressure-mattresses and sawdust beds can be used effectively to distribute pressure more evenly. In addition, keeping the skin dry, massage and lubrication are helpful. Cotton doughnuts are frowned upon because they usually do not stay in place and when they are tied there is a possibility that the tie or the doughnut will restrict circulation. Small pillows placed strategically are more effective. If talcum powder is used, it should be used sparingly to avoid caking in the creases and producing irritation.

The nurse should remember that paralyzed parts are often insensitive; heat should be used with extreme care because of the danger of burns. Nutritional needs of the patient are met by high-caloric and high-protein diets. Maintenance of the protein needs of the patient is of the utmost importance.

The dressings should be inspected for undue wetness, a sign of a leak of cerebrospinal fluid. This is a most serious complication because of the danger of meningitis, and the surgeon should be notified at once.

Elimination. Regularity is of prime importance in the rehabilitation of the bowel. A paraplegic or a quadriplegic will have to depend upon exercise, diet, medications and a planned schedule. In addition he may have to resort to enemas. The use of crutches and braces, as well as bed exercises, will provide activity. His diet should include high residue foods. Glycerin suppositories are helpful; however, in some people mineral oil taken each night may be all that is necessary. The time for defecation should be the same each day. Occasionally, it is necessary to give prostigmine to stimulate intestinal movements sufficiently to expel contents.

If there is retention of urine with overflow, efforts should be made to develop an automatic bladder (see p. 387). Catheterization must be done with the most scrupulous care because of the danger of cystitis. Supportive treatment also is given with antibiotics or chemotherapy. A flaccid paralysis of the bladder sphincter results in the continual dribbling of urine from an empty bladder. An inlying catheter may

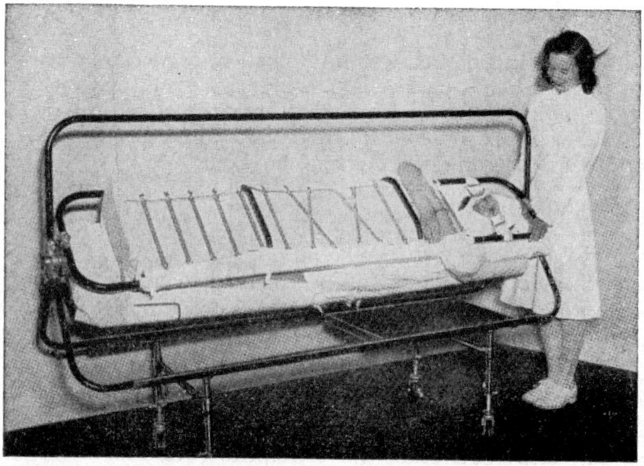

FIG. 215. Stryker frame.

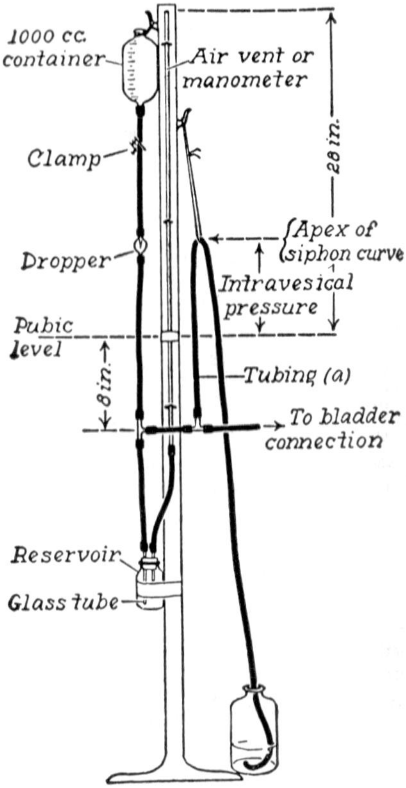

FIG. 216. Munro apparatus for irrigating and emptying the "cord bladder." For instructions as to working of apparatus, see below.

best be inserted. Munro's apparatus for tidal drainage of the bladder is an efficient method devised to avoid and treat the bladder complications of spinal cases. This apparatus alternately fills the bladder to a predetermined degree of intravesical pressure and then empties it by a combination of siphonage and gravity flow, the siphonage being interrupted when evacuation is complete. Dr. Donald Munro, of Boston, describes this method as follows:

The solution in the 1,000-cc. container flows about 40 to 60 drops per minute into the reservoir. During this filling, air escapes through the air vent. When the reservoir is filled to the level of the horizontal arm of the T tubes, the solution flows through the tubing to the bladder and rises simultaneously in the glass manometer and tubing (a). This continues until the solution, filling both the bladder and tubing, reaches the desired intravesical pressure determined by the height of the curved tubing (a). When the liquid reaches the apex of the curved tube, it begins to flow down into the waste bottle, thereby creating suction, the loop acting as a siphon to empty the reservoir of solution and to drain the bladder of its contents. Since the glass tube in the reservoir is one-half the size, or less, of that of the bladder connection, the reservoir empties only one-half as rapidly. When the reservoir is emptied, air enters the system through the manometer, thus breaking the siphonage system and starting a new cycle. It will be recognized that the size of the reservoir and the rate of the flow of the solution influence the length of the cycle. The complete cycle is usually regulated to last two to three hours. The distance of the loop above the bladder determines the maximum pressure to which the bladder is subjected.*

REHABILITATION

There is no group of patients in whom rehabilitation is more difficult and more dramatic than this. The personal tragedies, frustrations, fears and conflicts that beset the paraplegic lead to a feeling of safety in isolation, and of despair and detachment. An understanding doctor and nurse can do much toward helping these patients to rehabilitate themselves. They must help the patient first to realize the full meaning of his condition and then to accept it and be willing to begin life on a new but by no means hopeless plane.

Parts of the body that function normally, arms and shoulders, can be strengthened by exercise to serve partly in place of the paralyzed muscles. By the application of braces, and with the aid of crutches, these patients can learn to become completely ambulatory, and even drive manually operated automobiles. To help the patient give up his sense of futility and encourage him in the emotional adjustment that must be made before he is willing to venture into the "outside world" is a role that an intelligent and informed nurse can fill probably better than any other person. She must realize that a too sympathetic attitude may develop a dependence that defeats the purpose of the entire program. She should teach, help when necessary, but not take over activities that the patient can do for himself with a little effort. This type of nursing care more than repays itself in the satisfaction of seeing a completely demoralized and helpless patient again begin to live a happy and useful life.

SPINA BIFIDA

A condition that may result from congenital malformation or lack of development of the bony protection of the spinal cord is called a *spina bifida.* The rounded tumor of meninges and often cord tissue which outpouches through the opening is called a *meningocele* or *myelocele.* A spina bifida usually occurs in the sacral or lower lumbar region.

Often operative repair is attempted in infancy. The most important postoperative nursing measure is to prevent the contamination of the dressing with urine and feces. The most satisfactory position seems to be with the infant lying in the prone position with the hips slightly elevated. Diapers should not be used until the wound is completely healed.

* Munro, Donald: New England J. Med. **212**:229-239.

REFERENCES AND SUGGESTED READING

Unit Nine: Nursing in Conditions of the Nervous System

General

(See also those for Unit One, Page 205)

Barton, Betsy: The Long Walk, New York, Duell, 1948.

DeGutiérrez-Mahoney, C. G., and Carini, Esta: Neurological and Neurosurgical Nursing, St. Louis, Mosby, 1949.

Emerson, C. P., and Bragdon, J. S.: Essentials of Medicine, ed. 17, pp. 600-672; pp. 623-626 (special nursing problems), Philadelphia, Lippincott, 1955.

Hamby, W. B.: The Hospital Care of Neurosurgical Patients, ed. 2, Springfield, Ill., Thomas, 1948.

Klemme, R. M.: Nursing Care of Neurosurgical Patients, Springfield, Ill., Thomas, 1949.

Sachs, Ernest: The Diagnosis and Treatment of Brain Tumors and the Care of the Neurosurgical Patient, St. Louis, Mosby, 1949.

Brain

Baker, E. E., and Sokoloff, M.: Teaching aphasic patients to talk again, Am. J. Nursing **52**:831-832, 1952.

Behnken, P. B., and Merrill, E. G.: Nursing care following profrontal lobotomy, Am. J. Nursing **49**:431-434, 1949.

Carini, E., and Robinson, F.: Acute craniocerebral injuries, Am. J. Nursing **50**:423-427, 1950.

Dotter, E., and Wade, E.: Brain tumor, Am. J. Nursing **51**:300-303, 1951.

Emerson, C. P., and Bragdon, J. S.: Essentials of Medicine, ed. 17, pp. 601-614 and pp. 626-646 (cerebral disorders); pp. 658-662 (CNS syphilis); pp. 665-670 (toxic disorders), Philadelphia, Lippincott, 1955.

Ewald, F. R., Freeman, Walter, and Watts, J. W.: Psychosurgery: the nursing problem, Am. J. Nursing **47**:210-213, 1947.

Jeffries, E. O., and Wilson, J. H.: The management and nursing care of craniocerebral injuries, Trained Nurse & Hosp. Rev. **118**: 97-101, 417-421, 1947.

——: Prefrontal lobotomy and its nursing care, Trained Nurse & Hosp. Rev. **119**:268-275, 1947.

Lennox, W. G.: The epileptic patient and the nurse, Am. J. Nursing **46**: 219-223, 1946.

Manfreda, M.: The electroencephalogram, Am. J. Nursing **44**: 1144-1149, 1944.

Merritt, H. H., and Fedder, H.: Trigeminal neuralgia, Am. J. Nursing **48**:368-371, 1948.

Mitchell, H. C., and Danca, Eleanor: Streamlining the neurosurgical ward, Am. J. Nursing **47**:598-601, 1947.

Poppen, J. L., and Hansen, R. B.: Ventricular drainage, Am. J. Nursing **47**:161-162, 1947.

Trowbridge, L. K., and Trowbridge, W. V.: Measures used in controlling central hyperthermia, Am. J. Nursing **53**:1092, 1953.

Uihlein, A.: Aneurysms of the cerebral carotid arteries, Am. J. Nursing **51**:492-496, 1951.

Weston, M. L.: Devices to simplify neurological nursing, Am. J. Nursing **45**:22-24, 1945.

SPINAL CORD

Briggs, M. V.: Nursing care of injuries of the spinal cord, Am. J. Nursing **45**:103-106, 1945.

Bruck, H.: Nursing the laminectomy patient, Am. J. Nursing **51**:158-161, 1951.

Chandler, F. A.: Laminectomy, Am. J. Nursing **51**:156-158, 1951.

Clarke, McGovern and Lee: "Self-help aids" in rehabilitation of quadriplegic patient, Occup. Therapy **27**:167-174, 1948.

Emerson, C. P., and Bragdon, J. S.: Essentials of Medicine, ed. 17, pp. 614-623 and pp. 646-651 (spinal cord); pp. 651-658 (peripheral nerves), Philadelphia, Lippincott, 1955.

Jeffries, E. O., and Wilson, J. H.: Surgery of the spinal cord—special emphasis on the nursing care preoperatively and postoperatively, Trained Nurse & Hosp. Rev. **118**: 279-286, 341-343, 1947.

Lever, A. M.: The paraplegia patient, Am. J. Nursing **46**:701-704, 1946.

Mella, M. R.: The mental rehabilitation of patients with spinal cord injuries, Am. J. Nursing **45**:370-372, 1945.

Morrissey, A. B.: The procedures of urinary and bowel rehabilitation, Am. J. Nursing **51**:194-197, 1951.

Ryan, E. K.: Nursing care of the patient with spina bifida, Am. J. Nursing **51**:28-30, 1951.

Skinner, G.: Nursing care of a patient on a Stryker frame, Am. J. Nursing **46**:288-292, 1946.

——: Head traction and the Stryker frame, Am. J. Nursing **52**:694-697, 1952.

CLINICAL SITUATION: CRANIOTOMY

When Mr. Rossen became aware that he was listing to one side as he walked and that he was having visual disturbances, he sought the advice of his physician. The results of a physical and neurologic examination confirmed the suspicion that he had a space-occupying lesion of the brain. After more tests, Mr. Rossen submitted to a craniotomy.

1. Mr. Rossen is to have a ventriculogram. This procedure involves

____(1) replacing air in the ventricles with an opaque medium

____(2) injecting an opaque medium into the main arterial system of the brain

____(3) replacing fluid in the ventricles with air

2. Symptoms suggestive of an increasing intracranial pressure are

____(1) increase in blood pressure, increase in pulse pressure, decrease in pulse and respirations

____(2) falling blood pressure, increase in pulse pressure, increase in pulse and respirations

____(3) rise in blood pressure, decrease in pulse pressure, slowing of pulse and respirations

____(4) decrease in blood pressure, increase in pulse pressure, increase in pulse and respirations

3. Before operation, Mr. Rossen had a convulsion. The responsibility of the nurse is to

_____(1) try to stop the seizure by slapping him
_____(2) insert a padded tongue depressor between his front teeth
_____(3) cover him with blankets to prevent chilling
_____(4) observe the progression of the seizure and the condition in which it leaves him

4. Preoperative morphine sulfate for a patient with this condition is usually
_____(1) contraindicated
_____(2) indicated

5. The reason for the answer given in Question 4 is that morphine sulfate
_____(1) acts as a respiratory depressant
_____(2) relieves apprehension of major surgery
_____(3) masks pupillary signs
_____(4) decreases chances of increased intracranial pressure

6. Following his craniotomy, Mr. Rossen appeared to be going into shock. Without a doctor's order, the nurse may
_____(1) place him in Trendelenburg position
_____(2) apply hot-water bottles
_____(3) increase the rate of flow of intravenous fluids
_____(4) administer oxygen by mask

7. While Mr. Rossen is unconscious, desirable body posture can be maintained by
_____(1) using a padded footboard to keep each foot in dorsiflexion
_____(2) placing a trochanter roll under the femur of each leg
_____(3) spreading out the fingers and supporting them in this position with a folded bath towel
_____(4) keeping each arm in adduction, using a rolled towel for support if necessary

8. Psychological rehabilitation is just as important as physical recovery; therefore, it is important to
_____(1) remind Mr. Rossen that his persistent bedwetting is unnecessary
_____(2) do everything possible for Mr. Rossen so that his body reserve can be directed toward tissue repair
_____(3) help him to accept slow relearning of walking and talking
_____(4) provide activities for him which are just a step beyond his present abilities

UNIT TEN

Nursing in Conditions of the Musculoskeletal System

CHAPTER TWENTY-FIVE

Injuries of the Musculoskeletal System

INTRODUCTION

As the student begins her experience in orthopedic nursing, she soon will discover the extensiveness of this specialty and its obvious relation to all other forms of nursing. Patients are of all ages. Social, economic and psychological problems usually are present; many patients are faced with a long disability and are in need of mental, physical and spiritual rehabilitation. The nurse also will gain a greater realization of the importance of proper body mechanics. Her role as a case finder is a very significant one. The nurse is a teacher, too, as she provides continuity of care between the hospital, the clinic and the home. Her concept of comprehensive nursing care almost automatically will embrace preventive and curative aspects as they extend into the community.

ANATOMY AND PHYSIOLOGY

The musculoskeletal system is composed of bones, muscles, cartilage, ligaments and fascia. It is the bony framework of the body. It is made up of many bones, attached to each other by strong ligaments at joints. The ends of the bone are provided with smooth coverings of cartilage where they articulate with each other. At other sites, cartilage is found instead of bone where a flexibility instead of rigidity is desirable. Thus, cartilage is found as part of the framework of the nose and the rib cage and as a cushion between the vertebral bodies.

The bony framework can act as a support and a protective mechanism for body organs; also, it can move because the bones have attached to them a system of motor muscles which are fastened by strong fibrous cables called *tendons.* The muscles act as motors by reason of their ability to contract (shorten) and relax (lengthen) under control of nerve impulses arising in the cerebral cortex. The power of muscles permits the bones to act as levers with the joint as a fulcrum, to rotate with the joint as an axis, or to remain in a fixed position. In most places in the body the muscles are so placed as to have one set act as antagonist to the other group; thus, the biceps flexes the forearm on the upper arm, while the triceps extends it. The muscles are divided and surrounded by strong fibrous envelopes called *fascia.* In the extremities they surround and give support to the main blood vessels and nerves.

The joints have a smooth lining called *synovium;* this secretes a synovial fluid which lubricates the joints to prevent friction. At points where muscles glide over bony prominences, e.g., the greater trochanter of the femur, or where one bone glides under another, as at the shoulder, or where skin glides over a bony point, as at the elbow, nature develops a gliding mechanism called a *bursa,* a potential space in the *areolar tissue.*

The smooth working of this complex system is dependent upon all parts functioning normally and together. If the bones are broken, the muscles cannot function; if the nerves do not send impulses to the muscles, as in paralysis, the bones cannot move; if the joint surfaces do not articulate normally, neither the bones nor the muscles can function. Injury to one part of the system usually produces injury to other parts and to the structures enclosed or supported by them. Thus, a fracture also produces injury to muscles surrounding the injured bone and to blood vessels and nerves in its vicinity.

Treatment. In the treatment of injury to the musculoskeletal system, support is provided the injured part until nature has time to heal it. This may be accomplished by bandages, adhesive strapping, splints or plaster casts, applied externally. In some cases, support may be applied directly to bone, in the form of pins or plates. In others, it may be necessary to correct deformity and overcome overlapping by weight-traction.

After the immediate and painful effects of the injury have passed, consideration must be given to prevention of fibrosis and resulting stiffness in the injured muscles and joint structures. Active function, i.e., use of the part by the patient, is the best form of treatment to guard against this disability. In some cases the support applied may permit active function almost from the start, and modern treatment is directed toward this end. In other cases the nature of the injury may not permit function, and even in those cases where partial function is possible, we may aid nature in the healing process and hasten recovery of function by various forms of physical therapy.

COMMONLY USED TERMS AND PREFIXES

Adduction	movement of a limb toward the body's center
Abduction	movement away from mid-line of the body; turning outward
Eversion	turning outward
Inversion	turning inward
Extension	bringing the members of a limb into or toward a linear position
Flexion	bending
Dorsiflexion	bending backward
Arthr-	pertaining to joints
Coxa-	pertaining to the hip joint
Cubita-	pertaining to the elbow
Genu-	pertaining to the knee
Hallux-	pertaining to the great toe
Manu-	pertaining to the hand
Myo-	pertaining to muscle
Spondyl-	pertaining to the vertebrae

CONTUSIONS

A *contusion* is an injury to the soft tissues, produced by blunt force (a blow, kick, fall, etc.). There is always some hemorrhage into the injured part (ecchymosis), due to the rupture of many small vessels. This produces the well-known discoloration of the skin (black-and-blue spot), which gradually turns to brown and then to yellow, until it finally disappears as absorption becomes complete. When the hemorrhage is sufficient to cause an appreciable collection of blood, it is called a *hematoma*.

The local symptoms (pain, swelling and discoloration) are easily explained.

Treatment consists of elevating the affected part and applying cold, moist or dry, for the first 8 or 10 hours. Pressure in the form of an elastic or elastic adhesive bandage is also of distinct value in reducing hemorrhage and swelling. When the hemorrhage has stopped, moist or dry heat and massage promote absorption, thus hastening the cure.

SPRAINS

A *sprain* is an injury to the ligamentous structures surrounding a joint, caused by a wrench or a twist. As is the case with contusions, ruptures of blood vessels occur, with a resultant rapid swelling, due to the extravasation of blood within the tissues. The movement of the joint becomes painful. In order to be certain that there is no bone injury, all these patients should have an x-ray examination.

Treatment and Nursing Care

The treatment of a sprain is the same as that recommended for contusions. Some surgeons reduce the swelling by the immediate application of tight adhesive strappings which are renewed every few days until the swelling and the pain have disappeared.

DISLOCATIONS

A *dislocation* of a joint is a condition in which the articular surfaces of the bones forming the joint are no

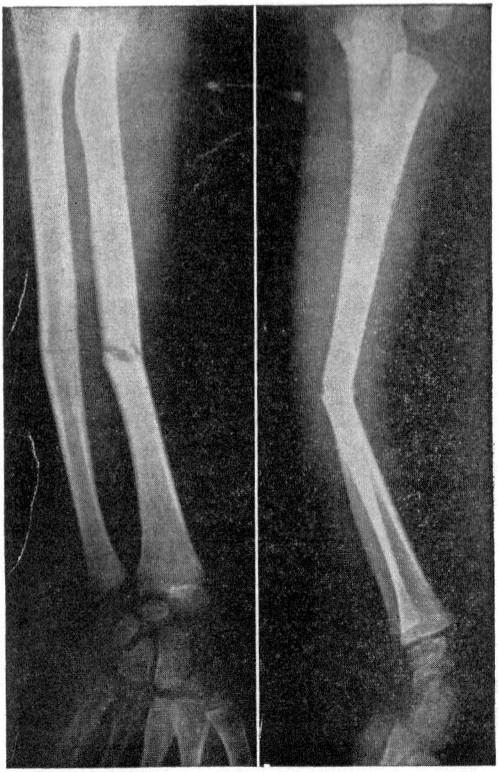

FIG. 217. Roentgenogram, showing greenstick fracture of both bones of the forearm.

longer in contact. Dislocations may be (1) congenital (present at birth, due to some maldevelopment, most often noted at the hip); (2) spontaneous or pathologic, due to disease of the articular or periarticular structures; and (3) traumatic, due to injury, such as the application of force in such a manner that the capsule of the joint is torn.

Symptoms. The cardinal symptoms of a dislocation are four in number: (1) change in contour of the joint, (2) change in the length of the extremity, (3) loss in normal mobility, (4) change in the axis of the dislocated bone. Roentgenograms will confirm the diagnosis and should be made in every case because not infrequently there is an associated fracture.

Treatment and Nursing Care

Irreparable damage can result when someone who is not trained attempts to reduce a dislocation. Immobilization of the part is the best first-aid procedure before medical aid is obtained.

Reduction of a dislocation is usually performed under general anesthesia. The head of the dislocated bone is manipulated back into the joint cavity through the rent in the capsule, and the joint is immobilized by bandages and splints for three or four weeks.

The nursing care following reduction of dislocations is essentially the same as that following the reduction of fractures. The part must be kept immobilized for a sufficient time to permit the ligamentous structures about the joint to heal. Therefore, splints and casts are the usual dressings. The nurse must watch for the complications that are common to such appliances, such as constriction due to tight dressings producing venous and sometimes even arterial obstruction. The cyanosis, pain and disturbance or loss of sensation should be familiar to the nurse, who should immediately notify the surgeon. Attention must be paid to the slightest complaint of the patient. The nurse must watch for signs of pressure, both within and outside the immobilization dressing.

FRACTURES

Any break in the continuity of a bone is called a *fracture*. The break may be *incomplete*, only a line or fissure in the bone, as frequently found in fractures of the skull. It may extend only part way through the bone, splintering the fibers on one side and bending them on the other. This latter form is spoken of as a *greenstick* fracture, and it occurs in children at an age when the bones are soft and pliable. On the other hand, the bone may be *completely* broken, transversely or in a spiral direction, and very frequently it is broken into several (more than two) fragments, when the fracture is said to be *comminuted*.

When the fractured surfaces are protected from contamination with the outside air, that is, when the skin remains intact, it is said to be a *simple* or *closed* fracture; but if a wound occurs at the time of the fracture, so that air and therefore bacteria may be admitted, the fracture is spoken of as being *compound* or *open*. Such a fracture is more difficult to treat than a simple fracture because the wound and possibility of infection must be considered as well as the fracture itself. At times, soft-tissue injury may be a greater problem than the fractured bone.

Not infrequently other structures such as nerves, blood vessels, joints, lungs, bladder and other organs are injured by the force causing the fracture or by the fracture fragments. When such injuries occur, the fracture is called a *complicated* one.

Growth in long bones in early life takes place from two lines of cartilage, called epiphyseal lines, which separate the main shaft of the bone (the diaphysis) from the articular extremities (the epiphyses). As full growth is attained, these lines of cartilage disappear, being transformed into dense bone.

In childhood and in early youth, an accident frequently occurs which is in effect a fracture, but actually is a separation of the epiphysis from the rest of the bone. These injuries, called *epiphyseal separations*, frequently pass undiagnosed or are called sprains. They are important because an accurate reposition of the epiphysis must be secured and maintained, otherwise the bone may

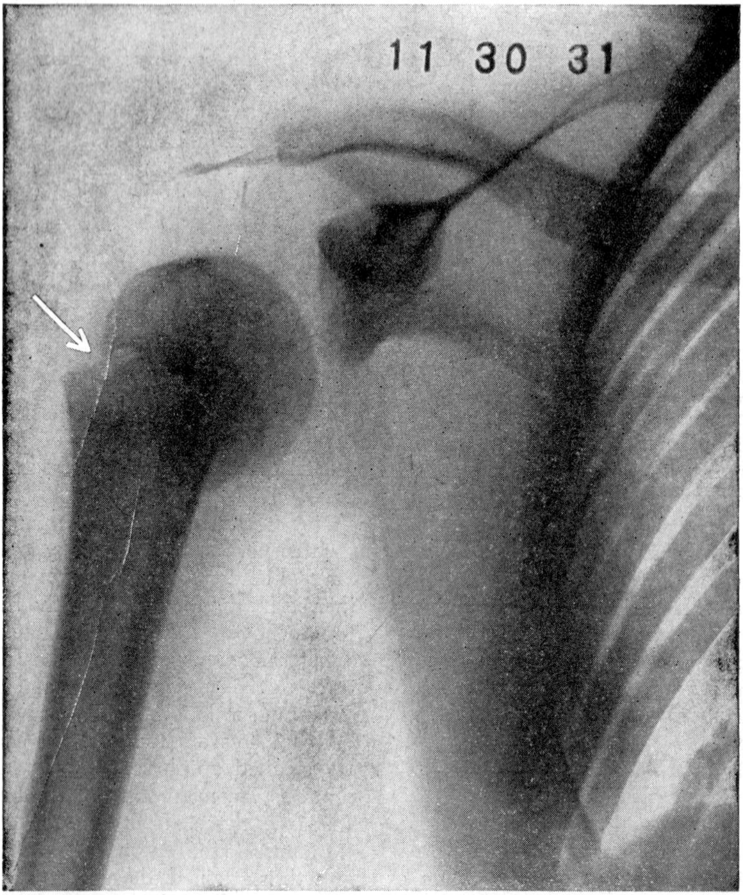

Fig. 218. Epiphyseal separation of the head of the humerus. The head of the bone with epiphyseal cartilage is displaced from its normal position on the shaft of the bone.

not attain its normal growth. Therefore, such separations are looked upon and treated as fractures.

Symptoms

The symptoms of a fracture may be learned easily by picturing what happens when a bone is broken. The break allows unnatural movement in a position which is normally rigid. The displacement of the fragments causes a deformity of the limb when compared with the sound member of the opposite side of the body. The limb cannot function properly because normal func-

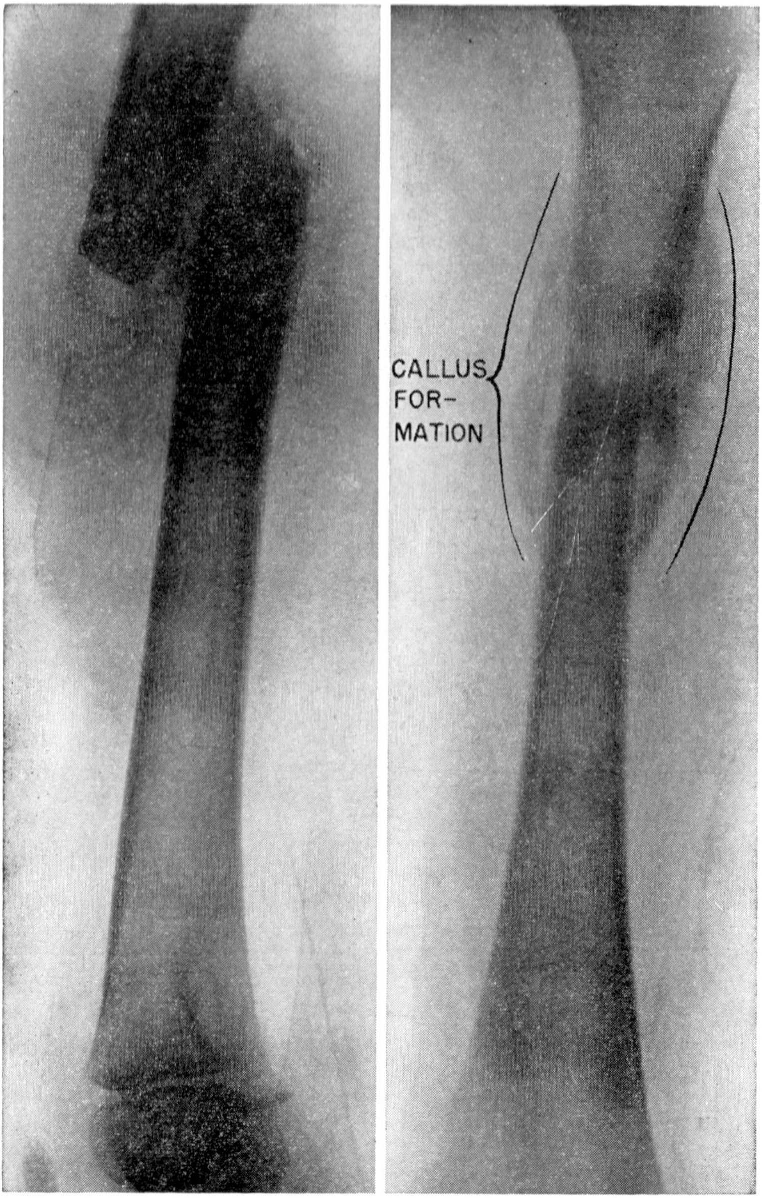

Fig. 219. Roentgenogram of a fractured femur of 4 weeks' duration. (*Left*) Lateral view. Note overlapping. (*Right*) Anteroposterior view. Note deposition of callus.

tion of the muscles is dependent upon the integrity of the bones to which they are attached.

Upon examination of the limb, a grating sensation, called *crepitus,* is imparted to the examining fingers, due to the rubbing of the fragments one upon the other. In fractures of long bones there is actually shortening of the limb, due to the contraction of the muscles which are attached above and below the site of the fracture. The fragments may often overlap as much as an inch or two. Finally, there are pain, tenderness, swelling and discoloration of the skin due to the trauma causing the fracture and the hemorrhage which follows it.

All of these symptoms are not necessarily present in every fracture. When there is a linear or fissure fracture, or in cases where the fractured surfaces are driven together (called *impacted* fractures), many of these symptoms may be lacking.

Diagnosis

In modern practice, the diagnosis and the treatment of fractures are not thought to be complete without at least one and often many x-ray examinations. By this means the position of the fragments may be determined accurately, and the indications for further treatment confirmed.

The *fluoroscope* is an apparatus by means of which the position of anything opaque to the x-rays may

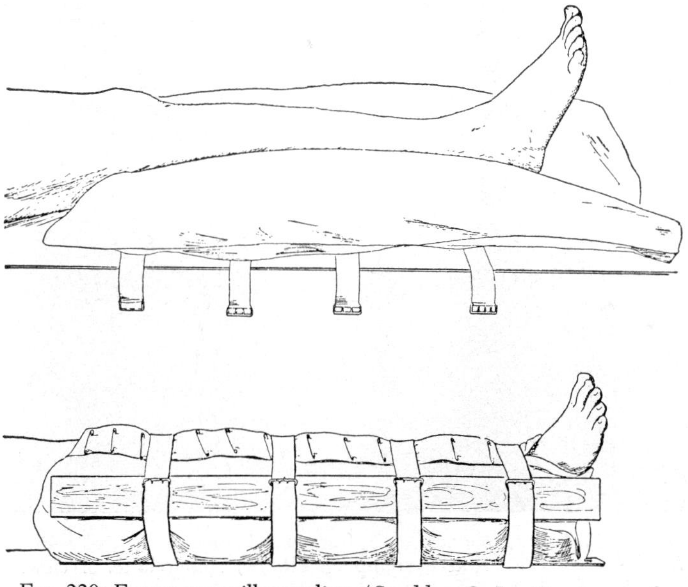

Fig. 220. Emergency pillow splint. (Scudder, C. L.: Treatment of Fractures, Philadelphia, Saunders)

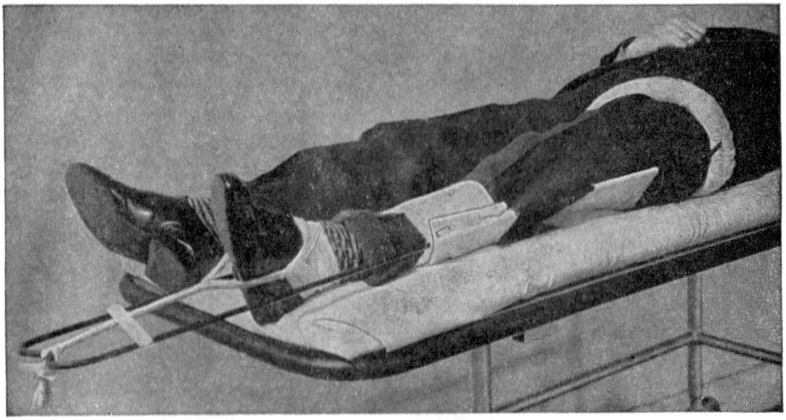

FIG. 221. Emergency splint for a fractured femur; a Thomas splint with traction applied by use of Collin's cinch of muslin bandage. Traction is produced by a windlass twisting of the bandage tied to the end of the splint. Slings of muslin bandage fastened with safety pins support the leg in the splint. A traction fixation never should be attempted by one unskilled in its application, unless under the guidance of a physician.

be visualized on a screen. By the aid of this apparatus the bone fragments may be brought into position with considerable ease and accuracy, but a roentgenogram always should follow to serve as a permanent record of the reduction.

Emergency Treatment

For transportation, the fractured limb should be rendered as immobile as possible by the temporary application of such makeshift splints as well-padded pieces of wood, cane, etc., firmly bandaged over the clothing. It must be remembered that the pain associated with a fractured bone is severe, and the surest way to decrease the discomfort of the patient and the possible shock is by fixing the bone so that the joints above and below the fracture are immobilized. Before transportation is attempted, morphine should be given if available.

In cases of compound fracture the wound should be covered with a sterile dressing, no attempt being made to reduce the fracture, even if one of the bone fragments is protruding through the wound. Splints should be applied as described above. Immediately following injury, a patient who is in a state of confusion may not be aware of the possibility of a fracture, i.e., he may walk on a fractured extremity. Therefore, it is important to immobilize that part of the body when a fracture is suspected.

Immediate Hospital Treatment and Nursing Care

When a patient comes to a hospital suffering from a fracture, at once he should be given morphine

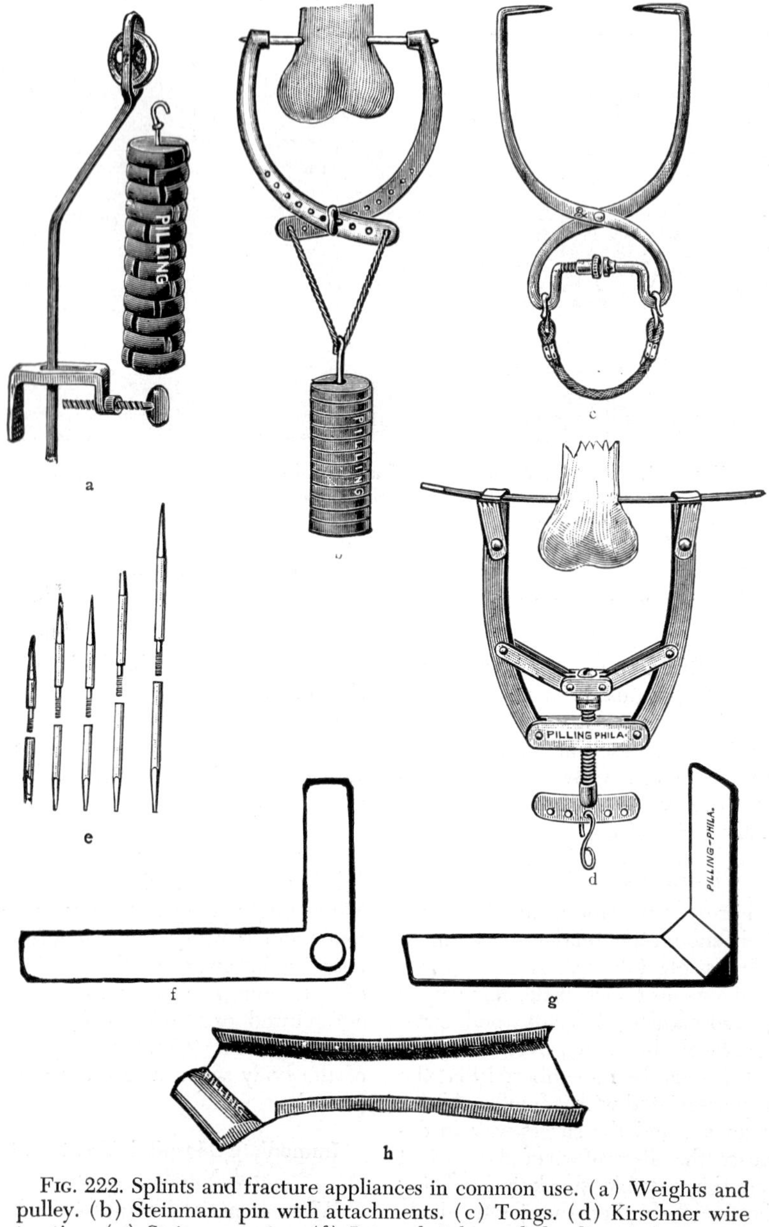

FIG. 222. Splints and fracture appliances in common use. (a) Weights and pulley. (b) Steinmann pin with attachments. (c) Tongs. (d) Kirschner wire traction. (e) Steinmann pins. (f) Internal right-angled splint. (g) Anterior angled splint. (h) Bond splint. (See also Fig. 223.)

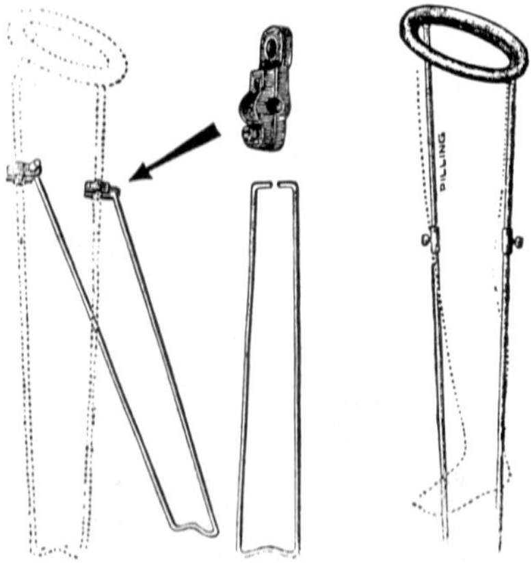

FIG. 223. Splints and fracture appliances in common use. (*Left*) Pearson attachment for Thomas splint. (*Right*) Thomas splint. (See also Fig. 222.)

or Demerol sufficient to relieve his pain. Then with all care and gentleness his clothes are removed, first from the uninjured side of his body, and then from the injured side. The fractured limb must be moved as little as possible to avoid disturbing it; sometimes the patient's clothing must be cut away on the injured side.

As a rule patients with fractures should not be moved until the injured part has been supported by temporary splints. However, there are times when moving is necessary. In those cases the limb should be supported both above and below the site of the fracture, and traction should be made in the line of the long axis of the bone in order to prevent rotation as well as angular motion.

Before reduction of the fracture, time enough usually elapses for the patient to be undressed, washed and made comfortable. A limb which is to be manipulated and dressed in a splint or a cast must not be dirty.

FRACTURE REDUCTION

In most cases anesthesia, either general or local block, is necessary to reduce a fractured bone properly without pain. Anesthesia also produces a relaxation of the muscles and this makes for an easier and quicker reduction. By manipulation and traction, the bone fragments are brought into apposition. Fractures should be reduced as soon as possible after the accident; swelling is no contraindication. The longer the interval before treatment, the greater is the possibility of complications.

Some fractures, especially those of the femur, are treated by weight traction. This method gives gradual reduction without an anesthetic.

FRACTURE DRESSINGS

After the fracture has been reduced, the bone fragments must be held in position until union has had time to take place. This immobilization may be accomplished by bandages, adhesive, splints, or by extension or traction. If the fragments have been properly reduced and immobilized, the swelling should disappear rapidly and the part should become less and less painful. If pain persists or increases, the nurse should suspect that something is wrong and call the surgeon at once. Increasing pain usually means an ill-fitting cast or splint. Early remedy is necessary to prevent necrosis.

Bandages, usually of muslin, are used commonly to immobilize cer-

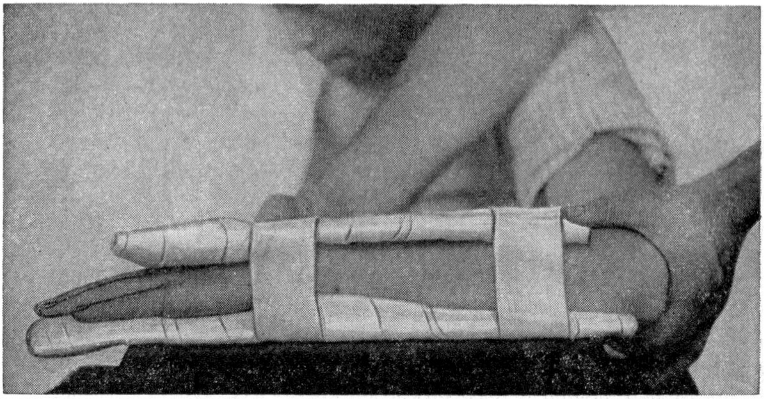

Fig. 224. Forearm splints, showing padding to fit the contour of the part. Note the wrinkles in the straps when the two splints are pressed together, thus illustrating the fact that the straps should retain the splints without undue pressure.

tain fractures. The Velpeau bandage dressing is applied by many surgeons for fractures of the clavicle. The Barton bandage is employed occasionally for fractures of the lower jaw.

Splints may be made of any rigid, firm material: wood, plaster of Paris, woven wire, cardboard, wire rods, etc.

Wooden splints are useful as temporary dressings for most fractures and occasionally as permanent dressings for many fractures, especially those of the arm. They are manufactured in various sizes and shapes for use as the occasion arises, to accord with a wide variety of uses. In addition, flexible splints of compressed wood are often incorporated in plaster casts to add stiffness with less plaster.

Wooden splints do not fit the curves of the limb; hence, they must be well padded with cotton and gauze to avoid pressure points. The padding should be applied only on the side of the splint which lies in contact with the skin; as a rule gauze bandage is used to hold the padding in place on the splint. It is important that the ends of the splint be well covered with padding. Bandages and adhesive strips are used to hold the splints firmly to the limb, but they should not be drawn tight enough to cause constrictions.

Plaster of Paris

Plaster of Paris is perhaps the most valuable of the materials used for fracture dressings. It is usually employed in the form of bandages of crinoline into the meshes of which powdered plaster of Paris has been rubbed. When the bandage has been wet, it becomes soft for a time, but soon sets as it dries and hardens, taking the shape to which it has been molded before setting.

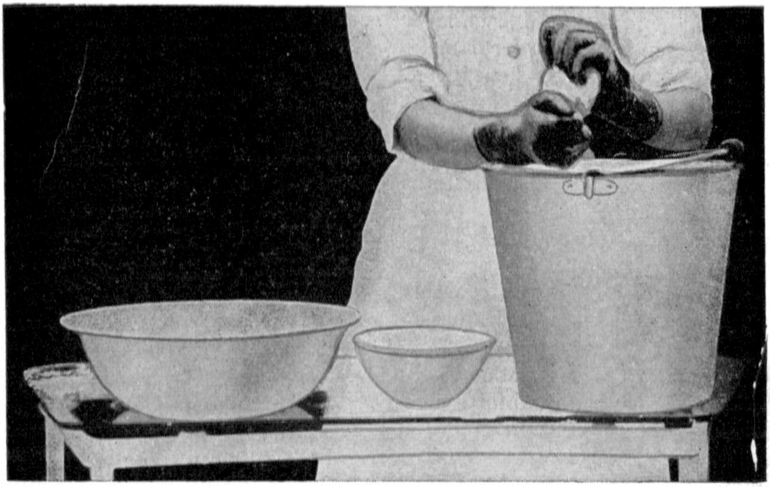

FIG. 225. Method of squeezing water from bandage.

Plaster Bandages. These are usually made in several widths (2, 4, 6 and 8 inches wide) and wrapped separately in crepe or waxed paper. For use they are stood on end in a bucket of warm water with their wrappings still in place but open partially at both ends. This procedure varies with different physicians. The addition of 3 or 4 teaspoonfuls of ordinary table salt to the water will hasten the subsequent hardening of the plaster. When bubbles of air cease to rise from the bandage, the nurse will know that the bandage has been wet through. She then takes the bandage so that the palms of the hands cover the ends of the roll and gently squeezes out the excess water (losing as little plaster as possible), removes the wrapper, finds the beginning of the bandage and passes the roll to the surgeon in such a way that the roller comes to his right hand and the free end to his left.

Plaster Casts. Before applying a plaster cast, the skin and soft tissue must be protected. Bandages of sheet wadding (cotton batting) are usually employed, and if considerable pressure is likely to result, felt pads are used. If the felt is to be next to the skin, the patient will be more comfortable if it is wrapped with a layer of gauze bandage before it is applied. Some surgeons use elastic tubular jersey sleeving (stockinet) with cotton batting; others apply the plaster directly to the skin without any padding.

Having protected the skin, some surgeons prefer to place zinc strips covered with waxed paper at the place where the cast must be cut. Rubber tubing may be used instead of the strips. The plaster bandage is then applied over them, turn upon turn, applying pressure to each layer with the open hand in order to make it unite with the one beneath it. Places where strain will take place, like the groin, back of the knee, etc., must be reinforced in one of three ways: there must be (1) many turns of the bandage at these points (which makes for an extremely heavy cast), (2) a wet piece of compressed wood-fiber may be incorporated in the cast, or (3) a reduplication of plaster bandages may be used.

"Reduplications" are made by rolling the bandage back and forth until a strip is obtained from 8 to 10 layers thick and of the desired length and width, the layers being well rubbed together with the open hand. The reduplication is then molded to fit the desired part of the cast and covered by several layers of plaster bandage. Such splints or "reduplications" are commercially available in various sizes. (Fig. 226.)

Before the cast is dry the operator should smooth it by rubbing with the open hand, at the same time making sure that it fits the limb. If the first few bandages have been applied firmly and smoothly, the cast usually will be well molded and without wrinkles.

In casts where zinc strips have been used, the following procedure is carried out. When the plaster has set, but before it is dry, incisions are made with a plaster knife through all the layers of the cast down to the zinc strips, leaving uncut about 1 or 2 inches at each end of the strip. The zinc strip may then be withdrawn, leaving its casing of waxed paper in place. When such incisions are made on each side of the cast, it may be removed with comparative ease or easily spread to relieve pressure should signs of constriction appear (cyanosis, coldness, or loss of sensation in fingers or toes). Any complaints by the patient of painful areas under the plaster should be reported or investigated.

The "hanging" cast can be used for certain fractures of the humerus. It consists of plaster applied from the axillary fold to the wrist with the elbow flexed at right angles. A sling is passed through a ring made with the plaster bandage at the wrist and this is then tied around the neck.

Plaster Splints. Plaster splints are reduplications made upon a pattern of lint. It is well to make the lint pattern about a full inch larger than the size desired. By making the plaster reduplications slightly smaller, enough lint remains to fold over the sharp edges which otherwise have a tendency to cause considerable pressure (see Fig. 246).

As soon as they are made, the plaster splints are bound firmly to the part with gauze bandage. As a general rule, plaster casts or splints are more comfortable if the joints which they enclose are slightly flexed. If casts are applied with traction, special tables are frequently employed.

Nursing Care

Application of Cast. When plaster is being used, the hands may be protected by rubber gloves, which are easily cleaned if washed in water before removing. A thin coating of petroleum jelly on the hands may be preferred to rubber gloves. The room in which plaster is applied should be one having a minimum of

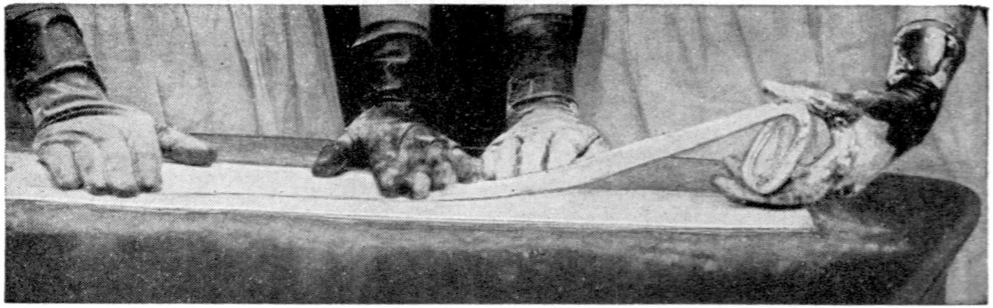

Fig. 226. (*Top*) Method of making a "reduplication" or splint.

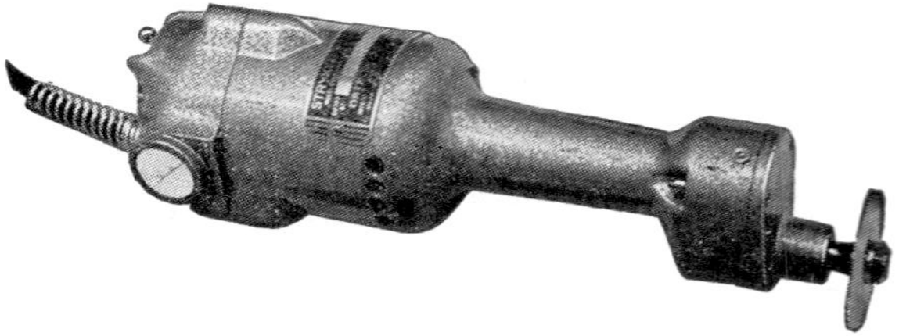

Fig. 227. (*Center*) Stryker electric cast cutter. The blade oscillates, cutting rapidly through rigid plaster with safety. (Orthopedic Frame Co.)

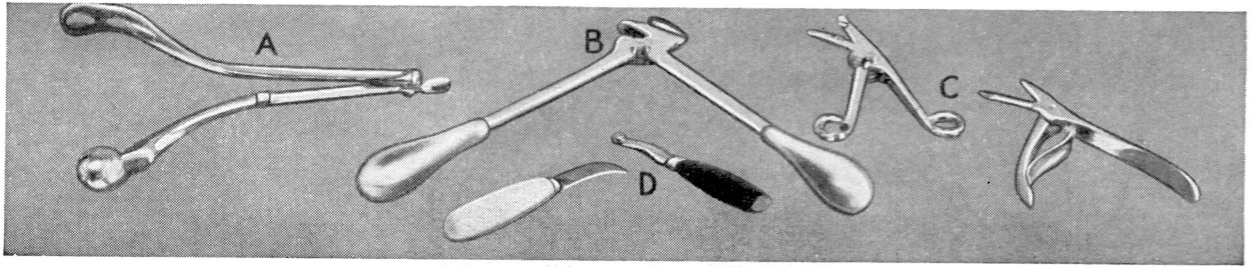

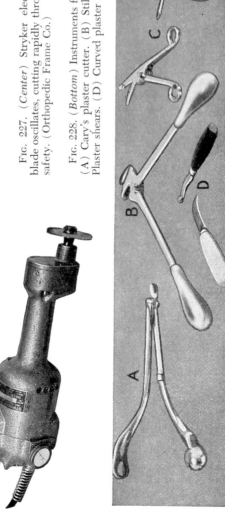

Fig. 228. (*Bottom*) Instruments for use in plaster work. (A) Cary's plaster cutter. (B) Stillé plaster cutter. (C) Plaster shears. (D) Curved plaster knives.

furnishings to facilitate cleaning. Some form of lubricant applied to the orthopedic table will make it easier to remove plaster and prevent rust formation. Plaster knives and shears are the only instruments needed (Fig. 227). They must be cleaned thoroughly and oiled after use. The plaster-laden water in which the bandages are soaked should not be poured into the ordinary drain basin, because a clogged pipe is almost sure to result. It is better to allow the plaster to settle in the bucket, then the water may be poured off, and the remaining plaster emptied into the waste can. In most modern hospitals, plaster traps are installed in the drain pipes of sinks in rooms where plaster is used. The trap will catch most of the plaster poured into the sink, but it must be cleaned frequently if it is to work efficiently.

Newspaper should be spread out so as to protect the furniture (tables, chairs, etc.); since these papers can be discarded after use, this makes the cleaning up after plaster application less burdensome. If a marble or board slab is used, this can be placed on newspaper so that plaster drippings are easily caught and discarded. If the bucket in which the plaster is soaked is placed on a table protected by newspaper, the plaster drippings that invariably occur when the plaster is taken from the water, and when water is expressed from the bandage, fall on the newspaper, which can be discarded readily. The use of sheets or other drapes to protect furniture from plaster is an expensive protection.

Care of the Patient in a Cast. A fundamental principle not to be lost sight of is that we are still caring for a patient as well as a cast. Experience has taught that any complaint of discomfort must not go unheeded. Two types of complications occur. One is due to pressure of the cast on tissues, especially bony points which give pain; the other is due to swelling underneath the cast which produces a circulatory impairment. Toes and fingers of extremities recently encased in plaster must be inspected frequently to note any signs of circulatory impairment. This is manifested by swelling, blanching or discoloration, tingling, numbness, or temperature change and *must be reported immediately,* for serious results such as paralysis and necrosis may occur. Conscientious observation should continue as long as the patient is in the cast; if there is swelling, the cast will seem tighter.

When a large cast is applied, such as a body or hip spica, the bed must be prepared before the patient is received. A board under the mattress will give the necessary firmness to the bed. To make allowances for the contour of the cast, 3 rubber-covered pillows placed crosswise on the bed will suffice for the body cast. For a hip spica, 1 pillow placed crosswise at the waist and 2 pillows placed lengthwise for the affected leg are necessary. If both legs are involved, 2 additional pillows are necessary. It is important that the pillows be next to each other, because any spaces in between will allow the damp cast to sag, become weak and possibly break.

In moving a patient from side to side in a large cast, at least 3 people are necessary. Only the palms of the hands are used to lift the cast; fingers make indentations in soft plaster. Support should be given to the entire cast and most particularly at such vulnerable points as the hip and the knee.

The nurse must remember that the patient receives first consideration and his cast is secondary in importance.

A freshly applied cast should be exposed to circulating air or a blower type drier so that it will dry.

Covers are not necessary for they restrict the escape of moisture. As the moisture evaporates and the cast hardens, heat is generated. In a warm room it may be necessary to use an electric fan to keep the patient comfortable. When a large cast is dried, it is often desirable to use mechanical aids, such as a heat lamp or hair dryer, to facilitate the process. This should not be placed closer than 18 inches and then it should be moved frequently from one area to another so that drying is achieved evenly. It is to be remembered that burns may occur under the cast from overexposure even though the skin is not exposed directly. If the patient is cold, those parts of the body not encased in plaster should be covered and kept warm. When the patient is in shock, the cast can be exposed piecemeal. It takes about 24 hours for a cast to become dry, depending upon the size of the cast and the moisture in the air; a dry cast is white and shiny, resonant and odorless as well as firm; a wet cast is gray and dull in appearance, dull to percussion, feels damp and has a musty odor.

Turning the Patient. While the cast is still in the process of drying, the patient should be turned every 6 hours to promote even drying of the cast and to prevent fatigue of the patient (this may vary with the physician or the hospital policy). The initial turning of a large cast is usually done on the evening of the day it is applied so that the posterior surface may be dried. This should be done with sufficient help. The patient is first moved to the side of the bed toward the leg encased in plaster. At this time fresh pillows and sheets can be placed on the vacant side so that it will be ready to receive the turned patient. The patient with a hip spica should be turned as one piece on the leg *not involved* and adequate support must be given to the uppermost leg, which is encased, especially at the groin. His arms may be placed above his head or kept at his sides, whichever is most comfortable. Two persons on the side of the bed to which the patient is closest and one person on the opposite side can turn a patient effectively without lifting him. When he is lying prone, a pillow placed crosswise under the dorsum of the feet will prevent the toes from being forced into the mattress. Sometimes allowing the toes to hang over the edge of the mattress is more comfortable. After the cast is thoroughly dry, pillows are used as necessary to maintain comfort and good body alignment. They are used also to bring the level of the cast up to that of the bed pan when the latter is used. A pillow under the abdomen often adds to the comfort of the patient.

A comfort measure which will be appreciated by the patient in a body cast is the "back scratcher." This can

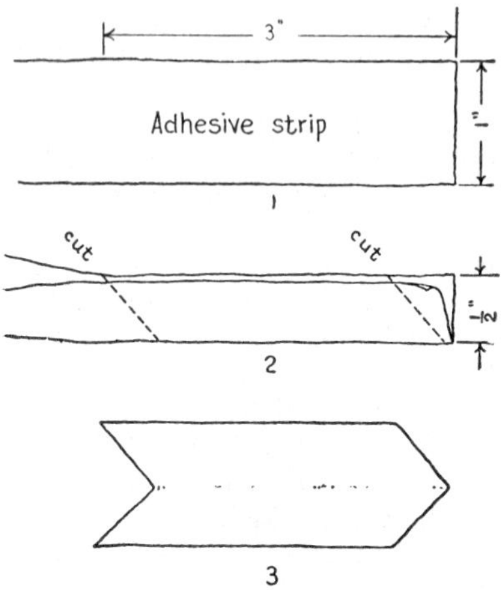

FIG. 229. Drawings to show method of cutting petals for covering edge of the cast. (1) A strip of adhesive is folded so that the adhesive side is out and cut as indicated in the diagram. (2) In cutting several petals from a strip of adhesive, only single cuts are necessary for each petal. (3) A finished petal. The petals are applied to the edge of the cast, as shown in Fig. 230. The length of the petal may be varied to suit the situation in which they are to be used.

be a length of 3-inch flannel which can be inserted inside the back of the cast by a long alligator forceps. (A thoughtful nurse can suggest this to the surgeon immediately before the application of the cast.) By holding each end of the flannel, the nurse can give the patient a friction rub.

Protection of the Skin and Care of the Cast. Pressure areas may develop over any bony prominence. A common site of pressure from a large cast is the buttocks. When the patient is turned on his abdomen, the exposed skin can be washed carefully and massaged. The rough edges of the cast here as well as elsewhere must be made smooth. Often pulling stockinet from inside the cast over the rough edge and fixing it to the outside with adhesive will eliminate cast crumbs and make the edge smooth. The nurse should reach up under the cast edges as far as possible with her fingers to remove plaster crumbs and to massage the skin area. Around the perineal area, it is often necessary to protect the cast against excretions. If the opening is inadequate for hygienic care, the nurse should report this. When the cast is dry, pliofilm, oiled silk, cellophane, or waxed paper can be cut in 4-inch strips and tucked under the cast; they can be fastened to the exterior, allowing for adequate coverage of the outside of the cast. These can be pulled out and cleaned or replaced daily.

To clean soiled parts of a cast, it is acceptable to rub the area with a damp cloth. It may be sufficient to apply a piece of plaster bandage ("patch" method) which is cut to cover the soiled area. Another effective method is to use a cloth which has been rubbed over a cake of a cleaning agent such as Bon Ami. The outside of a cast may be shellacked after the cast is thoroughly dry.

Cast edges can be molded satisfactorily by "petaling." One-inch or 2-inch adhesive tape can be cut as petals and applied (Figs. 229 and 230). This method is more economical of time and materials than circular petals. Measurements can vary according to need.

The skin around the edges of the cast must be inspected frequently for signs of irritation. All accessible

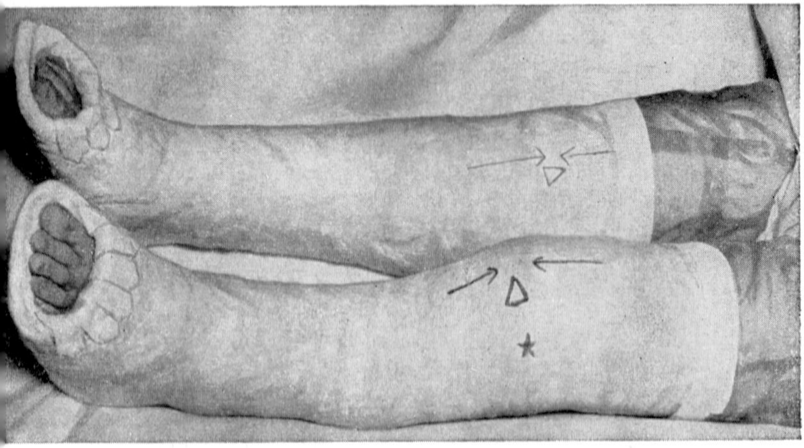

FIG. 230. Photograph showing casts, the edges of which have been covered by petals to protect the foot from the edge of the cast. In this case, the upper ends of the casts have been protected by waterproof plastic material. This type of protection is used frequently in incontinent patients.

skin should be massaged gently with alcohol. When there is irritation, the area must be treated as a potential decubitus.

Complications of Casts

Since many cases of fracture are treated by the application of plaster casts, it is well to note complications that may arise when casts are used. Constriction of the part may occur, especially when the casts are applied while the patient is under the influence of an anesthetic. Any signs of constriction developing at any time should be reported immediately.

Pressure is the chief cause of the complications which develop. The sites most frequently affected are over the sacrum, the outer and posterior aspects of the knee, and the posterior aspect of the ankle. Therefore, these points should receive special padding and attention. Pressure sores develop over the sacrum because the skin of this region is hard to keep clean, for the padding frequently becomes wrinkled and rough from crumbs or rolls of padding, and because this area bears the weight of the pelvis. Therefore, this region must be watched carefully. The patient may be turned, the legs supported with pillows, and an opportunity given to care for the skin.

Pressure beneath the knee is not so common, but frequent enough to make it advisable to bear it in mind as a possibility when padding is being applied. The peroneal nerve lies over the head of the fibula, a little below and to the outside of the knee, a location that makes it especially subject to injury caused by pressure from a cast. The pain associated with this complication may be very short-lived, but a paralysis of the nerve with a consequent foot-drop may develop and persist long enough to complicate convalescence, although such a condition is rarely permanent. To guard against this complication the cast should be well padded over the head of the fibula and not applied too tightly over that area. The patient's complaint of pain at the knee never should go unheeded. He should be reminded frequently to mention without fail and at once any discomfort. Relief measures can be instituted easily when discomfort is reported early. Later, the problems may be more serious.

Removal of the Cast and Care of the Patient. A cast can be removed by using an electric cast cutter or by making an incision with a plaster knife and cutting the cast with heavy shears. Acetic acid or hydrogen peroxide forced along the incision line from an aseptic syringe aids in softening the plaster. One of the most important things to remember when a cast has been removed is that the part or parts involved have been immobilized for a considerable period of time. When the support and protection of the cast have been removed, there are stresses and strains placed on tissue which has been resting. The patient complains of pain and stiffness, often much different from the original injury, and he is depressed and discouraged because the early anticipated release from the cast has only added further problems.

The responsibility of the nurse is to help to make the adjustment of the patient easier. This can be accomplished by supporting the part to maintain the same position as existed in the cast, with small pillow supports under the knee, the lumbar spine, etc., allowing for gradual removal of support. In moving an extremity, the nurse must provide adequate support and move the limb gently. Gradual movement on the part of the patient must be encouraged. This is often aided by proper exercises, supervised by a physical therapist.

The care of the skin is not a pressing problem. Its care is less important than the care to the muscles and the bones; therefore, careful washing with a mild soap, followed by oil or lanolin, is sufficient. Soap or oil poultices may be effective. The exudate noted on the skin should not be scrubbed with a brush, for it is a good protective agent. If a new cast is to be applied, some surgeons prefer that the skin be powdered only and that there be no washing of the skin which might be traumatizing. Briefly, the skin and the underlying tissues must be handled carefully until gradual restoration of normal function is achieved. Atrophy of the part may be noted but this will disappear gradually with the return of muscle function. Should the patient go home with a cast, he must be instructed as to the care of his cast. If the cast has been removed, the principles of skin care must be understood. He must know also the signs of impaired circulation and evidence of infection or skin breakdown. The nurse should stress the importance of his returning to his physician or clinic for follow-up care.

Turnbuckle Cast. In some cases casts are applied, not only for im-

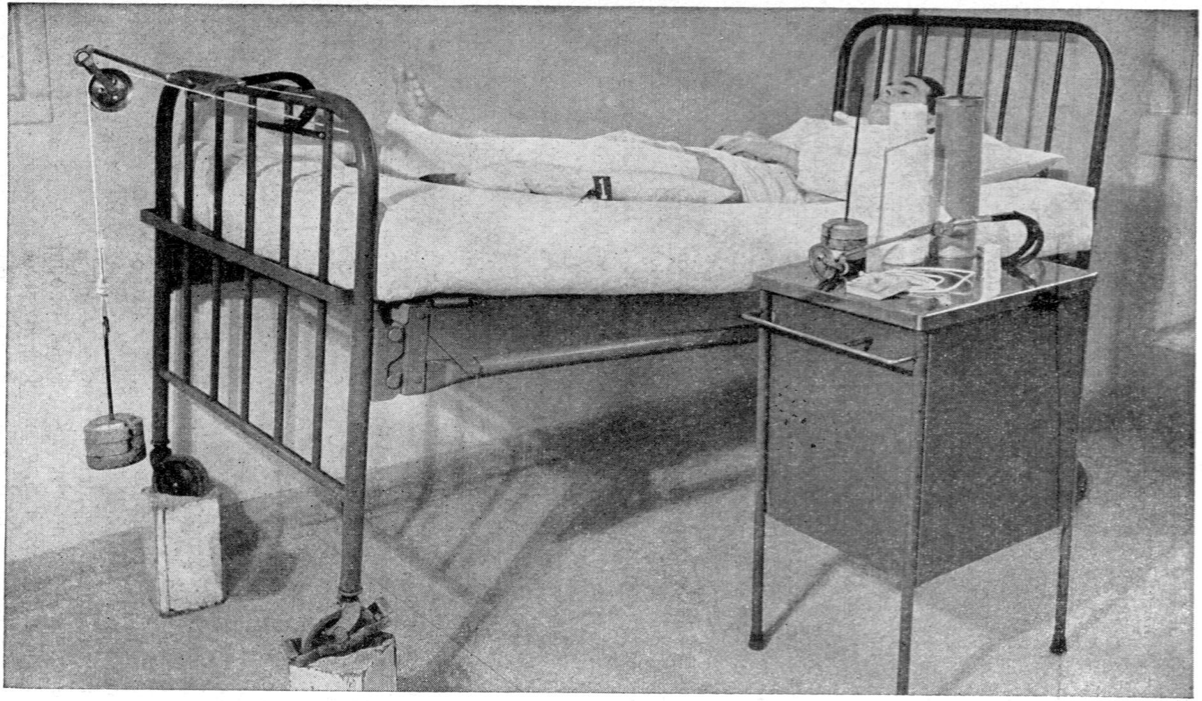

FIG. 231. Buck's extension for skin traction. The leg should be shaved and moleskin cut and applied with bandages as shown. Note (1) the small pillow under the leg. When traction is applied to the lower extremity, it is necessary usually to raise the foot of the bed by the use of bed pins or blocks. Note slots in which bed wheels fit. On the side table are placed materials for the application of a Buck's extension-pulley which may be attached to the bed and weights, moleskin adhesive rope and bandage.

mobilization, but also for the purposes of overcoming bony deformities and muscular contractures. Traction with weight pulleys is sometimes used for this purpose, but in many cases casts are applied which can be cut and the contracture overcome gradually by changing the angle of the cast. In such cases a gradual change may be brought about by incorporating a turnbuckle in the cast, usually across a joint. The part may be straightened by gradually turning the turnbuckle. The nurse must be extremely careful in turning the patient that this extra appliance is not pulled upon and displaced so as to break the cast and interrupt the patient's treatment. She also must be alert *constantly* for new signs of pressure with each manipulation of the turnbuckle.

Traction

Traction is the method of fixation used most often for fractures of the femur. This method is also employed by some surgeons for fractures of the humerus, the tibia and other bones. The traction developed by weights and pulleys is applied to the part by one of two methods: skin traction or skeletal traction with either wire, pins, or tongs.

Skin Traction. By this method adhesive "moleskin" strips are attached to each side of the limb, connected below to weights by a rope passing over a pulley wheel. For a fractured femur the strips should be cut long enough to extend about 4 inches above the knee on each side. In the center of the strip at the sole of the foot should be placed a piece of wood 3 inches high and an inch wider than the greatest distance between the two malleoli. This serves as a spreader and will prevent pressure along the sides of the foot. It should have a hole in the center through which the traction rope may be passed. Cut the moleskin the desired length and pattern before removal of the protective crinoline. After the block has been attached, it is held in place by a second strip of moleskin which should extend for 10 or 12 inches on each side of the wood to prevent adhesion to the malleoli. The adhesive is applied and then held in place by gauze or Ace bandage. Shaving the part and painting the skin with benzoin tincture will make the adhesive hold better; benzoin tincture also acts as a skin disinfectant and is said to prevent an itching skin and be more comfortable. The traction may be begun almost immediately. When skin traction (such as Buck's extension) is applied to the leg, pressure not infrequently develops on the Achilles tendon above the heel and should be inspected several times daily.

Skin traction is usually used with the Thomas splint for fractures of the femur. These patients have a tendency to slide down toward the foot of the bed, but this may be counteracted by elevation of the foot of the bed 12 or 15 inches. The pulleys may be of any kind, but the most suitable ones are those attached to the foot of the bed by a clamp (Fig. 231).

Weights may be ordinary traction weights of metal, or bags of shot or sand. Enough weight is applied at first to overcome the shortening tendency of the injured limb but is gradually lessened as the fracture becomes more fixed. *A nurse never*

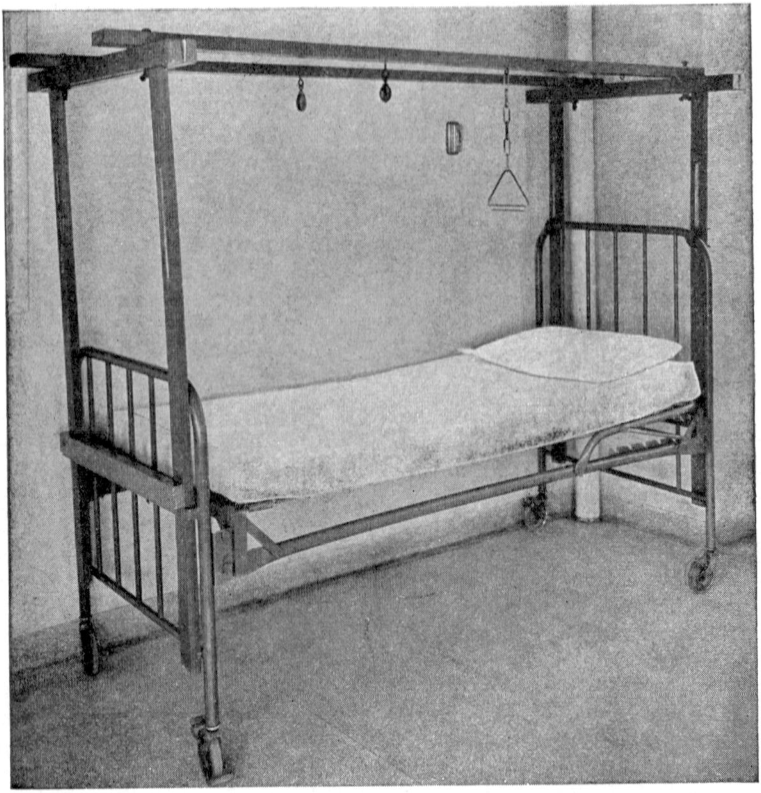

FIG. 232. Balkan frame attached to an ordinary hospital bed.

should remove weights from a fracture case under any consideration. Weight and pulley traction is applied to secure constant corrective extension. If, then, the weights are removed to move the patient from one department to another, the whole purpose of their use has been defeated. Many valueless x-ray films have been made because nurses have removed the weights from fracture cases while taking the patients to the x-ray department. In moving fracture cases, however, the weights should be steadied and kept from swinging.

Skeletal or Bony Traction. This method is used by many surgeons in the treatment of fractures of the femur, the humerus and the tibia. The traction is applied directly to the bones by the use of tongs (Fig. 222) or a pin driven through the bone. Instead of the tongs or pin, many surgeons use the Kirschner steel wire, which is drilled through the bone with a hand- or electric-driven drill (Fig. 222 b, c and d). Usually the tongs, pin or Kirschner wire may be inserted through a small opening in the skin made under local anesthesia. They should be sterilized and inserted with all the sterile precautions of an operation. The wound is covered with a small gauze square held in place by adhesive strips. If the wire or pin extends beyond the skin or beyond the caliper, a cork placed over the end of the pin will prevent the tearing of linen and other more serious accidents.

Traction is applied by weights and pulleys as described for skin traction. The Thomas splint with the Pearson attachment is usually used with skeletal traction in fractures of the lower part of the femur (Fig. 223). It may be used with skin traction and other balanced suspension apparatus. Because upward traction is required for these fractures, a Balkan frame should be fastened to the bed before the traction is applied. Instead of the wooden frame, hospitals are now being supplied with steel fracture beds having a metal framework and adjustable pulleys, which are more convenient (see Fig. 239).

When the apparatus has been properly adjusted, the fracture should become constantly more comfortable. At times one part of the tongs will slip from its bony anchorage and exert its traction on the soft tissues. As might be expected, considerable pain is caused by this accident. The surgeon in charge should be notified at once.

Nursing Care

The importance of frequent inspection of the fracture dressing in the first 24 hours after application cannot be impressed too strongly on the nurse responsible for the care of the patient. A bandage that appears sufficiently loose when applied may in a very few hours cause serious constriction which, if not relieved, may lead to gangrene of the extremity.

Dressings always should be applied in such a way as to leave the tips of the fingers and toes exposed. Any cyanosis, loss of temperature, tingling, or loss of sensation in these parts should warn the nurse that the dressings are too tight. If the condition is caused by a single turn of the bandage, the turn may be divided with the scissors, but it is usually advisable to notify the surgeon who has charge of the patient. After the first 24 hours, the fracture dressing should be inspected by the nurse at least three or four times daily. She should inquire whether there are any painful areas, look for evidences of constriction and see that there are no pressure points, e.g., heel is not on the bed, bedclothes do not rest on toes, there is no pressure on the Achilles tendon, etc. If traction is being used, the apparatus should be inspected to see that the ropes are in the wheel groove of the pulleys, that the weights hang free, that the patient has not slipped down in bed. The foot must be in a natural position; rotation outward or inward should be reported. The rope sometimes frays; therefore, it too must be inspected at least daily. An alert nurse will be sure to examine the skin around the traction for evidence of circulatory impairment.

A comfort measure is to place a firm thin pillow covered with oiled silk lengthwise under the leg in traction so that the pillow is under the thigh and extends to just above the heel (with permission of the physician). If the oiled silk is powdered it will eliminate bed friction; the heel will not be resting on the bedclothes and will be free of pressure, which is desirable.

Foot drop may be prevented in several ways: (1) A stockinet boot can be fixed at the ankle with several turns of bandage; the other open end, which is about two inches above the toes, is drawn together with stitching as in a pursestring. To this end is attached a metal ring, through which a rope is drawn to the top of the Balkan frame where it meets a pulley. A one-pound weight is sufficient to keep the foot in proper position. (2) A strip of adhesive attached to the plantar surface of the foot and extending beyond the toes can be attached to the same type of pulley arrangement as described above. A metal eyelet in the adhesive serves as a means of attachment for the rope. (3) Metal or wooden frames, some of which are hinged, can also be secured from instrument companies or can be made in the hospital maintenance department. When fracture beds or Balkan frames are used, rings or a trapezelike rod may be suspended overhead within easy reach of the patient (Figs. 232 and 239). This piece of apparatus is of great help in permitting the patient to move about in bed, on and off bedpans, etc. It is also a help to the nurse in caring for these patients. He is usually not permitted to turn on one side or the other or on his abdomen. Because of this, the nurse must make a special effort to give him good back care, keep the bed dry and free of crumbs and wrinkles. This can be accomplished without her straining her back, because the patient may raise his hips from the bed by holding onto the overhead trapeze. Often a patient uses the heel of his good leg to act as a brace when he raises himself. This digging of the heel into the mattress may be injurious to the tissues; hence, it must be massaged with lanolin and inspected for pressure areas. Some physicians wrap both legs of traction patients in Ace bandage in an attempt to decrease in the incidence of thrombophlebitis. If the patient is unable to raise himself, the nurse can push down on the mattress with one hand, leaving space for the other hand to massage the skin.

Internal Fixation

Methods of fixation applied externally, such as have been described, are suitable for many types of fractures. There are some fractures, however, which are treated by a rigid fixation directly across the fracture line from one fragment to the other. This type of fixation is spoken of as internal, and it may be provided by pins or nails applied through the bones as in fractures of the neck of the femur and in long bone fractures. The use of various types of metal rods (pins) to fix fractures has revolutionized the care of many fracture patients. There is a marked decrease in the length of immobilization and hospitalization.

Open Reduction

In some cases, the fracture may be reduced and internal fixation introduced through a small wound without a formal operation. In many fractures, however, reduction cannot be accomplished because of a separation of the fragments by muscle, fascia, or a detached bone fragment. In others, it may be impossible to hold the fragments in position even though reduction was accomplished by manipulation. Internal fixation may be achieved by the application of a plate to the cortex of the bone across the fracture line. The plate is held in place with screws inserted through holes in the plate into the bone shaft. This necessitates a formal incision and exposure of the fracture site and is called an *open reduction* of the fracture. After closure of the wound, external fixation is often used in addition by the application of splints or casts. The internal fixation may be removed after bony union has taken place, but in many cases it never is removed unless it produces symptoms.

After-care

The surgeon in charge of a patient with a reduced fracture will inspect the dressing daily for several days. If the fracture has been accurately reduced and immobilized, the patient should become increasingly more comfortable.

Redressings are required for many fractures dressed with splints, especially those which involve or are near the joints. The nurse should provide diluted alcohol for sponging off the skin, as well as talcum powder, bandages and adhesive. Fractures complicated by joint involvement, or those treated by the application of a cast, are often benefited by a regimen of baking and massage, after union is firm enough for external support to be discontinued. Under ordinary conditions with proper treatment, the fragments of the broken bone unite by the formation of a soft callus in which are deposited calcium salts, so that in time a patch of bone results which is as strong as the original part. (See Fig. 219.)

Healing Process

The rapidity with which union occurs varies with many factors. For instance, it is well known that fractures that occur during infancy and youth unite much more quickly than those occurring in old age. Fractures of the various bones require different periods of disability before active function can be resumed—thus fractures of the humerus on the average require from 6 to 10 weeks; those of the forearm, from 8 to 10 weeks; those of the femur, 6 months; and those of the lower leg, from 2 to 4 months.

Delayed and Nonunion. Occasionally, because of local causes or systemic disease, union does not take place within the usual period. In many of these cases union occurs if the patient is permitted the use of the limb supported by braces, and appropriate treatment is given the systemic disease which may be present. If union does not result at the end of from 10 to 12 weeks, the fracture is said to be ununited. In these cases the fragments have between them only fibrous tissue; no bone salts have been deposited. Such patients often develop a false joint (pseudoarthrosis) at the site of the fracture. When such an unfortunate result occurs, braces may be used to give the patient a useful limb, or by an operation the ends of the bone

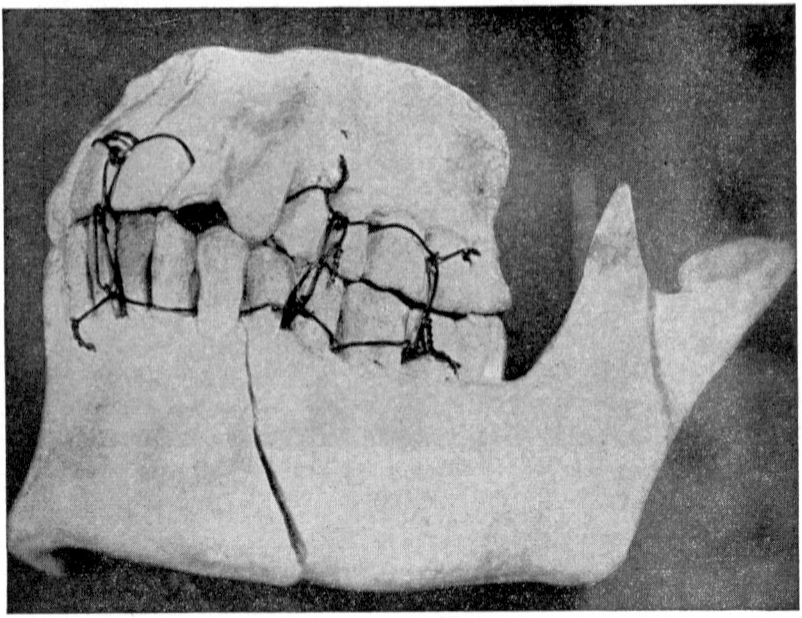

FIG. 233. Fracture of the mandible. Method of wiring teeth in occlusion on each side of the fracture. (Ivy: Surg., Gynec. & Obst. 34:670)

may be freshened, and an attempt made to unite them by means of a graft removed from another bone which is placed in position between the fragments. Fractures of the middle of the humerus, of the neck of the femur in old people, and of the lower third of the tibia most frequently result in nonunion.

Compound Fractures

Compound fractures are often associated with so much damage to the soft tissue that amputation of the member is necessary. If it is possible, however, that a useful limb may result, the surgeon will thoroughly débride the wound. After débriding or excising devitalized tissue and removing foreign material, he will place the fragments in position and repair the soft tissues (muscles, nerves and tendons) as well as possible. These wounds may be closed under favorable circumstances, otherwise left open, loosely packed with petrolatum gauze and a compression dressing applied. In these days of antibiotic therapy, compound fractures may be expected to heal primarily with primary closure if they have been treated early. When the wounds are grossly contaminated or when there has been delay of treatment, débridement and immobilization are carried out, with secondary closure in 5 to 7 days. When there has been much loss of tissue, skin grafting may be necessary.

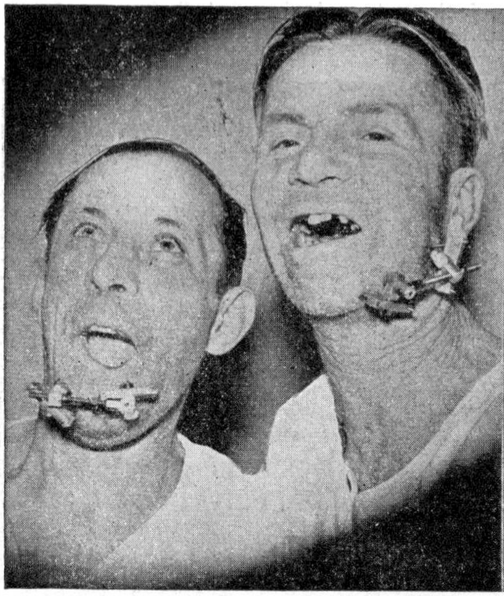

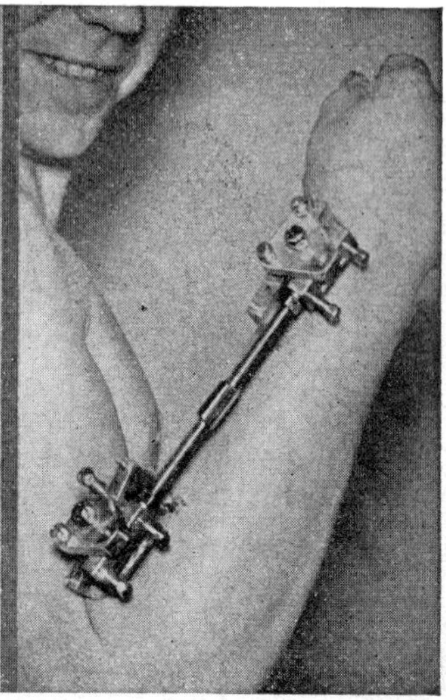

FIG. 234. (*Left*) The Stader splint, which permits ambulatory convalescence with maximum use of the afflicted part. Application of splint to fracture of the jaw. (Shaar, C. M., and Kreuz, P., Jr.: Manual on Treatment of Fractures by External Skeletal Fixation, Philadelphia, Saunders)

FIG. 235. (*Right*) Application of the Stader splint to fracture of the forearm.

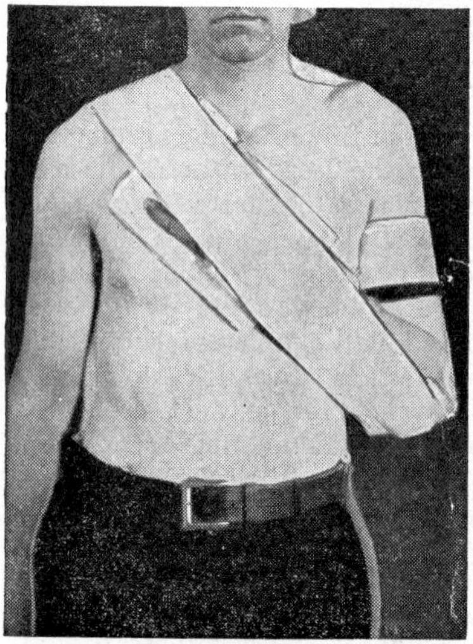

FIG. 236. Sayre's dressing, anterior view. Slits for the fingertips and the olecranon are helpful. (Magnuson, P. B., and Stack, J. K.: Fractures, ed. 5, Philadelphia, Lippincott)

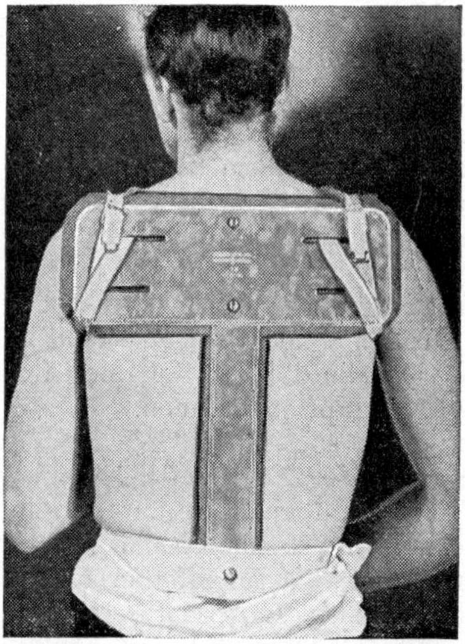

FIG. 237. T splint for immobilization in fracture of clavicle, posterior view. (Magnuson, P. B., and Stack, J. K.: Fractures, ed. 5, Philadelphia, Lippincott)

Individual Fractures

Treatment and Nursing Care

Skull and Spine. These have been considered in Chapter 22 on the nursing of neurosurgical diseases.

Mandible (Jaw Bone). These fractures are compound, opening into the mouth. They are treated by fixing the lower jaw against the upper by wires placed between the teeth, or by a firm bandage. The problem then is one of treating a fracture compounded into the mouth in a patient who cannot open his jaws. In other instances molded metal bars are wired to the teeth on both sides of the fracture line (Fig. 233). The Stader and other splints using multiple-pin fixation are popular (Figs. 234 and 235). With these splints it is necessary to protect the patient's neck or upper chest from irritation by the Stader splint. Occasionally, a patient has a fear of this apparatus. The nurse can do a great deal to allay such concern.

The nurse should be cognizant of the danger of vomiting in patients having the jaws wired together. She should know that the jaws may be opened by removal of the wire loops if this complication arises. By the use of a simple hemostat the wires which join the loops attached to the upper and the lower teeth may be untwisted. A wire cutter may have to be used if untwisting the wires takes too long.

Careful attention to the hygiene of the mouth must be insisted upon, using warm alkaline mouthwashes at least every 2 hours and after each feeding. In addition, the mouth should be inspected at least once or twice daily to ensure thorough cleansing. A flashlight and a tongue blade to retract the cheeks are essential equipment.

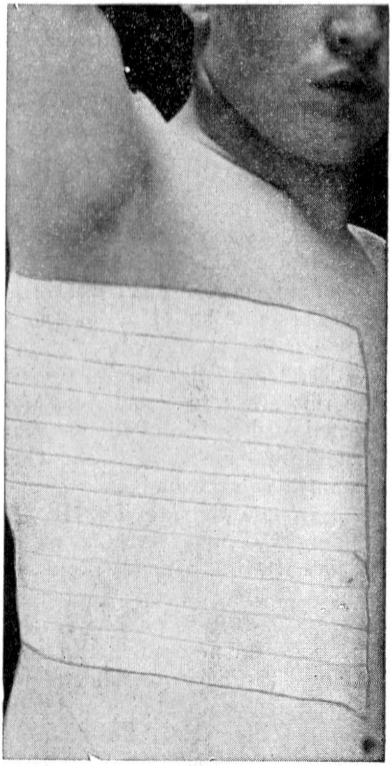

Fig. 238. Adhesive dressing for fractures of the rib.

The diet must necessarily be liquid, but sufficient caloric and fluid intake can be given easily to these patients. They can be fed through a straw without much difficulty and occasionally soft foods may be given with a spoon.

Clavicle (Collar Bone). This is one of the most common of fractures and it practically always unites.

A Velpeau or Sayre dressing may be used in ambulatory treatment. For both of these dressings, gauze or lint should be provided for placing in the axilla and between the arm and the chest.

The Velpeau requires muslin bandages 2 or 3 inches in width and a safety pin to secure them.

The Sayre dressing is applied with long adhesive strips cut as wide as the patient's forearm (Fig. 236). A clavicular cross is used as a dressing by many surgeons (Fig. 237). A figure-of-eight strapping or plaster bandage may be used also.

Ribs. Uncomplicated fractures of the ribs are very common and are treated easily by firm adhesive strapping 2 or 3 inches in width which should reach beyond the mid-line both front and back. This type of binding is applied as the patient exhales. These patients should be watched carefully for symptoms of pleurisy and other pulmonary complications. Before applying the strips it is well to shave the hairy regions to make removal of the adhesive less painful (Fig. 238). Injections of local anesthesia along the intercostal nerves of the injured area and about the fracture site are often given to relieve pain.

Humerus. SURGICAL NECK. The commonest fracture in the upper arm and the shoulder is that of the surgical neck of the humerus. It occurs most often in adults, and the patient comes for aid with the affected arm hanging limp at the side, supported with the uninjured hand.

Reduction is best accomplished with the aid of the fluoroscope while the patient is under gas or local anesthesia. The dressing applied is the one which will best hold the fragments in position. The simplest dressing is one which employs: (1) A well-padded shoulder cap. This may be made of wood, felt, cardboard, or plaster of Paris. (2) An axillary pad. This is a triangular pad of gauze with a base about 4 or 5 inches in width, a perpendicular equal to the distance from the patient's axilla to his elbow, and a little broader than the broadest part of the patient's arm. (3) A wrist sling of 4- to 6-inch muslin bandage. The sling is applied first, and the pad and the shoulder cap are held by bandages about the patient's body, placed so as to hold the arm to the side. The turn about the chest should include the sling in order to draw the hand and the forearm close to the body. This dressing is maintained for from 4 to 6 weeks.

SHAFT. These fractures are among the most difficult of all fractures to treat. The bone is surrounded by thick muscles which often become interposed between the fragments and make reduction difficult. The musculospiral nerve lies posterior to the bone, in the musculospiral groove, and not infrequently it is involved in shaft fractures or in the callus formed by their healing. It is important, therefore, to make frequent inspection for wristdrop, the sign of paralysis of this nerve, both before and after reduction of the fracture.

Many dressings are used for this fracture: the shoulder cap, axillary pad, and sling; many forms of traction with splints; the airplane splint.

A form of dressing known as the "hanging cast" is used. A plaster cast is applied to the forearm and the arm, holding the elbow flexed to a right angle. The cast is slung at the wrist, the weight of the cast producing traction upon the lower fragment. Movement of the arm at the shoulder is encouraged. Union occurs without the usual immobilization of the fragments.

Above the Elbow. These fractures are very common in childhood and adolescence. There are many varieties, the most common being the supracondylar type. They are usually attended with considerable swelling, and, because the lower fragment is displaced posteriorly in most cases, the forearm appears to be shortened. The fragments are best maintained in position by holding the arm acutely flexed, and the usual dressings are applied with the arm in this position. In the "Jones position," which is frequently used, a sling from the wrist draws the hand close to the neck.

A very important nursing measure in caring for a patient with an elbow fracture treated by acute flexion of the arm is to observe the hand for swelling and blueness of the nails. These signs may indicate a disturbance of blood supply and should be reported immediately.

Forearm. Both Bones of Forearm. These fractures are most common in the middle third. Since it is almost impossible to tell which dressings are indicated until the fracture reduction has been completed, the dressings which should be provided are:

1. Two plain board splints, long enough to reach from elbow to finger-tips and padded higher in the middle than at the sides (Fig. 224).
2. Internal right-angled and anterior-angled splints (Fig. 222 f and g).
3. Plaster bandages 2 to 4 inches wide and lint.
4. Muslin or gauze bandages and adhesive.

Above the Wrist. These fractures result very often from falls on the outstretched hand. The Colles (suprastyloid) type is the most common. This is a fracture of the radius from ½ to 1 inch above the wrist, with a posterior displacement of the lower fragment. The hand is deviated to the thumb side. The position is often spoken of as the "silver-fork deformity." These fractures are dressed in many ways, most often by the use of Bond splints (Fig. 222 h) or of molded plaster splints. Bandage and a sling are always necessary.

Pelvis. Pelvic fractures are commonly found following severe trauma. They are serious injuries because frequently they are associated with injuries to the intrapelvic structures. The bladder, the urethra, or the intestine may be ruptured and prove to be of more serious import than the fracture itself.

Treatment and Nursing Care

The urine and the stools should be examined daily for several days for evidences of blood and the patient must be watched carefully for signs of intra-abdominal trouble. The fracture is usually treated by rest in bed, with weight traction applied to one or both legs to immobilize the hips. The Bradford frame contributes largely to the comfort and the ease of handling these patients, because they need not be removed to use the bedpan, etc. (Fig. 251). Another type of fracture bed is made so that a bedpan may be used without disturbing the position of the patient.

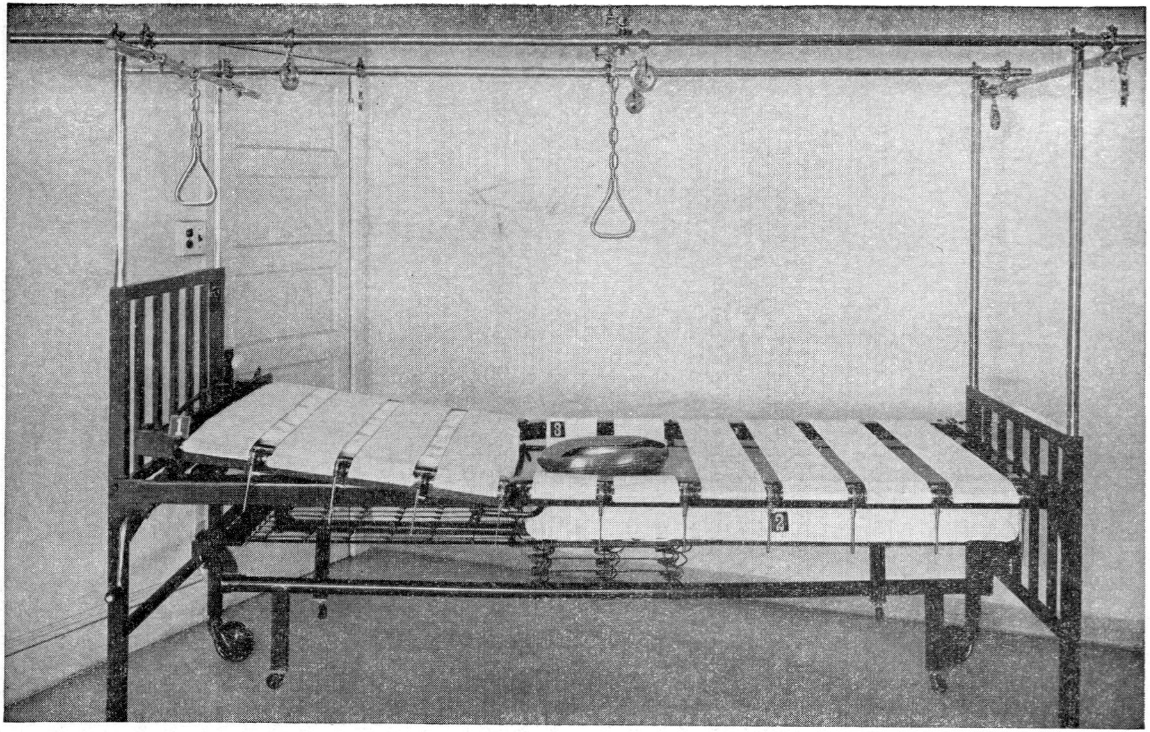

Fig. 239. Modern type of fracture bed. Note (1) the adjustable back rest, (2) the adjustable canvas straps across the bed, on which the patient's weight may be maintained while the bed is lowered, (3) the canvas straps which may be lowered in sections for use of the bedpan without disturbing the patient and (above) the adjustable pulleys and hand rings.

This is made possible by mechanical adjustments of the bed (Fig. 239). The nurse must frequently inspect all traction apparatus and watch carefully for signs of pressure. Good care of the skin and gentle handling of the patient do much to prevent complications and to make his difficulties more easily borne.

Femur. NECK. These fractures occur most frequently in old people, especially in women, and are due often to very insignificant injuries. The patient is unable to move the leg, which lies characteristically with the foot turned outward flat on the bed, knee fully extended. If the limb is compared with its fellow by inspection or by actual measurement, there is found to be considerable shortening. A measuring tape should be at hand in order to estimate and record this finding accurately.

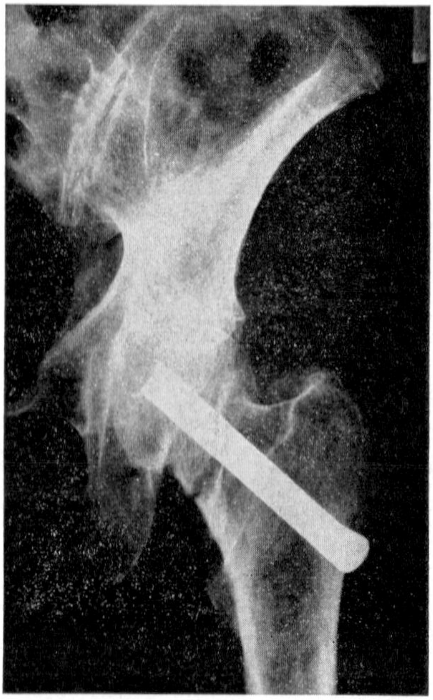

FIG. 240. Smith-Petersen nail inserted for fracture of the neck of the femur.

Treatment and Nursing Care

Surgeons usually treat fractures of the neck of the femur by the use of pins or nails (Fig. 240). After reduction of the fracture, the nails are introduced through the tronchanter along the neck of the femur into the head. The pins are inserted under local or spinal anesthesia through a very small wound made on the outer side of the thigh. Patients so treated may be up and in a chair within a very few days. As soon as possible, they may be taught to use crutches, bearing weight on the uninjured leg only.

These patients, because of their age, are particularly prone to develop complications which may become more important with regard to treatment than the fracture itself. The shock of the injury may be fatal. Shock also is known to cause bladder incontinence; control is gradually regained later. Other complications are disorientation in the elderly patient, fecal impaction, thrombophlebitis and pulmonary emboli. Because of the necessity for these patients to remain in one position for long periods of time, bedsores frequently develop. The nurse may do much to avert their occurrence by attention to the skin on the back, especially under the hips and the shoulders, and by relieving constant pressure by airfoam pillows, etc. Many hospitals use rubber mattresses routinely for these patients. A trapeze suspended from the Balkan

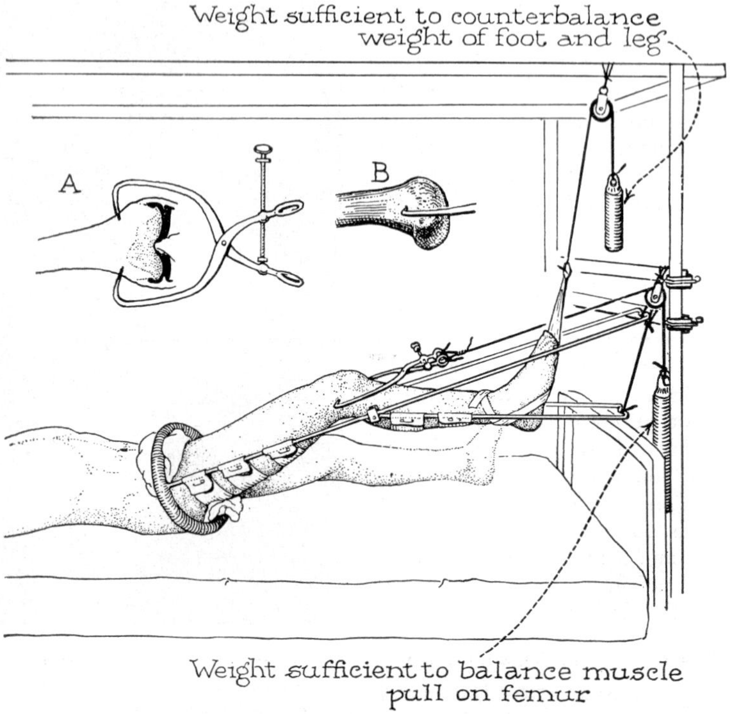

FIG. 241. Diagram of the method of use of ice-tong calipers with the Thomas splint and the Pearson attachment in fracture of the femur. (A) Point of application (anteroposterior). (B) Point of application (lateral view). (Magnuson, P. B., and Stack, J. K.: Fractures, ed. 5, Philadelphia, Lippincott)

frame or fracture bed permits the patient to lift himself; this is a great aid in the nursing care. During the first few weeks it may be impossible to turn the patient, but after the fracture has begun to unite it is often possible to turn him at least partially on the side, supported by pillows under the shoulder and the hip.

Renal calculi and other kidney problems may arise. Pulmonary complications such as hypostatic congestion of the lungs and bronchopneumonia can occur and may be fatal. Deep-breathing exercises, change of position at least every 2 hours and protection of the chest with a shoulder blanket are measures which may help to prevent the development of these complications (see p. 140). The nurse should be familiar with the precautions which are to be observed in treating patients with traction or casts (see pp. 542, 545, and 550).

SHAFT. These fractures occur most commonly in youth and middle age. There is marked swelling of the

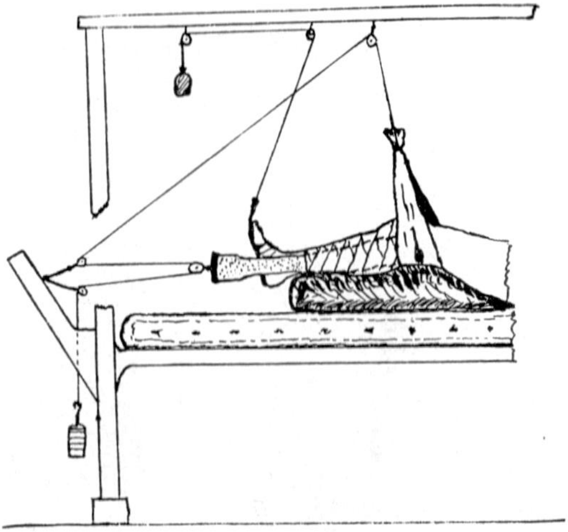

FIG. 242. The Russell method of treating a fracture of the shaft of the femur. A small spring scale sometimes is inserted between the pulley and the traction block so that the amount of traction may be estimated accurately.

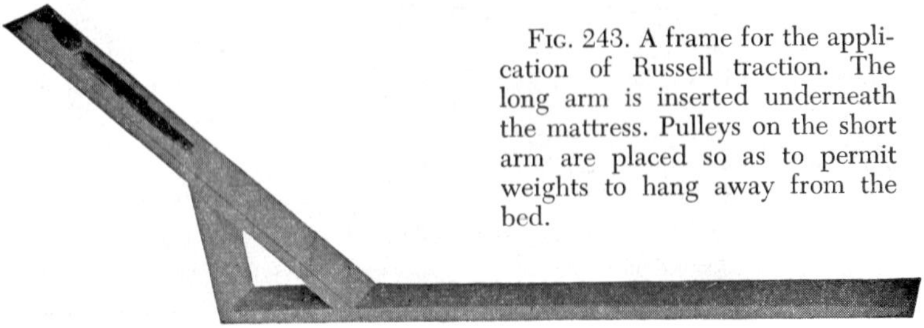

FIG. 243. A frame for the application of Russell traction. The long arm is inserted underneath the mattress. Pulleys on the short arm are placed so as to permit weights to hang away from the bed.

thigh, with shortening. The use of intramedullary pins is becoming increasingly popular. Frequently, reduction is accomplished by traction, using a Thomas splint and Buck's extension, or by the use of a Thomas splint (Fig. 223 j) and a Pearson (Fig. 223 i) attachment, applying tractions to the lower fragment by means of a Kirschner wire, a Steinmann pin, or tongs (Fig. 241). Some surgeons apply upward as well as horizontal traction on the lower fragment by the Russell method (see Figs. 242 and 243). A spica cast may also be used.

In the treatment of most cases of fractured femur, a fracture bed or Balkan frame is necessary to which the pulleys for traction may be attached. The fracture must be immobilized for 7 to 8 weeks, at the end of which time the patient may be allowed to get up and to walk with the aid of crutches. Full weight bearing must not be allowed for at least 6 months.

Fractures which occur in children under 10 years of age are frequently treated by the Bryant method of vertical suspension. Adhesive traction is applied to both legs equally,

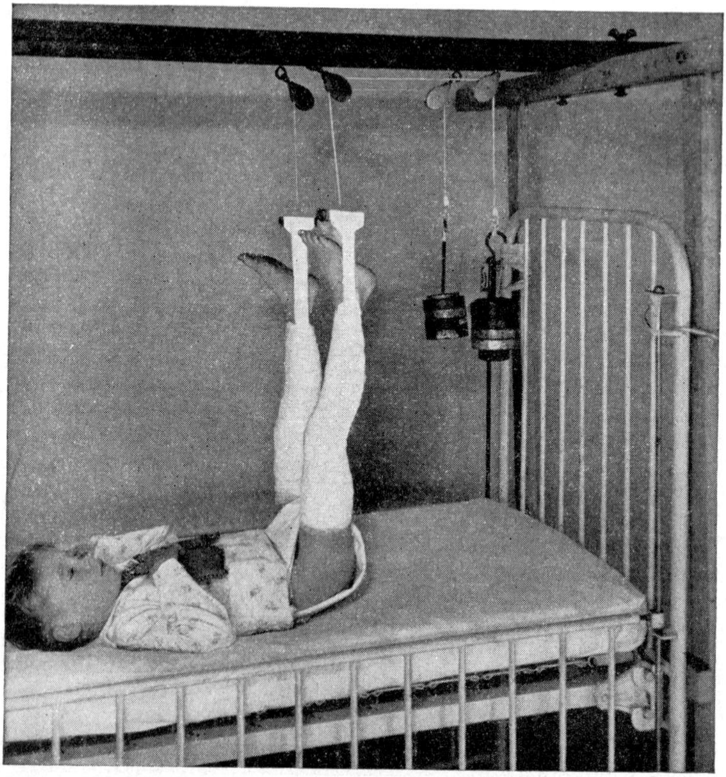

FIG. 244. The Bryant method of vertical traction for fractures of the femur in children. Note that both legs are suspended by skin traction with weights sufficient to lift the pelvis from the bed. The fractured limb requires the heavier weight.

sufficient weights being employed just to lift the buttocks off the bed. This dressing is maintained for 6 weeks (Fig. 244).

MEDULLARY PIN. The medullary pin is used in some clinics in approximating fractures of the shaft of the femur. The patient usually has skeletal traction for a week preoperatively, which allows time for systemic studies and for the reduction of any swelling. The medullary nail may be introduced by the open or the closed method. The chief advantage of such nailing is that the patient can be up and out of bed to begin weight bearing by 3 weeks. Prior to this time, he has opportunity to move his leg, thereby preventing stiffening and muscular atrophy. Disadvantages are (1) there is believed to be some destruction of bone marrow with resultant hemoglobin and red blood cell reduction, (2) there is a possibility of producing bone infection and (3) there is a chance for the formation of a fat embolism in the closed method. After

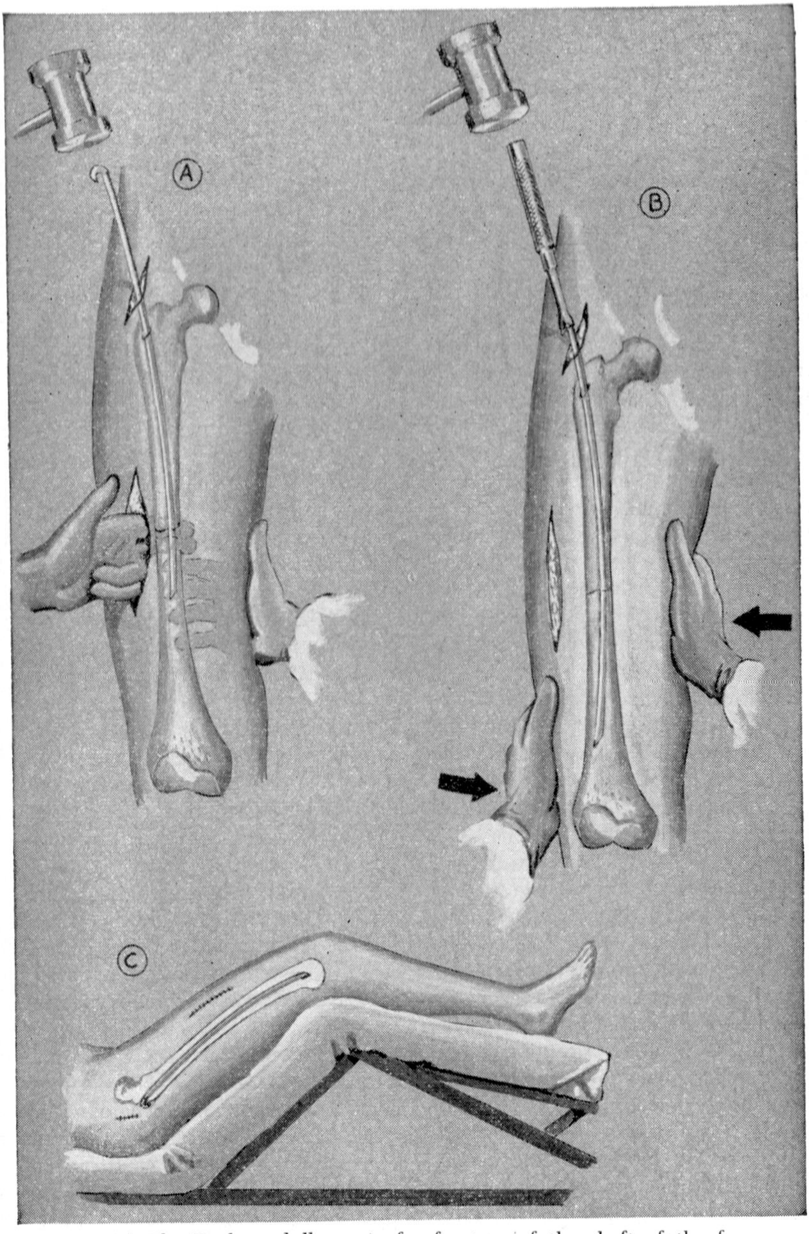

FIG. 245. The Rush medullary pin for fracture of the shaft of the femur. (Berivon Co.)

about a year, the stainless steel nail is removed through a small incision.

Internal Derangement of the Knee. Injury to most joints consists of a tear of its supporting ligaments. In the knee joint, however, there may be also a displacement or tear of the semilunar cartilages. These are two crescent-shaped cartilages attached to the edge of the shallow articulating surface of the head of the tibia. They normally move slightly backward and forward to accommodate for the change in the shape of the condyles of the femur when the leg is in flexion or extension. In sports and falls, the body is often twisted with the foot fixed. Since no torsion movement is normally permitted in the knee joint, an injury results which very often is either a tear of the cartilage from its attachment to the head of the tibia, or an actual tear or fracture of the cartilage itself. These injuries leave a loose cartilage in the knee joint which may slip between the femur and the tibia and so prevent full extension of the leg. If this happens when the patient is walking or running, he often describes his disability as his "leg giving way" under him, and there are times when the cartilage gets caught between the articulating surfaces so that the knee "locks." The patient may hear or feel a click in his knee when he walks, especially when he extends his leg bearing his weight, as in going upstairs. When the cartilage is attached front and back, but torn loose laterally (bucket-handle tear) it may slide between the bones to lie between the condyles and prevent full flexion or extension.

These various types of injury arising from a common cause are spoken of as an internal derangement of the knee joint, and they produce a disturbing disability because the patient never knows when the knee will give him trouble. The treatment of this disability is removal of the injured cartilage, which can be done with relative ease through an incision into the knee joint. The joint function is thereby returned to normal, and no apparent disability results from the loss of the cartilage.

Preparation for operation consists of a shave of the entire leg. Some surgeons desire a "sterile prep" in addition.

Postoperative Nursing Care

After suture of the wound, a pressure dressing is applied, and at times a posterior splint. The leg should be elevated on pillows with a slight bend at the knee. The most common complication is an effusion into the knee joint which produces marked pain. The physician should be called. Relief can be obtained by cutting the pressure dressing and reapplying it more loosely. Frequently, the joint may be aspirated under local anesthesia and pressure relieved by withdrawing the fluid in the joint. To prevent atrophy of the thigh muscles, often these patients are instructed to "set" their muscles while in bed. After one or two days the patient may be up with crutches bearing weight by touching only his toes on the operated side. In a short time, 1 to 2 weeks, full weight-bearing is possible, but the knee usually is supported for another few weeks by an elastic bandage. Full and normal function may be looked for in from 6 to 8 weeks from the time of operation.

Tibia and Fibula. Fractures of the

shafts of these bones are often associated. There usually is considerable swelling which disappears readily if reduction and immobilization are accomplished early. Reduction is best done under the fluoroscope by traction and manipulation, and the leg dressed in a plaster cast extending from toe to thigh, or better by the use of molded lateral plaster splints, which include the foot and the thigh. Here again, an intramedullary pin may be used.

Pott's fracture, the commonest below the knee, is a fracture of the lower two or three inches of the fibula due to "twisting the ankle." There is also a fracture of the internal malleolus and of the posterior portion of the articular surface of the tibia, frequently associated with it. Swelling and discoloration about the ankle are marked.

Fluoroscopic reduction is recommended. The dressing used is a plaster cast, or lateral plaster splints. Elevation of the leg for several days reduces the swelling very rapidly.

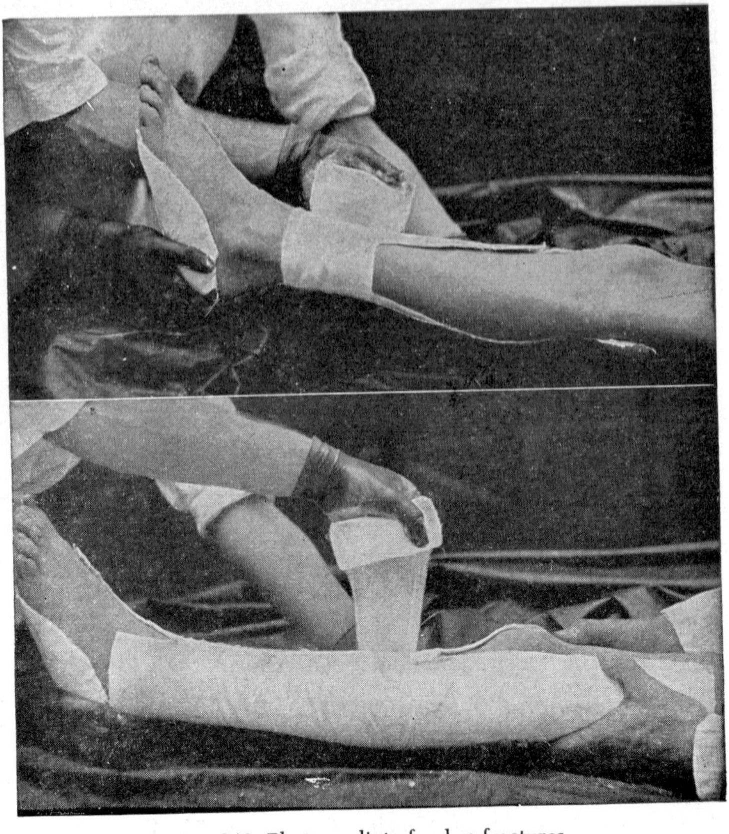

FIG. 246. Plaster splints for leg fractures.

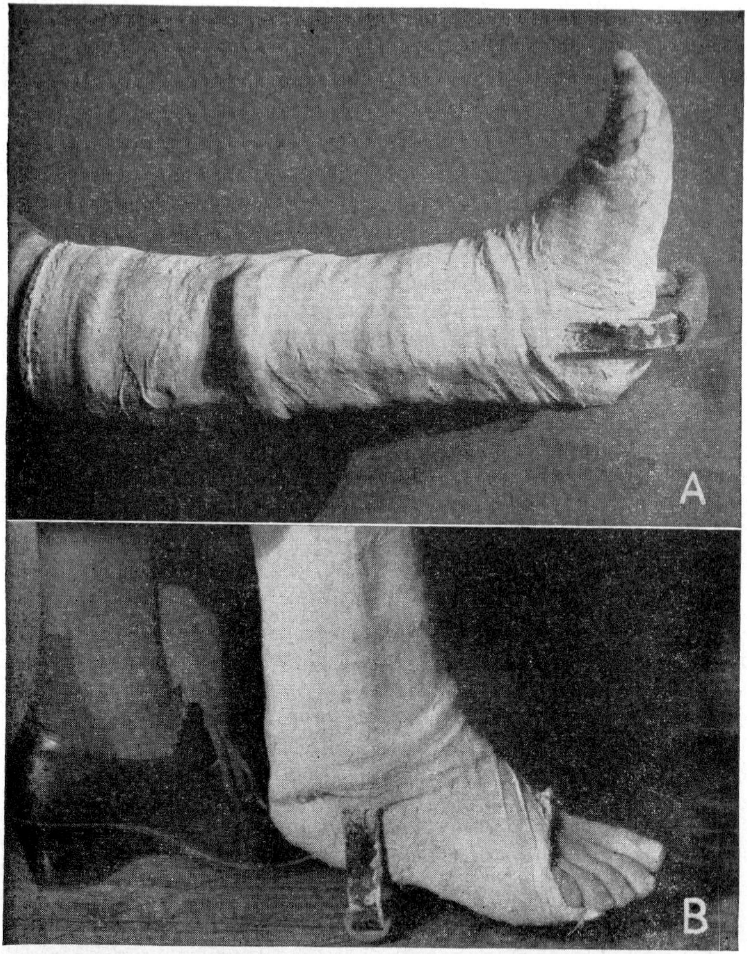

FIG. 247. Fracture of the lower tibia and fibula treated with a cast in which a walking iron is incorporated.

Function may be renewed in four months.

Crutches. All fractures of the lower extremity require the use of crutches during convalescence. Adjustable crutches are the most practical. They should be about 1 inch longer than the distance from the axilla to the heel and should be fitted with rubber suction tips. Soft padding of cotton under the armpit, held in place with gauze, serves to make their use more comfortable. (See also Crutches, p. 569.)

Walking Iron. In many clinics these fractures are treated by the application of a cast in which is incorporated a walking iron. This treatment cannot be employed until after the swelling has disappeared. By the use of the walking iron the patient may be able to walk fairly easily without any support or with the aid of a cane (Fig. 247).

AMPUTATION

Amputation of extremities is frequently necessary in the treatment of gangrene, tumors, deformities, septic wounds, compound fractures and severe crushing injuries, gas gangrene, etc. In severe trauma, an amputation is done to save a patient's life. The nurse will be aware that this is a major adjustment for the patient to make. One day he is a perfectly normal individual and the next day he must accept his loss. For the individual who has a longstanding disease which causes him pain and restricts his ability to get around, the acceptance of an amputation is not as difficult.

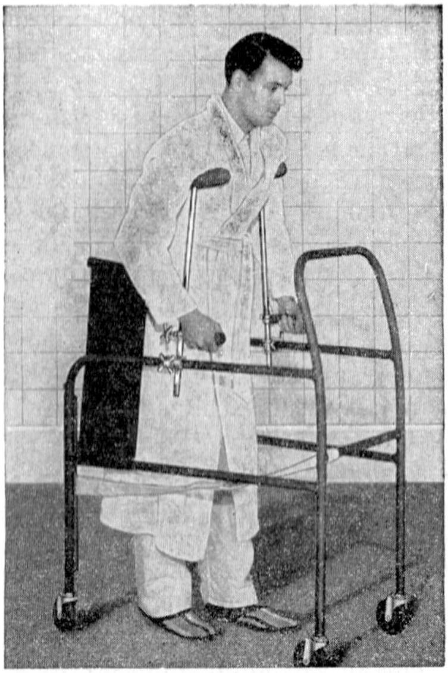

FIG. 248. The Comper Invalid Walker is of clinical and economic value on ambulatory service for orthopedic, fracture, paralytic and postoperative patients. (The Surgical Supervisor, American Sterilizer Co., Erie, Pa.)

Nursing Care

Preoperative Care. Often before surgery, the physician will perform tests to determine the patency of circulation. These will include surface temperature, color changes when the limb is elevated or dependent, and oscillometric readings. His state of nutrition must be recognized and improved if necessary. Psychological preparation cannot be neglected. The physician and the nurse can help to build a healthy optimism in this patient by making him realize that he can overcome his handicap and be independent. Preparation for the operation when possible should consist in shaving of the part and thorough cleansing with soap and water. Intravenous fluids are administered to combat dehydration; blood is made available. Before the operation the limb should be elevated continuously for at least 5 minutes to allow the venous blood to drain as completely as possible from the part. This procedure is aided in many clinics by the application of a pneumatic tourniquet or an Esmarch bandage, an elastic bandage of 2-inch rubber applied in the direction of the trunk, to compress the extremity. A tourniquet of heavy rubber is then applied and drawn tight enough to compress the blood vessels.

Refrigeration of the part before operation is being used with much success. (See p. 79.)

Postoperative Care. Amputations are usually performed by making soft-tissue flaps, which are used to cover the bone stump. The site of the amputation is determined by two factors: circulation in the part and the requirements of an artificial limb (prosthesis). In many amputations, especially of the leg, when performed for gangrene of the foot due to vascular impairment, a high amputation (midthigh) must be done because the circulation of the leg below is insufficient to bring about healing of an amputation site at a lower level.

Experience with artificial limbs has shown that stumps of some certain length function best in these appliances. If the stump is too long, it may be awkward and hard to fit; if it is too short, the adjacent joint cannot function well. When they are made below the knee and the elbow joints, it is well to splint the part for a time to prevent contractures. These patients should be watched carefully for any signs or symptoms of hemorrhage. As a precaution, a tourniquet should be in plain sight at the foot of the bed, and, if bleeding occurs, should be applied to the stump and pulled sufficiently tight to stop the bleeding. It should be left in place until the surgeon can be notified. The stump should be elevated for the first day on a pillow protected with a rubber or plastic pillow case. Such a pillow should support the entire stump from the hip down, in order that knee flexion be prevented. This pillow is removed as soon as possible, by physician's order, to avoid hip contracture. In some hospitals it is required that the stump remain uncovered and in full sight for the first 24 to 48 hours, the period in which hemorrhage is most likely to occur. Oozing usually appears at the bottom of the dressing, and linen may be spared by placing the stump upon a sterile cellucotton pad. The dressings should be reinforced rather than changed. A footboard should be used to keep the remaining foot in dorsiflexion.

During the first 24 hours, especially in older patients, a shocklike state is frequently present, and the patient does not fully realize that he has had an amputation. Often the realization may come as a shock to him, even though he knew before his operation that an amputation was to be performed. Frequently, these cases are complicated by the production of pulmonary emboli and so must be watched carefully for such findings as cough, chest pain, hemoptysis, severe sudden collapse, cyanosis, or even sudden death. On occasion, especially when the amputation has been done for infection, a guillotine type may be performed without any attempt to suture the skin. In such cases, to prevent the retraction of the skin, traction may be applied and eventual healing brought about. The principles given under Nursing Care of the Patient in Traction (p. 550) apply here.

After the first 24 to 48 hours, depending upon physician's orders, the patient should be encouraged to turn from side to side and to be on the abdomen to prevent flexion contracture of the hip. A pillow can be placed under the abdomen and the stump; the forefoot can be placed over the edge of the mattress. He must learn to recognize the value of moving the stump so that contractures are avoided. Sometimes patients use an overhead trapeze when changing their position in bed; this will strengthen the biceps. Unfortunately, this set of muscles is not as necessary in crutch walking as are the triceps. These can be strengthened by pressing with the palms against the bed when moving the body. Exercises under the supervision of the physical therapist, such as hyperextension of the stump, will also aid in strengthening muscles as well as increasing circulation, reducing edema and preventing atrophy. In getting the patient out of bed, regard must be given to maintaining good posture.

After the wound has healed, the nurse should learn from the surgeon how he wishes the stump to be bandaged. Thereafter, the nurse can teach the patient or some member of his family the correct method of bandaging. Usually, an Ace elastic bandage is used. It should be laundered frequently in tepid water and placed on a flat surface to dry so that its elasticity is retained as long as possible.

When amputations of the leg have been performed on old, debilitated patients, especially diabetics and arteriosclerotics, particular care should be taken to protect the stump against external infection. Such patients frequently become incontinent of urine and feces, and not infrequently the dressing and wound of the stump may become soiled. Rubber tissue or plastic material secured by a wide adhesive strip about the leg above the dressing has proved to be a good prophylactic measure.

Often during the convalescence while the muscle stumps are adjusting themselves, twitchings and spasms occur. Heat, massage, change of position to procure relaxation, a light sandbag on a thigh stump to counteract the psoas action—all will help. During this stage, and often for an indefinite period to follow, the patient may complain as though the pain were in the amputated limb —the "phantom limb" complication so often very difficult to cure. An Ace compression bandage is a comfort and at the same time it helps by compression to prepare the stump of a leg or a thigh for the prosthesis to follow.

CRUTCHES

In the treatment of most fractures of the lower extremity, of various forms of arthritis and after operations on the leg, especially after amputation, crutches provide a convenient method for getting from one place to another. Many patients look forward to the day when they might walk again; others are not so optimistic. At any rate, crutch walking is not a skill which is inherited. A patient must be taught; and this learning process must begin early. It includes psychological preparation which can be developed long before the physical need is present. Each patient must be considered from his individual needs and the method of approach directed to this end. The age of the patient, his interests and future intentions, as well as his prognosis, are essential factors.

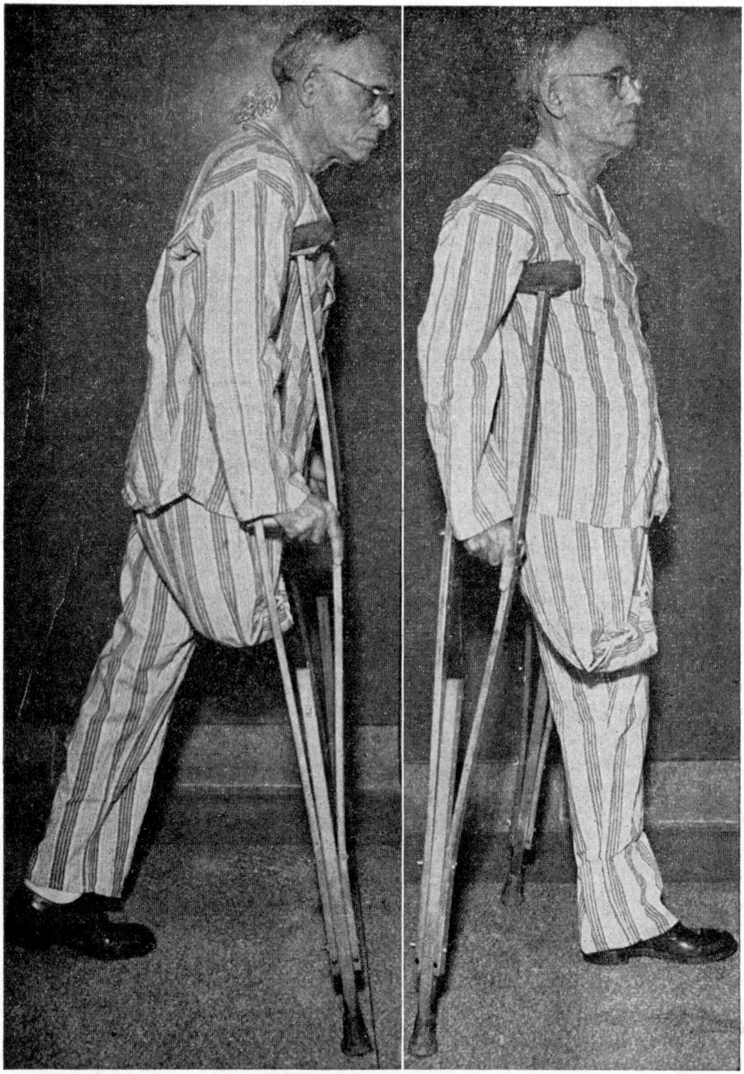

FIG. 249. Crutch-walking. (*Left*) Note that the patient's weight is borne not in the axilla but on the palm of the hand, with the arm extended. The weight of the patient's body should be inclined forward to be supported by the crutches. (*Right*) The well leg should swing through the crutches, and the foot should be placed in a position in front of the crutches. (Note adjustable type of crutches.)

Early exercises such as pressing the palms of the hands against the bed ("push-ups" to strengthen triceps muscle and shoulder depressors), "dangling" and getting up to sit in a chair, help in conditioning the patient for the use of crutches. At all times, good body posture should be practiced. Incorrect shifting of body weight can cause undue strain on muscles and organs. Invariably, such a patient has difficulty and tires easily.

Adjustable crutches are more practical than the nonadjustable type. The measurements which are most important are the length of the crutch and the position of the hand bar. The most serviceable measurement for the length of the crutch is about one inch longer than the distance from the armpit to the sole of the foot. It is best made with the patient standing if possible and with his shoe on. The hand bar should allow for almost complete extension of the arm when the patient places his weight on his palms. Crutches should have suction tips to prevent slipping. Padding of the axillary rest is optional if the crutches fit correctly, for there should be no pressure under the arm. Padding may be desirable in protecting the clothing from the wooden bar. Sponge or air-foam rubber affords good protection if covered with a washable material.

It is wise to tell and demonstrate to the patient how he should manipulate his crutches before he attempts it. Here again, maintaining good posture is emphasized. Crutches should be placed wide enough apart to allow a broad base of support. The most convenient placement varies with individuals, but they should not be so close to the body as to interfere with walking, nor so far away as to permit slipping. Weight should be borne by the palms of the hands and not the axilla. Crutch paralysis may develop if the weight is borne in the axilla and not on the hands and extended arms, since the pressure of the crutch is exerted on the superficial radial nerve.

Ability to shift body weight is the next step and can be done only after determining the patient's condition and the doctor's orders. In some conditions, the patient is not permitted to bear weight on a leg. Of the several technics for crutch walking, that which is easiest and meets the needs of the amputee or the patient with a fractured leg is the *swinging method* or *tripod walking*. The patient bears weight on his good leg, places the crutches at an equal distance ahead of him and then swings to a position just ahead of the crutches. Weight is shifted to the palms of the hands and then back to the good leg. The elevation produced by a medium-heeled shoe on the good leg may permit the affected leg to swing through without touching the floor and without unnecessary flexion.

The teaching of crutch walking is usually delegated to the physical therapist. In many institutions, this responsibility rests with the physician. A nurse can be of help if she recognizes the need for preparing the patient as described above and assists in helping the patient to practice correctly what he has been taught. The nurse should not permit patients to walk for too long, especially those who have been bedridden for a long time. Such signs as cyanosis, sweating, or shortness of breath should be indications that the lesson on crutches should be stopped and the patient permitted to rest or go back to bed.

PROSTHESES

The fitting of artificial appliances to replace lost limbs has advanced very rapidly in the last decade or two so that now the most astonishing aids to function are available for almost any need. Various materials (aluminum, plywood, papier-mâché, willow wood, plastics, etc.) are used in their manufacture.

Design of the apparatus should be considered from the point of view of age, weight, height and occupation of the patient. For a leg, it is now unusual to see a shoulder harness. Instead, the pelvic band is being used. The suction socket is a more recent method whereby suction is created during the application of the socket to the stump.

A below-knee amputation stump is much more difficult to fit than the above-knee stump. The reason is that the skin over the new bony prominences is not prepared for weight-bearing. Therefore, a good limb fitter will attempt to devise a prosthesis which will spread the weight-bearing pressure over a wide area rather than a small spot.

Every stump should be fitted with a stump cotton sock. This must be kept clean. It acts as a buffer between the socket and the stump and also acts as a ventilating mechanism to absorb perspiration.

Every amputee should have a prosthesis for social reasons so that he may appear like a normal person. If the cost, interference with routine activities, etc., outweigh the social advantages, then this may not be necessary.

A reliable firm should be employed early in these cases to help in a speedy rehabilitation and readjustment directed toward a psychological and economic return to normal, thus preventing that inferiority complex so hard to combat. The salesmen for these appliances are often wearers of artificial limbs, and when the patient is introduced to them a mutual understanding is easily accomplished, with, as a rule, excellent results.

Throughout the entire period of physical and mental trial, which is so hard on the morale, an interested, understanding and sympathetic nurse can produce astonishing results. She can teach the patient early to be self-reliant and helpful. Among other things, she can induce him to move about in bed, to get into a chair and to learn to balance himself. However, she must not be oversolicitous, overhelpful and overanxious, as this will make the situation more difficult and may result in a useful limb but a patient full of self-pity and no self-reliance.

When prostheses are first being used, they should be tried only for short periods, for not only is the unaccustomed position and balance in lower limb cases most difficult and tiring, but the straps, pressure spots, and lost co-ordination rendered worse by twitchings and spasms make the performance a real workout.

Nursing Care of Orthopedic Surgical Patients

Preoperative Care. In general, the principles of preoperative care are the same as in the care of any surgical patient. Only the differences will be stressed.

Psychological. Many orthopedic patients experience a curious mixture of fear and anticipation before surgery. Will I be able to walk again? Or is this too much to hope for? If an individual has been handicapped and dependent for most of his life, he faces reconstructive surgery with added concern. Some patients have faced repeated operations; patience and hope are almost gone. These are the people who need much help from an understanding nurse.

Following surgery, if the patient is to be placed in a different type of bed with special apparatus such as traction or a plaster cast, he should have some preparation for this preoperatively.

Physical. Whatever the method used in preparing the skin of the orthopedic patient for surgery, the principles remain the same. The procedure usually is more painstaking because of the difficulty in controlling infection in the bone, should that occur. A meticulous nontraumatizing cleansing of the skin with soap and water, followed by careful shaving, is done first. Then, soap-and-water washing is repeated, and a fat solvent can be used, followed by a mild antiseptic.

Disability can result, should infection occur within a bone or a joint. In no instance should one rely on the antibiotics to control infection and thereby justify slipshod preoperative preparation.

It is well to remember that, when a cleansing enema is ordered, it should be given before the skin preparation is begun. Some orthopedic surgeons do not require a preoperative enema for surgery on the extremities.

Adequate hydration is always an essential objective in orthopedic patients, particularly those immobilized for a long period of time. Kidney complications and breakdown of pressure areas will result if this is neglected.

Postoperative Care. Patients who have bone and joint surgery experience real *pain*. Many times, the person who has had surgery to correct a foot condition is much more uncomfortable than one who has had extensive abdominal surgery. Narcotics and other pain-relieving measures should be administered liberally. However, in the long-term patient it is well to remember that habit-forming possibilities can be a considerable problem. It should be pointed out that even though a patient has had an orthopedic operation, the pain may not necessarily be the result of the wound and of the operative trauma. Swelling frequently follows, and when it occurs under tight bandages or casts, there may be interference with the blood supply, which also produces excruciating pain. This type of pain can be suspected when there is blueness and swelling beyond the limits of the cast and they can be relieved by cutting the cast or the bandages. Another type of pain occurs in orthopedic patients when there is prolonged pressure over bony prominences such as areas of the heel, the head of the tibia on the lateral side of the leg just below the knee and the tuberosity of the tibia. Even though they have been well padded before the cast has been applied, these areas eventually may become painful. The pain is characteristically of a burning type. It is wise not to treat this with narcotics but to call it to the attention of the surgeon, who may wish to cut away areas of the cast to relieve the pressure. In major orthopedic surgery, *shock* also is a common problem, and the nurse must be on the alert for its symptoms.

Bone does not mend so readily as soft tissues. Therefore, even though the skin incision is well healed, bony structures underneath still need time to repair. This is especially important to remember in surgery of the lower extremities, for in addition to normal movement, bone must be able to bear weight in ambulation.

Other complications which may occur are similar to those of general surgical patients. They are oozing and bleeding, abdominal distention, wound infection and pulmonary and circulatory problems.

Rehabilitation of Orthopedic Patients. In allowing the patient to help himself, he must be taught the best way. The physical therapist working with the physician and the nurse can guide the patient in the proper use of his muscles and joints. Emphasis is placed on activities of daily living so that he will be able to perform those functions which will allow him independence. He will need patience and constant encouragement. He may want to perform a certain activity but fear that self-inflicted injury may result. The extent to which a patient may progress safely must be understood clearly by him as well as all who care for him.

When he goes home, the patient should have explicit instructions which he understands, indicating those activities which he may and may not perform. It is not enough to bid him "good-bye, and take it easy." The patient must know any untoward signs and symptoms which should be reported to his physician. He must be aware of the importance of follow-up visits. If he has any difficulties, he ought to know where and how to get help. The nurse has a major part of the responsibility for instructing her patient before he leaves the hospital.

CLINICAL SITUATION: FRACTURE OF THE FEMUR

Mr. Reilly was admitted to Tompkins East I with a diagnosis of an intertrochanteric fracture of the left femur. Upon admission he was placed in Russell's traction. Two weeks later he was taken to the operating room, where the fracture was reduced, he was encased in a hip spica cast and returned to the floor.

1. Points to be observed in the daily care of Mr. Reilly while he is in traction are as follows:

_____a. Be sure that adhesive is secured down over the lateral malleoli.

_____b. Remove weights while changing the sheets on the bed.

_____c. Be sure that the spreader is in contact with the foot of the bed.

_____d. Turn Mr. Reilly frequently to avoid pneumonia.
_____e. See to it that the weights are hanging freely.

2. If Mr. Reilly had a comminuted fracture of the femur, it would be one in which the bone:
_____a. was splintered.
_____b. penetrated the skin.
_____c. was fractured on one side and bent on the other.
_____d. was broken across entirely.

3. When Mr. Reilly returned to the ward in his cast, signs which might be indicative of impaired circulation were:
_____a. Swelling.
_____b. Cyanosis of the toes.
_____c. Decreased temperature.
_____d. Redness of the skin and a feeling of warmth.
_____e. Pain.

4. When turning Mr. Reilly in his hip spica cast:
_____a. his arms should be at his sides.
_____b. he should be moved to the side of the bed closest to his unaffected leg.
_____c. traction should be maintained on the leg that is affected.
_____d. his affected leg should be on top.
_____e. his unaffected leg should be on top.

5. When drying Mr. Reilly's cast, the points to be observed in using an electric drier are:
_____a. Keep the drier 18 inches from the patient.
_____b. Keep the drier 36 inches from the patient.
_____c. Direct the drier to one area until it is dry and then move to another area.
_____d. Keep covered with a blanket the part of the cast which is not being dried.
_____e. Keep covered the exposed parts of the patient not encased in plaster.

CHAPTER TWENTY-SIX

Diseases of Bones, Joints and Bursae

DEFORMITIES
INFANTILE PARALYSIS
OSTEOMYELITIS
TUBERCULOSIS
OSTEITIS FIBROSA CYSTICA
BONE TUMORS
DISEASES OF JOINTS
DISEASES OF BURSAE

The word orthopedia is derived from two Greek words meaning "straight" and "child." The original scope of this branch of surgery was very narrow, being restricted, as the name implies, to the care of deformed children. With the advent of asepsis, the x-ray and skillful manipulation, orthopedics has become a highly specialized but much broader branch of surgery. Today orthopedic surgery has to do with the cause, the prevention and the correction of deformities of all the apparatus of locomotion, and in some localities it embraces bone and joint diseases, as well as fractures. Early recognition of signs of deformity is a significant factor in the successful treatment of these patients. Many have conditions that require prolonged hospital and convalescent home care. Here the emphasis must be placed on the close co-operation of the physician, the physical therapist, the medical social worker and the nurse with the family. These people also must continue their schooling, childhood training and guided recreation during rehabilitation. Further, in adults occupational therapy is of great help to their morale. They must be taught the use of braces and crutches, and how to work and to play. A good observant and understanding nurse can do much for them physically and mentally.

DEFORMITIES

Deformities may be divided into two great classes: (1) congenital—those that occur before or during birth; or (2) acquired—those that occur after birth, due to injury, paralysis or disease.

Congenital Dislocation of Hip

Congenital dislocation of the hip probably is one of the most frequent of these deformities. It is due to a malformation of the head of the femur and of the socket in which it rests (the acetabulum). Girls are affected much more frequently. Both

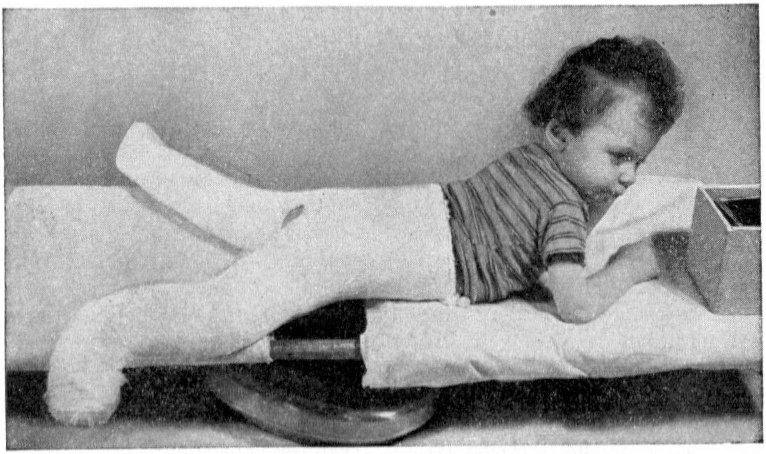

Fig. 250. Frog position for congenital hip dislocation. Note child on Bradford frame.

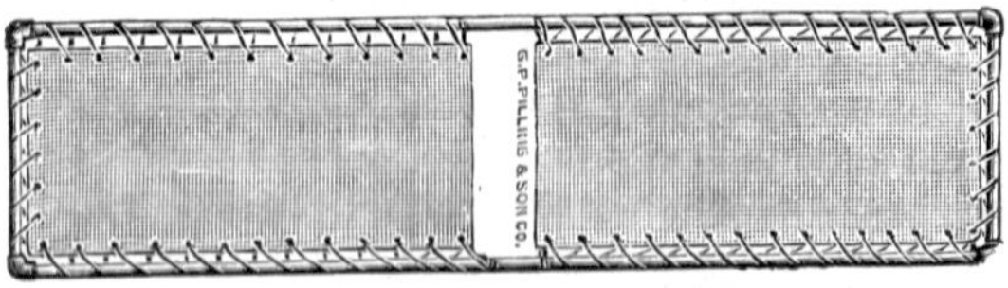

Fig. 251. Bradford frame.

hips may be dislocated, but more often the deformity is limited to one side.

A partial or a complete displacement of the head of the femur, an extra fold of skin near the gluteal region on one side, unequal leg length and limited movement of one leg are very early signs that suggest a congenital hip dislocation. However, in the usual case, no abnormality is noted until the child begins to walk. Then it is observed that one leg appears shorter than the other and the child walks with a decided limp. If the dislocation is bilateral, a decided waddle is a characteristic symptom. Other deformities (for example, curvature of the spine) develop as the child grows older, so that, unless the dislocation is reduced, the child must face a future of semi-invalidism. Every child who walks with a limp at the hip joint should be examined by x-rays, which will show whether or not the hip is dislocated.

Treatment. The treatment of this condition is easier and more successful if it is begun early (between 2 and 5 years of age). As the child grows older, reduction becomes more and more difficult; often, even with operation, only a partial cure can be effected.

Two methods of treatment have

been employed. In one, the "bloodless" method, by manipulation under anesthesia, an effort is made to place the head of the femur in the acetabulum, holding it there by the application of plaster casts or splints. The leg is dressed in the extreme abducted position, frequently spoken of as the "frog position." This position is maintained for from 4 to 6 months. Smaller children are kept on an elevated frame (Bradford frame) made of small gas piping, between which canvas is stretched. The patient is so placed that the bedpan may be used without moving him. Elevation of the head of the frame will prevent seepage of urine. The plaster cast should be kept dry and clean. The principles outlined in the preceding chapter on cast care will apply here. In addition, the shellacking of the cast (with the permission of the physician) or the use of tubular stockinet to cover the cast will help the nurse and, later, the mother to keep the cast clean. As with all patients in plaster casts, constant vigilance is necessary to avoid pressure sores at the edge of the cast, and the skin must be kept clean and dry at these points. This is especially important in the perineal region, where urine and feces are apt to cause maceration of the skin. If the area of perineal exposure is not conducive to maintaining cleanliness, the nurse should notify the physician. The cast may be supported by pillows or rolled blankets to prevent chafing of the skin from pressure of the cast edges round the extremities.

Older children may be encouraged to walk with support, as use of the legs tends to deepen the socket for the head of the femur. If, at the end of from 4 to 6 months, it is found that the head of the femur will not stay in place, open operation usually is necessary, even in young children. At the end of the 6-month period of immobilization in plaster, the leg is straightened gradually by a succession of plaster casts. After about a year or 18 months, weight-bearing with or without support may be permitted. Normal motion in the hip joint will be impaired for a considerable period, but this disability may be relieved gradually by a period of baking, massage and supervised exercises carried out in an orthopedic gymnasium.

In patients over 6 years of age, operation usually is necessary, replacing the femur in the acetabulum or, if this is impossible, forming a new socket in which the head of the bone may rest. Casts are applied after operation, including the involved foot, lower extremity and the pelvis, and holding the extremity in extension, abduction and internal rotation. This position is maintained for at least 3 months, after which the extremity is brought down gradually into the normal attitude. The patient then may be permitted to get up without support of any kind, and he is encouraged to use his leg gradually.

Nursing Care

After operation, the care of the child is largely in the hands of the nurse. The long period of ether anesthesia necessary for these operations often predisposes to dehydration and, at times, acidosis. These conditions are characterized by persistent vomiting, red dry tongue, and, in cases of acidosis, by a fruity odor of the breath (the odor of acetone) and the appearance of acetone in the urine. Treatment consists of the maintenance of adequate fluid and nutritional levels. The nurse should be able to recognize the symptoms of this complication in order to notify the surgeon when it appears. The patient's general condition must be checked carefully. Temperature, pulse, respirations and blood pressure should be taken periodically and recorded on the nurse's chart. Shock should be watched for carefully (see p. 136) and its presence reported at once to the surgeon. Hemorrhage in the region of the operative site may escape detection because of the cast, but periodic examination should be made at the bottom of the cast, and any increasing blood-staining of the cast should be reported to the surgeon immediately. (See Care of the Patient in a Cast, pp. 542-548.)

Birth Palsy

This is a paralysis of the arm caused by injury to the brachial plexus during birth. (Erb's paralysis involves the shoulder muscles only.) The nurse may notice the flaccidly hanging arm during the infant's first bath. If only the shoulder is involved, the prognosis is good. By splinting or the application of a cast, the arm can be maintained in abduction and external rotation. The length of treatment varies directly with the severity of the paralysis.

Torticollis (Wryneck)

Probably due to hemorrhage in the sternocleidomastoid muscle caused by trauma during delivery, the child's head may incline to one side. This is brought about by a shortening of the muscle on the side involved. Palpation of the neck reveals a mass in the muscle, and attempts to straighten the head on the trunk are unsuccessful. This is called *torticollis* or *wryneck*. As healing takes place in the injured muscle, fibrosis and contraction occur and the child keeps the head turned to the opposite side and inclined toward the shoulder on the involved side. If uncorrected, this deformity leads to marked facial asymmetry.

Treatment of torticollis usually is successful if discovered soon after birth. Heat, massage and carefully regulated stretching as a rule bring a return to normal in a month or two. In untreated cases, the fibrosis and resulting contracture of the muscle result in a deformity that cannot be relieved by conservative means. A cutting of the tendon at its insertion to the clavicle and the sternum is performed. After operation, a plaster cast that includes head, neck and upper chest is applied. The head thus is held in an overcorrected position for a time and brought gradually to its normal position.

Nursing Care

Nursing problems which result from adhesive traction, a brace or a plaster cast applied as a corrective device for torticollis are similar. During the immediate postoperative care, the nurse must be aware of the danger of aspiration because of the restricted movement brought about by one of the above-mentioned devices. Observation of those areas which are in contact with close-fitting apparatus is a necessary nursing function. In addition, cleanliness must be maintained. The use of bibs, waterproofing materials, cleaning agents and deodorants (described in preceding chapter under Cast and Traction Care) should be used. Diversional activity suited to the preferences of the patient will make time pass more quickly. The role of the nurse as teacher here is important. She can help to educate the mother in ways to help the child to help himself; for example, encourage the child to turn his head in the corrected position by the placement of toys or other such devices.

Clubfoot (Congenital Talipes, Equinovarus)

Clubfoot is a deformity thought to be due to arrested growth, a defect in the ovum, familial tendencies or malposition in the uterus. It may involve one foot or both feet. The foot is turned in and, in extreme cases, so deformed that the child walks on the outside of the foot with the heel elevated and the sole turned backward.

Soon after birth the deformity may be recognized and, if treatment is instituted at that early date, a complete cure usually results. If untreated, the tendons become shortened, the bones and the calf muscles are ill-formed, and a cure is effected with much more difficulty. Treatment may be done in mild cases by means of manipulation and strapping. The nurse can help a great deal by convincing the parents that such treatment must be continuous and adhered to faithfully. Generally this is accomplished best by applying a series of plaster casts to correct the deformity. The forefoot adduction, heel inversion and, finally, the equinus attitude are corrected in that order. The casts are changed weekly at first and, as the condition improves, they may be left in place for longer intervals. The casts are made by applying plaster-of-Paris bandages over snugly fitting flannel or cotton wadding that extend from the tips of the toes to just below the knee. The Kite method is the use of a plaster cast that is wedged at intervals as the correction progresses. With this method, the nurse must be on the alert for new pressure areas. During this period of treatment it is of the utmost importance to guard against impairment of circulation and the development of pressure sores, which may require splitting or trimming of the cast and even its removal and the application of a new cast. When the foot has been corrected satisfactorily, as verified by clinical x-ray examinations, the foot may be removed from plaster and manipulated several times daily. The child then may be fitted with clubfoot corrective shoes and allowed to walk. However, it may be necessary to maintain the corrected position at night by means of the appropriate splint.

The Denis-Brown apparatus is another method of treatment, in which the feet are strapped to footplates attached to a cross-bar; correction is obtained by the force of the child's kicking in the splint. There are several disadvantages to this method, and when it is used it is usually in treating infants less than 1 year old.

If correction cannot be secured in this manner, especially in older children, anesthesia is administered and the foot is brought into position by forcible manual correction. Casts then are applied as described above to hold the foot in a position of overcorrection. For 24 hours after this operation, the child should be confined to bed with the foot and the leg elevated to prevent undue swelling. After two or three days, walking is permitted in the plaster cast. After three or four weeks another dressing similar to the first is applied. Following a series of casts, changed about every three weeks, the treatment may be continued with exercises and special shoes. In some cases, elastic traction bands may be used instead of cast or after cast treatment.

Cutting operations—cutting tendons or ligaments—or operations involving the bones of the foot are reserved for those late cases in which correction cannot be obtained by the above methods. Recurrence of the deformity is not uncommon, and the child should be re-examined by the surgeon periodically for many months.

Infantile Paralysis

Paralytic deformities frequently appear following infantile paralysis. This disease affects children and adults, and results in a destruction of anterior horn cells of the spinal cord. Paralysis appears in the muscle groups enervated by the destroyed cells. It involves most commonly the muscles of the extremities, and often is bilateral; but any part may be affected, including the muscles of the spine and the abdomen. The paralysis is of the flaccid type, leaving the limb flail-like. Contractures of the unparalyzed muscles may cause increasing deformities.

As soon as the paralysis becomes evident, it is necessary to prevent, so far as possible, the development of deformity and protect weak musculature. The usual method of accomplishing this is by means of splints or molded plaster casts that maintain the affected extremities in the neutral position (for example, the foot should be at right angles to the leg). The bedclothes are supported with pillows or a cradle.

Sister Kenny's method of treatment consists of the periodic application of hot packs to the affected parts and painstaking re-education of the involved muscles as soon as the patient's condition permits it. For its proper use this treatment requires specially trained nurses and physiotherapists. Physiotherapy measures should be used to maintain the range of motion in the joints.

After the acute symptoms subside, carefully supervised physiotherapy (bathing, massage, electrical treatments, hydrotherapy and exercises) may be beneficial. Swimming exercise in pool or otherwise still is a most valuable adjunct of the rehabilitation treatment in many cases of paralyses, when muscle action is to be restored. Often some form of supportive brace or appliance is indicated, and the nurse should see to it that these are in the proper position at all times. Considerable improvement may be observed under this treatment. Usually, after the lapse of a year or two, no further improvement will be evident.

Operation is indicated in many of

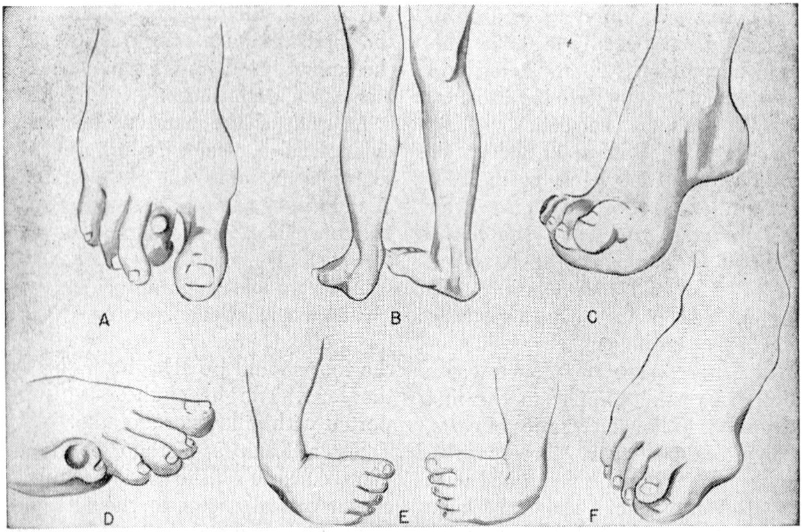

FIG. 252. (A) Second hammer toe. (B) Pronated flatfeet. (C) Clawfoot. (D) Congenital hammer toe. (E) Congenital talipes equinovarus–clubfoot. (F) Hallux valgus.

these cases for the relief of deformities that develop from neglect of, or in spite of, proper supporting apparatus and for optimum functional return. Tendons may be transplanted so that functioning muscles may act in place of paralyzed ones or, when paralysis is extensive, the flail-jointed "dangle foot" may be converted into a much more useful member by producing an artificial union of the bones forming the joint. This is done by an operation called an *arthrodesis*. The leg must be encased in a plaster cast for a time (usually twelve weeks) to give the bones a chance to form a solid union.

After operation, the leg should be elevated to prevent undue swelling. Even with this precaution, the toes must be watched carefully for signs of interference with the circulation, i.e., swelling, cyanosis and numbness. Often it is necessary to spread the cast enough to permit an adequate circulation.

Other Foot Conditions

Hallux valgus is an inward deviation of the great toe at the first metatarsophalangeal joint. This is associated with an exostosis on the head of the first metatarsal and a bursa overlying the exostosis, which is called a *bunion*. Bunions may be acquired or congenital. Properly fitting shoes and support of the metatarsal arch usually relieve pain and discomfort.

Flatfoot deformity in children frequently is found with bowlegs or knockknees. Usually, prescribed shoes with heel lifts are recommended; these are changed as the child grows. Flat feet are common also as an adult deformity.

Hammer toes may be congenital or acquired and result from the spasmodic contracture of the extensors of the toes. The first interphalangeal joint is usually prominent; it is flexed and often has a corn on top. The treatment is any measure to release the contracture of the muscle.

Clawfoot is a contracture of the muscles and the ligaments of the plantar arch and is seen following infantile paralysis. Treatment may involve arch supports and probably a tenotomy of the extensor tendons to the toes.

Nursing responsibility in relation to foot conditions is primarily a teaching one. It is for the nurse to relay important information to her patients regarding foot exercises, the proper selection and care of shoes, the care and the use of foot pads and plates, the care of boot casts and the significance of symptoms of circulatory constriction. The socioeconomic factors must not be ignored.

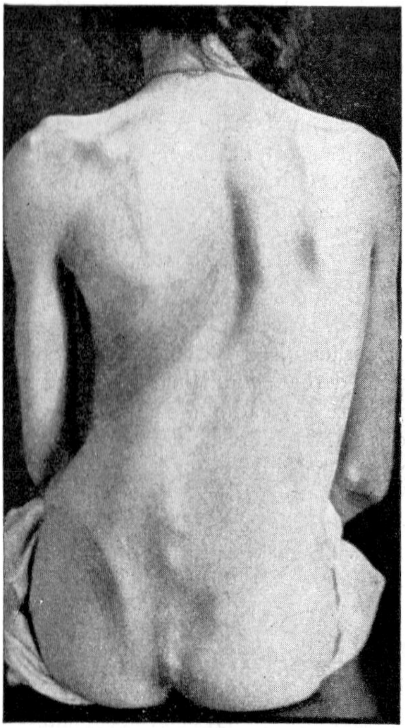

Fig. 253. Scoliosis of the spine. (Indiana University Department of Illustrations)

Spinal Curvatures

Curvatures of the spine may be of 3 types: (1) *kyphosis*, anteroposterior curvatures, or hunchback, of which more mention will be made in the discussion of tuberculosis of the spine (p. 589); (2) *lordosis*, or exaggerated hollow back; and (3) *scoliosis*, or lateral curvature.

Scoliosis. This condition may be a secondary result of deformities of other parts—for example, the shortening of one leg, thoracic disease such as empyema, rickets or habitual faulty posture. The last produces what is known as postural or functional scoliosis. It begins merely as a faulty attitude in the decade between 5 and 15 years of age. The spine is curved slightly to one side and there usually are coexistent round shoulders and round back. Statistics show this minor deformity to be present in from 20 to 25 per cent of schoolchildren. While the condition appears to be of little importance, it should not be neglected, because the tendency is toward an increase in the deformity as growth progresses. The lateral curvature becomes more noticeable, the shoulder (usually the left) droops and the right hip becomes prominent. If the condition goes untreated, structural (bony) changes occur.

Treatment. The treatment of this condition often falls to the school or "district" nurse, in association with the surgeon. It requires a thorough investigation of the hygienic practices of the patient. Overwork in school and after school should be prevented. An examination of the eyes is indicated if visual error is suspected that would lead to improper posture in reading. The schoolroom desk and chair should be inspected with the child seated at the desk. If the desk is too far from the chair, or if it is too small for the child, habitual faulty posture can hardly be prevented (Fig. 254). A patient's family can be taught to help the child in maintaining good posture. Often it is difficult to sell the idea of the need for corrective exercises to the patient. Emphasis on the cosmetic result often is effective. Many orthopedic surgeons relieve weight on the shoulders by having the patient wear clothes that hang from the waist as much as possible. Habitual malposture and functional scoliosis may be corrected by spinal gymnastic exercises that are continued for one or two years.

In those cases in which there is marked rotation of the ribs associated with the lateral curvature, support often is applied in the form of a plaster jacket having large windows over the compressed portion of the thorax to allow for its expansion.

Fig. 254. (*Left*) Showing child sitting at desk in improper position. Desk too small for child. (*Right*) Showing child sitting at desk in proper position.

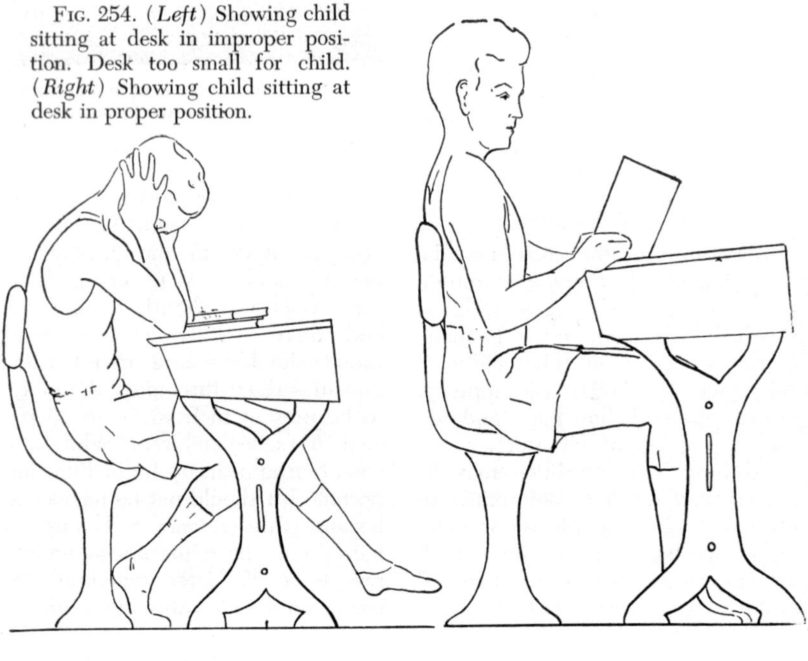

Adequate correction may have to be obtained by applying a cast with wedges cut in either side (Risser jacket), so that the spine may be straightened by the use of hinges and turnbuckles (see p. 546). In many cases, an operation (spinal fusion) may be necessary to hold the spine in the corrected position. When the desired result is obtained, a spinal brace often is employed to maintain the overcorrected position for a time.

Backache

A common and annoying problem experienced by many people is backache. Oddly enough, in most instances this discomfort can be prevented. From the nursing and the public health point of view, one must be aware of the many causative aspects: improper body mechanics employed in lifting, twisting and turning, poor walking, sitting and lying posture and improperly fitting shoes, including heels that are too high, too flat or worn down. Many back pains are referred from some other part of the body. Gynecologic conditions, psychosomatic complaints or obesity may be the reason for back discomfort.

Correction of any of the above factors may relieve back pain. Perhaps the use of a properly fitting brace will help. All mechanical defects must be investigated and corrected before any more radical procedure, such as fusion, is attempted.

Rickets (Rachitis)

The treatment of rickets really belongs to the pediatrist but, because of the bony deformities that occur, it is of interest also to the orthopedic surgeon and nurse. It is a disease of young children (under three years of age). It is found most often in children who have been brought up under poor hygienic conditions and who have had improper feedings and little sunlight, fresh air or exercise. Research has shown that the lack of vitamin D (found in fish oils, vegetables and certain other types of food) will cause this condition. Exposure of the child to the ultraviolet rays of the sun or a special mercury arc lamp will prevent the condition and benefit it if it has occurred.

Symptoms. The symptoms of the disease usually begin in the first or the second year. The mother notices fretfulness, head-sweating and a "backwardness" in walking, crawling and sitting. The ends of the long bones become swollen. This is especially marked at wrist and ankle joints and where the ribs join the sternum. The enlargement at the last-mentioned site often is called the *rachitic rosary*. The bones are soft, due to a lack of lime (calcium) deposit, that results in various types of deformities. "Bowlegs," "knock knee" and kyphosis are a few of the common types.

Treatment. The treatment of these cases is directed toward the cure of the constitutional disease and the prevention and the relief of disabling deformities. The child should be fed a diet rich in fresh vegetables and vitamins, especially vitamin D, and adequate milk. Open air and direct sunlight are therapeutic agents of more merit than most medicines. Sunlight is of value because of the ultraviolet rays it contains. These rays are lost largely by passage through glass; therefore, the child should be out of doors. Practically the whole body should be exposed. Instead of sunlight, or combined with it, most surgeons use the ultraviolet rays obtained from a mercury arc lamp. The children are exposed to the rays without clothes for increasing periods. Several precautions must be taken in the use of these rays. The eyes of both patient and nurse must be protected by dark glasses or goggles. Overexposure must be avoided to prevent skin burns. A nurse always should be present during the exposure, and a time clock should be set that will ring at the end of the prescribed period.

In the early stages of the disease the treatment is directed toward the prevention of deformities. Braces or plaster-of-Paris splints are used to overcome mild deformities. After the age of 3 years, little improvement can be expected from the brace treatment, and operations have been devised to relieve the deformities. The bones are divided deliberately with a sharp instrument and the limbs are placed in a plaster cast in an overcorrected position for from 6 to 8 weeks. The ordinary precautions taken in any postoperative plaster cast are indicated.

OSTEOMYELITIS

Acute osteomyelitis is an acute infection of the bone marrow that rapidly involves other bony structures. It affects the long bones most frequently, and is caused most commonly by the *Staphylococcus aureus*. The infection usually is blood-borne from other foci of infection, but it may follow slight trauma or exposure to cold and wet. It is essentially a disease of childhood and adolescence. However, osteomyelitis may occur, by direct infection of the bone resulting from compound fractures. The onset of the disease usually is sudden, occurring often with a chill, high fever, rapid pulse and general malaise. In children, in whom the disease usually begins as an acute epiphysitis, these constitutional symptoms at first may overshadow the local signs completely. As the infection extends from the marrow cavity through the cortex of the bone, it involves the periosteum and the soft tissues, and the limb becomes painful, swollen and extremely tender. Thus an abscess of bone is formed. In the natural course of events, the abscess may point and drain but, more often, incision and drainage are done by the surgeon. The resulting abscess cavity has in its walls areas of dead tissue, as in any abscess cavity; however, in this case the dead tissue is bone, which cannot liquefy easily and be discharged as pus. This dead bone is called a *sequestrum.* Healing in a bone abscess is more difficult than in an abscess in soft tissue, because the cavity cannot collapse and heal. New bone, the *involucrum,* forms in nature's attempt at repair. Often it grows so as to surround a sequestrum. Thus, even though healing appears to take place, a chronically infected sequestrum remains that is prone to produce recurring abscesses throughout the life of the individual. This is the so-called chronic type of osteomyelitis.

Treatment. Acute osteomyelitis begins as a staphylococcic septicemia,

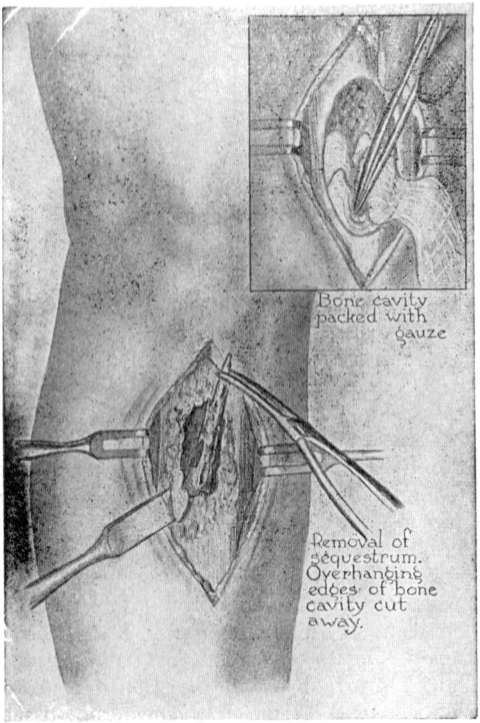

Fig. 255. Method of sequestrectomy and saucerization. Inset shows bone cavity packed with petrolatum gauze. (Steindler, A.: Orthopedic Operations, Springfield, Ill., Thomas)

and formerly the acute toxemia frequently was fatal. Since the sulfa drugs and penicillin became available, early and intensive treatment usually produces a rapid recovery. The development of an abscess of the bone, with the resulting marked and prolonged morbidity, thus can be avoided. In neglected or untreated cases, aspiration or incision and drainage of an abscess may be necessary. Often penicillin is used locally in addition to its systemic administration.

In chronic osteomyelitis, the dead, infected bone must be removed before permanent healing takes place. This operation, called a *sequestrectomy* (Fig. 255), consists of the removal of enough involucrum with mallet and chisel to enable the surgeon to remove the sequestrum. Often sufficient bone is removed to convert a deep cavity into a shallow saucer (saucerization). Muscle sometimes is used to help obliterate the resulting wound. These operations are becoming increasingly rare since the advent of penicillin. Primary healing may be obtained frequently by the use of penicillin if the cavity can be closed and the skin approximated. Sometimes the granulating wound may be covered by a split-thickness skin graft.

When osteomyelitis occurs in a

compound fracture by direct implantation of the offending organisms, there is no preceding septicemia, but the treatment is in general as outlined above, except that the fracture must be treated in addition.

Nursing Care

Osteomyelitis is in the group of diseases in which good nursing care is absolutely necessary. The wounds themselves frequently are very painful and require great care and gentleness in their handling. Pillow support to the adjoining joints and maintenance of good alignment are comfort measures. Careful handling also is essential because of the possibilities of cross infection and pathologic fracture. Hot packs may be prescribed for indurated areas. Less pain is experienced if petrolatum gauze is used in the dressing. Scrupulous care of the skin is required to prevent bedsores. Fresh air, sunlight and a high caloric diet rich in vitamins will hasten the convalescence of these patients. They should be watched carefully for any development of painful areas or sudden rises in temperature, as these symptoms usually indicate the formation of a secondary abscess. A frequent problem encountered is an unpleasant odor due to the foul drainage. A deodorizer near the patient's unit may help. Some physicians use a specially prepared charcoal plaster which absorbs the odor. For the most part, to reassure the patient that this is a usual result of bone infection will help. Because of the long period of hospitalization and frequent readmissions sometimes necessary in the treatment of these patients, their morale often is low and they need stimulation and diversion. During their hospital stay the occupational therapy department and the hospital school teacher often are able to find interesting and useful employment suited to their ability.

TUBERCULOSIS

Tuberculosis is a chronic infectious disease caused by the *Bacillus tuberculosis* (*Mycobacterium tuberculosis*). The organisms gain entrance through the respiratory or alimentary tract and may spread to almost any tissue in the body. In childhood and in youth, tuberculosis of bones and joints and of lymph nodes is most common. In adult life, the peritoneum, the lungs and the meninges also are involved. The disease is slow and insidious in its onset, associated rarely with the marked fever, tenderness, redness and edema that have been mentioned (Chap. 2) as characteristic of the onset of an acute infection. It slowly destroys the tissues infected by a process known as *caseation*, so named because of the cheeselike appearance of the pus formed. A chronic inflammatory granulomatous tissue, associated with pus formation, result. In the later stages of the disease there is a characteristic afternoon rise of temperature of 1° or 2°. Unless secondary infection occurs, the leukocytes are reduced (leukopenia).

Treatment. In the treatment of all forms of tuberculosis, constitutional rest is a requisite. Rest in bed is essential so long as there is any elevation of temperature. These patients should live, day and night, in the open air and sunlight because of their tonic effect. In hospitals these facilities are obtained usually in the form of roof gardens or balconies. The patients can be wheeled there and remain the greater part of the day in the open. In addition, a wholesome diet, rich in vitamins, does much to build up resistance against the infection.

In addition to these hygienic measures, streptomycin has assumed a place of importance in the treatment of tuberculous lesions. Often it is combined with penicillin when a mixed infection is found. Isoniazid is used with success in some hospitals.

Tuberculosis of Bones and Joints

Among the commonest forms of surgical tuberculosis is that involving the bones and the joints. It occurs most often in children up to twelve years of age, and is characterized by more or less pain, wasting of surrounding muscles, loss of weight and the formation of cold abscesses. These last are so called to distinguish them from acute inflammatory abscesses associated with acute infectious processes. A discussion of the bones and the joints most frequently involved follows.

TUBERCULOSIS OF SPINE POTT'S DISEASE

This is one of the most frequent forms of secondary tuberculosis. It occurs usually in children from 2 to 10 years of age. The thoracic vertebrae are involved most often. The bodies of the vertebrae undergo caseous softening and, because the weight of the trunk is borne by these parts, a kinking or a knuckling (*gibbus*) of the spine results. This deformity is called *kyphosis* or hunchback by the laity. As the process goes on, cold abscesses form, and often symptoms of the nervous system develop due to injury to the spinal nerves or cord.

Symptoms. The symptoms appear slowly. The child may be listless and fretful. In moving about he tries to protect his back, supporting himself by holding on to chairs and avoiding bending over whenever possible. At night he may be awakened by sharp pains that make him cry out. These are due to the unguarded motion of affected areas. Such "night cries" are a characteristic symptom of tuberculous disease of the bones and the joints. Later, when the body of the vertebrae has undergone caseous necrosis, deformity appears.

Treatment and Nursing Care

Rest and Drug Therapy. In addition to streptomycin supplemented with para-aminosalicylic acid, complete rest is an important part of the treatment. By this means the vertebrae may be protected from weight-bearing and, by the aid of proper constitutional treatment, the child is able to overcome the infection. These children are placed on their backs on a Bradford frame or a curved Bradford (Whitman) frame in such a position that the affected vertebrae are directly over the bend in the frame and held in that position by a jacket applied over the chest and the shoulders. This position of hyperextension is maintained to relieve pressure and to prevent possible collapse of vertebrae on the spinal cord structures. The frame should be covered with tightly stretched canvas made in two pieces, leaving a space about 4 inches wide at the buttocks, so that the bedpan

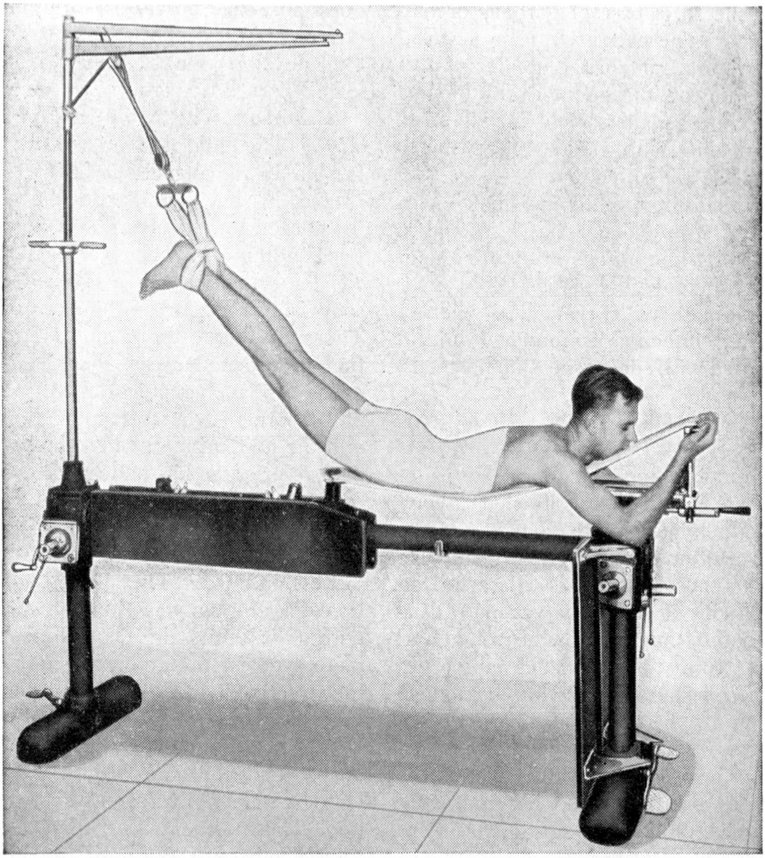

Fig. 256. Orthopedic table with patient arranged for application of body cast.

may be used without disturbing the hips. After removing the bedpan, a canvas strip should be placed under the buttocks and fastened to the frame to prevent sagging. The canvas should be covered with folded sheets. If there is marked kyphosis, pillows or felt should be used in such a way as to remove the weight from the hump.

Because of the prolonged period of treatment, many hospitals have accommodations whereby the schooling of the child is continued.

Extension. Extension usually is applied to the legs (Buck's extension) and the head to ensure immobility. Many surgeons employ the arched or inclined frame for treating these patients, applying extension to the legs. The child should remain in one of these two positions for a considerable period of time—at least until all symptoms have disappeared.

The essential part of the treatment (which the nurse must know) is the avoidance of any motion of the spinal column.

The patient should be clothed with gowns and sweaters that open in the back and fasten only at the neck. Feeding and drinking may necessitate the aid of a nurse at first, but the child soon learns how to manage his spoon and fork, even though he is lying flat on his back. Fluids are given through a tube or by the use of the "feeding duck."

The daily bath is given with the patient in the same position. When the child must be turned to be bathed and have his back rubbed, the turning must be done in the same manner as rolling a log. This is accomplished best by two nurses. One nurse places one hand on the pelvis and the other hand at the back of the shoulders and rolls the patient toward her. The pillows should be prepared to maintain the same degree of hyperextension. The other nurse, standing on the opposite side of the bed, quickly bathes and rubs the back.

The hygienic and constitutional treatment—wholesome diet, sunlight and fresh air—is as important as the fixation. The children should be on a sun porch or balcony from 7 A.M. to 7 P.M. daily. On days when sunlight is not available, the ultraviolet lamp may be used.

When traction is being used, the nurse must guard against the development of a "pointed-toe deformity." This may occur if the foot is kept constantly in the extended position by the weight of the bedclothes and is not supported. A bed cradle over the feet and a foot board will prevent this complication, also called "foot-drop."

Treatment as described is necessary until all symptoms of the disease have been absent for 2 or 3 months. Often this may take from 6 months to a year. When the child is allowed out of bed, a body brace is applied so that treatment may be continued. If a cast is necessary, it is put on with the patient lying prone on a canvas sling or suspended from the neck and the shoulders. Sufficient padding must be used to prevent pressure over bony prominences, and large windows are cut anteriorly to reduce the weight of the cast and to allow free breathing and feeding. The cast may be worn for from 3 to 6 months without changing, but at frequent intervals it should be inspected thoroughly. The distinctive smell of an excoriated area often is the first indication of pressure. The finding of such signs requires removal of the cast and the application of a new cast or braces. Braces always should be used for a considerable period.

Operation. Tuberculosis of the spine may be treated by operation in some cases, the principle of all the types of operation being to fix the spine in one position. In some types, a bone graft, usually from the tibia, may be removed from the leg and transplanted so as to unite the vertebrae. In such cases it is necessary for the nurse to prepare the leg as well as the back for operation. Some bone grafts come from the posterior iliac crest. The absolute necessity of scrupulously careful preoperative preparation of the skin cannot be overemphasized. An accepted procedure includes two separate preparations of the site of operation within 24 hours of surgery and the application of sterile cloths to the prepared regions (for Sterile Preparation Tray, see p. 57). These operations often are quite shocking to the patient, so that the nurse must always prepare a warm bed, hot fluids and so forth. (See Chap. 6.)

After operation, the patient is kept in bed for at least 10 to 12 weeks. The usual precautions against bedsores must be taken. When the patient is allowed out of bed, braces or a plaster jacket should be worn for a time.

This patient needs careful care of the skin area around the gibbus; pressure must be prevented when he lies on his back. In caring for patients with Pott's disease, the nurse should be on the lookout for the appearance of masses (cold abscesses). These usually appear below the groin, but they may develop in the back or the loin and the surgeon's attention should be drawn to them at once. They should be protected from pressure as much as possible. The treatment of cold abscess usually is aspiration rather than incision and drainage, because of the danger of secondary infection through an open wound. However, despite this precaution, infection usually occurs eventually and necessitates later incision and drainage.

TUBERCULOSIS OF HIP JOINT

Tuberculosis of the hip joint is probably the second most common type of tuberculosis involving the bones and joints. It occurs mostly in children under 10 years of age. The patients as a rule are in poor general health. The first symptoms noticed are stiffness in the hip joint, and pain often referred to the knee, that is due to irritation of the obturator nerve, which often lies in contact with the capsule of the joint but supplies sensation to the knee joint. The stiffness of the hip often is apparent only in the morning when the child gets out of bed. Gradually the limp and pain increase, and "night cries" are common, due to pain caused by the relaxation of the muscle spasm while the child sleeps and to the unguarded motion at the affected site. The leg is held in continuous partial flexion, and walking is on the ball of the foot on the side affected. If the condition goes on without treatment—and even at times with treatment—cold abscesses appear, usually on the outside of the thigh or in the gluteal region (buttocks).

Treatment. The object of treatment, as for Pott's disease, is to give the part absolute rest. The patient is placed in bed, often on a Bradford frame, and Buck's extension or Russell's traction is applied to relax muscle spasm and keep the joint surfaces apart. It may be impossible, because of the pain and spasm, to give traction in the horizontal direction. Then, extension is applied with the thigh somewhat flexed, the legs being supported with a series of pads that are reduced gradually in number until the leg reaches the horizontal. The pads should extend for the entire length of the leg. The bedclothes must be supported and the foot so held that the deformity of pointed toe does not develop.

The care of these patients is simi-

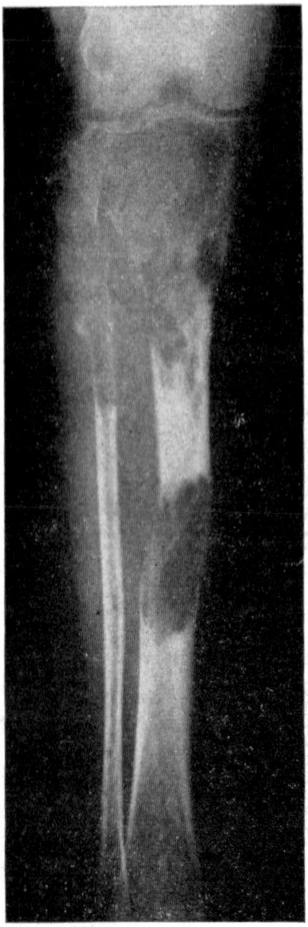

FIG. 257. Roentgenogram showing marked destruction of tibia by metastatic carcinoma. The carcinoma in this case occurred primarily in the breast.

lar to that recommended for Pott's disease.

Bed treatment may be continued for from 6 months to 2 years, until all symptoms, pain, fever, limitation of motion and so forth have disappeared. After the patient has remained symptom-free for from 2 to 3 months, a fusion may be done or a brace may be applied from axilla to foot and the patient is permitted to be about with crutches, wearing a high-soled shoe on the unaffected side, so that the diseased limb may swing free of the ground. The nurse must watch at all times for any signs that suggest a relapse. Finally, gradual weight-bearing with crutches may be permitted with the brace in place. If, after 8 months or a year, no further joint involvements are evident, crutches are used without a brace until by gradual stages full weight-bearing is proved to be safe.

The healing of tuberculous lesions usually results in a fusion of the bones forming the joint (ankylosis). Experience has shown that more rapid healing can be obtained by operative fusion of the involved bones (arthrodesis). Then the patient is immobilized in a cast until solid union takes place. When there are secondary tuberculous sinuses, the administration of streptomycin is especially valuable.

The treatment of tuberculosis of other bones and joints is carried out in essentially the same manner as has been outlined already for Pott's disease and tuberculosis of the hip.

OSTEITIS FIBROSA CYSTICA (VON RECKLINGHAUSEN'S DISEASE)

This is a disease of bone produced by an increased secretion of the parathyroid glands, due either to a parathyroid hyperplasia or an adenoma. The bone changes, the multiple cysts, the benign giant cell tumors and the generalized decalcification (osteoporosis) are a prominent manifestation of the disease. There are associated symptoms of weakness, pain in the legs and the thighs, backache and occasional pathologic fractures through a cyst or decalcified bone. When the disease is advanced, marked deformity results. Kidney stones form as a result of the large amounts of calcium mobilized by the excess parathormone. Blood studies show an increased calcium and a decreased phosphorus. Operative removal of the parathyroid tumor results in a return to normal. (See p. 474.)

BONE TUMORS

Benign tumors of bone are not uncommon, but they are not important unless they develop symptoms such as interference with or restriction of motion of an extremity or cause unsightly cosmetic defects. Bones frequently are the seat of sarcomatous growths. They occur usually in young adults and are characterized by rapidly increasing swelling, pain and disability. An x-ray usually will be necessary to confirm the diagnosis, and early amputation is the only treatment of any avail. (See Amputation, p. 567.)

Bone is a frequent site of metastatic growths in carcinoma of the prostate, the breast and the thyroid, in renal carcinoma and hypernephroma and less often, in other carcinomas (Fig. 257). And bone may be involved, but the spine, the pelvis and the femur are common sites. A constant, dull ache is the usual early manifestation. This later becomes such severe pain that almost continuous sedation is necessary. The destruction of the affected bone may result in a pathologic fracture after minimal trauma. These fractures differ from the usual fractures in that they are associated with relatively little pain.

It is important for the nurse to recognize the significance of the appearance of pain in patients having carcinoma. In most cases the carcinoma is far advanced and the problem is one of terminal care. Metastatic carcinoma of bone produces an added pain that necessitates added sedation. Hormone therapy frequently is helpful in prostatic carcinoma and sometimes in breast carcinoma. In prostatic carcinoma, the removal of the source of male hormones, orchectomy, frequently relieves the pain within 24 to 72 hours. The administration of female hormones, estrogens, appears to inactivate the male hormones and, therefore, achieves the same result as orchectomy within 7 to 10 days. In many cases both treatments are used. Male hormone, testosterone, also may give relief of pain and recalcification of bone in some cases of breast carcinoma. The results are less constant than with hormone therapy of prostatic cancer.

Two common forms of malignant bone tumors usually requiring radical treatment are osteogenic sarcoma and Ewing's tumor.

DISEASES OF JOINTS

Synovitis is the term given to an inflammation of the synovial membrane of the joint. It may be due to trauma: traumatic synovitis. It is characterized by a swelling and pain in the affected joint. The knee is the joint injured most commonly, and "water on the knee" is the descriptive term applied to it by the laity. The pain is due in most part to distention of the joint capsule and can be relieved by aspiration of the joint. If the fluid is bloody, an associated fracture or other injury is suspected. As a rule, restriction of motion, pressure bandages and application of heat result in a rapid recovery.

Joint Mice

Loose bodies called joint mice not infrequently are found in joints. The knee is the joint most often affected. These bodies may lie free in the joint, or they may be attached by a pedicle to the capsule. Often they may be palpated and frequently are shown by x-rays. They cause symptoms when they slip between the bones, causing the joint to lock in semiflexion.

Treatment. An *arthrotomy* (incision into the joint) and removal of the bodies will give relief. After the operation, the limb is kept elevated and is splinted with a plaster trough for about 2 weeks.

Arthritis

When all parts of a joint are affected (synovium, cartilage, bone) the affection is called an *arthritis*. Arthritis may arise from various types of infection. Gonorrhea is characterized at times by a monoarticular inflammation, usually of the knee joint. Rapid recovery takes place with appropriate sulfa and penicillin therapy. Locally, rest provided by splints and elevation on pillows under a bed cradle are employed.

When the bacteria infecting the joint form pus, a *pyarthrosis* or *suppurative arthritis* results. Aspiration of the pus with instillation of antibiotics may be sufficient at times to overcome the infection. Usually, the joint must be drained, immobilized by splints or extended by traction and treated in the same way as any infection elsewhere in the body. If the infection is drained early, an almost normal joint may result. If the drainage is instituted late, the joint cartilages may be destroyed largely, with the result that fibrous or bony adhesions form between the bones and produce a stiff joint or, as it is technically called, an *ankylosis*.

Chronic arthritis (arthritis deformans) is a large group of joint diseases exhibiting atrophic and hypertrophic changes in the x-ray. Multiple joints are affected, usually in older people. The etiology is not known definitely. These patients usually are treated medically, but when conservative measures fail and the person is unable to use the part, operation is recommended at times. Occasionally, restoration of joint function may be attempted by an operation called an *arthroplasty*. This consists of removal of the damaged joint surfaces and adjacent bone. In some cases fascia may be used to form a new joint surface, and in others the bone end may be covered with a smooth-shaped surface of vitallium. Often a metallic prosthesis may be inserted where the grossly deformed head and neck of the femur have been resected. Fusion of the joint may be done in still other cases. The ankylosis produced may cause a disability that is less than the painful arthritis.

DISEASES OF BURSAE

A *bursa* is a small fluid-filled sac occurring between muscles, tendons and bones. Its function is to promote muscular movement with the least possible amount of friction. These sacs frequently are the seat of inflammation due to trauma or infection, or to calcareous deposits that form in their walls, with the result that muscular movement becomes painful. Rest for the part, removal of focal infection and dry heat frequently will effect a cure. If the inflammation becomes acute, or is not relieved by conservative treatment, operation with drainage or excision of the bursa will be necessary.

Subdeltoid Bursitis

The bursa most commonly giving symptoms is the one which lies between the deltoid muscle and the greater tuberosity of the humerus. This bursa may be injured by falls on the outstretched hand so that the bursa is pinched between the head of the humerus and the overlying acromium process of the scapula. However, most commonly, the bursa becomes painful as a result of degeneration. Often a calcium deposit appears in the tendons which lie underneath it over the head of the humerus. The calcified area may be the seat of an inflammation producing tension in the dense supraspinatus tendon. This produces acute pain when the shoulder is moved and is spoken of as *acute bursitis.* The chronic form of bursitis often follows repeated use of the arm above the head. There is pain produced by certain abduction movements of the arm, as in putting on a coat, and often pain is noted at night when the patient rolls over on the arm of the affected side. These affections really involve the bursa secondarily but produce marked disability in shoulder motion.

The acute form of bursitis may be relieved by x-ray therapy or by operative removal of calcium deposit. Some forms of the chronic type may respond to conservative therapy, x-ray therapy and, more recently, the injected hydrocortone.

REFERENCES AND SUGGESTED READING

Unit Ten: Nursing in Conditions of the Musculoskeletal System

General

Bailey, Jean: Care of the patient with a Taylor spine brace, Am. J. Nursing **44**:665-668, 1944.

Colonna, P. C.: Regional Orthopedic Surgery, Philadelphia, Saunders, 1950.

Emerson, C. P., and Bragdon, J. S.: Essentials of Medicine, ed. 17, pp. 677-715; pp. 707-715 (muscle diseases), Philadelphia, Lippincott, 1955.

Ghormley, R.: Specialization in medicine: what is orthopedic surgery, J. Bone & Joint Surg. **31-A**: 459-463, 1949.

Knocke, F. J., and Knocke, L. S.: Orthopaedic Nursing, Philadelphia, Davis, 1951.

Larson-Gould: Calderwood's Orthopedic Nursing, ed. 3, St. Louis, Mosby, 1953.

Magnuson, P. B., and Stack, J. K.: Fractures, ed. 5, Philadelphia, Lippincott, 1949.

Mercer, Walter: Orthopedic Surgery, Baltimore, Williams & Wilkins, 1952.

Newton, Kathleen: Orthopedic problems of older people, Am. J. Nursing **48**:508-511, 1948.

Stevenson, J. L.: Orthopedic Conditions at Birth—Nursing Responsibilities, New York, Joint Orthopedic Nursing Advisory Service, 1943.

——: Posture and Nursing, ed. 2, New York, Joint Orthopedic Nursing Advisory Service, 1948.

Posture and Body Mechanics

Fash, Bernice: Body Mechanics in Nursing Arts, New York, McGraw-Hill, 1946.

Leavitt, D. G., and Leavitt, H. L.: Scoliosis: prevention, control, corrections, Am. J. Nursing **50**:198-200, 1950.

Stevenson, Jessie: Posture and Nursing, New York, Joint Orthopedic Nursing Advisory Service, 1948. (Pamphlet.)

Winters, M. C.: Protective Body Mechanics in Daily Life and in Nursing, Philadelphia, Saunders, 1952.

Foot and Back Conditions

Emerson, C. P., and Bragdon, J. S.: Essentials of Medicine, ed. 17, pp. 693-694 (backache and spinal deformities), Philadelphia, Lippincott, 1955.

Howorth, M. B.: Your feet and your shoes, Am. J. Nursing **52**:1368, 1952.

Stimson, B. B.: Backache, Am. J. Nursing **51**:672-674, 1951.

Fractures—Traction—Casts

Bonfiglio, M., and Batchelet, A. E.: Slipping of the upper epiphysis of of the femur, Am. J. Nursing **53**: 1191-1195, 1953.

Calderwood, Carmelita: Internal derangement of the knee—nursing care, Am. J. Nursing **47**:22-23, 1947.

——: The patient comes out of his cast, Am. J. Nursing **44**:202-205, 1944.

——: Russell traction, Am. J. Nursing **43**:464-469, 1943.

Gibson, A.: Vitallium cup arthroplasty of the hip joint, J. Bone & Joint Surg. **31-A**:861-868, 1949.

Godecke, Janet: Traction and you, Am. J. Nursing **48**:123, 1948.

Hacker, G. I.: The medullary nail, Am. J. Nursing **50**:104-106, 1950.

Magnuson, Paul, and Stack, James: Fractures, ed. 5, Philadelphia, Lippincott, 1949.

Miller, B. L.: Well-leg and well-hip splints, Am. J. Nursing **48**:572-576, 1948.

Moore, Moore: Ambulation following fractures of the lower extremity, Am. J. Nursing **53**:174-175, 1953.

Shaar, C. M.: The Stader-splint, Am. J. Nursing **44**:215-220, 1944.

Wilde, O.: The patient in a spica—abed and afoot, Am. J. Nursing **51**:429-432, 1951.

——: Traction and suspension, Am. J. Nursing **53**:1465-1468, 1953.

Amputation

Glover, J. R.: The major amputations, Am. J. Nursing **50**:544-550, 1950.

Moskopp, M. E., and Sloan, J.: Nursing care for the amputee, Am. J. Nursing **50**:550-555, 1950.

Schwartz, O. R.: A year after—, Am. J. Nursing **46**:820-823, 1946.

Shimberg, M. M. D.: Amputation stumps and prosthesis, Pub. Health Nursing **37**:138-145, 1945.
Spittler, A. W., Woodward, G. S., and Cleland, C. K.: Cineplasty for arm amputees, Am. J. Nursing **53**: 802-805, 1953.

CONDITIONS OF BONE, JOINT, BURSAE

Allen, I. E.: Congenital dislocation of the hip, Am. J. Nursing **47**:722-726, 1947.
Anderson, H. C.: Nursing the patient with bone and joint tuberculosis, Am. J. Nursing **48**:215-220, 1948.
Emerson, C. P., and Bragdon, J. S.: Essentials of Medicine, ed. 17, pp. 679-697 (joint, bursae, arthritis); pp. 698-706 (bone); pp. 824-831 (poliomyelitis), Philadelphia, Lippincott, 1955.
Jones, M. H.: The cerebral palsy child, Am. J. Nursing **46**:465-468, 1946.
Kerr, Marion: Nursing responsibilities in cerebral palsy, Am. J. Nursing **46**:469-474, 1946.
Kilham, B. A.: Nursing patients with osteomyelitis, Am. J. Nursing **50**: 19-21, 1950.
Kottke, F. J., and Kubicek, W. G.: The patient with bulbar—respiratory poliomyelitis, Am. J. Nursing **49**:374-377, 1949.
Leavitt, H. L.: Bone and joint tuberculosis, Am. J. Nursing **48**:213-215, 1948.
Lowman, C. L.: Poliomyelitis. I. The management of poliomyelitis, Am. J. Nursing **47**:307-369, 1947.
Margolis, H. M.: Rheumatoid arthritis, Am. J. Nursing **47**:787-793, 1947.
Newton, Kathleen: Poliomyelitis. II. Psychological considerations in poliomyelitis care, Am. J. Nursing **47**:369-370, 1947.
Niemeier, V.: The child on a Bradford frame, Am. J. Nursing **45**: 1025-1026, 1945.
O'Brien, R. M.: Osteomyelitis, Am. J. Nursing **50**:17-19, 1950.
Seidenfeld, M. A.: Poliomyelitis. III. The nurse in poliomyelitis care, Am. J. Nursing **47**:371-372, 1947.
Stevenson, J. L.: Nursing for the poliomyelitis patient, Am. J. Nursing **48**:290-293, 1948.
Young, H. H.: Surgical treatment of arthritis, Am. J. Nursing **48**:27-29, 1948.

REHABILITATION—PROSTHESES

Barton, Betsy: The Long Walk, New York, Duell, 1948.
Clarke, C. D.: Facial and body prosthesis, Am. J. Nursing **48**:82-83, 1948.
Covalt, D. A., and Buchward, E.: Aids to ambulation, Am. J. Nursing **53**:1085-1088, 1953.
Covalt, N. K.: Early exercise for the convalescent patient, Am. J. Nursing **47**:544-546, 1947.
Henriksen, H. L., and Wilder, W. S.: The worker with a prosthesis, Am. J. Nursing **48**:444-448, 1948.
Jones, F. T.: The nurse's responsibility in rehabilitation, Am. J. Nursing **48**:76-79, 1948.
Knocke, L. S.: Role of the nurse in rehabilitation, Am. J. Nursing **47**: 238-240, 1947.
——: Some common types of braces, Am. J. Nursing **52**:868-869, 1952.
Morrissey, A. B., and Zimmerman, M. E.: Helps for the handicapped, Am. J. Nursing **53**:454-456, 1953.
Morrissey, A. B.: The nursing technics in rehabilitation, Am. J. Nursing **49**:545-551, 1949.

Olmsted, Lois: Crutch walking, Am. J. Nursing **45**:28-35, 1945.
Rusk, H. A.: Implication for nursing in rehabilitation, Am. J. Nursing **48**:74-76, 1948.
Rusk, H. A., and Taylor, F. J.: New Hope for the Handicapped, New York, Harper, 1949.
Soden, W. H.: Rehabilitation of the Handicapped, New York, Ronald, 1949.

CLINICAL SITUATION: CONGENITAL DISLOCATION OF THE HIP

Penelope was 15 months old when she began to walk. Her mother noticed an abnormal gait and called it to the attention of the pediatrician. He suggested that "Penny" be hospitalized for the correction of a congenital dislocation of the right hip.

1. Penny's unusual gait could be described best as
____(1) a waddle
____(2) a limp on the right side
____(3) a limp on the left side
____(4) typical of the toddler

2. Congenital dislocation of the hip might be discovered early if the nurse in the nursery notes
____(1) an extra fold of skin near the gluteal region on one side
____(2) a tendency to keep one leg flexed and the other extended
____(3) limited movement of one leg
____(4) inversion of the foot and adduction of the forefoot

3. Congenital hip dislocation probably can be corrected if treatment for Penny is instituted
____(1) immediately
____(2) between the ages of 2 and 5
____(3) between the ages of 6 and 10

4. Following manipulation under anesthesia, the child usually is placed in the following position:
____(1) The leg is placed in adduction, 45° to 90°.
____(2) The leg is placed in abduction, 45° to 90°.
____(3) Any position is permissible; no cast or splint is required.

5. If surgery is done, the objective of the operation is to
____(1) replace the femur in the acetabulum
____(2) replace the deformed femur with a vitallium prosthesis
____(3) create a new socket in which the head of the femur may rest
____(4) insert a jointed medullary bar into the femur and the acetabulum

UNIT ELEVEN

Nursing in Conditions of the Reproductive System

CHAPTER TWENTY-SEVEN

Diseases of the Female Reproductive Organs

INTRODUCTION

The gynecologic patient often calls for more understanding than other patients because, in addition to physical conditions, there are many emotional factors governing the situation. She may resent any reference to her genito-urinary system, feeling that she is suspected of questionable social or sexual habits. A real fear of venereal disease or of cancer may exist. All or any of these thoughts may manifest themselves in her conversation with the nurse, who by an understanding attitude can do much to dispel such anxieties.

Mixed emotional upsets can result from other fears. The suggestion of surgery as a means of treatment may raise a fear of disturbance of the reproductive process. Perhaps an explanation of the anatomy and the proposed treatment will clarify the situation. Any intention of sterilization must be explained carefully to the patient and her husband by the physician. Perhaps religious belief is more important to a patient than physical treatment. The decision rests with the patient and, when made, it must be respected and supported.

Psychic factors may present themselves at the menopausal period. The loss of the reproductive capacity may cause disappointment if the woman has had no children. For a woman with a grown family, it may mean that she feels there is no further need for her. Present methods of mass production have left the individual with much less to do than formerly, and leisure time may hang heavily on her hands. But the nurse will continue to practice the principles of good nursing care and bend her energies to helping her patient to orient herself to any change that may be necessary for her to make at this period.

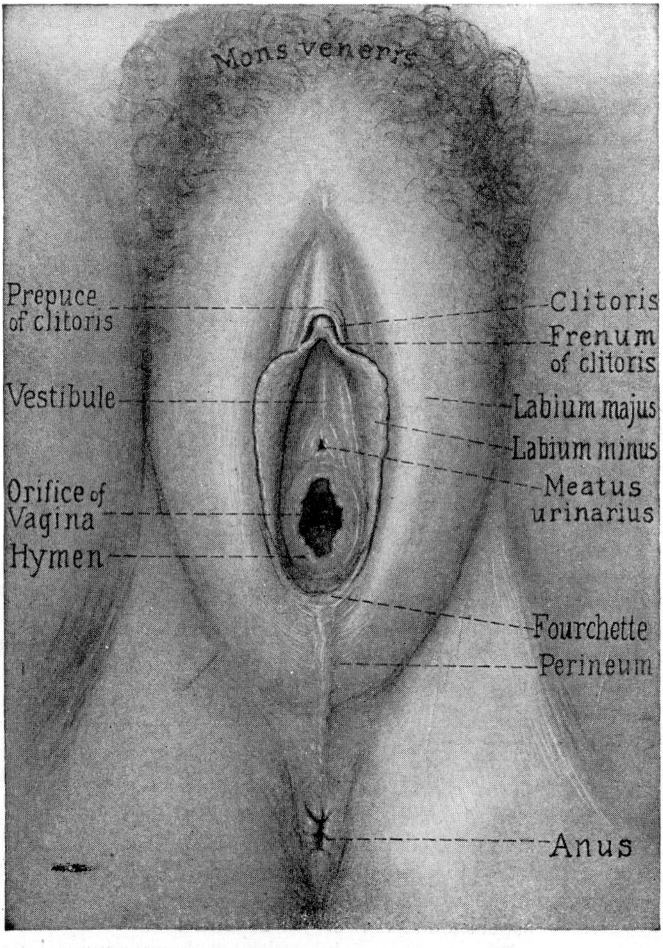

FIG. 258. External genitalia in the female.

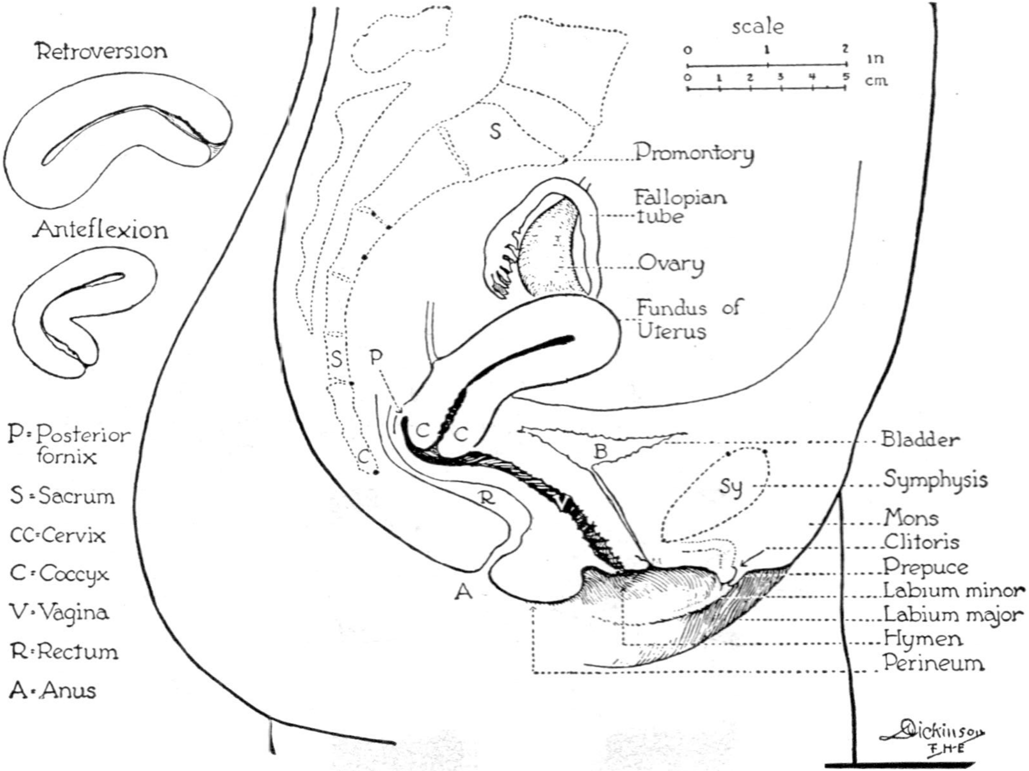

Fig. 259. Female pelvis and contents, standing, median section. (Robert L. Dickinson, M.D., New York City)

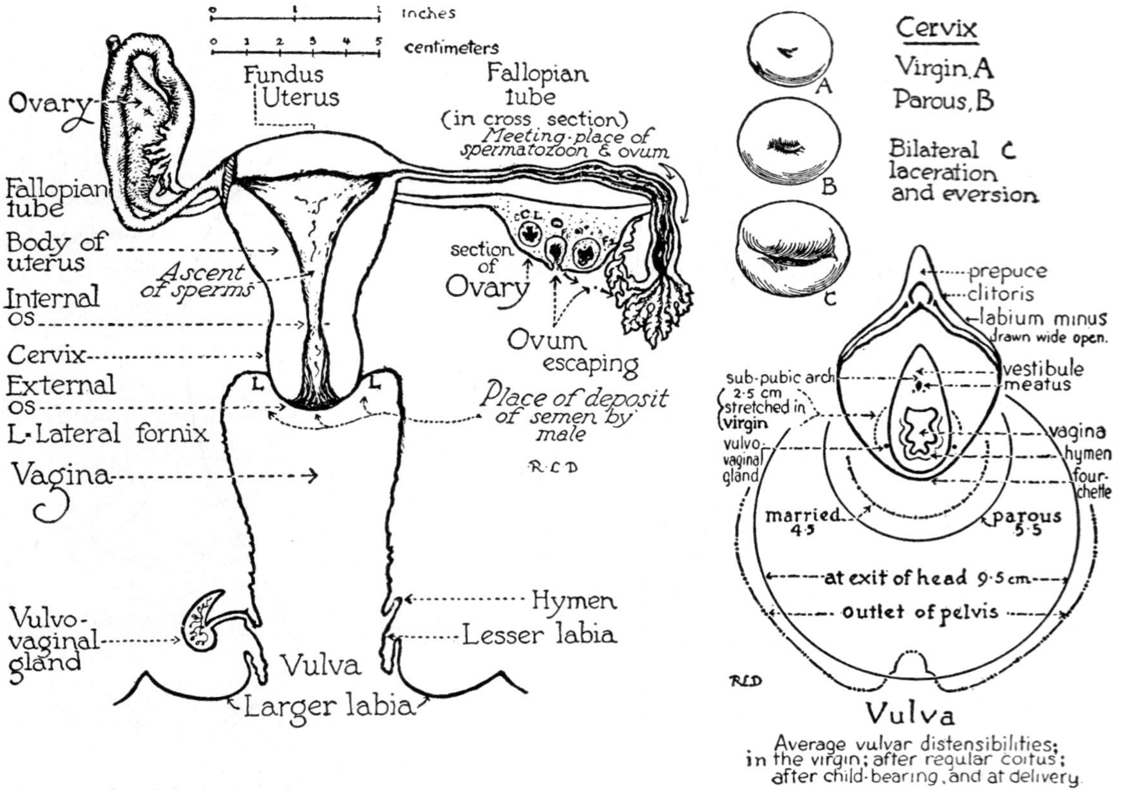

FIG. 260. Diagram of internal genitals. (*Left*) the ovary and the tube in true position; (*right*) spread out and cut in two to show inside structure. (Robert L. Dickinson, M.D., New York City)

ANATOMY AND PHYSIOLOGY

Anatomy

The nursing of the gynecologic patient requires a certain knowledge of the anatomy of the female organs. The external genitalia (vulva) are enclosed by the *labia majora*, two thick folds of tissue. They extend above from the hairy eminence over the pubic bones and the mons pubis, and are united below by a fold of tissue called the *posterior commissure*. The *labia minora* are two smaller lips of tissue covered with delicate skin within the labia majora. They unite above to form a partial covering for the *clitoris*, a highly sensitive organ made up of erectile tissue. Between the labia minora, below and posterior to the clitoris, is the external urinary meatus, the external opening of the short (1½ in.) female urethra. Below this orifice is a larger opening, the vaginal orifice, made smaller in the virgin by the *hymen*, a thin fold of tissue stretched across the lower part of the entrance to the vagina. It disappears largely after childbirth.

On each side of the vaginal orifice is located a *Bartholin's gland*, a small bean-sized gland that empties its mucous secretion by a small duct, the orifice of which is to be found within the labia minora, external to the hymen.

The tissue between the external genitals and the anus is called the *perineum*.

The *vagina* is the canal lined with mucous membrane, about 3 or 4 inches long, that extends downward and forward from the uterus to the vulva. Anterior to it are the bladder and the urethra, and below it lies the rectum. The anterior and the posterior walls normally lie in contact with one another. The upper part of the vagina, called the fornix, surrounds the cervix or the neck of the uterus.

The *uterus* is a pear-shaped muscular organ that in the virgin is about 3 inches long and about 2 inches wide at its upper part. Its walls are about ½ inch thick. It is divided into a narrow neck or cervix that projects into the vagina and a larger upper part, the fundus or body, that is covered posteriorly and partly anteriorly by peritoneum. It lies posterior to the bladder and is held in position in the pelvic cavity by several ligaments. The *round ligaments* extend anteriorly and laterally to the internal inguinal ring and down the inguinal canal, where they blend with the tissues of the labia majora. The *broad ligaments* are folds of peritoneum extending from the lateral pelvic walls and enveloping the fallopian tubes. The uterosacral ligaments extend posteriorly to the sacrum, and the uterovesical ligaments pass anteriorly. The cavity of the uterus is triangular in the fundus. It narrows to a small canal in the cervix that has a constriction at each end, the external and the internal os. The upper lateral parts of the uterus are called the *cornua*. From them extend outward the oviducts or fallopian tubes, the lumen of which is continuous internally with the uterine cavity.

The *ovaries* lie behind the broad ligaments, behind and below the tubes. They are oval-shaped bodies, from about 1 inch to 2 inches long, and they contain thousands of tiny egg cells or ova. The ovaries and the fallopian tubes are called the *adnexae.*

Physiology

The ovary, which normally contains from 30,000 to 40,000 ova, remains quiescent in early life, but at the time of puberty, usually between the twelfth and the fourteenth years, a new function appears. The ova begin to ripen or mature, enlarging as a sort of cyst known as a *graafian follicle.* The cyst enlarges till it reaches the surface of the ovary, where rupture occurs and the ovum is discharged into the peritoneal cavity. This function of periodic discharge of matured ova is called *ovulation.* The ovum usually finds its way into the fallopian tube, where it is carried to the uterus. If it meets a spermatozoon, the male reproduction cell, a union occurs and *conception* takes place. Following the discharge of the ovum, the cells of the graafian follicle undergo a rapid change. Gradually they become yellow in color (the corpus luteum) and produce a secretion that has the function of preparing the uterus for the reception of the fertilized ovum.

If conception does not occur, the ovum dies and the mucous membrane lining the uterus (the endometrium), which has become thickened and congested, becomes hemorrhagic. The upper layer of lining cells and the blood that appears in the uterine cavity are discharged through the cervix and the vagina. This flow of blood, mixed with mucus and cells, which occurs as a rule every 28 days during the sexual life of females, is called *menstruation.* The period of flow lasts usually from 4 to 5 days, during which time from about 50 to 60 cc. of blood is lost. After the cessation of the menstrual flow the endometrium returns to an inactive state until stimulated again by ovulation. It is believed that ovulation usually occurs midway between menstrual periods. During the menstrual periods there is often a physical as well as a mental depression.

Between the ages of 45 and 50 years, there is in most women a cessation of the menstrual flow, which period is called the *menopause* (change of life). This period is associated with atrophy of the breasts and genital organs, and often with psychic and vascular disturbances. At this time malignant disease often develops in the uterus and the breasts. If ovarian secretion is terminated suddenly by removal of the ovaries or by irradiation, an artificial menopause may be induced. This may produce even more marked symptoms than the normal menopause. Substitution endocrine therapy often is helpful to tide the patient over this distressing period of physiologic readjustment.

DISTURBANCES OF MENSTRUATION

There is a definite interrelation between the hormonal secretions of the ovary, the thyroid and the pituitary glands. A disturbance of this relationship, an increased or decreased function of one or more of these glands, may have an influence on the menstrual function. This is probably the most common cause of menstrual disturbances.

Dysmenorrhea, or painful menstruation, is a common condition found most often in unmarried women. The pain probably is due to uterine spasm. This may be caused by a narrowing of the cervical canal, but is more probably a result of endocrine gland dysfunction. The symptoms, acute cramplike pains in the lower abdomen, often associated with headache and vomiting, are most severe during the first day of the period. Pregnancy and childbirth often cure the condition.

TREATMENT. The treatment of dysmenorrhea may be medical, surgical and/or psychological. The medical treatment comprises rest in bed, the application of heat over the lower abdomen and the administration of such drugs as aspirin, benzedrine, atropine and glandular extracts. In the surgical treatment an effort is made to correct the conditions causing the narrowing of the cervical canal. Displacements of the uterus (pp. 621-622) are corrected, and the cervical canal is dilated or stretched. Perhaps correction of poor hygienic and dietary habits is all that is necessary. Emotional upsets must be investigated and corrected. Some physicians prescribe pelvic exercises and others have treated the condition by cutting nerve fibers (presacral neurectomy).

Amenorrhea, or the absence of menstrual flow, occurs normally during pregnancy and lactation. However, extreme anxiety, acute or chronic disease, anemia or disease of the ductless glands (especially of the thyroid and the pituitary and certain ovarian tumors, particularly arrhenoblastomas) may cause amenorrhea.

TREATMENT. The treatment is directed toward the correction of the cause. Often there is a hypopituitary or thyroid function that may be helped by appropriate glandular extracts.

Menorrhagia is excessive bleeding at the time of the regular menstrual flow. Its cause in early life may be due to endocrine disturbances, but menorrhagia with increase in duration of the menstrual periods in later life usually is due to inflammatory disturbances or tumors of the uterus.

Metrorrhagia is the appearance of blood from the uterus between the regular menstrual periods or after the menopause. It is always the symptom of some disease, often cancer or benign tumors of the uterus; therefore, it merits early diagnosis and treatment.

Leukorrhea is the name given to a whitish or yellowish vaginal discharge. It may be the result of one or more vaginal or uterine diseases, acute or chronic infections, lacerations of the cervix and neoplasms.

NURSING CARE. The nursing care comprises cleansing antiseptic douches. Correction of the cause of the discharge is necessary for cure.

DIAGNOSTIC TESTS

Examination of Patient. The patient who is to have a gynecologic examination often has many fears and worries. She needs reassurance, understanding and tactful regard for her emotional as well as her physical problems. Preparation includes voiding and evacuation of the bowels. Sufficient clothing should be removed to allow adequate exposure of the genitalia. All bands about the waist

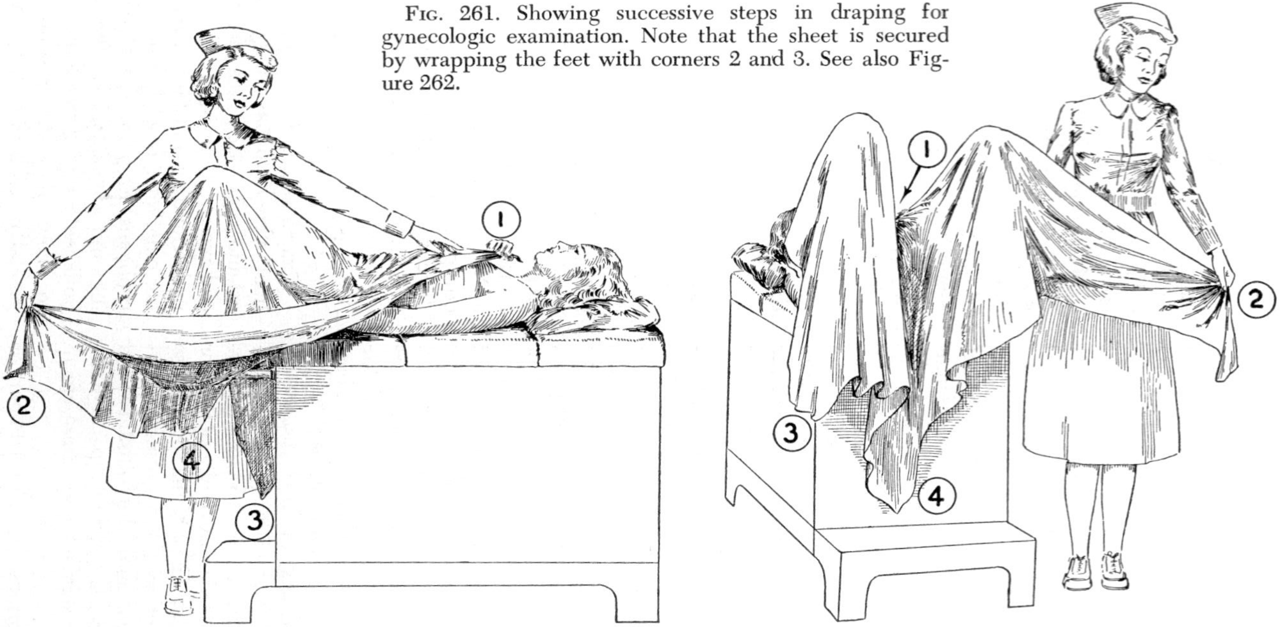

Fig. 261. Showing successive steps in draping for gynecologic examination. Note that the sheet is secured by wrapping the feet with corners 2 and 3. See also Figure 262.

must be loosened and corsets removed to permit examination of the abdomen. In the preparation for the examination and in placing the patient on the examining table, the nurse should take special precautions to avoid exposing the patient. The nurse should be in attendance during the examination.

Positions. The examination of the patient for gynecologic disease is made best with the patient on the examining table. Three positions are employed commonly for these examinations. The most common is the dorsal position, with the knees and the hips flexed and the heels resting in foot rests. A sheet is draped diagonally over the patient, the lower corner being caught in the hands and gathered up so as to expose the vulva. A small towel then may be used to cover the exposed parts until the surgeon is ready to make the examination (Fig. 263).

In Sims's position, the patient lies on one side, usually the left, with her left arm behind her back. The

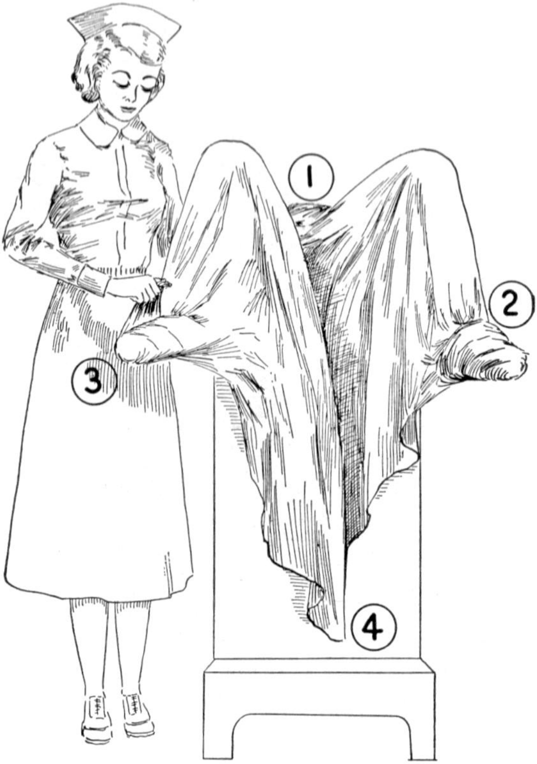

FIG. 262. See also Figure 261.

right (uppermost) thigh and the knee are flexed as fully as possible, and the left leg is partly flexed. A sheet then is draped over the lower extremities and hips in such a way as to expose the genitalia (Fig. 264).

In the knee-chest position, the patient kneels on the table so that the feet extend over the end. The knees should be separated and the thighs at right angles to the table. The head is turned to one side and the arms grasp the sides of the table; the chest and the side of the face rest on a soft pillow (Fig. 265).

If for any reason an examining table is not available, or the patient

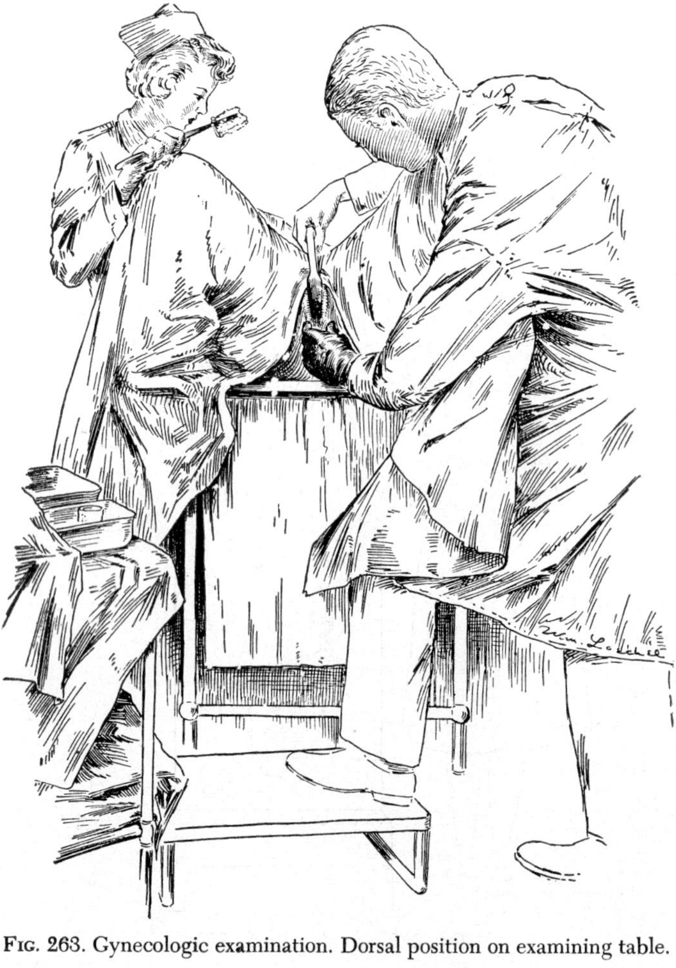

FIG. 263. Gynecologic examination. Dorsal position on examining table.

cannot be moved conveniently, these positions may be assumed in bed. Many surgeons prefer to make the examination in the dorsal position with the patient across the bed, the hips extending slightly over the edge and the feet on the examiner's knees or on two chairs placed beside the bed. The cross-bed position must be used if instruments are to be used in making the examination. A sheet drape is used to cover the patient in the same way as for the table examinations.

Examining Tray. For examining patients the nurse should prepare a tray containing the following sterile supplies and instruments:

Specula—one small and one large of each kind
Sims, bivalve speculum
2 Double tenaculum forceps
1 Speculum forceps
1 Uterine sound
1 Probe
1 Pair gloves
1 Basin with an antiseptic solution
Receptacle containing cotton balls
Culture tube and glass slides
Tampons
Lubricant

The tray should be covered with a sterile towel and kept out of sight of the patient.

The Examination. This includes first an inspection of the external genitalia, then an examination of the vagina and the cervix, the speculum being used to expose the parts. Finally, a bimanual examination is

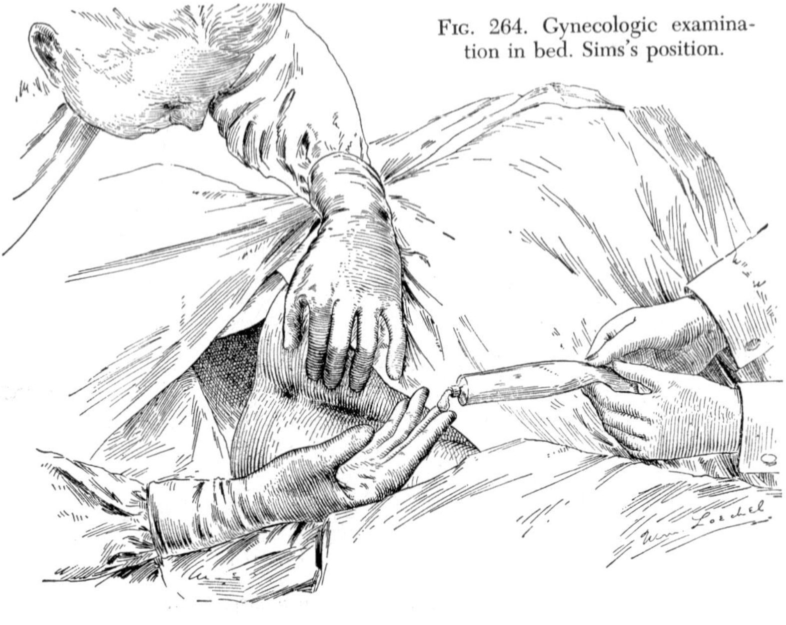

FIG. 264. Gynecologic examination in bed. Sims's position.

made by inserting one or two fingers of the left hand in the vaginal canal and palpating the abdomen with the right hand. In this way the uterus and the adnexa may be more or less accurately examined.

Cytologic Test for Cancer (Papanicolaou). This test is done for the purpose of diagnosing genital cancer. It comprises the aspirating or the swabbing of vaginal secretions from the posterior fornix and making a smear on a glass slide. The secretion usually is "fixed" immediately by immersing the slide in equal parts of 95 per cent alcohol and ether. The slides then are sent to a laboratory, where they are stained and read by skilled pathologists.

Dilatation and Curettage. For this procedure, the patient usually is sent to the operating room, and preoperative preparation is determined by the nature of the anesthetic agent. With the patient in the lithotomy position, the cervix is dilated with an instrument and scrapings of the endometrium are obtained by means of a curette. Tissue for biopsy also may be obtained by cutting with an electric needle or by using a punch biopsy forceps. After operation, the

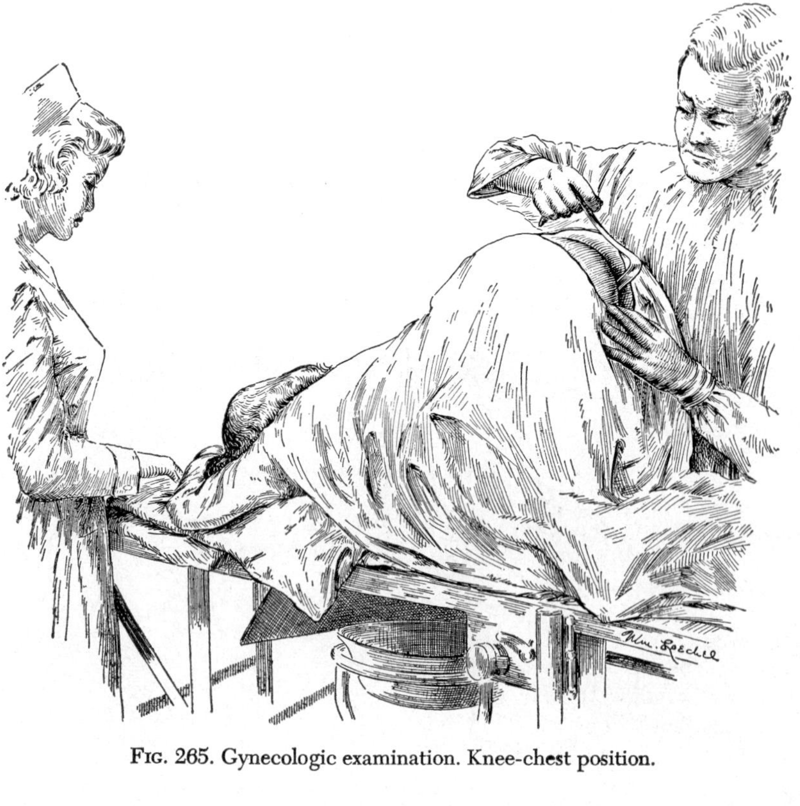

FIG. 265. Gynecologic examination. Knee-chest position.

patient usually prefers to rest the remainder of the day. Her diet is as she desires. Hemorrhage and inability to void must be watched for and a sedative given for discomfort.

Nursing of Gynecologic Patients

Because many gynecologic diseases may be caused by highly infective organisms, especially the gonococcus, it is absolutely imperative that all instruments and apparatus (catheters, douche nozzles, bedpans, rectal tubes and so forth) used in the treatment be sterilized both before and after their use. The nurse may protect herself by the use of rubber gloves, which should be cleansed and resterilized after treating each patient. If gloves are not available, or the procedure does not require their use, it is wise to scrub the hands thoroughly, especially after having had anything to do with an infected patient. When possible, dressings, vulvar pads and so forth should be handled with forceps, and forceps should be sterilized between cases.

The spread of an infection from one patient to another, or to the nurse, is evidence of extreme laxity and carelessness in the nursing personnel, and its possibility should be constantly in mind in gynecologic work.

A second admonition to the gynecologic nurse is this: Never talk about your patient or her disease. Gynecologic diseases often are of such a personal and private nature that no patient would wish her nurse to tell other nurses, friends, or even her own family, the details of her operation or treatment. All such questions must be referred to the surgeon in charge of the patient. He alone is responsible. It is up to him to decide what information to give concerning his patient and which person should get it.

PREPARATION OF PATIENT FOR GYNECOLOGIC OPERATIONS

This differs little from the details described for the preparation of a patient for a laparotomy. The lower half of the abdomen and the pubic and the perineal regions should be carefully shaved and cleansed with green soap and water. The bowels and the bladder should be empty before the patient is sent to the operating room. This is most important.

Douches

Douches are common therapeutic measures in the treatment of patients with gynecologic diseases. They are used both before and after operation and are of two types: (1) vulvar and (2) vaginal.

Vulvar Irrigations. These are indicated chiefly after operations on the perineum. They should be given after each urination or bowel movement in an effort to keep the incision free from infection. The patient should be brought to the right side of the bed and placed on the douche pan in the dorsal position, with the knees apart and the labia separated. The bed should be protected by placing a rubber or plastic sheet under the pan. Warmed sterile water then is poured gently over the vulva from a sterile pitcher. The area is dried with sterile gauze or cotton, and a sterile dressing or pad is applied and held in place with a T binder.

Vaginal Douches. Vaginal douches are used therapeutically to cleanse or disinfect the vagina and adjacent parts both before and after operation. They may be used also to soothe inflamed tissues and to stimulate relaxed tissues. Occasionally hot or cold douches are indicated in the treatment of oozing from the parts.

The patient is prepared for a vaginal douche in the same manner as for a vulvar douche. The equipment necessary is as follows:

Infusion pole on which douche bag may be hung
A Kelly pad or plastic sheet with douche pan
Sterile gloves, used for protection of both patient and nurse
Sterile douche tray containing:
Irrigating outfit:
Enamel can or rubber douche bag, rubber tubing with shutoff clamp and curved douche nozzle
Curved basin
Container with cleansing solution
Cotton sponges (small and large)
Solution as ordered

The solutions commonly used are:
(1) For simple cleansing:
Sterile water
Normal saline solution
Boric-acid solution (1 tsp. to 1 qt. of water)
(2) For disinfection:
Potassium permanganate, 1:4,000 solution
Bichloride of mercury, 1:8,000 solution
Vinegar (4 tbsp. to 1 qt. water)
(3) For astringent action:
Alum or zinc sulfate (1 tsp. to 1 qt. of water)

All these douches should be given at a temperature of 110° F. or as ordered.

Douche Procedure

To give the douche, the patient is placed in the dorsal position on the douche pan and covered to prevent chilling. The tube leading from the douche bag is clamped, and the end of the tube with the douche nozzle is inserted into the reservoir, which then is hung on the standard. The reservoir should be not more than 2 feet above the level of the patient's hips. The nurse then puts on the sterile gloves and, separating the labia with the thumb and the forefinger of the left hand, the vaginal orifice is cleansed and the douche nozzle is inserted gently into the vagina for a distance of 2 inches, the tip being directed toward the hollow of the sacrum. The clamp then is removed from the tube, and the solution is allowed to flow. Pressure should be avoided to prevent douche fluid refluxing through the uterus and the tubes. This can be done intermittently until at least one liter of solution has been used. The procedure should not be done hastily if therapeutic benefits are to be achieved. It should take from 20 to 30 minutes. At this time, the nozzle may be removed and the patient should be asked to strain as if trying to move the bowels. This act tends to expel the fluid remaining in the vagina. The douche pan then is removed and the parts are dried with cotton. The patient should be instructed to remain flat on her back for at least an hour after a hot douche. After the douche has been completed, the apparatus should be cleansed and sterilized again, including the bedpan.

Vaginal Antiseptic Jellies

Since the advent of chemotherapy, sulfa and penicillin jellies have been available for local application.

By means of an applicator, the patient is able to administer such medication. Creams or jellies can be used before and after operation, and in many instances they are substituted for the therapeutic and cleansing douche. It may be necessary for the patient to wear a perineal pad during the course of the application.

CONDITIONS OF EXTERNAL GENITALIA AND VAGINA

Vulvitis and Abscess of Bartholin's Glands

Vulvitis, an inflammation of the vulva, may occur as a result of uncleanliness or irritating discharges, but most often it is the result of a gonorrheal infection. The infecting organism, the gonococcus, "is infectious only in the moist state and grows only on moist surfaces. Under dry conditions it soon dies. Gonorrhea is therefore, an almost purely contagious disease and is rarely transferred indirectly except in the case of young children. With this last exception, gonorrhea of the genitals is transmitted almost exclusively by sexual contact." (Graves.) (See p. 634.)

Symptoms. The symptoms of the disease may be very slight, but in the typical case the patient complains of a constant burning pain that is worse during urination and defecation. The genitalia become red and edematous, and there is a profuse purulent exudate, in which the gonococci may be found by examination of a smear.

The infection usually involves Bartholin's gland, the glands in the floor of the urethra and those in the cervix of the uterus. Not infrequently, the infection of Bartholin's gland leads to the formation of an abscess (vulvovaginal) that is characterized by more acute throbbing pain and swelling between the labia.

Treatment. In the treatment of such a condition, the antibiotics (especially penicillin) are most effective. Not infrequently, the inflammatory reaction may subside, but there usually is a recurrence later if the gland is not excised. The duct of the gland often may be occluded after subsidence of the inflammation. As the gland continues to secrete, a Bartholin's cyst is formed. These cysts usually are removed surgically.

Once the acute stage of the infection has passed, the disease tends to become chronic. The organisms lurk in the infected glands and the patient becomes a constant source of infection for others, often innocent persons. She is likely to have recrudescences of the disease with extension of the infection to the uterus, the fallopian tubes, and even the peritoneal cavity. (For additional treatment, see p. 624.)

Vaginitis

Vaginitis is an inflammation of the lining of the vaginal wall. *Trichomonas vaginalis* and *Monilia albicans* are two very common parasitic invaders. They produce intense itching and characteristic discharges.

Trichomonas vaginalis can be controlled by using Floraquin, which restores the glycogen, the *Döderlein bacilli* and the acidity which are characteristics of normal vaginal tissue. A more recent treatment is the insertion of gelatin capsules of chlortetracycline every other night for a period of 2 weeks. *Monilia albicans* is treated successfully by swabbing with gentian violet. Certain medi-

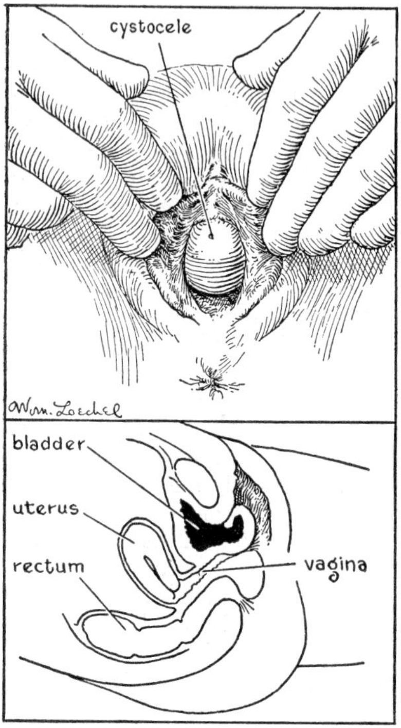

FIG. 266. Cystocele. Relaxation of the anterior vaginal wall permits downward bulge of bladder on straining.

cated jellies are also effective and more convenient to apply.

GONORRHEAL VULVOVAGINITIS

This occurs often in infants and in little girls by indirect infection through towels, diapers, thermometers and the hands of attendants. It is not uncommon for an epidemic of this disease to occur in babies' and children's wards in hospitals or institutions; for this reason, every female child admitted to such an institution should be examined and a smear taken from the vulva for microscopic examination.

Treatment. The treatment of acute gonorrheal vulvitis and vulvovaginitis is carried out best with the patient in bed. Soft diet, especially plenty of fluids, and urinary antiseptics comprise the early treatment. Female sex hormone has been used with success. This may be given hypodermically or by vaginal suppositories. Penicillin is used with excellent results.

The nurse must employ every possible precaution against spreading the infection to other patients by instruments, dressings, bedpans and towels, and, in addition, especially in children, care must be taken against infecting the eyes. (See p. 449.)

CONDYLOMATA

Condylomata are warty papillary excrescences that appear on the external genitalia. They are the result of irritation and infection. There are two usual types: those of the pointed type are associated with gonorrhea; the flat condylomata usually are considered to be syphilitic in origin. The condylomata of themselves cause few symptoms, but nearly always there is an associated leukorrheal discharge that causes maceration and irritation.

CYSTOCELE

Cystocele is a downward displacement of the bladder toward the vaginal orifice. It is caused occasionally by tissue weakness, but most often it is a result of injuries received during childbirth. The condition appears as a bulging downward of the anterior vaginal wall that causes a sense of pelvic pressure, easy fatigue and, often such urinary symptoms as incontinence, frequency and urgency of urination.

Treatment. The treatment of the condition is surgical, the operation for the repair of the anterior vaginal wall being termed *anterior colporrhaphy*. Perineal exercises sometimes are prescribed and help to strengthen the weakened muscles. These are more effective in the early stages of a cystocele.

Kraurosis

This is a disease of the vulva in which the skin over these structures becomes thin and white and easily fissured. As the disease advances, the structure of the vulva may be shrunken and leathery in appearance. The chief symptom is marked itching. Often it leads to the development of cancer of the vulva.

Treatment. Ovarian extract, antihistaminics and vitamin A have been used with some success in the treatment of these patients, but in advanced cases vulvectomy often is performed.

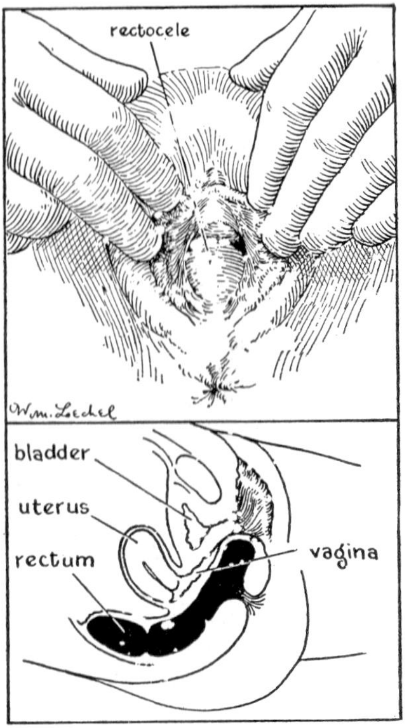

Fig. 267. Rectocele. Relaxation of the posterior vaginal wall permits bulging of the rectum with the vagina on straining.

Rectocele and Lacerations of Perineum

Injuries to the muscles and the tissues of the pelvic floor frequently occur at the time of childbirth. Due to tears in muscles below the vagina, the rectum may pouch upward, pushing the posterior wall of the vagina in front of it. This condition is termed a *rectocele*. The lacerations may extend at times so as to sever completely the fibers of the anal sphincter (complete tear). The symptoms of this condition are similar to those given for cystocele, substituting for the urinary symptoms those of constipation and incontinence of gas and liquid feces in cases with complete tears.

Treatment. The operation for the repair of these cases is called a perineorrhaphy or a posterior colporrhaphy. Anterior and posterior colporrhaphies often are classed together under the term *plastic operations*.

Nursing Care After Perineal Operations

The patient always is urged to void within a few hours after operation, and every 4 to 8 hours thereafter. The bladder should not be allowed to accumulate more than 5 ounces of urine for the first few days, especially after operations for cystocele and complete tear. If the patient does not void within the above period, or if she feels uncomfortable or has pain in the region of the bladder before 6 hours, catheterization should be performed. Some physicians prefer to have an indwelling catheter in the patient for from 2 to 4 days. There are various other methods of bladder care.

After each urination or bowel movement, the perineum should be irrigated with warm sterile saline (see vulvar douche) and the area dried with sterile cotton.

There are two methods used in caring for the stitches: one by which the stitches are left alone until healing occurs, i.e., for from 5 to 10 days, and daily vaginal douches of sterile saline given thereafter during the period of convalescence; the other, the wet method, in which small douches of sterile saline are given twice daily, beginning on the day after operation and continuing throughout convalescence. The method to be used depends, of course, on the preference of the surgeon.

The routine postoperative care is much like that after an abdominal operation. The patient is placed in bed with the head and the knees elevated slightly. Liquid diet (many surgeons omit milk) is given for the first day and then full diet as soon as desired.

Patients after operations for a complete perineal laceration (through the rectal sphincter) require special care and attention. The bladder should be emptied by catheterization if the patient is having discomfort. The patient should be kept flat in bed with the head raised on a pillow. Most surgeons prefer no bowel movements for from 5 to 7 days. A rectal tube should not be introduced during this period, and enemas never are used. Liquid diet without milk is given and, in order to reduce peristalsis and "lock the bowels," opium pills or tincture of opium (15 minims) may be administered. On the sixth or the seventh day, the bowels are opened by giving 1 ounce of mineral oil, followed at the first inclination for a bowel movement by a small oil enema (3 or 4 ounces) that should be retained for a few minutes.

Throughout the convalescence of all plastic patients, liquid petrolatum, oz. i, is given each night after soft diet is begun.

CONDITIONS OF UTERUS

Lacerations of Cervix

Lacerations of the cervix often occur as a result of childbirth. When healing takes place, a considerable portion of the mucous membrane, which normally lies in the cervical canal, is everted. It practically always becomes infected and causes an annoying leukorrhea. Most surgeons believe that cervical lacerations predispose to cancer of the cervix, and for this reason these lacerations should be repaired, particularly in the fifth decade, the time when cancer is most likely to occur.

Endocervicitis

Endocervicitis is an inflammation of the mucosa and the glands of the cervix. In the majority of cases, the inflammation is caused by the ordinary pyogenic organisms, but gonorrheal infection of the gland occurs not infrequently. The chief symptom is a thick purulent leukorrheal discharge, at times associated with sacral backache, low abdominal pain and disturbances in menstruation.

Treatment. Palliåtive treatment consists of douches and the application of antiseptics to the cervix, but often a cure is effected only after destroying the cervical glands with a cautery or excising the diseased tissue. Bacitracin in combination with penicillin is proving effective in the treatment of chronic cervicitis and cervical erosion.

Cancer of Cervix

Cancer of the cervix may occur at any age, but most commonly it is between the ages of 30 and 50. (Review Chap. 11, pp. 195-204.) It is found most often in patients with cervical lacerations due to childbirth. It may become a large cauliflowerlike growth or a deep ulcerating crater before giving many symptoms of its presence.

Symptoms. The two chief symptoms of early carcinoma are leukorrhea and irregular vaginal bleeding. For a long time the leukorrhea may be the only abnormal symptom. The discharge increases gradually in amount, becomes watery and, finally, dark and foul-smelling when there are necrosis and infection of the tumor mass. The bleeding occurs at irregular intervals, between the periods or after the menopause (metrorrhagia). It may be very slight, just enough to spot the undergarments, and it is noted usually after some form of trauma (intercourse, douching or defecation). As the disease continues, the bleeding may become constant and increase in amount.

As the cancer advances, the tissues outside the cervix are invaded, including the lymph glands anterior to the sacrum. The nerves in this region become involved, so that there is excruciating pain in the back and the legs that is relieved only by large doses of morphine. The final picture is one of extreme emaciation and anemia, often with irregular fever due to secondary infection and absorption from the ulcerating mass.

Treatment. Except in a few clinics, surgical removal of the cervical cancer has been abandoned in this country in favor of radium and roentgen therapy. By this method of treatment a cure may be effected in about 40 per cent of all cases and in from about 50 to 80 per cent of the cases in which the growth still is confined to the cervix. Because early diagnosis and treatment are the only hope of a permanent cure, the nursing and the medical professions have a real responsibility in informing the public that leukorrhea or bleeding from the vagina at abnormal times and in abnormal amounts, especially in a woman past the menopause, should lead to an immediate examination by a competent physician. Periodic examinations also should be encouraged.

Nursing Care

Whether a woman has a *simple hysterectomy* (removal of the uterus) or a *radical panhysterectomy* (entire uterus, both tubes and ovaries), the psychological factors are significant. Often, she has fears regarding the ultimate effects of such surgery. These concern the possibilities of not becoming pregnant, of having satisfactory marital relations, of having a recurrence of the malignancy and of facing uncontrollable weight gain. By developing an atmosphere of confidence, the nurse can encourage her patient to share her concerns. When medical advice is necessary, it should be sought.

Physically, the preoperative preparation and postoperative care of this patient are the same as for abdominal surgical patients. Following a hysterectomy, the patient probably will experience *surgical menopause.* The symptoms vary in different patients; they are manifested by "hot flashes," irritability and palpitation of the heart. Estrogens usually are prescribed and may be administered orally, intramuscularly or implanted as pellets in the rectal muscles.

Radium. Radium is being used by many surgeons in the prophylatic treatment of operable cases and in the palliative treatment of many inoperable cases. It is applied in small tubes encased in metal and rubber filters that have heavy silk threads tied to them. These should be anchored to the thigh with adhesive. Another device used in applying and directing radium to a particular area is the Ernst applicator. Radium applications may last from several hours to 3 or 4 days.

Nursing Care for Patients Receiving Radium Treatment

The responsibilities of the nurse are the same as for any postoperative case. She should give special attention to keeping the patient in the dorsal position and see to it that the radium tubes are not dislodged. Plain or medicated packing usually is inserted to stabilize the position of the radium. Often an indwelling catheter is inserted in the operating room. This catheter should be inspected frequently to make sure that it is draining properly. The chief hazard of improper drainage is that the bladder may become distended and be in the path of radiation.

A linen bag is kept in the patient's unit, and any soiled linen is stored there until the radium has been removed and accounted for. The patient is observed for evidence of temperature elevation, nausea or vomiting. These symptoms should be reported to the physician, as often they are indicative of radium sickness; newer drugs are appearing on the market for their relief. These patients often have poor appetites and need to be encouraged to eat and drink.

At the end of the prescribed period (the nurse should know the duration of the application), she should notify the surgeon in charge that it is time for the removal of the radium. Sterile gloves, long forceps and a waste basin should be provided for his use.

Radium is the most expensive metal in common use today. The tiny amount used in the application often is valued at thousands of dollars, so that extreme care is necessary in handling the tubes after their removal from a patient. The number of tubes applied should be noted on the operating sheet, and the nurse should be sure that the same number is removed. After removal from the filters, the tubes should be placed in small lead or brass bottles supplied for the purpose and taken immediately to the hospital repository. Burns may be obtained by an overdosage; that is, by not removing the radium at the end of the prescribed time or by too frequent handling of radium tubes. For this reason they should be removed promptly from the patient at the end of the prescribed period and handled as much as possible with long forceps, preferably behind a lead shield. After the patient has had the radium removed, usually she is given a cleansing enema and then may be out of bed. (See p. 200, Radiation Therapy.)

Nursing Care for Patients Receiving Roentgen Therapy

Unfortunately, before x-rays can reach the tissue which requires treatment, they must pass through healthy tissue. The skin is especially vulnerable, and caution must be practiced in order to avoid burns. Following large doses of x-rays, the patient may show anorexia, nausea and vomiting. These should be reported to the physician, who will decide whether treatment should continue.

During treatment, the nurse should encourage her patient to drink citrus-fruit juices. Small, frequent servings may be more appetizing than large servings. The skin usually is kept dry; when very red or denuded areas occur, a bland ointment may be prescribed. Pyridoxine orally is helpful in minimizing discomfort.

Displacements of Uterus

The uterus lies normally with the cervix at right angles to the long axis of the vagina and with the body inclined slightly forward. However, it is freely movable, owing to the requirements of pregnancy. The strain of this physiologic function, the formation of adhesions or a weakening of its natural supports may produce changes in the normal position that usually cause no trouble to the patient but may give rise to many troublesome symptoms.

Backward Displacements. The backward displacements (retroversion and retroflexion) may give rise to such symptoms as backache, a sense of pelvic pressure, easy fatigue, and leukorrheal discharge. More retrograde displacements are asymptomatic rather than symptomatic.

Treatment. The treatment of backward displacements is surgical only if the condition is incapacitating. The uterus is brought forward into its normal position by way of an abdominal incision and maintained by shortening its ligaments. Some patients with retroversion may be treated by the use of pessaries. These are S-shaped instruments of hard rubber or crystal-clear Plexiglas that keep the uterus forward by exerting pressure on ligaments attached to the posterior wall of the cervix. They are of great value as a test of the patient's symptoms and often effect a cure. Pessaries must be removed and cleaned by the surgeon at frequent intervals.

Prolapse and Procidentia. Due to the weakening of the supports of the uterus most often brought about by childbirth, the uterus may work its way down the vaginal canal (prolapse) and even appear outside the vaginal orifice (procidentia). In its

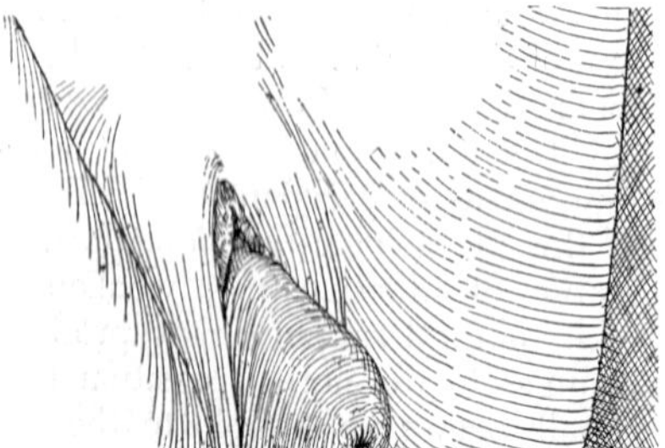

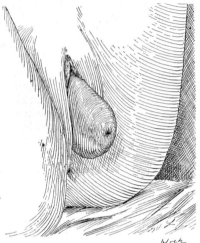

FIG. 268. Procidentia uteri. This is really a vaginal hernia caused by relaxation of the uterine ligaments. The vagina turns inside out and protrudes through the vulva. The opening in the center of the prolapsed vagina is the cervix.

descent the uterus pulls with it the vaginal walls and even the bladder and the rectum. The symptoms caused are similar to those mentioned for backward displacements, plus urinary symptoms (incontinence and retention) due to displacement of the bladder.

TREATMENT. The best treatment is operative; the uterus is sutured back into place. In patients after the menopause, the uterus may be removed (hysterectomy). Many patients may be treated by pessaries when, because of age or disease, operation is not feasible.

Patients with prolapse or procidentia should be kept flat in bed for 2 or 3 days with a vaginal pack or pessary in place. This treatment serves to take the tension off the strained ligaments and allows the surgeon to proceed with greater ease.

Anterior Displacements. Anterior displacements of the uterus may give no symptoms, but often they are associated with dysmenorrhea or sterility, or both.

TREATMENT. This may be operative. Or a stem pessary may be used, a rubber or glass rod being introduced into the uterus for about 6 weeks to hold it in position.

MYOMATA OR FIBROID TUMORS

Myomatous or fibroid tumors of the uterus are benign tumors arising from the muscle tissue of the uterus. They are very common, occurring in at least 40 per cent of all women (Graves). They develop slowly between the ages of 25 and 40 and often attain large size after this period. They produce symptoms due to pressure on surrounding organs—pain, backache, constipation and urinary symptoms—and they often cause menorrhagia, metrorrhagia, and even sterility.

Treatment and Nursing Care. The treatment of uterine fibroids depends to a large extent upon their size and location. Large tumors producing pressure symptoms should be removed as a rule. Usually the uterus is removed (hysterectomy), the ovaries being preserved if possible. If the tumor is small, it may be removed (myomectomy), the wound in the uterus being closed. This is the procedure of choice in young women. If the tumor is producing excessive bleeding, the uterus and the tumor are removed above the cervix (hysteromyomectomy). In

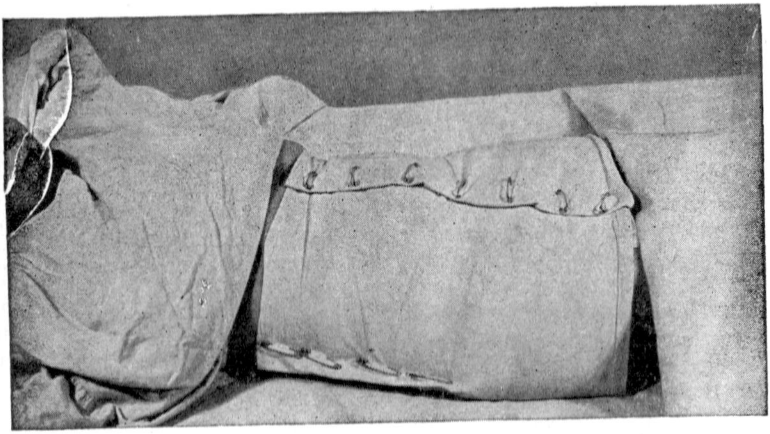

FIG. 269. Showing how abdominal binder is fitted to patient with safety pins.

some cases, radium or x-ray treatment is successful in reducing the size of the tumor and in checking the menorrhagia.

The postoperative care after removal of the uterus does not differ in the ordinary case from that described for any laparotomy. In patients in whom there is anemia due to the loss of blood caused by the tumor, convalescence may be hastened by a high caloric diet that is rich in liver. If the tumor has been so large as to produce marked relaxation of the abdominal walls, often it is wise to advise the patient to wear a supporting belt for a time after operation. In these patients it is well to apply an abdominal binder immediately after operation to be worn until a belt is obtained.

Cancer of Fundus

Cancer of the fundus of the uterus is seen only about one-eighth as often as cancer of the cervix. About 50 per cent of all patients with postmenopausal bleeding have cancer of the fundus. Its progress is slow, metastasis occurs later, and the symptom of irregular vaginal bleeding often appears early enough in the disease to allow cure by the removal of the uterus. In late cases, radium and x-ray are the usual therapeutic measures.

CONDITIONS OF OVARIES AND BROAD LIGAMENTS

Ovarian Cysts and Tumors

The ovary is a frequent site for the development of cysts. These may be simply pathologic enlargements of normal ovarian constituents, cysts of the graafian follicle or corpus luteum, or they may arise from abnormal growth of ovarian epithelium, when they are to be considered as benign tumors with a possibility of becoming malignant.

Dermoid cysts are tumors that are

believed to arise from parts of the ovum that disappear normally as ripening (maturation) takes place. As their origin is unsettled, all that can be said is that they are tumor growths of undifferentiated embryonal cells. They are slow-growing and at operation are found to contain a thick yellow sebaceous material arising from a skin lining. Hair, teeth, bone, brain, eyes and many other tissues often are found in a rudimentary state within these cysts.

When the cysts are small and uncomplicated, few symptoms are produced. When the cysts become large, or are fixed in the pelvis, symptoms develop due to pressure on the surrounding structures: constipation due to pressure on the rectum and sigmoid; edema of the legs due to pressure on the veins; backache and pain in the legs due to pressure on the nerves. Large tumors produce a marked distention of the abdomen, often larger than that due to pregnancy. Gradual emaciation occurs, and the patient takes on a characteristic drawn, haggard look, commonly referred to as the "ovarian facies."

If the tumor is pedunculated, it may become twisted and give rise to acute sudden pain, often shocking in its severity.

Treatment and Nursing Care

The treatment of ovarian cysts is surgical removal. However, if malignant degeneration has taken place, with invasion of the abdomen and emaciation (general carcinomatosis), operation is of little benefit. The patient may be given x-ray therapy and testosterone. The abdomen may be tapped to relieve distention from ascites.

The postoperative nursing care after cystectomy needs no special mention, except for one particular. The marked decrease in intra-abdominal pressure incidental to the removal of a large cyst often leads to considerable abdominal distention. This complication may be prevented in a measure by the application of a pad and an abdominal binder.

CONDITIONS OF FALLOPIAN TUBES

Acute Salpingitis

Acute salpingitis (acute inflammation of the fallopian tubes) may be due to infection by streptococci or staphylococci but most commonly by the gonococcus. (See p. 634.) This organism reaches the tubes via the uterus, and the pus formed may escape from the abdominal opening and involve the ovary and the peritoneum of the pelvis. The extension of the inflammation gives it the name *pelvic inflammatory disease.* As the acute process subsides, widespread adhesions may form between intestines, ovaries, tubes, and even within the tubes themselves. These tubal adhesions are frequent causes of sterility and ectopic pregnancy.

Symptoms. The symptoms of acute salpingitis arise somewhat suddenly, and often a considerable time after the primary infection. There is an acute attack of abdominal pain, associated with tenderness across the lower abdomen, moderate fever and, usually, vomiting. With symptoms more pronounced on the right side, the diagnosis of the disease must be differentiated from appendicitis.

Treatment and Nursing Care

It has been found by experience that the inflammation tends to subside under conservative treatment. Penicillin and the sulfa drugs have been used with great success in producing an early subsidence of the acute inflammation. Therefore, these patients are placed in the Fowler position and given hot vaginal douches twice daily and hot applications to the abdomen. Within 1 to 4 weeks the acute symptoms subside and the patient enters into the stage of chronic pelvic inflammatory disease. The residual adhesions may produce a variety of symptoms—pelvic pain, disturbances of menstruation, constipation, sterility, neuroses and so forth. However, many patients recover completely after one or two attacks if reinfection is prevented. Patients with large bilateral masses may be cured completely and even have children.

In young women, operation is deferred as long as possible. Surgical intervention is considered only when symptoms persist after douching, rest, continence, and diathermy have been tried.

The surgical treatment of these patients is to free adhesions and remove as much of the pelvic organs as appears beyond repair. Very frequently a removal of the uterus with both tubes and ovaries—bilateral salpingo-oophorectomy and hysterectomy—is necessary to effect a cure.

The nursing care of these patients presents no special difficulty. The douches in the acute stage should be given at 120° F., and usually 4 liters of solutions are used. The nurse should bear constantly in mind the necessity for observing strict precautions against infection when caring for these patients (see p. 613).

After operation, the chief complications are distention (see Chap. 8), constipation and urinary retention.

Ectopic Pregnancy

Ectopic pregnancy is a pregnancy in which the fertilized ovum does not reach the cavity of the uterus but becomes caught and embedded in the fallopian tube or, occasionally, in the ovary or the abdomen. As the fertilized ovum increases in size, the tube becomes more and more distended until finally, from 4 to 6 weeks after conception has occurred, rupture takes place and the ovum is discharged into the abdominal cavity. The symptoms may start with attacks of colicky pain on the affected side due to distention of the fallopian tube. When tubal rupture occurs, the patient experiences agonizing pain, faintness, shock and air hunger. It is recognized at once that the patient is desperately ill; all the signs of hemorrhage—rapid, thready pulse, subnormal temperature, restlessness, pallor, sweating—are in evidence. By vaginal examination the surgeon is able to feel a large mass of clotted blood that has collected in the pelvis behind the uterus.

Treatment. The treatment of ectopic pregnancy always is surgical—removal of the tube (and ovary if necessary) on the affected side. However, many patients are in such a shocked condition that immediate operation cannot be performed. Measures then should be instituted to combat the shock and hemorrhage (see Chap. 8) by elevation of the foot of the bed, transfusions and so forth. When the operation is performed early, practically all such patients recover with remarkable rapidity, but without operation the mortality ranges from 60 to 70 per cent.

After operation the treatment is the same as for any laparotomy, plus transfusions to combat the acute anemia.

INFERTILITY

Infertility is the inability to conceive. It may be remedied. However, should the condition persist, it is referred to as *sterility*. It becomes a gynecologic condition because it may be caused by many gynecologic diseases, among which may be mentioned displacements and tumors of the uterus, genital infantilism and inflammations.

Treatment. The treatment of these conditions varies with the causative disease. In arriving at the correct diagnosis, the *Rubin test* often is used. This procedure is to determine the patency of the fallopian tubes, which so frequently become closed after inflammation, especially of the gonorrheal type. A gas (oxygen, carbon dioxide) introduced into the uterus through a cannula should escape under normal conditions through the tubes into the abdominal cavity. If no gas escapes, the tubes are believed to be closed and point to the probable cause of sterility. Lipiodol, a radiopaque substance, often is used to determine the site of tubal obstruction. This oily material is introduced through the uterus to fill the tubes. Then an x-ray picture is taken to show the outline of the tubal lumen (salpingogram).

As the secretions of the endocrine glands, especially the thyroid and the pituitary, are so closely related to ovarian function, the investigations often include a basal metabolic test and examination of the urine for female sex hormone. It is known that sterility often is due to a hypofunction of the thyroid, the pituitary and the ovary.

It should be stated that extensive investigations of the female should not be attempted until the husband has been examined. In about 35 per cent of sterile marriages, the male is at fault.

The treatment of sterility is a difficult matter because it may be caused by a combination of several factors. Efforts are made to build up the general health of the patient, supplying the lacking glandular hormones as indicated. Operative treatments include removal of obstructions and plastic operations to restore tubal patency.

REFERENCES AND SUGGESTED READING

Unit Eleven: Nursing in Conditions of the Reproductive System

Anderson, M. H., and Reich, W. J.: Dysmenorrhea, Am. J. Nursing **49**: 220, 1949.

Baer, J. L.: Carcinoma of the reproductive organs in women, Am. J. Nursing **49**:78-80, 1949.

Best, N.: Radiotherapy and the nurse, Am. J. Nursing **50**:140-143, 1950.

Bickers, W., and Woods, M.: Premenstrual distress and what to do about it, Am. J. Nursing **52**:1087-1089, 1952.

Clark, C. W.: When patients ask you

about sex, Am. J. Nursing **53**:73-76, 1953.
Emerson, C. P., and Bragdon, J. S.: Essentials of Medicine, ed. 17, pp. 719-725, Philadelphia, Lippincott, 1955.
Ferguson, Elizabeth: New procedures in gynecological nursing, Canad. Nurse **45**:517-519, 1949.
Gamble, C. J.: Human sterilization, Am. J. Nursing **51**:625-626, 1951.
Greenhill, J. P.: Office Gynecology, ed. 5, Chicago, Yr. Bk. Pub., 1948.
Hirst, D. V.: The "simple cleansing douche"; how dangerous is it, Am. J. Obst. & Gynec. **64**:179, 1952.
Jones, G. W.: We have to watch for ectopic pregnancy, Trained Nurse & Hosp. Rev. **114**:204-205, 1945.
McVay, L. V., Jr., et al.: A new method of treatment of Trichomonas vaginalis vaginitis, Surg., Gynec. & Obst. **93**:177-184, 1951.
Miller, N. F., and Hyde, Betty: Gynecology and Gynecologic Nursing, ed. 2, Philadelphia, Saunders, 1949.
Peck, Elizabeth: Perineal care, Am. J. Nursing **47**:170-172, 1947.
Pratt, J. H., and Lahre, Grace: Care of patients with vesicovaginal fistula, Am. J. Nursing **48**:239-241, 1948.
Ranney, B.: Endometriosis, Am. J. Nursing **52**:1465-1467, 1952.
Stone, Abraham: Infertility, Am. J. Nursing **47**:606-608, 1947.
TeLinde, R. W.: Operative Gynecology, ed. 2, Philadelphia, Lippincott, 1953.
Walker, Elizabeth: Cytologic test for cancer, Am. J. Nursing **49**:43-45, 1949.

CLINICAL SITUATION: RADIUM IMPLANTATION

Mrs. Tanté had a subtotal hysterectomy for fibroids 8 years ago. Now this 50-year-old woman was admitted for radium insertion in the cervix. She was referred by the Gynecologic Outpatient Department when her Papanicolaou test revealed cells suggestive of cancer.

1. A Papanicolaou test is a
_____(1) biopsy of cervical tissue
_____(2) smear of vaginal secretions
_____(3) dilatation and curettage

2. Early symptoms which Mrs. Tanté probably experienced are:
_____(1) leukorrhea–metrorrhagia
_____(2) sacral backache – lower abdominal pain
_____(3) burning pain on urination–slight swelling between the labia

3. Check the correct statements regarding radium.
_____(1) Radium is expensive because it is used only once, inasmuch as the beneficial rays have expended themselves.
_____(2) Radium must be sterilized by autoclaving since it is inserted in a cavity of the body.
_____(3) Radium should be handled with long forceps, preferably behind a lead shield.

4. In preparing Mrs. Tanté for radium insertion, it is
_____(1) unnecessary to do a perineal shave since no incision will be made
_____(2) routine to administer a

colonic irrigation and a vaginal douche

_____(3) likely that an enema and a perineal shave will be ordered

5. While the radium is in place, Mrs. Tanté may notice

_____(1) that she has developed a voracious appetite

_____(2) that her mouth is dry and she perspires frequently

_____(3) a slight fever and occasional nausea or vomiting

6. Cancer of the cervix is treated **most** often by

_____(1) surgical removal

_____(2) radium implantation

_____(3) a combination of (1) and (2)

7. Radium implantation is

a. very expensive therapy because

_____(1) the element is expensive to obtain

_____(2) it is expensive to "re-charge" it after each use

b. not very expensive therapy because

_____(3) the American Cancer Society pays for it

_____(4) the element can be used over and over again

UNIT TWELVE

Nursing in Surgical Communicable Diseases

CHAPTER TWENTY-EIGHT

Treatment and Nursing Care of Patients with Surgical Infections

TETANUS (LOCKJAW)

Etiology. Tetanus is a disease caused by *Bacillus tetani (Clostridium tetani)*. The bacillus cannot live in the presence of oxygen (air); therefore, it is found most commonly in wounds with small external openings. It may occur in any deep wound that is contaminated with soil or harbors foreign bodies. It happens not infrequently that the wound of entrance is so insignificant that it cannot be found. (See Chap. 2, p. 13.)

Signs and Symptoms. The toxins formed in this disease have an especial affinity for nervous tissue. They are absorbed by the peripheral nerves and carried to the spinal cord, where they produce what amounts to a stimulation of the nervous tissue. The sensory nerves become sensitive to the slightest stimuli, and the hypersensitive motor nerves carry impulses that produce spasms of the muscles that they supply.

The muscle group first affected is that of the jaws, and the patient is unable to open his mouth. This characteristic symptom has given the name *lockjaw* (trismus), which is used commonly by the laity.

Other groups of muscles are included rapidly in the spasms, until the whole body is involved. The spasm of groups of muscles is continuous, but the least stimulus—a door banging or a loud voice—may add a generalized convulsion, with every muscle in violent contraction. Because the extensor muscles are stronger than the flexors, the head

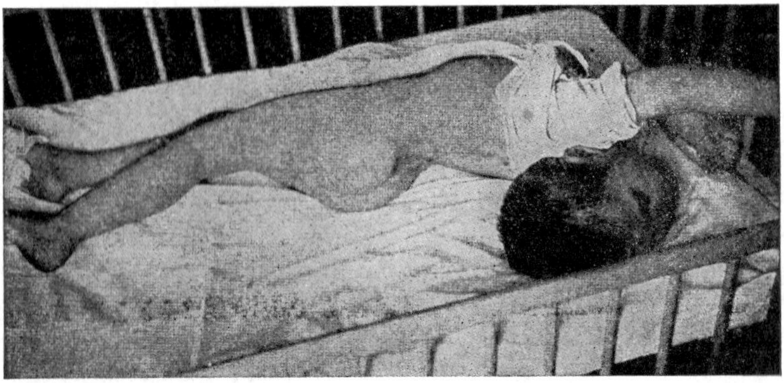

FIG. 270. Opisthotonos of tetanus. (Jeans, Wright and Blake: Essentials of Pediatrics, ed. 5, Philadelphia, Lippincott)

is retracted, the feet are extended fully and the back is arched, so that during a convulsion the whole body may be supported on the back of the head and the feet. This condition is called *opisthotonos* (Fig. 270).

The spasms of the facial muscles produce a so-called sardonic grin, which is quite characteristic for this disease and persists even during convalescence (Fig. 271).

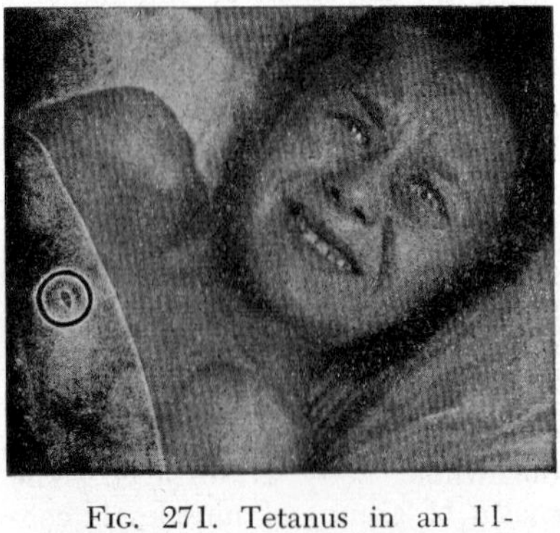

FIG. 271. Tetanus in an 11-year-old girl. Wound between the toes contained pieces of decayed wood. Mouse inoculation with this wood produced tetanus. (Pfaundler and Schlossmann: The Diseases of Children, Philadelphia, Lippincott)

Death may occur from asphyxia due to spasm of the diaphragm and, more frequently, from exhaustion due to loss of sleep and lack of nourishment, and excessive fatigue due to the constant muscle spasms.

Tetanus Toxoid. The danger of tetanus is so widespread that prophylactic measures as for smallpox, diphtheria and so forth have been developed. By immunization with tetanus toxoid, an active immunity may be built up in the patient so that the danger from tetanus is very slight. Experience in World War II has demonstrated the effectiveness of toxoid prophylaxis. The injection of a "booster" dose of toxoid produces a rapid increase in the active immunity, and is used instead of, or with, antitoxin in case of injury.

Treatment and Nursing Care

Prevention is the best method of treatment of this disease. Every primarily infected wound, especially a septic puncture wound, should be treated as if it were infected with the tetanus organism. Thorough cleansing of the wound, usually with wide incision, and removal of foreign bodies are the important procedures in the primary treatment of the wound. In addition, a prophylactic dose of 1,500 units of tetanus antitoxin should be given hypodermically. (See Serum Reaction and Treatment, p. 14.)

If the disease already has developed when the patient is first seen, the same care of the wound is indicated. To neutralize the toxins that have formed, large doses (as much as 100,000 units daily) of the antitoxin are given round the wound, intramuscularly, intravenously and intraspinally. These measures are to be supported by most careful nursing of the patient. Since the slightest stimulation may excite convulsions, absolute silence must be enforced. Even such apparently insignificant disturbances as a draught of cold air, the jarring of the bed, bright lights, squeaky doors and cold hands are to be avoided.

Avertin has been used by rectum to control the convulsive spasms. Usually the initial dose is from 80 to 100 mg. per Kg. of body weight. Succeeding doses, which are always administered before the effects of the previous dose have worn off, are given in smaller amounts. No opiates or other narcotics need be used when avertin is given. Other barbiturates may be used by mouth or hypodermically, as well as other sedatives, but their effects seem to be less valuable in controlling these convulsions.

The bowels should be cleared by an enema early in the disease, and a careful watch should be kept for retention of urine and the development of bedsores. Feeding is a difficult problem in these cases but, by constant attention, sufficient food and fluids usually can be given. If the jaws are not locked completely, and even if they are, high caloric liquids may be given by straw or spoon. Frequently, however, it may be necessary to feed a patient through a nasal catheter (Fig. 272).

When the muscles of the patient are in such continuous tension as to interfere with respirations, curare may be given cautiously, and the patient may be placed in a respirator. By supplying artificial respiratory movement, gas exchange may be accomplished. Oxygen also may be given at this time.

GAS BACILLUS INFECTION (GAS GANGRENE)

Etiology. Gas bacillus infection is observed frequently as a complication of severe contusions, often associated with compound fractures, and

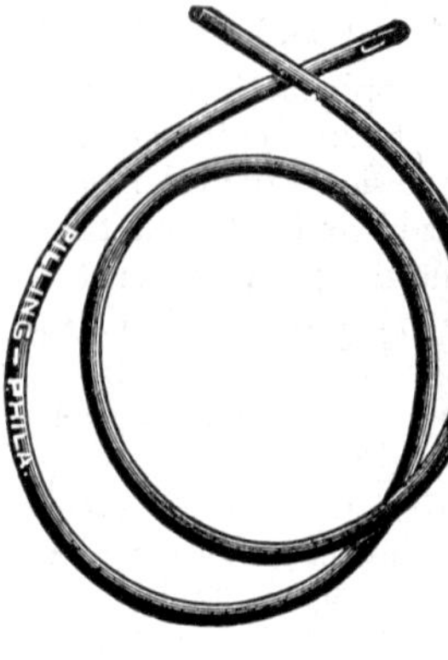

Fig. 272. Tube for nasal feeding.

it may be found in supposedly clean wounds, especially after amputations for gangrene. The gas bacillus—*Bacillus welchii (Clostridium welchii)*, *B. oedematiens (Clostridium oedematiens)*, and vibrion septique *(Clostridium septicum)*—like the bacillus of tetanus, is an anaerobe, and a spore former; therefore, it occurs in wounds in which the oxygen supply is reduced by reason of injury or disease of the blood vessels.

Signs and Symptoms. The wounds infected by the gas bacillus are characterized by an extreme tenderness, swelling and a bronzed discoloration of the surrounding skin. These signs are associated with a rapid pulse and respiration and some temperature elevation. As the disease progresses, gas forms in the tissues due to the action of the bacteria on the tissues, and the area about the wound crackles under the fingers. If the wound is opened, a frothy fluid and malodorous gases escape, and the muscles form a purple pultaceous mass. Death from toxemia usually results if the process is at all advanced.

Treatment and Nursing Care

The prophylactic treatment here, as in tetanus, is most important. Early excision (débridement) of all devitalized and infected tissue with wide incisions will prevent the disease in most traumatic cases. Once the infection has developed, amputation of the extremity often is necessary, although the combination of local excision of the affected muscle plus the introduction of chemotherapy often suffices. These cases often are treated and operated upon under refrigeration anesthesia.

Because the gas bacillus is an inhabitant of the human intestinal tract, it is liable to be the infecting organism in wounds of thigh amputations, especially if the patient is incontinent. Gangrene, incontinence and debility often are combined in patients with diabetes, and it is in the amputation stump of diabetic patients in which gas gangrene is most prone to occur.

The prophylactic treatment in this instance consists of special care in keeping the bed clean and dry and in protecting the wounds and the dressings against contamination. Oiled silk applied over the dressing and sealed to the skin by a wide strip of adhesive at its upper margin accomplishes this purpose. Many surgeons give prophylactic doses of an antitoxin (perfringens antitoxin) before operations for diabetic gangrene.

The disease is important from the nursing point of view because of the extreme care that is necessary to nurse these patients properly. The danger, of course, is the spread of the infection to other wounds. To guard against this, both doctor and nurse should wear gloves when dressing these patients. The contaminated dressings should be disposed of immediately, and the instruments and the trays used should be washed with gloves on and autoclaved after each dressing. It is advisable to isolate the patient and to keep a single dressing tray for that patient alone.

Gas bacillus infection produces an intense toxemia. The essentials in nursing care are the adequate administration of fluids, either by mouth or intravenously, and an easily assimilated high caloric diet. Attention should be paid to elimination by the bowels, enemas being given as needed. In these extremely sick patients there is always danger of the development of a decubitus ulcer, and it may tax the ingenuity of the nurse to give proper attention to the back and other sites of pressure. Although amputation is performed less frequently now than formerly, the care of an amputated stump may be a part of the nursing attention. (See p. 567.)

ACTINOMYCOSIS

This lesion is caused by the ray fungus that affects man, cattle and swine and develops later into tumors associated with fistulae. The common sites are the head, the neck, the thorax and the abdomen. An inflammatory swelling is produced. This tends to suppurate and discharge the characteristic sulphurlike granules. The most widely used treatments are excision, potassium iodide and irradiation. Chemotherapy and antibiotics have been used with favorable results, especially when the lesion is inaccessible to surgery.

CLINICAL SITUATION: TETANUS

Miss Sue Schmaltz, while working in her garden, pierced her hand accidentally with a small hand rake. The chief concern of the physician was to prevent tetanus.

1. This condition is known also as:

______a. Tetany.
______b. Gas gangrene.
______c. Lockjaw.
______d. Trismus.
______e. Opisthotonos.

2. Miss Schmaltz probably was given prophylactic injections of:

______a. Toxin-antitoxin.
______b. Tetanus toxoid.
______c. Avertin.
______d. Perfringens antitoxin.
______e. Tetanus antitoxin.

3. Symptoms of tetanus are:

______a. Acute sensitivity to noise.
______b. Trismus.
______c. Sardonic grin.
______d. Opisthotonos.
______e. Emphysema.

4. Anyone who develops tetanus presents such nursing problems as:

______a. Violent reactions to slight stimuli (for example, the sudden jarring of a door).
______b. Urinary retention.
______c. Feeding difficulties because of a locked jaw.
______d. Intense toxemia.
______e. Acute diaphoresis.

CHAPTER TWENTY-NINE

Venereal Diseases

Gonorrhea and syphilis are infective diseases obtained in most instances by sexual intercourse. However, the infection may be obtained in innocent ways (see below).

GONORRHEA

Etiology. This disease is caused by the gonococcus, a tiny organism that may be found within the pus cells from the discharge of an acute case. It is a true parasite, being cultivated with difficulty and dying soon when discharged from the body. It is unlikely that the genital form of the disease is communicated in any other manner than by direct inoculation. But, occasionally, infection may be transmitted by towels, hands, toilet seats and so forth. Examples of such infection may be found in the vulvovaginitis in little girls and the gonorrheal infection of the eyes in adults. Because of the possibility of this mode of carrying the infection, patients with the disease must be warned not to touch the eyes, and extreme precautions must be taken by the nurse in caring for such patients not to transmit the infection innocently to herself or to others.

Symptoms. The acute symptoms appear within 2 to 6 days after the infection has been acquired. The organism produces an acute purulent inflammation of the mucous membrane of the urethra and the vagina, with swelling and pain of the adjacent parts. Burning or smarting pain is experienced on urination. In some patients, especially females, these symptoms may be slight and of short duration. As the disease progresses, the organism leaves the mucous membrane but tends to lurk in the small glands opening into the urethra (prostate in the male, Skene's tubules in the female) and the vagina (cervical glands and Bartholin's gland). The profuse discharge decreases gradually in amount and the acute symptoms disappear. However, this more or less quiescent stage does not always mean a cure; the infected glands always remain a source of infection that may lead to other complications—prostatitis, epididymitis or stricture of the urethra in the male (Chap. 16); endocervicitis, salpingitis, pelvic abscess and so on in the female (Chap. 25) and gonorrheal infections in the joints of both sexes.

Treatment. The antibiotics, penicillin and chloramphenicol have supplanted largely other methods of therapy for acute gonorrhea.

The treatment of the chronic stage of the disease in the female has been discussed in Chapter 25, page 624.

In the male, the prostate gland is the chief lurking place of the gonococci. Massage of this gland through the rectum with the gloved finger tends to evacuate the secretion and wash out with it part of the organisms. Vaccines and sera have been used, but not with marked success, except, perhaps, in the treatment of the arthritis that sometimes occurs in the later stages of the disease.

An essential part of the treatment of this disease is the instruction given the patients. They should be told of the infective nature of the disease, the danger of gonorrheal ophthalmia (Chap. 19) and the possibility of complications unless instructions are obeyed strictly.

Many innocent wives are infected by husbands who contracted the disease in earlier years but retained a chronic infection. Early treatment is the best preventive of the more serious and long-standing complications of the disease.

SYPHILIS (LUES)

Syphilis is an infectious disease caused by a parasite, the *Treponema pallidum (Spirochaeta pallida)*. The organisms enter the body through some abrasion in the skin or the mucous membrane, directly from a syphilitic sore in another person, usually during sexual intercourse. However, it may be transmitted by kissing or by means of soiled towels,

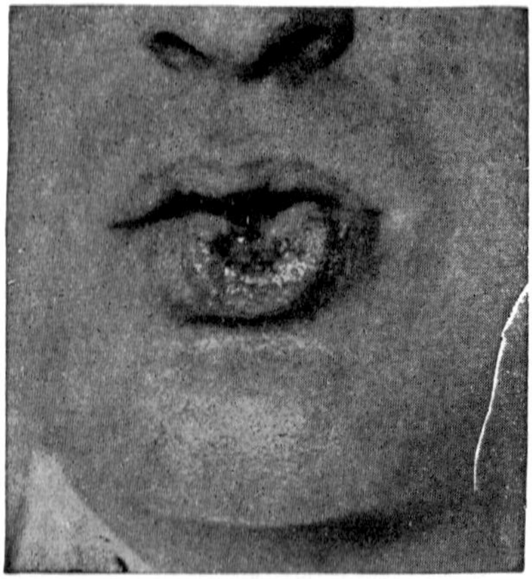

Fig. 273. Chancre, initial lesion of syphilis. (Dr. Hartzell)

pipes, nail files, combs, brushes, lipsticks or eating utensils.

Besides the sore, the blood of syphilitics may transmit the organisms. It is not rare for surgeons and nurses to become infected innocently due to the entrance of syphilitic blood into cuts or abrasions during the performance of an operation. Syphilis acquired after transfusion from an infected donor is seen not infrequently. With proper clinical and serologic examination of donors, this tragic accident can be prevented, and its occurrence under present-day conditions is inexcusable.

Besides these means of acquiring lues, the disease may be inherited (congenital syphilis) by children from syphilitic parents. The congenital forms are similar to the acquired type, except that there is no primary stage (see below).

The disease has three stages, so divided because of the various manifestations that occur at different times in its course.

Primary Stage

The characteristic lesion of the primary stage is the chancre. This lesion appears within 2 to 5 weeks after inoculation as a hard, half-pea-shaped papule at the site of infection. The papule ulcerates but forms no pus, leaving an open sore from which material can be obtained that will show the spirochete when examined under the microscope (darkfield). (This method is used widely in the diagnosis of early syphilis.) The lesion occurs at the site of inoculation, so that it may be on the lips, the anus or even the finger of a surgeon. The regional lymph nodes become enlarged, the patient may feel out of sorts and have a slight fever, but in the large majority of cases there are no subjective symptoms. The lesion may heal without treatment in 4 or 5 weeks, leaving a scarcely detectable scar. However, this does not mean that the patient is cured. The organisms have become diffused throughout the body and an examination of the patient's blood serum by means of the Wassermann technic will show a strongly positive (4 plus) reaction within 2 to 12 weeks after the development of the primary lesion (Fig. 273).

Secondary Stage

As the infection extends throughout the body, the patient may experience vague rheumatic pains, malaise, fever and headache. Within 6 to 8 weeks, the secondary manifestations of the disease appear. The lymph nodes all over the body become enlarged and various lesions appear in the skin and the mucous membranes. The skin lesions may take almost any form—papules, macules, acnelike eruptions and so forth—but never vesicles or bulla, except in congenital syphilis. These various types of eruptions may appear all at once and are characterized by a lack of itching or other subjective symptoms, a symmetrical appearance all over the body and a coppery red color. Wartlike growths called condylomas appear on warm, moist skin surfaces (for example, round the anus, the scrotum and the labia). Often the hair falls out in patches. This is called *alopecia syphilitica.*

Lesions corresponding to those found on the skin may develop in the mucous membrane of the mouth, the pharynx and the nose. Sore throat is a common symptom, due to ulcerative lesions of the pharynx. Whitish patches called mucous patches occur in the mouth or the vagina. These eruptions are teeming with the spirochetes, and from them infection occurs by means other than intercourse.

"The occurrence of the above in combination with skin rashes, lymphatic enlargement, falling out of the hair, and sore throat, is almost pathognomonic of secondary syphilis."

Tertiary Stage

After an interval of a few or many years, following the disappearance of the secondary lesions, the symptoms of the tertiary stage appear.

The disease may affect any tissue or organ of the body in this stage. The lesions are slow to develop and do not form pus, but, like those of tuberculosis, contain a cheeselike material so that these two diseases are classed together with several other conditions in that class of infections called granulomata. These syphilitic manifestations are given the name gumma. Often they grow to considerable size and are in any tissue of the body, but most frequently in the skin, the liver and the mucous membranes. The blood vessels frequently show changes, aneurysms (dilatation of arteries) appear, and apoplexy (rupture of a blood vessel in the brain) may occur before the patient is past middle age. Apoplexy in a young adult without hypertension is very suggestive of syphilis.

Interstitial keratitis and iritis are common manifestations in the eye. Skin lesions–deep ulcerations–develop frequently. Ulcerations of the mucous membrane of the nose and the pharynx may progress and involve the bones, producing a falling in of the bridge of the nose (saddle nose). The nervous system is a frequent site of tertiary lesions. Almost any form of disease may appear, the commonest types being tabes dorsalis (locomotor ataxia) in the spinal cord and "general paralysis of the insane" when the brain is attacked.

The spinal cord lesions often are followed by joint changes (Charcot's joint) and other lesions due to lack of normal nerve supply.

This multitude of manifestations of tertiary syphilis often includes many lesions that demand surgical treatment.

Hereditary syphilis is the result of infection of the ovum or fetus while still in the uterus. The pregnancy usually terminates in abortion or miscarriage, or stillbirth (birth of a dead child) at term. If a living child is born, lesions corresponding to the secondary stage of acquired syphilis usually appear very early. Skin eruptions, blisters, mucous patches and so forth are seen commonly. The baby may have the appearance of a "little old man with a cold in his head," but more often than not he seems to be well developed and nourished. The child often survives without treatment, and certain characteristic lesions such as interstitial keratitis, Hutchinson's incisors, eighth-nerve deafness, syphilitic hepatitis and saber tibiac may develop. Blindness frequently occurs, but the late lesions of congenital syphilis do not often cause death unless the nervous system is involved (juvenile tabes and paresis).

Treatment

Formerly, the treatment of syphilis was by a combination of drugs that were mostly heavy metals, such as arsenic, bismuth and mercury. Since the advent of penicillin, these methods seldom are used. The penicillin therapy of syphilis has proved to be so successful, not only in primary syphilis but also in all forms of congenital and late syphilis, that it has practically supplanted all other forms of therapy. Peroral chloremycetin also is showing promise in the control of syphilis. Whereas many of these patients used to be treated in hospitals, now many of them can be treated as ambulatory patients.

Tests for Syphilis. A large number of serologic tests for syphilis are available. They are of two types: the Wassermann or complement-fixation reaction and the flocculation or precipitation type. The Kolmer-Wassermann is a widely used example of the former and the Kahn test an excellent precipitation reaction. The Kline slide test is a convenient method for rapid diagnosis in emergencies, as in testing the blood of a donor, and it may be performed in about 45 minutes.

REFERENCES AND SUGGESTED READING

Unit Twelve: Nursing in Surgical Communicable Diseases

General

Emerson, C. P., and Bragdon, J. S.: Essentials of Medicine, ed. 17, pp. 729-755 and 870-873 (infection, immunity, chemotherapy); pp. 756-791 (bacterial); pp. 792-814 (tuberculosis); pp. 815-839 (viral); pp. 840-843 (rickettsial); pp. 844-860 (spirochetal and protozoan); pp. 861-870 (parasitic), Philadelphia, Lippincott, 1955.

Greenberg, M., and Matz, A. V.: Modern Concepts of Communicable Disease, New York, Putnam, 1953.

Pillsbury, M. E., and Sachs, E. J.: Nursing Care of Communicable Diseases, ed. 7, Philadelphia, Lippincott, 1952.

Stokes, J. H., and Taylor, J. B.: Dermatology and Venereology, ed. 4, Philadelphia, Saunders, 1948.

Tetanus

Emerson, C. P., and Bragdon, J. S.: Essentials of Medicine, ed. 17, pp. 777-780, Philadelphia, Lippincott, 1955.

Harris, Isabel, and Shapiro, S. K.: Tetanus—a challenge to nursing, Am. J. Nursing **50**:362-364, 1950.

Venereal Disease

Emerson, C. P., and Bragdon, J. S.: Essentials of Medicine, ed. 17, pp. 681-682 and 781-782 (gonorrhea); p. 836 (lymphogranuloma inguinale); pp. 844-850 (syphilis); pp. 658-662 (neurosyphilis), Philadelphia, Lippincott, 1955.

Eslick, Mildred: The rapid treatment center, Am. J. Nursing **46**:543-544, 1946.

Heller, J. R.: The rapid treatment center program, Am. J. Nursing **46**:542-543, 1946.

Nelson, N. A.: Modern venereal disease control, Am. J. Nursing **50**: 75-77, 1950.

UNIT THIRTEEN

Operative Aseptic Technic

CHAPTER THIRTY

The Operating Room and Its Equipment

INTRODUCTION

An operating room is a place where surgery, be it diagnostic, therapeutic or palliative, is done. The chief objective of operating room personnel is to perform a surgical procedure as quickly and as technically perfect as is humanly possible without losing sight of the fact that the individual being cared for is one who has feelings, be they expressed or not. To satisfy such an objective, the student nurse learns that the simple virtues are a "must" in the successful functioning of this department because the life of a patient is often held in the balance. Such attributes are honesty, punctuality, alertness, ability to work quickly and quietly, and an understanding of the reasons for doing things in a prescribed way.

In the operating room, harmful organisms are reduced to a minimum by such personnel practices as wearing a mask over the nose and the mouth, changing from street clothes to cleaner garments, keeping the number of persons in the operating room at the barest minimum, maintaining the cleanliness of all equipment, etc. Safety and efficiency are also maintained by eliminating unnecessary furnishings. If equipment is necessary, it must be placed where it can be used most effectively at the desired time. All apparatus should be checked periodically and repaired when necessary to avoid anesthetic hazards and other accidents.

From experience in an operating room, a student gains much which will make her a better nurse. The basic principles of aseptic technic are best learned where they are carried out consistently. The nurse becomes more acutely aware of the numerous significant details which must be prepared and checked for every surgical patient. She becomes conscious of the cost and the proper care of equipment. She soon realizes that every member of the team is dependent upon every other member; therefore, teamwork is essential. She is able to appreciate fine workmanship and artistic precision as she observes the surgeon and his assistants operate. Lastly, she gains a fuller meaning of the complete care of a surgical patient, because she develops a more intelligent understanding of the reasons for giving preanesthetic care and its effect on postoperative convalescence.

OPERATING SUITE

The arrangement and the location of the operating suite necessarily depend on the size and the general construction of the hospital. Generally speaking, however, the operating room should be isolated sufficiently from the rest of the hospital to prevent annoyance or disturbance by its sights, sounds or odors, and yet easily and quickly accessible from all surgical wards and private rooms, x-ray department and pharmacy. In modern structures, this is usually accomplished by air-conditioning and soundproofing the suite. When it is necessary to employ elevator service, there should be a system of signals or special elevators to avoid delay in the coming and going of patients.

The number and the size of the operating and accessory rooms vary considerably with the size of the hospital and the character and the amount of work done. For every operating room, there should be at least one sterilizing and one anesthetizing room. In addition, there should be dressing rooms for doctors and nurses, instrument and sterile supply rooms, scrub-up rooms, utility rooms with sinks and hoppers, workrooms, and adequate space for storage of apparatus and unsterile supplies not in constant use, such as fracture tables, splints, plaster bandages, etc. The outstanding feature of an operating suite should be simplicity, noted primarily in its architectural details and construction and, further, in its equipment.

Operating Room

Size and Construction. The size and the construction of the operating room come first in importance. Its dimensions should not be unnecessarily large and yet not so small as to interfere with perfect aseptic technic. Walls should be free from corners and ledges and of such construction as to permit easy cleaning. Washable paint, enamel, or tiling are the materials in general use. A floor of terrazzo is usually the most satisfactory, especially when impregnated with metal and grounded. It should be graded downward slightly to the center, where there should be a drain to allow for flushing.

Color Scheme. At the present time, various color schemes are found in the operating room rather than the former spotless white. One of the most popular color combinations consists of terrazzo floor, six-foot wainscoting of sage-green tile, with walls and ceiling painted in a softer tone. Other hues that find favor are battleship gray, buff and dull blue. White gowns and covers have also been displaced by colored ones, the shade depending on the individual preference of the chief surgeon.

Ventilation and Heat. These are factors to which great importance must be attached. The temperature of an operating room should be maintained at 78° F., with ample facilities provided for raising it to 80° F., or higher, when desirable. There should be an abundance of fresh air, without strong draughts, free from dust or other gross contamination. In modern operating rooms, air conditioning is being used as a method of supplying clean air at a constant temperature. If radiators are still being used, they should be constructed to allow for easy cleaning.

Illumination. Illumination of the operating room is one of its most essential features. General lighting is often adequate from diffusing globes near the ceiling. Reflecting lights, so constructed as to preclude shadows, are often employed for the operative field. In addition, pedestal and hand lights are required occasionally for satisfactory illumination of body cavities, such as the pelvis, the chest, and the brain.

There should be several sets of lights in an operating room, each on different circuits and connected with separate fuses. Such an arrangement avoids confusion and delay when a fuse blows out. Floor sockets with safety outlets for attaching the cautery, pedestal lights, etc., should be of sufficient number and situated conveniently near the location of the operating table. Dust-collecting wires and fixtures over the operating table must be avoided. Storage batteries should be provided for emergency lighting. These must be inspected and tested at frequent intervals.

Accessory Rooms

Accessory rooms, adjacent to the operating room, are essential. Their size and number are variable, although those already mentioned seem to be the minimum for the highest degree of efficiency. When space is lacking, various accessory rooms may be combined quite satisfactorily. Construction throughout the operating suite should be, in general, the same as that of the operating room proper.

Dressing rooms for doctors and nurses need not be large but should be provided with lockers, toilet facilities, showers and such other furnishings as may be desirable and necessary.

Instrument rooms should not be connected directly with the sterilizing rooms since the doors of such cabinets must be absolutely airtight for the exclusion of moisture and dust. Built-in cases or cabinets with glass doors are the most satisfactory for storage of instruments.

Sterile supply rooms likewise should be equipped with cases similar in construction to those of the instrument rooms for storage of sterile packs, sponges, linen, etc. No unsterile supplies should be kept in these rooms.

Scrub-up rooms, opening directly from the operating room, should have a sufficient number of washbasins for surgeons and nurses. These should be of customary construction, with hot and cold "gooseneck" faucets controlled by foot or knee valves. Provision should be made for containers for soap or skin detergent, brushes, sterile solutions and towels. The sterile gown and glove packages may also be placed in these rooms. Sometimes there are no separate scrub-up rooms, in which case one end of the main operating room must serve this purpose.

Sterilizing rooms should contain all sterilizing apparatus—autoclaves, water, instrument and utensil sterilizers—and be constructed in such a manner as to be impervious to moisture. In addition, there should be exhaust fans to reduce the heat and steam rising from sterilizers if these rooms are not air-conditioned. Doors should lead from these rooms into the main operating clinics and also into the sterile supply rooms.

Utility rooms may be combined with sterilizing rooms and should be well provided with sinks and hoppers for washing and scrubbing of instruments, utensils, gloves, etc. There should be at least one large closet for floor brushes, mops, scrubbing brushes, buckets, etc.

Workrooms should be well lighted, naturally and artificially, thoroughly ventilated, and, if possible, have a floor that is easily cleaned. Equipment should include suitable work tables. There should be a sufficient number of high stools and chairs for such tasks as can be done while sitting down. Cupboards or cabinets must be provided in this room for the storage of unsterile gauze, cotton, bandages, linen, adhesive, and the innumerable odds and ends necessary for carrying on the work of a busy operating room.

Anesthetizing rooms, with their equipment, have already been described in detail (Chap. 5). It seems superfluous to add that the anesthetizing room must be scrupulously clean, neat and quiet at all times. The patient enters this room first.

Storage rooms for infrequently used apparatus and supplies are also necessary.

In addition to the accessory rooms enumerated, there may be recovery rooms, laboratories, surgeons' offices, etc., along with special operating rooms, cystoscopic rooms, waiting rooms, record room and the like. Galleries for visitors and students are desirable.

Housekeeping

The housekeeping of the operating suite must be flawless. The operating room proper must be spotless and absolutely free from dust. In the morning, before "setting up," the floor should be mopped and all furniture dusted with a damp cloth. Following this, nothing should be placed on tables or basin racks until they are draped with their sterile coverings. Between cases, the floor should be mopped to remove any blood stains, water, etc. Buckets should be emptied and cleansed. When the day's operations have been completed, the operating table and all equipment, such as suture and instrument tables, stools, basin racks and floor, must be washed with soap and water and scrubbed if necessary to remove stains.

All doors, windows and doors of cabinets or built-in cupboards and all the sterilizers must be damp dusted at least once daily. Windows and all glass doors should be washed weekly. Wooden doors require polishing at rather frequent intervals. Sterilizers and any brass or nickel fixtures should receive a thorough polishing with one of the commercial cleaners at least once a week. In addition, all cupboards, closets, cabinets and storage space must be cleaned and their contents gone over and rearranged every week. Each article—instrument, utensil, sterile dressing, or whatnot—in the operating suite should have its definite place and always be kept in that spot. If the above roughly outlined routine for daily and weekly cleaning is adhered to, a rigid check can be kept on everything in use or in reserve, the operating suite will be neat and clean at all times, and more efficient work will be accomplished as a result.

At least once a year, and more often if necessary, all painted articles in the operating suite should receive a fresh coat of paint. The walls and the ceilings should be painted yearly. Every alternate year may be sufficient for the repainting of walls and ceilings provided that they are thoroughly washed in the interim.

Equipment of Operating Room

The equipment of the operating room should be adequate but not excessive and so arranged as to permit maximum efficiency with a minimum expenditure of energy. Exact details must be worked out for each operating room according to individual needs and preferences. An x-ray view box is a necessity. One or two built-in cabinets are desirable. A clock is essential, as is a blackboard in a teaching hospital where the surgeon lectures to medical students. Further than this, the operating table, tables for instruments and dressings, receptacles and stands for basins and drums, several stools for seats and two or three low stools to stand on comprise sufficient furniture even in the busiest of clinics. All operating-room furniture, with a few exceptions, should be of the standard make —monel metal preferably or metal with a white, or preferred color, enamel finish. Such a finish is not only durable but also easily cleaned.

Operating Table. There may be one or several. The type and make vary considerably with the funds available and the preference of the surgeon. Most operating tables are rather complicated in construction and manipulation. The anesthetist should be responsible for the arrangement, the adjustment and the proper position of the patient. However, every nurse in the operating room should be taught how to manipulate the table during her first few days there and should be required to give a satisfactory demonstration of all the various positions and adjustments not later than the end of her first week's operating

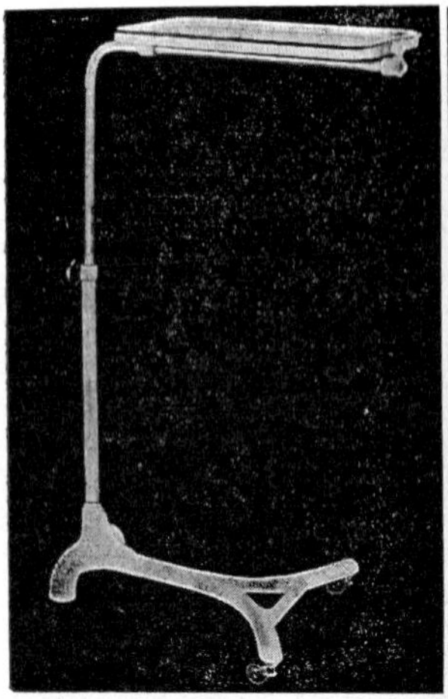

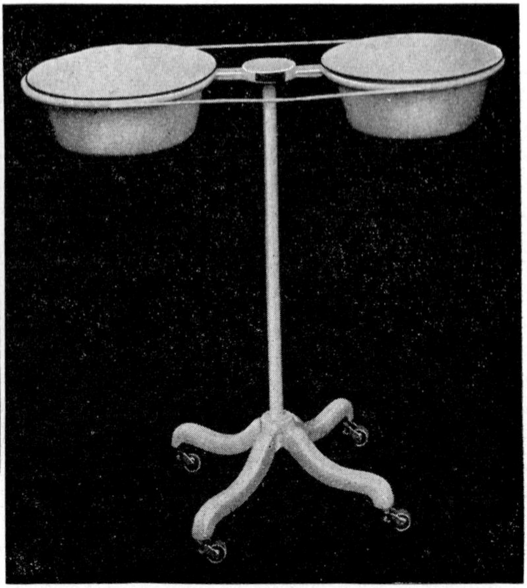

FIG. 274. (*Left*) Mayo stand.

FIG. 275. (*Right*) Double-basin rack.

room experience. Various kinds of pads are used for operating tables, usually of sponge rubber. Water-cooled mattresses are available to help prevent heat retention in surgical patients during hot weather. If serial spinal anesthesia is used, special pads are necessary when malleable needles are used. This is unnecessary when an indwelling catheter is the channel through which the anesthetic is administered.

Instrument Tables. The number of these differs with the size of the operating room and the number and kind of operations performed. Figure 274 illustrates the type of adjustable instrument table that can be extended across the operating table and placed within easy reach of the surgeon. There should be, also, reserve tables for supplementary instruments and supplies. These may be used in addition to those on the nurse's table.

All instrument and suture tables should have padded rollers so that they may be moved quickly, quietly and easily. When operations follow in rapid succession, much time can be saved between cases by having extra suture and instrument tables. Two of each, however, are usually enough—one for the case being operated on and another in readiness.

Accessory Tables. There are many occasions in which an accessory table the height of the operating table is necessary or convenient. Such a table is often of use for operations on the hand, open reductions of fractures of the arm, and for many other operations on the upper extremity. It should not be too wide, and should be fitted with rollers. Often one of the supply tables may be used if they are of the correct height, and if not, pads may be added. The table always should be covered with a sterile rubber sheet or duck canvas before it is draped for the operation.

Basins, Racks and Stands. One double-basin rack for hand solutions, 3 or 4 single racks, and perhaps two triple racks, where these are used for abdominal sponges, are usually sufficient. A soiled-sponge rack facilitates the counting of abdominal sponges. Drum and drum stands are not as desirable as sterile packs; however, if they are used, this is additional equipment. Duplicates are not absolutely necessary but are advisable when possible to save time between cases. One or two irrigator stands will be useful.

Stools. Adjustable stools for surgeons and anesthetist are essential. There should be 2 or 3 of these, depending on the character of the work to be performed. In vaginal operations, for instance, the surgeon often prefers to sit. There should also be 2 or 3 stools of varying heights on which the surgeon and his assistants may stand if necessary.

Drums. Drums are being used in many operating rooms; however, they are largely being replaced by packs, such as laparotomy packs, thyroid packs, etc. (Fig. 278, p. 648.) Drums are round, metal containers which are perforated at intervals with or without sliding bands for covering portholes. Under no condition should the drum load be compressed into tight masses. The drum load must be arranged very loosely to allow for satisfactory sterilization and must be protected by two layers of muslin with the same care that is practiced for exposed packs.

Utensils. The assortment and number of metal and glass utensils depend of necessity on the size of the operating room. There should be a sufficient supply of the following articles:

1. Basins, various sizes and shapes
2. Pitchers, preferably large size
3. Trays, various sizes
4. Buckets, large, for soiled sponges
5. Hampers, large, for soiled gowns, etc.
6. Glass bottles with corks for small specimens
7. Glass graduates, various sizes
8. Flasks, various sizes
9. Medicine glasses, cups

Suction Apparatus. A suction apparatus is employed for removing blood or other fluids from the field of operation. The suction tips and the noncollapsible rubber tubing leading from the vacuum chamber should be sterilized, and the entire apparatus tested immediately before each operation.

Sterilizers

Of all the equipment in the operating suite, the sterilizers are the most important. They should be the best obtainable and must be kept in perfect repair, otherwise the operating room will be a menace instead of a benefaction.

All sterilization must be timed accurately. Sometimes nurses are busy and neglect to look at the clock when the required temperature is secured or the proper amount of pressure obtained. To guess that the sterilization process has continued for a sufficient length of time is almost a criminal offense. To do so

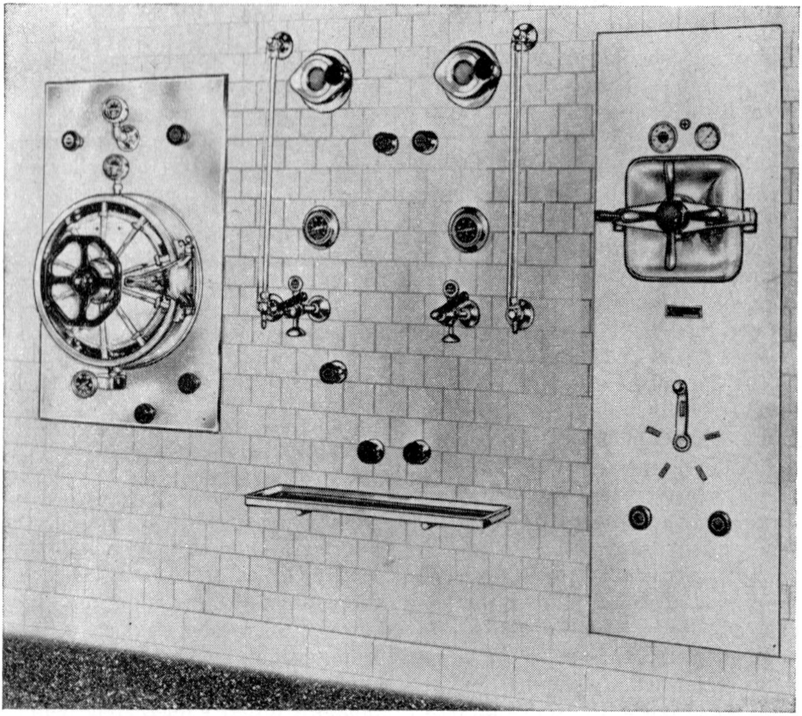

FIG. 276. Modern sterilizer arrangement. (The Manual of Sterilization, Disinfection and Related Surgical Techniques **12**:35–American Sterilizer Co.)

may cost the life of one or more persons. If a nurse forgets to look at the time when she should, the sterilization period should be counted as only beginning when she does remember to look at the clock. All timing of sterilization should be done by a clock in the sterilizing room, and not by nurses' watches.

Autoclave. The autoclave, with its construction, operation and care, has been described in detail in Chapter 3, and will, therefore, not be elaborated on here. Of all the sterilizers, the autoclave is the most important and the most complicated. Student nurses never should be entrusted with its operation until the head nurse has made certain that they are completely familiar with all the various details and their significance.

Testing for Sterility. The most comprehensive method for testing sterilization involves the careful use of a potentiometer, an instrument for

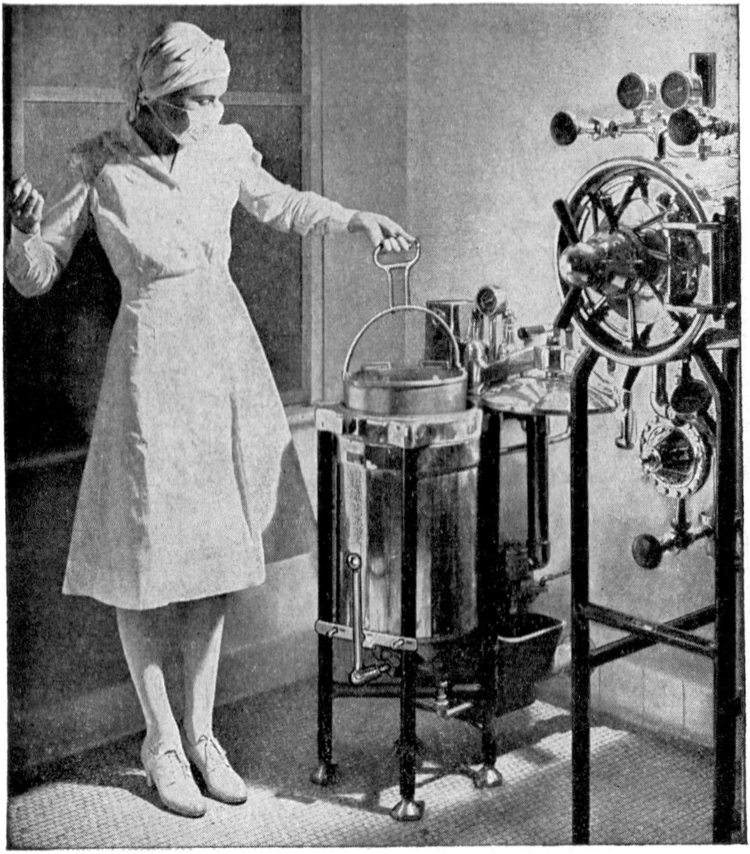

FIG. 277. Instrument washer sterilizer. (Wilmot Castle Co., Rochester, N. Y.)

measuring temperature in the heart of the load during sterilization.

Reliable sterilization indicators can also be used to denote whether a given performance is or is not adequate for sterilization. They have a disadvantage in that they do not indicate the actual build-up of temperature in a pack nor do they indicate how much overexposure may have been applied. The type indicator recommended consists of a formed pellet of chemical substance contained in a small hermetically sealed glass tube, available under the trade name of Diack control. The change in the pellet that occurs when it indicates sterilization is definite and easily distinguishable. It fuses or melts if subjected to heat uniformly applied to the glass container at 250° F. for 5 minutes. It

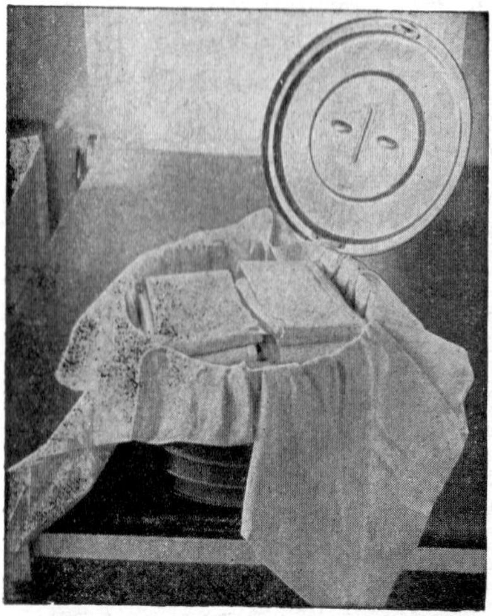

Fig. 278. If drums are to be used, the load must be planned carefully, as suggested in this picture, to avoid filling in the open spaces round the walls of the drum. If these spaces are filled in, the port openings in the sides will be closed off so effectively that prolonged exposure will be necessary for safe sterilization. (The Surgical Supervisor, American Sterilizer Company, Erie, Pa.)

will also change color from a faint yellow to a bright pink or red, but the color change alone is not significant and should not be considered as indicative.

The delay entailed in determining the results of culture tests makes them generally impractical except for an occasional check. If they are not properly planned they may be distinctly misleading. *B. subtilis* should be used because it is not pathogenic and quite safe to use. It should be prepared in small pledgets about the size of a postage stamp. Plant several of them in the load, locating them in the heart of the pack. Run them through the sterilizer and return them to the laboratory for incubation and examination. The results should be known in about 48 hours. This method is somewhat unwieldy because of the time required to determine the results.

Instrument Washer Sterilizer. The cleansing and the sterilizing of instruments can be done effectively in the pressure instrument washer sterilizer (Fig. 277), provided that certain conditions are met. All jointed instruments must be open. After instruments have been used, it is essential that they be placed in a basin of water. This will prevent excessive drying of blood or organic matter. A liquid detergent rather than one of powder or crystal will prevent the accumulation of a residue on the instruments. After going through a mechanical cleansing process and then reaching a temperature of 270° F. at a pressure of 27 lbs., instruments are ready for use.

Water Sterilizers. There should be 2 large tanks, one for hot and one for cold water, so that a sufficient supply of both may be available. Water sterilizers are constructed in such a manner that the water that fills them flows first through a filter. Both tanks of water must be resterilized once every 12 hours, whether any water has been withdrawn since sterilization or not. A gauge on the tanks clearly indicates the amount of water present. Tanks never should be filled to the very top. At least 1 inch should show on the gauge, otherwise the tanks will overflow during the sterilization process. Present models of water

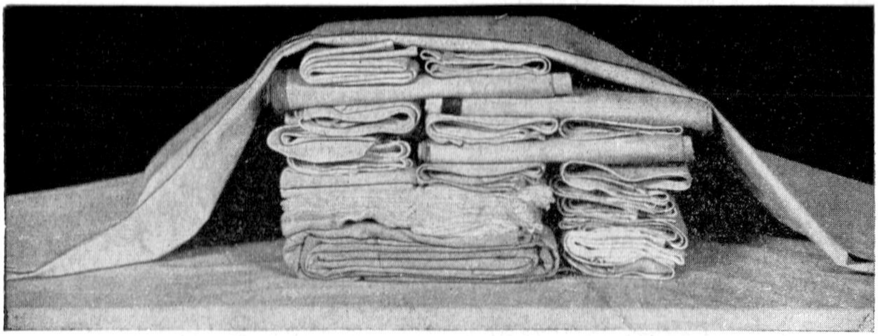

FIG. 279. A model heavy pack arrangement. None should be larger or more densely arranged. Note how alternate layers are crossed to promote free circulation of steam through the mass. Note also that gauze sponges are located near center of pack to break up close contact between masses of more tightly woven fabrics. (The Surgical Supervisor, American Sterilizer Co., Erie, Pa.)

sterilizers have very effective percolating devices by means of which the water in the reservoirs circulates continuously through the gauge glass for complete sterilization.

Following the filling of both tanks with sufficient water, the steam should be turned on and the temperature of the water permitted to advance until the temperature shows 240° F., and the pressure regulation for the tank should be adjusted so that the maximum temperature does not exceed 254° F. The period of exposure after the thermometer shows 240° F. with this regulation need not exceed 10 minutes. At the end of the required time, water and steam should be allowed to flow through the faucet for about 15 seconds. This will ensure a sterile outlet. After this, the cooling valves on the cold-water tank are opened so that the temperature may be reduced. The construction and the operation of water sterilizers are complicated and intricate. The instructor should explain their operation to the new nurse and, following instruction, require the inexperienced pupil to go through the various steps of sterilization and explain the uses of the different valves.

Instrument Sterilizers. These are similar in construction to the utensil sterilizers, only smaller. Another instrument sterilizer which not only sterilizes but washes the instruments has been devised. Such an autoclave or pressure steam sterilizer has been found to be very satisfactory for instrument sterilization and has replaced boiling.

MAKING AND STERILIZING DRESSINGS AND LINEN SUPPLIES

Linen supplies (sheets, gowns, covers and towels particularly) must be checked carefully on their return from the laundry before they are folded and packaged for sterilization. Holes and tears must be mended, tapes and buttons sewed on. Threads and ravelings must be removed. Usually all linen, including caps and masks, are dyed gray, blue or green, which eliminates the glare and reflection produced by bright lights on white linens.

Sheets and covers are folded to facilitate their use, such as fan-folding, etc. Such foresight will prevent undue handling and flourishing of sterile drapes. Covers and towels should be folded so that the edges

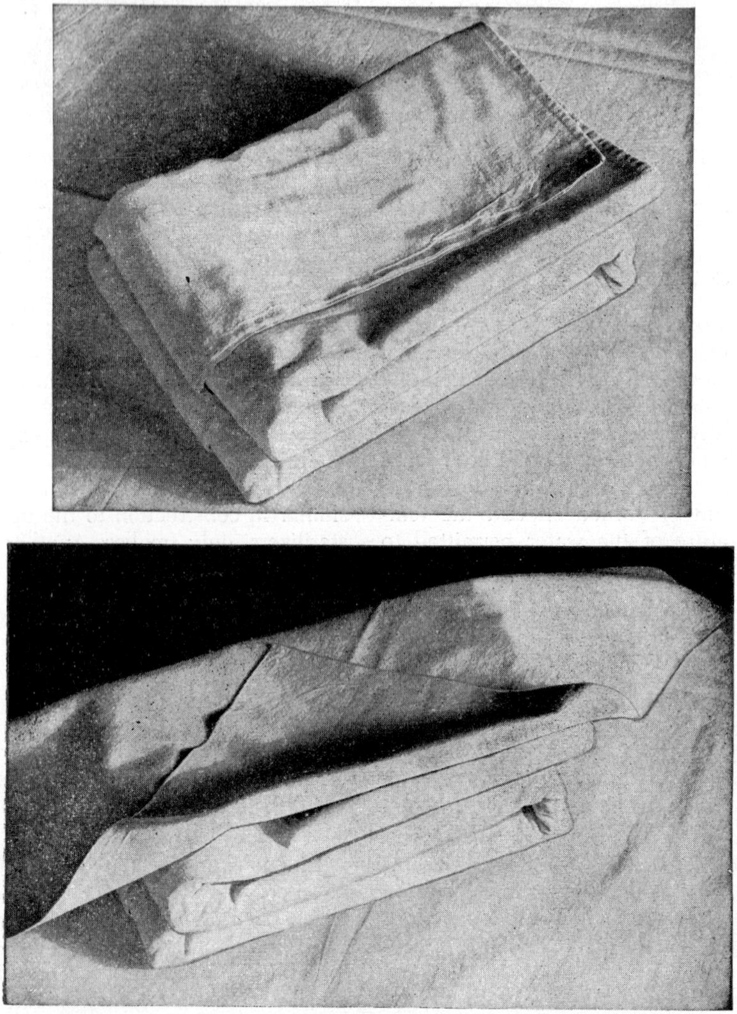

FIG. 280. (*Top*) The article folded loosely in place on a wrapper. (*Bottom*) The first fold in wrapping. See also Figure 281.

and not the center part will be handled when opened. Gowns must be folded wrong side out, so that the inner side only is touched by the ungloved hand when they are put on by the surgeon and his assistants. This is very easily accomplished by first folding the gown lengthwise and then, starting at the hem, rolling it into a compact bundle. A 5-inch length of 2-inch stockinet makes a very comfortable cuff for operating

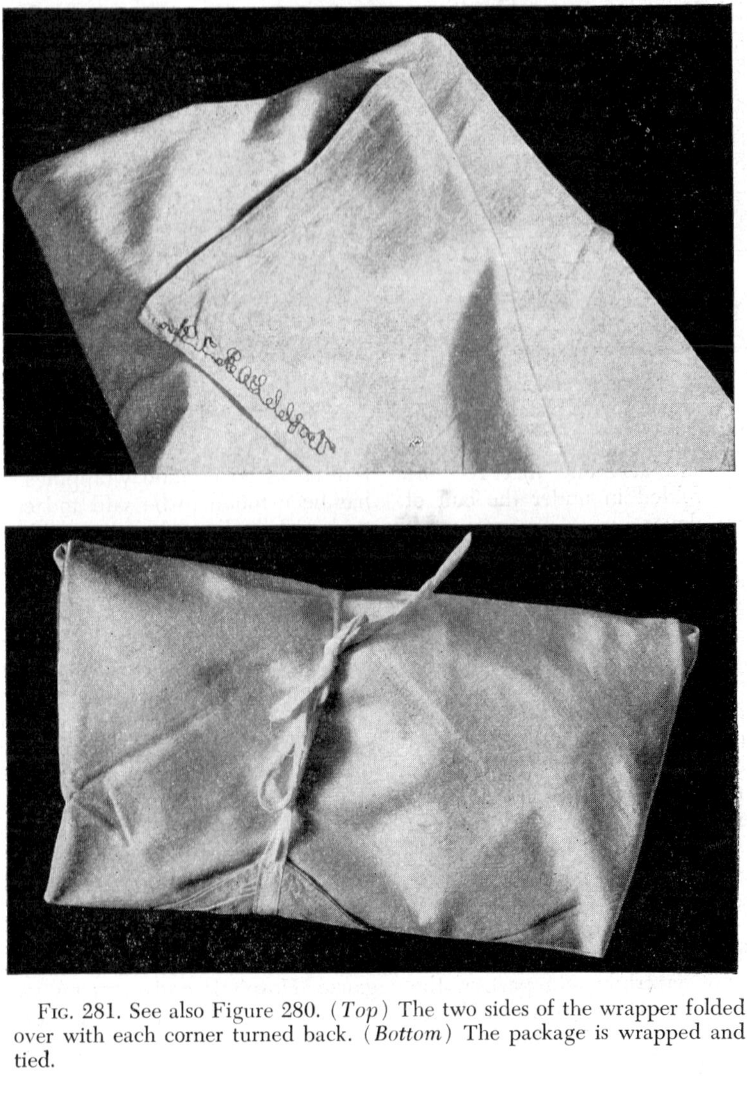

FIG. 281. See also Figure 280. (*Top*) The two sides of the wrapper folded over with each corner turned back. (*Bottom*) The package is wrapped and tied.

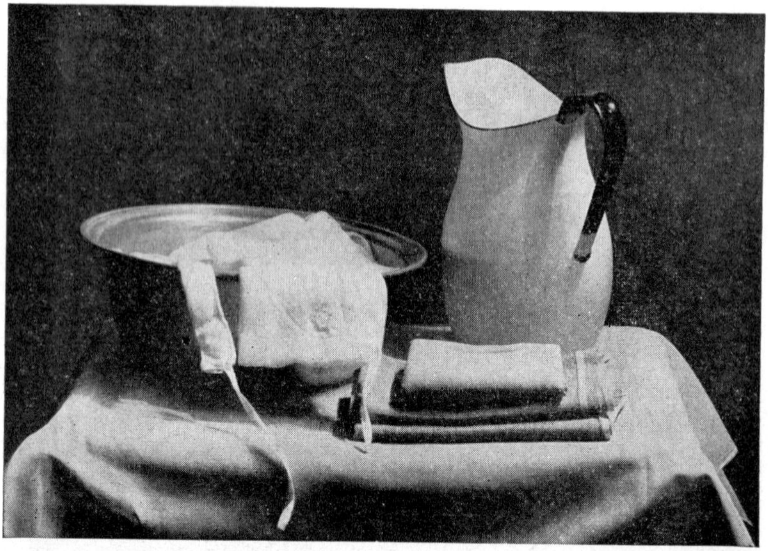

FIG. 282. Sponge table. Note narrow and small sponges with tapes. These sponges have metal rings sewed in them for x-ray identification.

gowns and also one that is more readily folded in under the cuff of rubber gloves.

The contents of a pack are arranged in such a way that the articles which are used first appear on top. The arrangement should facilitate steam penetration (Fig. 278). All gauze and linen supplies are packaged so that they can be handled by unsterile individuals and stored until needed. They are wrapped securely and neatly in clean, double-thickness covers so that they will not become undone in the usual handling.

Strings to fasten packages are preferred to straight pins. However, if pins are used, care must be taken in placing the pins so that the point does not protrude. No part of the pin must be visible except the head. In some hospitals heavy brown paper is used as covers and wrappings. It has been found to be safe and easy to handle. All packages should be legibly marked on the outside covering. The date of the sterilization should be marked on the package, in order to prevent packages being kept too long before use. Freshly sterilized supplies of all kinds should be placed on the bottom of the pile or in the rear of the cupboard. This method usually avoids an accumulation of stale supplies. If supplies are kept longer than two weeks after sterilization, they should be resterilized before use. This also applies to drums.

Dressings and Sponges. These are made from loose-meshed, bleached gauze. Hospitals and surgeons vary considerably in their specifications concerning the size and the shape of

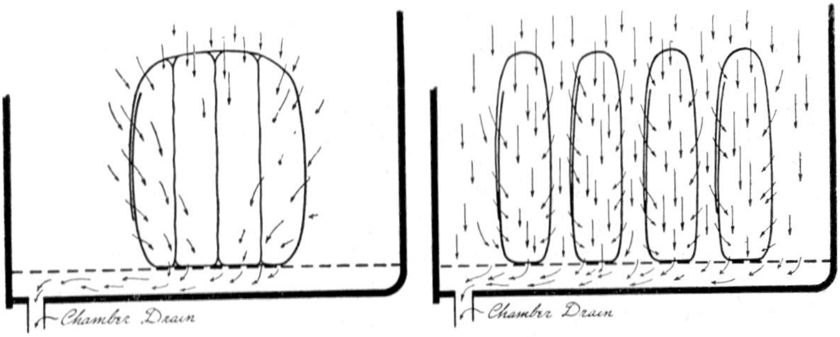

FIG. 283. (*Left*) One large pack. (*Right*) Same pack broken down into four small packs, and these are separated slightly from each other in the sterilizer. The single large pack shows why there is oversterilization of the outer portions when exposure has continued long enough to permit steam to penetrate adequately to the interior for sterilization. In the smaller packs, steam permeates the entire mass quickly and in the much shorter period of exposure needed.

sponges and the folding of gauze for dressings. The most essential feature in their making is to have all cut edges turned or stitched in so that there may be no ravelings. This is especially necessary in making gauze sponges. Sponges or pads for abdominal operations may have tapes or rings securely sewed in one corner. Commercially made abdominal sponges are available with a radiopaque filler. All abdominal sponges must be counted before being done up in packages for sterilization. The number in the packages depends on the method of counting in the particular operating room. Some supervisors prefer 5 sponges of one kind together, while others use 10 or 12. The exact arrangement is immaterial, but there must be some definite number adhered to without the slightest deviation. Before packaging, the sponges should be counted by 2 persons and again counted by 2 persons just before use. In this way, a rigid check can be kept and an incorrect sponge count avoided.

Eye dressings and sponges require special gauze and cotton (very fine-meshed gauze and the finest grade of absorbent cotton) and are made according to the taste of the individual surgeon. Dressings are often cut in an oval shape and no attempt is made to fold them.

Absorbent cotton is used for many purposes in the operating room.

Sterilization of Gauze and Linens. Gauze, cotton, covers, towels, etc., are sterilized in the autoclave for 30 minutes at 250°-254° F. The tighter the autoclave is packed, the longer it takes the steam to penetrate, causing destruction to some of the fabrics (Fig. 283). Goods should be wrapped in packs small enough that 30 minutes' exposure is adequate, and the temperature in the autoclave never should exceed 254° F.

Caps and Masks. Many different types of both doctors' and nurses' caps are satisfactory. The chief requisite of either should be to cover the hair completely. Doctors' caps are usually made of twilled muslin or stockinet, while nurses' caps are generally of lawn. Masks should be made of several thicknesses of lawn or gauze. From 4 to 6 layers of lawn, about 6 by 4 inches, with 4 tapes, 2 to tie on top of the head and 2 around the neck, make a simple but effective mask (Fig. 284). The mask should cover the nose. A pad of cotton and gauze fastened around the forehead is a comfort to those who perspire freely.

STERILIZATION AND CARE OF VARIOUS ARTICLES

Utensils

Basins, instrument trays and pitchers may be sterilized by autoclaving. If they are wrapped in muslin covers, sterilizing time is 30 minutes at a pressure of 15 lbs./sq. in. and a temperature of 250° F. *All containers must be placed on their sides to permit escape of air and entrance of steam.* If several basins are to be sterilized at one time, the same principle regarding position must be followed. Utensils necessary for one case usually are wrapped together in one package.

Instruments

Bright, shining and faultlessly working instruments should be one of the greatest delights of every good operating-room nurse. All instruments are expensive, not only in initial cost but in upkeep and repair if personnel are thoughtless or neglectful in their care of them. Instruments are made of stainless steel or

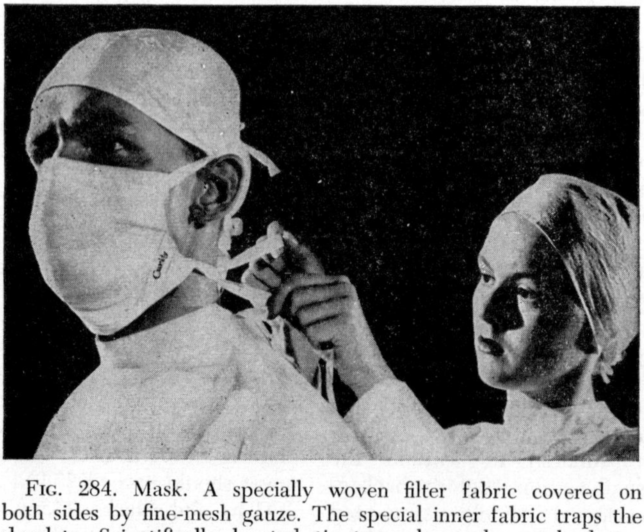

Fig. 284. Mask. A specially woven filter fabric covered on both sides by fine-mesh gauze. The special inner fabric traps the droplets. Scientifically located tie tapes keep the mask drawn tightly against the cheeks and the chin, and a flexible metal nosepiece keeps its upper edge tight against the nose and helps to prevent glasses from fogging. (Bauer & Black, Chicago)

chrome plated to prevent rust. Replating is particularly expensive and should not be necessary except at long intervals, provided that instruments are given the proper daily attention, not weekly or monthly. If adequate care is taken in the sterilization, cleansing and drying of instruments each time they are used, their life will be lengthened materially. Each instrument should be used only for the purpose for which it is intended; for example, a surgeon's dissecting scissors never should be used to cut bandage or dressings.

Metal Instruments. The process of sterilizing instruments by pressure steam (Fig. 277) is rapid, carries a greater margin of safety, is far less injurious to instruments and permits no scale formation. Regulation of temperature and exposure are the same as for all other surgical supplies, but, unlike all other loads, there is no lag factor in steam penetration because we are interested only in sterilizing surfaces. Routine exposure of ten minutes is advocated, timing the exposure when the thermometer indicates 250° F.

In extreme emergency when time is of the utmost importance, the period of exposure to steam under pressure can be reduced to 3 minutes at 270° F. This applies to single instruments rather than whole kits. If it can be assumed that the instruments are perfectly clean, with respect to dried particles in grooves and joints, this short exposure provides for perfect sterilization with a very small margin of safety factor.

After use, all instruments should be soaked for a few minutes in cold water and a detergent and then scrubbed with a brush under lukewarm running water. When steel instruments are covered with water they will not rust. If allowed to stand exposed to air in a moist condition they surely will rust. Various blood-dissolving solutions may be used to assist in the cleaning. Particular attention must be paid to teeth, crevices, joints, etc. All jointed instruments should be separated, cleansed and immediately reclamped. Sandsoap never should be used for scouring instruments, as it will remove nickel plating. Spots may be removed by gentle rubbing with a small amount of cleansing powder or soap. Instrument washing machines are gradually replacing hand washing of instruments.

Instruments used on **infected** cases should be washed clean by the scrubbed nurse while she still has her contaminated gloves on. Then the instruments may be soaked for 1 hour in an antiseptic, such as Zephiran Chloride. However, the steam-pressure method of washing and sterilizing is preferred.

All instruments should be well rinsed in hot water after thorough cleansing and should be dried immediately before putting them away. Forceps, scissors, etc., should be opened so that both blades may be thoroughly dried. If any instruments seem stiff, they should have a drop of high grade oil at the joint. Instruments that are seldom used should be wiped off once every week with a flannel cloth slightly moistened with the same kind of oil. This treatment will not only keep the instruments bright but will also prevent rust and corrosion spots. *Oil should be removed before sterilization.*

Cutting Instruments. Knives, scissors, chisels, etc., may be sterilized in the autoclave in such a way that each sharp edge does not touch any other instrument. This is best done by spreading the sharp-edged instruments on a towel in the sterilizer. Very delicate cutting instruments—cataract knives, tenotomes, urethrotomes—may be sterilized by immersion for 20 minutes in Zephiran Chloride 1:1,000 to which sodium nitrate has been added. Some surgeons prefer their cutting instruments to be autoclaved and then to be sharpened more frequently rather than run the risk of all organisms not being destroyed by soaking in disinfectant solutions. With the more expensive grade of instruments made from noncorrosive steel, this is both possible and satisfactory. Scissors, particularly, made from this steel retain their edge after repeated autoclaving and require sharpening comparatively infrequently, depending, of course, on the amount of use. If detachable knife blades are used, the handles should be sterilized with the instruments and the blades sterilized by soaking in a germicide or placed in the autoclave so that

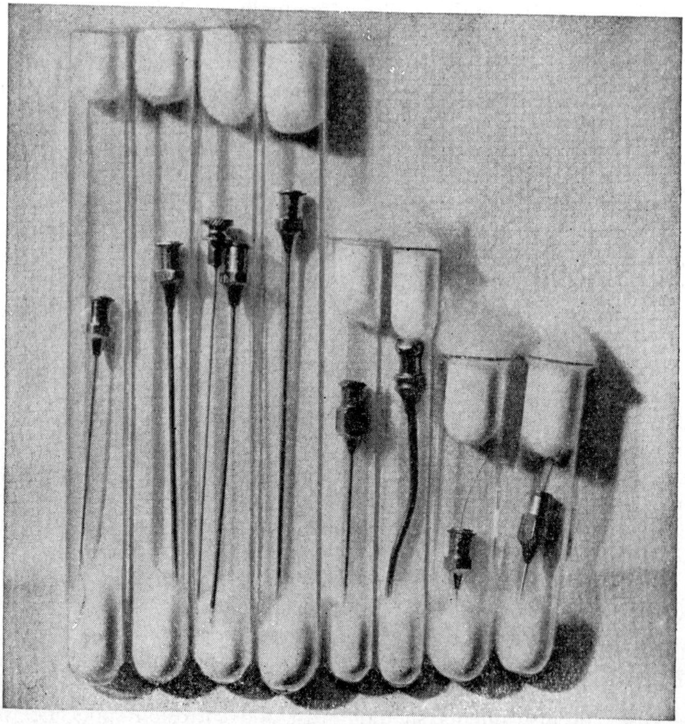

FIG. 285. Needles sterilized in autoclave in test tubes. Note cotton plugs and cotton in bottom of tubes.

they will not be injured by mechanical contact with others.

The after-care of cutting instruments is essentially the same as for other instruments. Precautions must be taken, of course, to protect the edges. All cutting instruments should be tested after use to determine whether or not they require sharpening.

Needles. Suture needles should be arranged in some definite order, according to personal taste and convenience, in a sufficiently large piece of gauze or a needle rack made of coiled wire which is fastened on a flat piece of metal. The latter method is preferable. Hot air of 320° F. for one hour is recommended because it leaves the needles free from rust. A safe method of sterilization is by autoclaving with the instruments. Hollow needles may be sterilized in the autoclave or hot-air oven. They should be sterilized with the wire or stilet inserted and projecting slightly beyond the point of the needle. The needles should be placed in the autoclave so that they lie on their side, in order to allow air to escape and steam to enter their containers.

For both hot-air and autoclave sterilization a small amount of cotton is placed in the bottom of the test tube to protect the needle point. The needles are then placed in the tube with or without stilets in place. The tube is closed and its rim protected with a gauze and/or cotton plug. After use, hollow needles should be washed at once both inside and outside with cold water. A cotton applicator should be used to clean the hub of the needle and the wire should be passed through repeatedly in order to dislodge any particles of dirt, blood clot, etc. When the needle is absolutely clean, alcohol and ether should be forced through it with a syringe and the wire inserted and withdrawn a sufficient number of times to dry the inside thoroughly. If needles are used infrequently, it is wise to place a small quantity of petrolatum or oil on the stilet before its final insertion. Stilets always should be inserted well beyond the point of the needle for adequate protection.

Both suture and hollow needles require occasional scouring. Bon Ami or Sapolio may be used for this purpose. Care should be taken always to rub toward the point of the needle. The proper way to scour needles is to place the needle directly on the cake of Bon Ami and to use a small piece of moistened cloth for rubbing it. Rubbing with a cloth, wet with waste ether and dipped in emery powder, not only cleans the needles but sharpens them as well. Trocars and cannulae may be sterilized with the instruments. Cannulae should have the same care after use as hollow needles. Trocars are treated in the same way as cutting instruments.

Cystoscopes, urethroscopes, proctoscopes and other such instruments containing delicate lenses cannot be sterilized by heat, owing to the unequal expansion of glass and metal. They should not be subjected to contact with alcohol, which will loosen the cement with which the lenses are fixed. They should be disinfected in a solution of Zephiran 1:1,000 for a half hour. Scopes should be rinsed thoroughly in sterile cold water before use. If the scope has the lens held in place by a newly

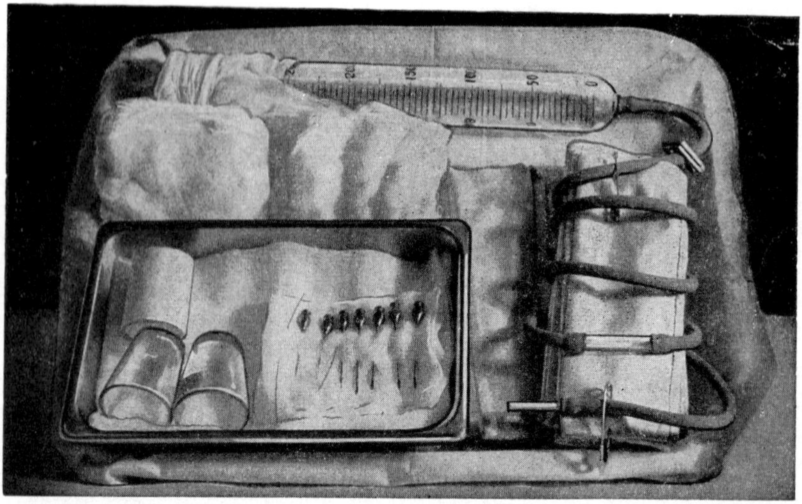

FIG. 286. Suggested arrangement of rubber tubing for sterilization. Fold 2 or 3 towels into a cylinder. Spiral the tubing, with both ends free—avoiding kinks—round the cylinder, securing both ends of the tube, without collapsing, to the cylinder with safety pins. Place the cylinder loosely in the tray, wrap with double muslin, sterilize the tray resting on its side in the sterilizer so that the cylinder rests vertically. Avoid tight packing in the sterilizer. (The Surgical Supervisor, American Sterilizer Company, Erie, Pa.)

developed heat-resistant plastic compound, such an instrument can be autoclaved.

Catheters. Silver catheters should be autoclaved. After use, they should be cleansed with cold running water followed by hot water and soap.

Gum elastic, woven silk and filiform bougies or catheters are best disinfected in Zephiran Chloride 1:1,000 for 30 minutes. After the sterilization period rinse thoroughly with sterile water. (See footnote, p. 384.)

Soft rubber catheters may be boiled or autoclaved.

ARTICLES OF RUBBER

Proper Care. Rubber tubing, drainage tubes, rubber dam, may be sterilized best in the autoclave. After thorough washing of the tubing, immediately before wrapping for sterilization, rinse the tubing thoroughly inside and outside with freshly distilled water. *Do not dry.* Leaving the rubber wet brings about the sterilization of the interior, whereas if the rubber tubing is put into the autoclave with the inside dry, steam will not permeate the interior, and sterilization will be highly questionable. Wrap immediately in muslin and sterilize in the autoclave for not more than 15 minutes (Fig. 286). All rubber deteriorates with repeated sterilization and always must be tested before use.

After use, rubber should be washed under cold running water, followed by tepid water and a little soap and then rinsed thoroughly in cold water and dried.

Acids corrode rubber. Oil and grease partially dissolve it. Lysol never should be used for disinfecting rubber goods. Metal instruments and soft rubber never should be sterilized close together in the same container, as the instruments will become discolored.

Rubber gloves and finger cots are sterilized in the autoclave. They should be well powdered, inside and out, protected by wrapping in muslin covers and arranged according to size or wearer. Properly wrapped gloves should be sterilized in the autoclave at 240° to 250°-254° F. for 15, definitely not to exceed 20, minutes of exposure. Longer exposure to the intense heat of the autoclave tends to destroy or greatly deteriorate glove fabric.

Considerable investigative work is reported on the use and abuse of talcum as a powder for hands and gloves (see References, p. 698). Although there appears to be some evidence that talcum may produce peritoneal irritation, this danger can largely be avoided by washing the gloved hands in sterile water before going to the operating table. There are available lubricating powders made of starch derivatives which appear to be free from the reported disadvantages of talcum.

Gloves, of course, are more easily cleansed when they are washed under running water before removal from the hands. For this reason, a period of soaking is recommended for operating-room gloves in order to loosen any adherent blood. Automatic glove washers are available. When done by hand, gloves must be washed thoroughly on both sides under cold or tepid running water, following which they should be well rinsed in cold water and hung up to dry in such a manner that the water can readily drain from the fingertips. When gloves have dried on one side, they must be turned inside out and permitted to dry on the other.

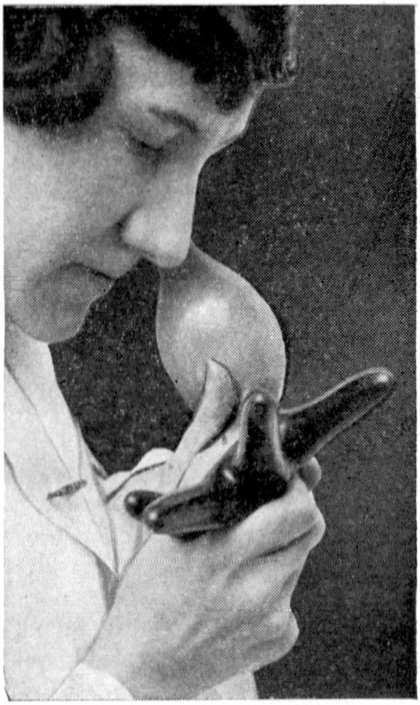

FIG. 287. Testing rubber gloves.

One of the most important tasks in the operating room is the testing, mending and mating of the rubber gloves. A tiny, almost invisible needle prick is as much of a menace as a readily discernible tear. Each finger, as well as the body of the glove,

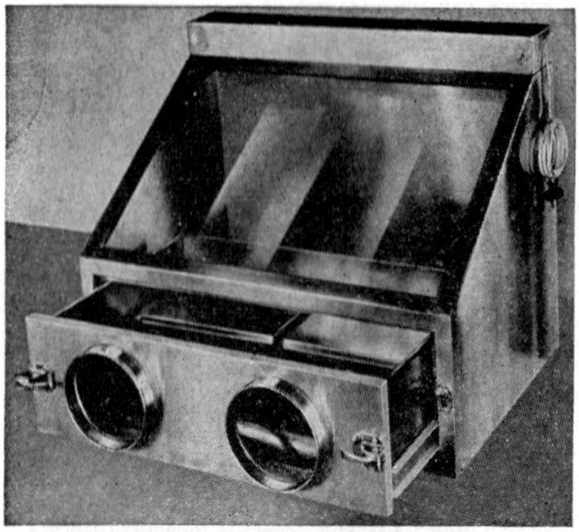

FIG. 288. A glove-powdering cabinet. (The Surgical Supervisor, American Sterilizer Company, Erie, Pa.)

must be tested thoroughly for defects. To do this, the glove should be well inflated with air, the air confined by grasping firmly the edges of the cuff, and the glove held close to the cheek in order to detect the escape of any air through perforations. If the glove is in good condition otherwise, the holes should be mended, using rubber cement and patches cut from strong parts of old gloves. Care must be taken to patch gloves on the wrong side. Different sizes should be kept together as the gloves are tested and mended, so that when the patching has been completed the various sizes may be taken separately for sorting, mating, powdering and subsequent placing in covers. Operators should rarely be given gloves that are patched, and never gloves that are patched at the fingertips, since this impairs their sense of touch. Gloves that are old and lifeless should be discarded, as should those that are badly torn. It is considered poor economy to use overly patched or mended gloves.

Special pains must be taken in the mating of gloves to be sure that there is one glove, right side out, for each hand. It is also most important to be very sure that no powder has been left in the fingertips. To prevent this, gloves should be powdered on one side, then turned and powdered on the other, following which they should be held up by the fingertips and slightly shaken to dislodge any excess powder (Fig. 288). The cuff of each glove should be turned back over the outside for approximately three to four inches, but not far enough to prevent seeing which is the right-hand and which the left-hand glove. Each pair of gloves should be put in a separate cover. Various types of covers are used, some having a small pocket for each glove, the whole folding over like a book. Whatever the type, the chief requisites are that they allow for adequate sterilization, that the material be sufficiently heavy (twilled muslin is most satisfactory), and that the covers be clean. Each packet of gloves should be marked with either the name of the wearer or the size, and should include a small amount of powder in a paper dispenser for powdering the hands immediately before putting on the gloves. A starch derivative powder rather than talcum should be used, inasmuch as talcum may cause adhesions. A sufficient number of gloves always should be sterilized to provide for accidents of tearing, contamination, etc.

Glass and china are of many types; therefore, the best method of sterilization is the one recommended by

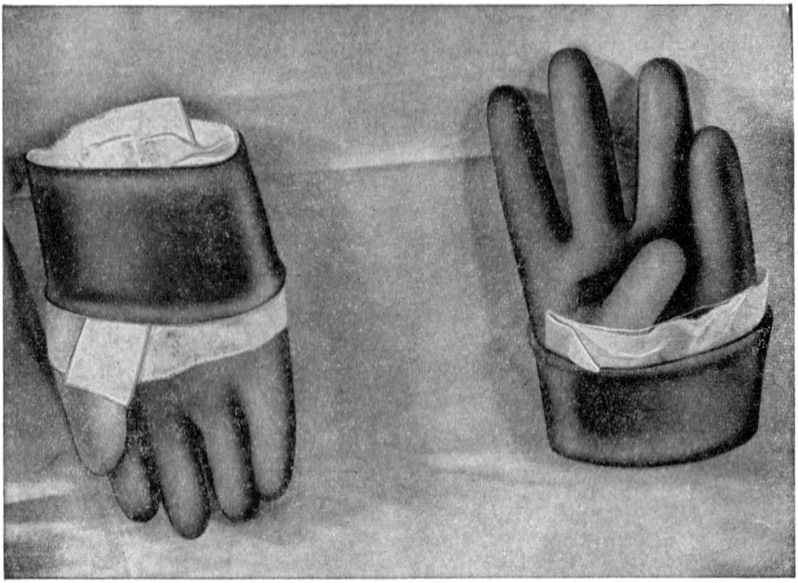

Fig. 289. A pad of gauze, muslin or crinkly paper should be inserted between the wrist surfaces of the glove, as the fold is made, to permit the free entrance of steam to these folded-over surfaces. It is less important—but a close approach to the ideal condition—to insert a similar pad as far in as the fingers in the hand of each glove. This permits steam to reach the inner walls of the glove. (The Surgical Supervisor, American Sterilizer Co., Erie, Pa.)

Fig. 290. (*Bottom, left*) "Right" and "Left" are embroidered on the two glove pockets to eliminate fumbling in removing the gloves from the envelope.

Fig. 291. (*Bottom, right*) The envelope shown in Figure 290 contains a pocket on the back, as indicated, for the powder envelope.

(The Surgical Supervisor, American Sterilizer Co., Erie, Pa.)

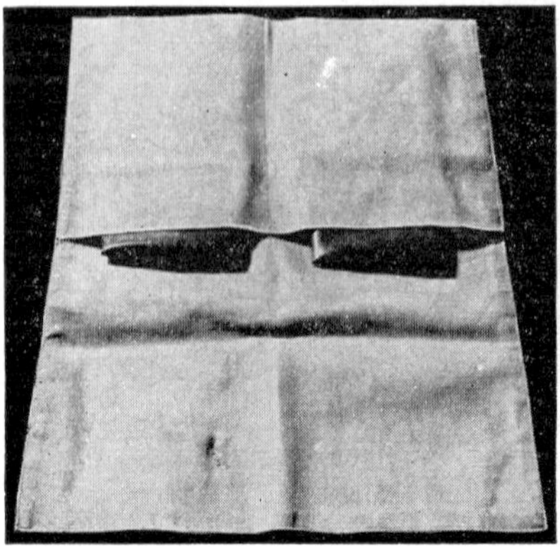

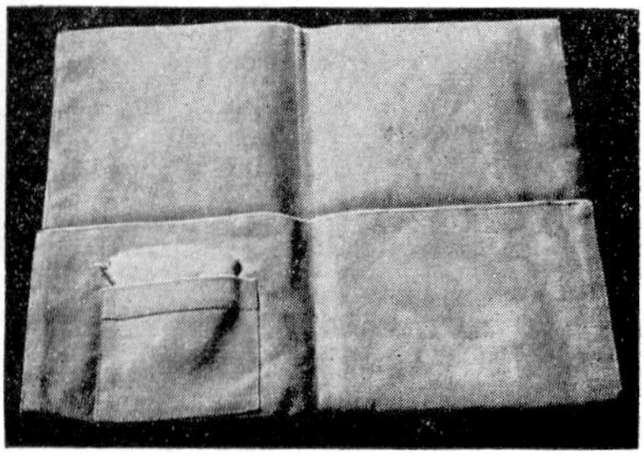

the manufacturer. Some are made to withstand heat and others are not. Some chemicals attack glass and cause corrosion. The most satisfactory method of sterilizing glass and china is to wrap and autoclave for 30 minutes. Another method of sterilizing glass and china is to soak the articles for at least 30 minutes in some disinfectant solution. Zephiran Chloride 1:1,000 may be used for this purpose.

Syringes. Glass syringes must be rinsed in cold water immediately after use and then cleaned thoroughly with soap and water. A small bottle brush is effective in this cleaning process. Mechanical washers are available to clean syringes. Neglect to care immediately for used syringes and needles often results in a needle's being firmly stuck to the ground-glass tip or the plunger's being locked in the barrel. Many syringes are broken from this neglect. Recommended methods of taking care of this difficulty are shown in Figures 293 and 294. Barrel and plunger are separated with gauze and wrapped in a double layer of muslin. Sterilizing time in the autoclave is 30 minutes, pressure 15 lb./sq. in., and temperature is 250° F. If boiling is used, again the barrel and the plunger should be separated. They are boiled for 20 minutes, preferably in distilled water.

Transfusion and Intravenous Trays

Special precautions are necessary in the care and the preparation of transfusion and intravenous trays. Transfusions and intravenous infusions are often given as emergency measures during or following an operation, and to find an instrument missing, or one which does not func-

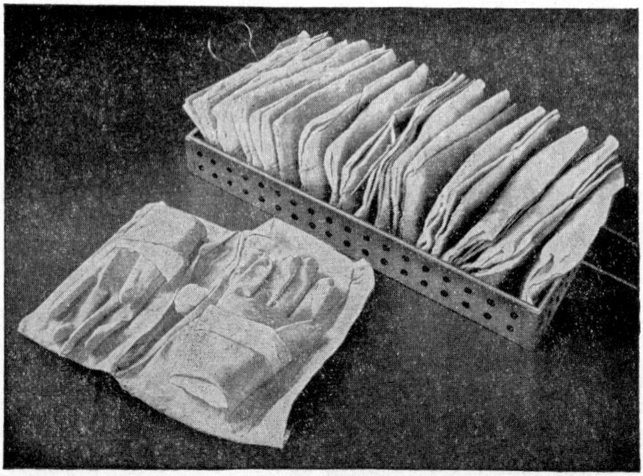

Fig. 292. An instrument tray used as shown for containing glove envelopes in the sterilizer is thoroughly practical. Note that there is no crowding. (The Surgical Supervisor, American Sterilizer Co., Erie, Pa.)

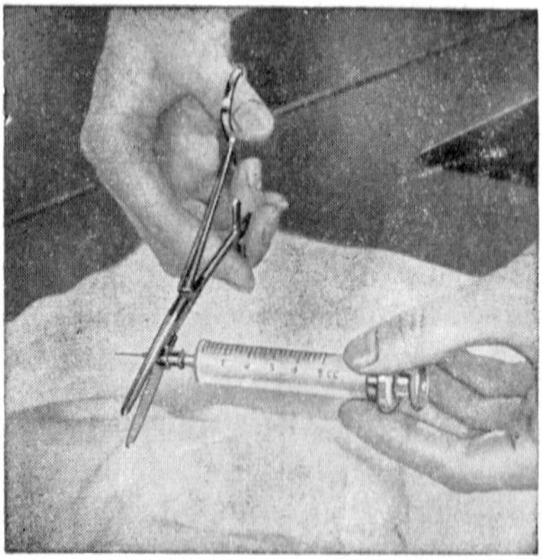

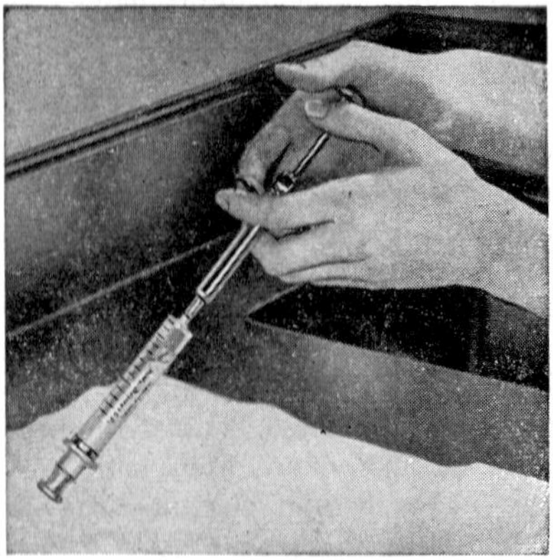

FIG. 293. (*Left*) In removing a stuck needle, grasp the square part of the needle hub firmly with a pair of pliers or with forceps. Rotate the syringe gently.

FIG. 294. (*Right*) An all-metal syringe equipped with a female Luer slip can be used to separate a stuck syringe by exerting steady, gentle pressure.

(Beckton, Dickinson & Co., Rutherford, N. J.)

tion, often means unnecessary delay. After each use the contents of the tray should be washed carefully to remove all traces of blood. The needles, the cannulae and the tubing demand special attention. The needles must be not only clean but also sharp. The large "donor's needles" should be sharpened after each use. The rubber tubing deteriorates with sterilization and should be replaced at frequent intervals. The scissors on the tray must be tested after each use to make sure that they cut well at the tip. (See p. 173 for further instructions.)

Radium Tubes

Tubes containing radium are sterilized when necessary by soaking for 30 minutes in 70 per cent alcohol or Zephiran 1:1,000. Tubes should be rinsed in sterile water before use. Radium in any shape or form always must be handled with forceps, never with the hands, even though gloved. Unprotected undue exposure of any part of the body may result in a burn.

Cautery Points

Cautery points are sufficiently sterilized by their own heat. After use, the point should be brought to "white heat" for a minute to burn off any adherent organic matter, then cooled, removed from the cautery box, washed, scoured if necessary, dried and replaced. Many types of electrocautery knives and connecting wires may be sterilized by autoclaving or by immersion in an antiseptic solution.

To facilitate the handling of the cautery in a sterile manner by the surgeon, a sterile mitten made of heavy muslin or canton flannel is placed over his gloved hand by the suture nurse.

There are two kinds of electrical currents: direct (DC) and alternating (AC). Some electrical appliances are made for use with only one type of current; others may be used with either type. In using electrical appliances it is important for the nurse to know which type of current is required. Cauteries, electrical diathermies and motors are often made useless if the wrong current is used. When both AC and DC currents are used in the operating room, the outlets should be plainly marked, and it is a good plan to have different types of safety plug-ins for the different systems so that there will be no confusion.

Operating Motors

Motors for bone surgery are contained in removable outer shells that can be sterilized by autoclaving. The chuck, all drills, doweling apparatus, saws, etc., can be autoclaved. The motor must not get wet. No attempt is made to sterilize it. Oil should be applied as directed. Motors that can be autoclaved in toto are most generally used.

CHAPTER THIRTY-ONE

The Nurse in the Operating Room

INTRODUCTION

(Review Chap. 5, The Patient in the Operating Room.)

When a patient arrives in the operating room, essentially 4 different groups have prepared for their role in his care. The first group is the anesthesiologist and his assistants, who greet the patient, administer the anesthetic agent and place him in the proper position on the operating table. The second team is the nurse or nurses who prepare the operating room for the reception of the patient and assist throughout the operation. Such a nurse does not scrub but remains unsterile and is often referred to as the circulating nurse. The third group is the nurse or nurses who scrub, set up the sterile tables to include all the instruments, sponges, sutures, etc., that will be necessary for the particular operation. The fourth group is the surgeon and his assistants who scrub and perform the operation. Auxiliary personnel who are called surgical technicians are being trained to take over some of the lesser functions of the nursing group.

Inasmuch as we are concerned primarily with the responsibilities of the nurse in the operating room, this section will be devoted to her role as a circulating (unsterile) nurse and as a scrubbed (sterile) nurse. Regardless of the particular responsibilities of each worker, the concept of team work should be practiced. Every member of an operating room group must work together so that the corps of workers may function, not as individuals, but as one unit, having one common interest—the welfare of the patient.

The responsibilities of everyone associated with the operating room should be outlined clearly. This avoids many errors and fixes responsibility at all times. If lists enumerating the duties of each person are placed where all may see and read them, endless difficulties will be avoided. More work will be accom-

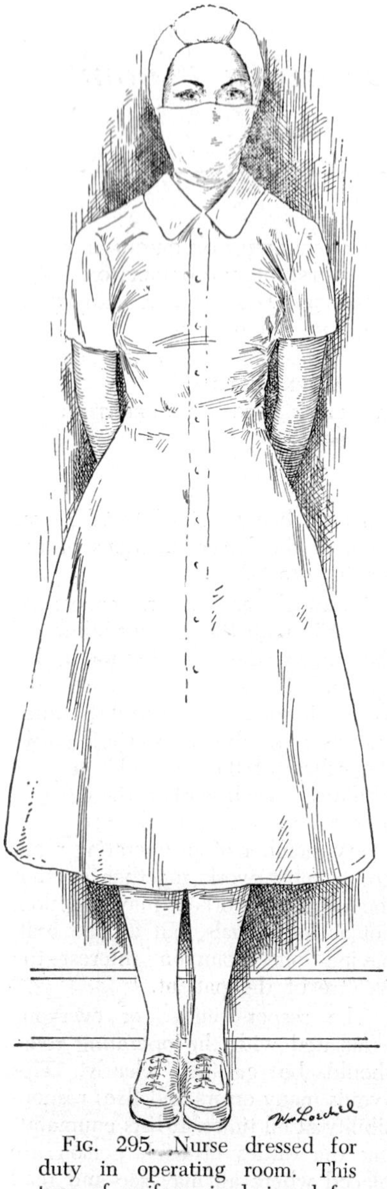

FIG. 295. Nurse dressed for duty in operating room. This type of uniform is designed for cleanliness, personal comfort and working efficiency.

plished in a shorter length of time, one person will not wait for another to do some task if she knows it to be part of her own particular duties, and, if something has not been done or has been done improperly, the head nurse knows at once with whom the fault lies.

Operating room nurses always should be clean and neat in appearance. A dirty or untidy gown or uniform not only looks bad but decreases the cleanliness of the operating room. The best of health is also essential. Colds, sore throat and infected fingers are a distinct menace and must be reported at once to the nurse in charge. A series of wound infections in clean cases was traced in one instance to a mild throat infection among the operating room nurses. Therefore, it can be understood readily how very important it is for nurses to report any seemingly slight ailment without delay.

RESPONSIBILITIES OF THE CIRCULATING NURSE BEFORE THE OPERATION

If aseptic technic is to be carried out, there is much to get ready for every surgical procedure. Many preparations are done some time before, and others are completed just prior to the operation. The long-term preparations include packaging and sterilizing dressings and linens, testing instruments for optimum function, checking supply closets for drugs, suture materials, adhesive, etc. Within the hour before the operation, the circulating nurse has the following more specific functions:

1. Regulate the temperature of the rooms to 78° F.

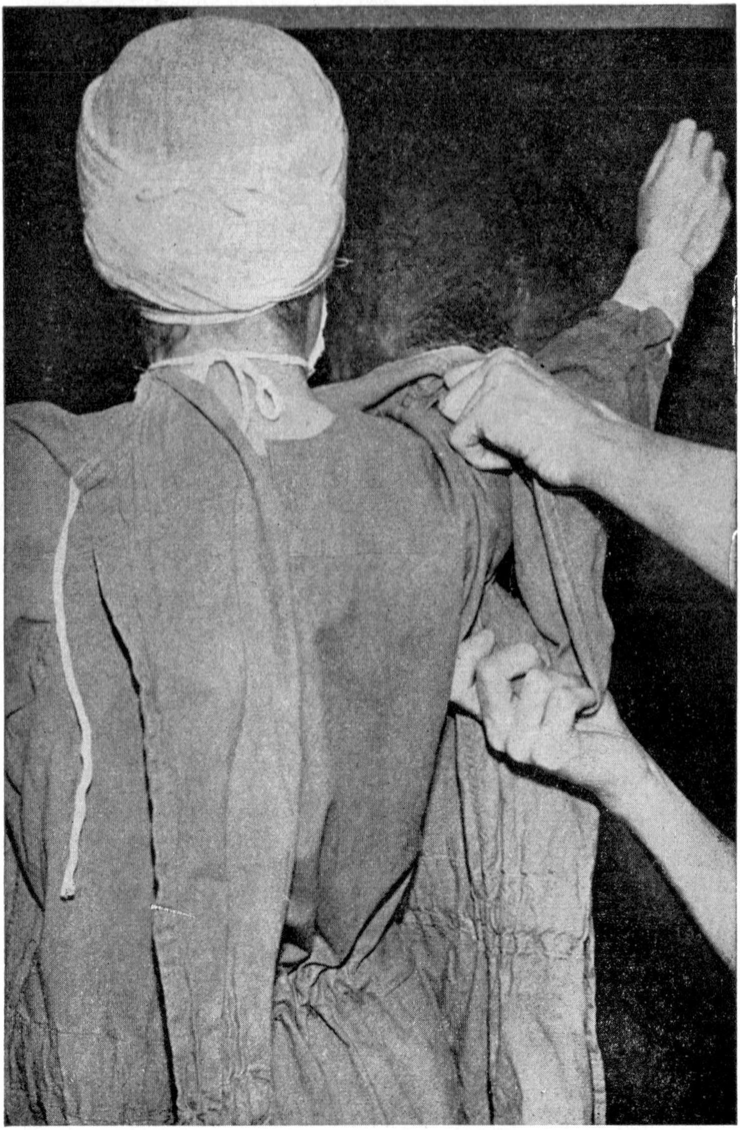

Fig. 296. Method of putting on sterile gown. The unsterile nurse at the back of the scrub nurse or doctor grasps the axillary seam from within the gown. By pulling on this seam toward the chest wall, the sleeve is drawn easily over the damp hand to its proper position.

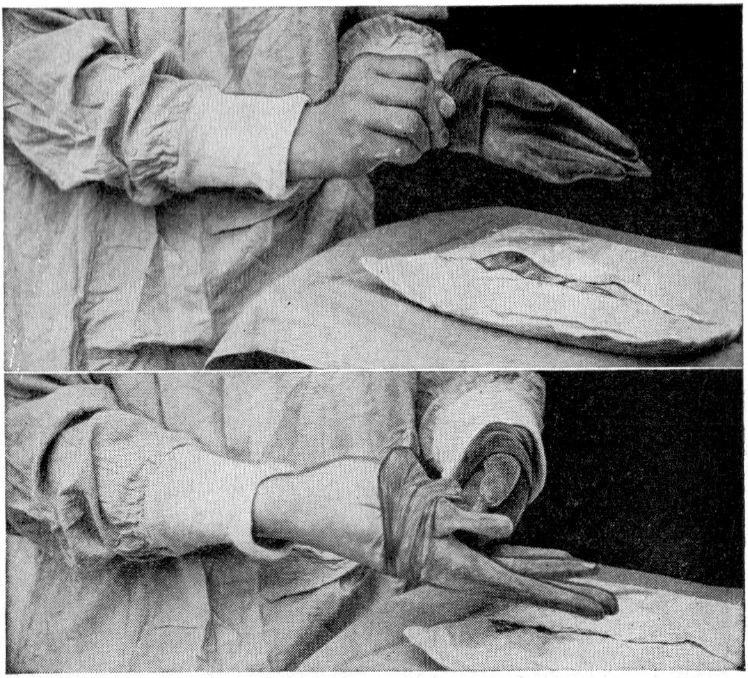

FIG. 297. (*Top*) Pulling on left glove without touching outside. (*Bottom*) Pulling on right glove by inserting gloved fingers into cuff.

2. Check tables and equipment for their cleanliness, freedom from dust, etc.

3. See that the steam supply on the necessary sterilizers is turned on. Note whether or not there is sufficient hot and cold water.

4. Inspect the scrub rooms for adequate supplies.

5. Check the instruments which have been selected for the case and see that they are sterilized.

6. See that the operating table is prepared and in working order. The pad should be securely strapped in place, sufficiently inflated (if the air-mattress type is used), and the whole protected with a mackintosh and a sheet. Shoulder braces, ether screen, stirrups and sandbags should be available.

7. Test all lights, suction apparatus, x-ray view box and any electrical equipment which may be used.

8. Select and arrange tables and stands likely to be used.

9. Gather sterile packages and place them conveniently so that they can be unwrapped quickly.

TECHNIC OF SCRUBBING, PUTTING ON GOWN AND GLOVES

About 1 hour previous to the scheduled time of the first operation, the nurse whose duty it is to set up the tables puts on her cap and mask and scrubs up, following which she dons sterile gown and gloves and proceeds with her duties.

Caps and Masks. These always should be adjusted properly before starting to scrub. Nurses must remember that the chief purpose of an operating cap is to cover the hair and that no hair should protrude from underneath the cap. The mask should completely cover the nose and the mouth.

Hands and Arms. The preparation of the skin is done for the purpose of removing dirt, fats, transient and resident bacterial flora in the most convenient time. Nails should be trimmed short and cleaned thoroughly with a sterile orangewood stick during the early process of scrubbing. A firm bristled, sterile brush, soap which emulsifies and lathers well, and warm water should be used to scrub the hands and the arms to at least two inches above the elbows. There should be a definite system of scrubbing: inner and outer surfaces of the thumb and the fingers, palm and dorsum of the hand, anterior and posterior forearm, with special attention to the interdigital spaces.

Intermittent rinsing should be done by allowing the water to flow from the hands to the elbows so that all water flows off at the elbow. The usual length of time for scrubbing has been 10 minutes. With the advent of more effective cocoanut oil or castor oil soaps and synthetic phenol compounds, the time element can be shortened. The trend is toward scrubbing with a definite number of strokes for each part rather than haphazardly for a definite period of time. Hands and arms must be as effectively cleaned as if no aseptic coverings were available, to provide protection when gloves are torn, pricked, etc. It is impossible to sterilize skin but it is possible to make it "surgically clean." After thorough scrubbing, all soap should be completely washed off with water, and some antiseptic should be used for chemical disinfection of the hands and the arms. Various solutions are used for this purpose. Some of the more common are bichloride of mercury, Zephiran Chloride, 1:1,000, or isopropyl alcohol, 70 per cent. Friction during immersion increases the germicidal action.

Gown and Gloves. Following scrubbing, disinfecting and drying the hands and the arms, the sterile gown should be put on, using great care to touch only the inside with the ungloved hands. The circulating nurse can help the scrubbed person with his gown by getting back of him and pulling the axillary seam from within the gown. This is the easiest way to pull the sleeve over the hands to its proper position on the arms. After both arms are well in their sleeves, she can tie the strings at the back of the gown. If the gown is "bunched up," she can pull it down firmly by getting hold of the bottom hem. All contact by the unsterile nurse should be limited to the inner part of the gown, the tie strings and the hem. After the gown is on, the packet of gloves may be taken and put on in the following manner.

Gloves should be prepared with the cuff folded back. If the hands are moist and require powdering, powder should not be applied di-

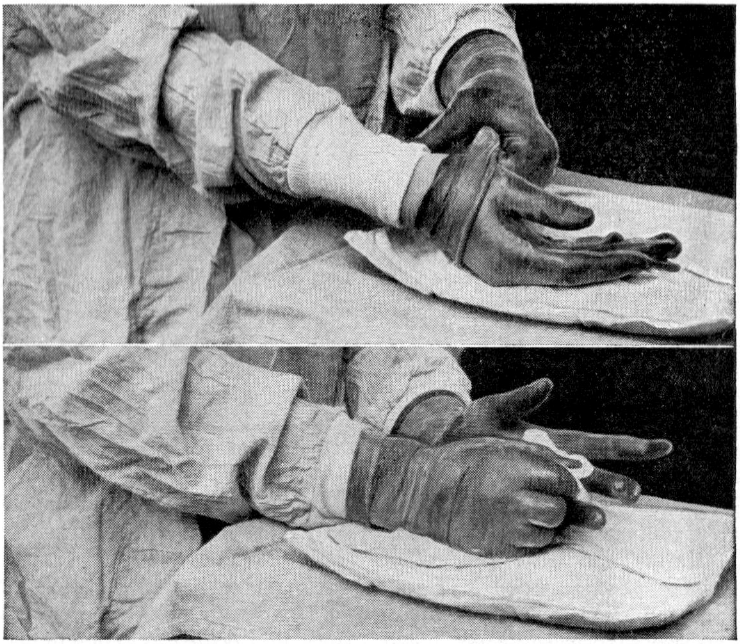

FIG. 298. (*Top*) Folding glove cuff over gown cuff. (*Bottom*) Working on glove fingers with sterile gauze.

rectly over the glove packet. The hands should be fairly well powdered, especially in hot weather, as otherwise gloves may be torn in the attempt to pull them on over a moist skin surface. The turned-back cuff of the left glove should be grasped with the right hand in putting on the left-hand glove. The gloved fingers of the left hand should then be placed inside the turned-back cuff of the right-hand glove and the right hand slipped into the glove. When both hands are gloved, the gown cuff should be folded snugly to the wrist and the glove cuff pulled up over it. If the hands have been well dried and powdered, gloves should slip on without difficulty. If the fingers do stick, no attempt should be made to pull the glove snug until both gloves are entirely on. Then, with a small piece of gauze, the glove fingers may be adjusted readily. The scrubbed nurse recognizes that certain parts of her gown are to be considered "dangerous areas" and should not be touched by her gloved hands. These are the back of the gown and the lower areas near the hemline. Hence, she will keep her hands in front of her at the waist line when she is not using them. Under no circumstances should her hands be at her sides because danger of contamination is too great.

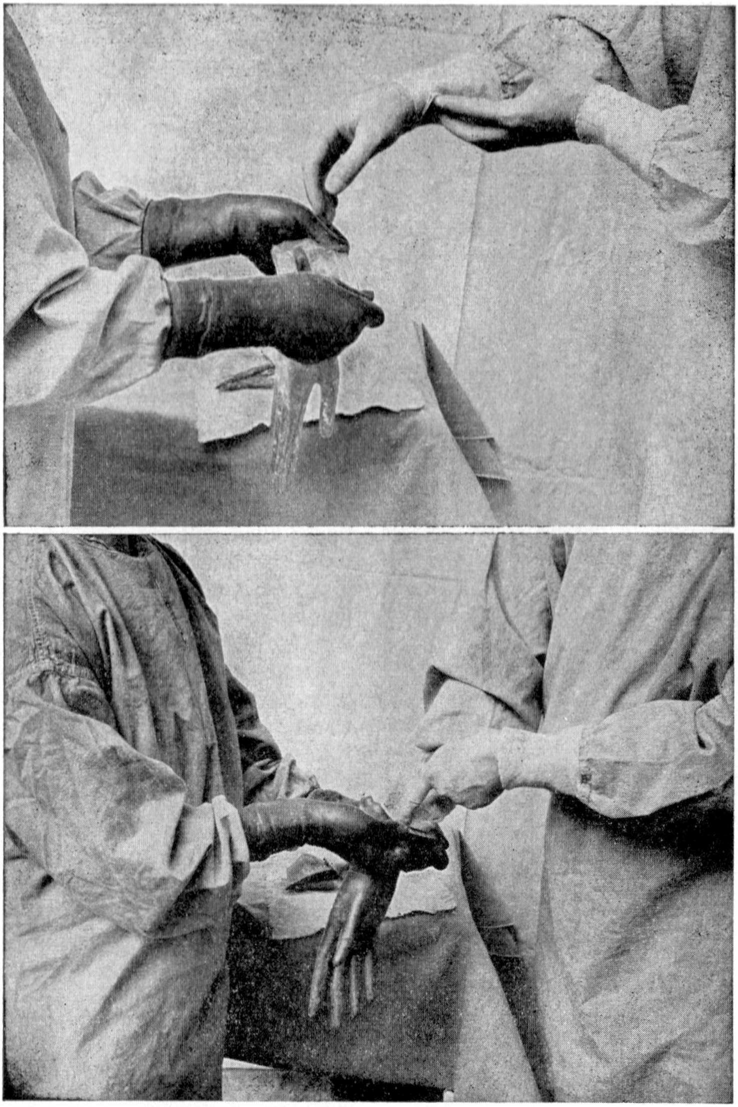

FIG. 299. (*Top*) Method of holding gloves for surgeon. Fingers of both hands are placed on inside of turned-back cuff (the outside of the glove), thumb up. Cuff then is stretched slightly to allow surgeon's hand to slip in freely. (*Bottom*) Holding gloves for surgeon. Surgeon has inserted hand into glove with quick thrust, nurse is pulling cuff of glove over surgeon's sleeve.

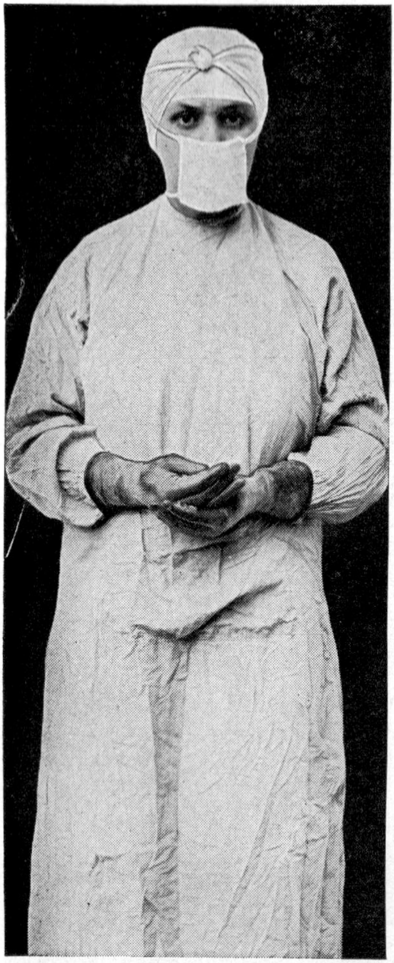

FIG. 300. Operating room nurse scrubbed up.

SETTING UP THE TABLES

At this time, the responsibility of the circulating nurse is to assist the scrubbed nurse in setting up the necessary sterile tables. Much time and effort can be saved during the process of "setting up" if all covers for tables, basin racks, etc., are done up for sterilization in one bundle. Sterile packs containing sponges, packing, extra covers, towels, etc., also greatly facilitate the procedure of preparing the operating room.

The handling of sterile material by the circulating nurse must be done in such a way that she does not touch or contaminate them. Packages have been wrapped to facilitate careful unwrapping (Figs. 301-305).

For equipment which must be transferred from sterile stock container to the sterile instrument table, the circulating nurse must use a transfer or pick-up forceps. Such a forceps is usually kept in a container filled with an antiseptic solution. Only that portion of the forceps is considered sterile which is immersed in solution. Therefore, when it is lifted from the container, care must be taken to prevent touching the side with the sterile tip. When using such a sterile forceps, the tips must point downward at all times. If they are inadvertently turned up, the solution will run to the unsterile part of the forceps and contaminate the sterile portion.

New forceps and containers are now available which eliminate the aforementioned possible ways of contamination. They are recommended (Fig. 306).

When pouring solutions, the flask or pitcher must be held high enough so that the unsterile outside of the container or the hand of the pourer will not touch the receiving sterile basin. On the other hand, it should not be held so high that the solution will splash. In removing a lid from a sterile container or pitcher, it should

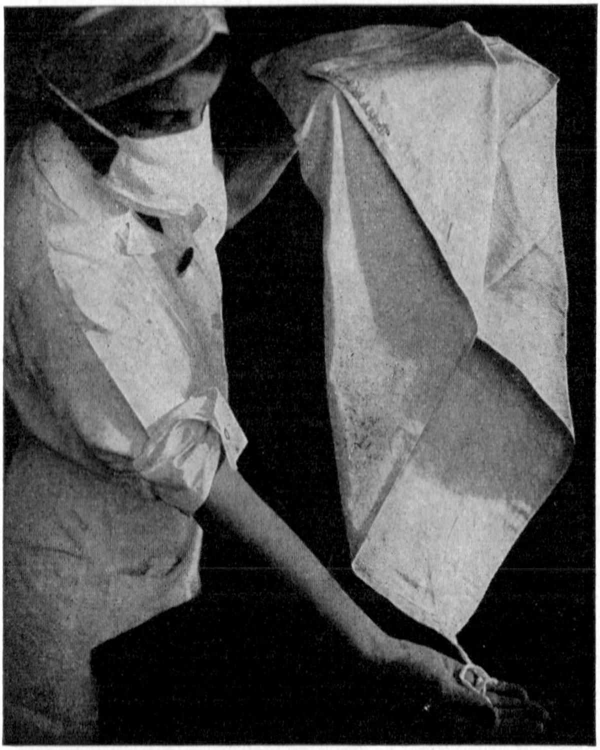

Fig. 301. (*Top*) The first step in unwrapping the package.
Fig. 302. (*Bottom*) The package completely unwrapped and ready to hand to a sterile nurse or to place on a sterile table.
(The Surgical Supervisor, American Sterilizer Co., Erie, Pa.)

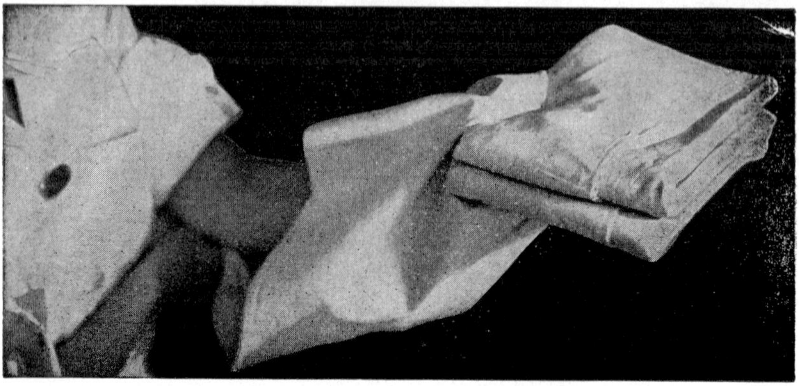

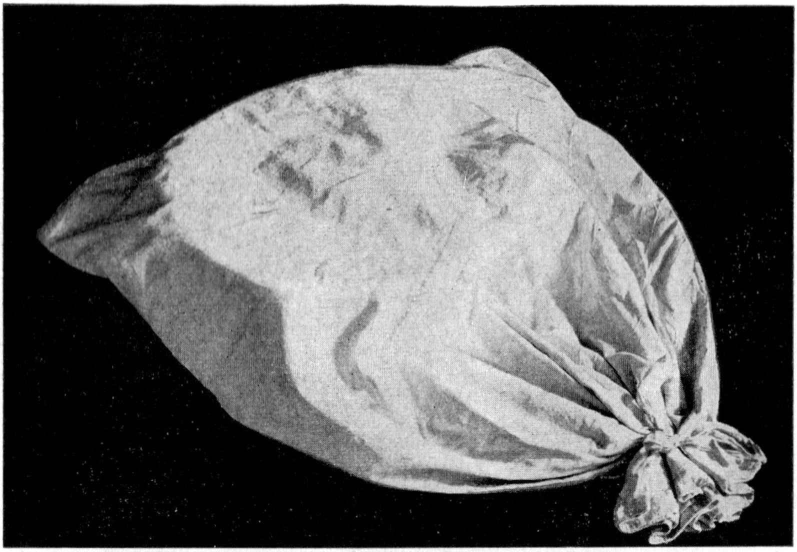

FIG. 303. (*Top*) A basin set enclosed in a bag.

FIG. 304. (*Bottom*) Suggesting the first step in removing the bag in the surgery. The open edge is held away from the individual. A cuff is turned back along the entire surface of the bag. The left hand holds the set while the right hand peels the bag away from the set over the left arm.

(The Surgical Supervisor, American Sterilizer Co., Erie, Pa.)

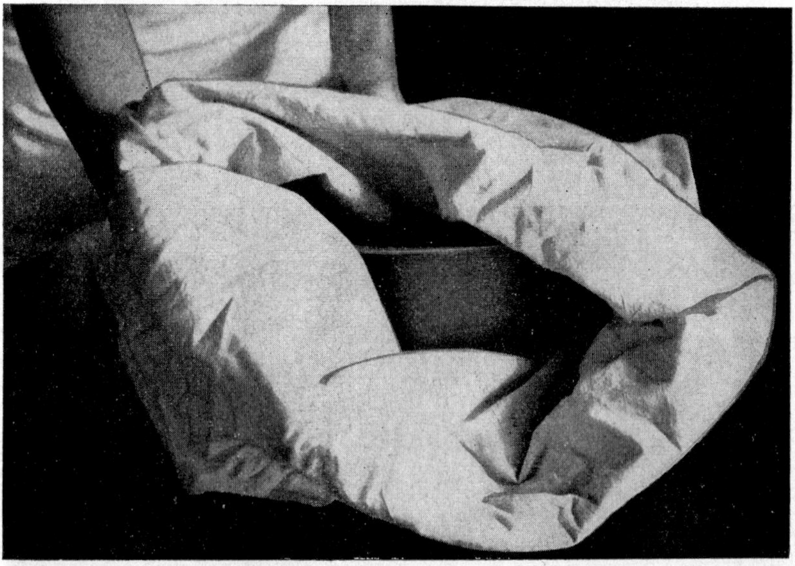

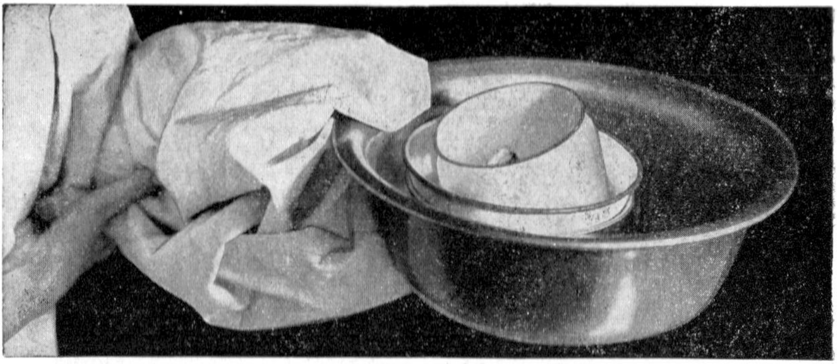

FIG. 305. (*Top*) The basin set is ready to hand to the sterile nurse or to place on a sterile table. (The Surgical Supervisor, American Sterilizer Co., Erie, Pa.)

FIG. 306. (*Bottom*) Use of transfer forceps. On the left is the container filled with antiseptic solution. The nurse has removed the top of suture container without contamination and transfers sutures with the forceps. (Ethicon Suture Laboratories, New Brunswick, N. J.)

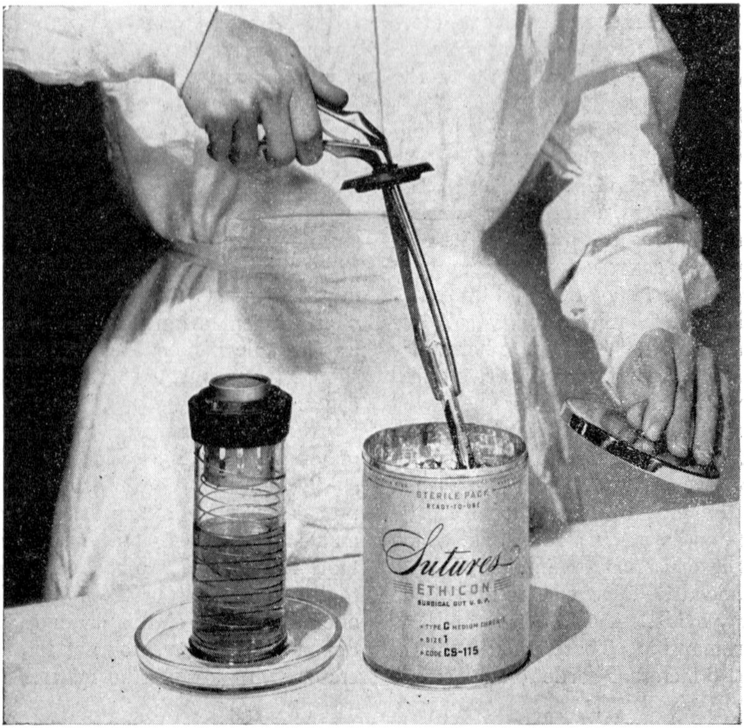

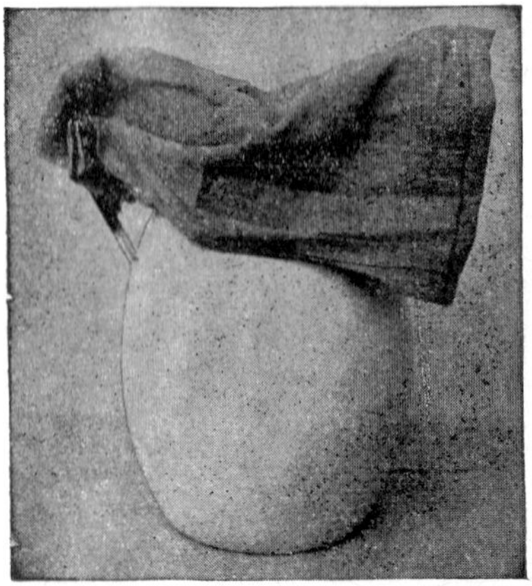

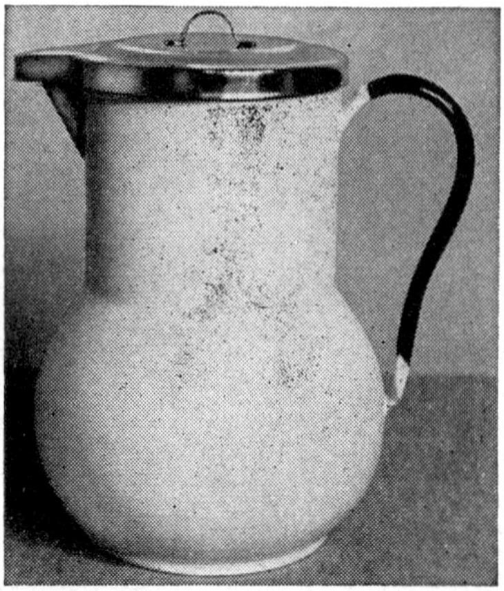

FIG. 307. (*Left*) Cloth-covered sterile pitcher.
FIG. 308. (*Right*) Metal-covered sterile pitcher.

be held in the hand in such a way that the sterile undersurface faces downward. However, if it is necessary to set the lid down, the sterile undersurface faces upward.

If a cloth cover is used, it should be doubled so that the nonsterile nurse may slip her hand between the folds to raise the cover without contaminating the pitcher or its contents. The cover is pinned securely to the handle (Figs. 307 and 308).

The first responsibility of the scrubbed nurse is to drape her tables with sterile covers; at least two thicknesses are used. Covers are held well in front of her so that they do not touch the lower part of her gown or the unsterile table. They are placed on the table from the front to the back and are never flourished, which might cause contamination. Evenly balanced table covers are one of the many evidences of neatness and fine workmanship. There should be at least 6 inches of border on any sterile table. From this point on, the scrubbed nurse receives the necessary supplies from her teammate, the circulating nurse (Fig. 309).

A definite routine for setting up must be carried out. Each article must have its specific place. No exact rules can be given for the placing of supplies, suture material, basins, instruments and the like. Individual preference, experience and judgment must be the deciding factors in the most efficient arrangement. As soon as the table is completely set up, it should be protected by a sterile cover.

Instruments, needles and suture material should be placed on the sterile tables as the final step in the procedure of setting up. The instruments on the surgeon's instrument table should be arranged according to the individual preference of the operator. Much of this arrangement depends on whether or not the operator will pick up the instruments

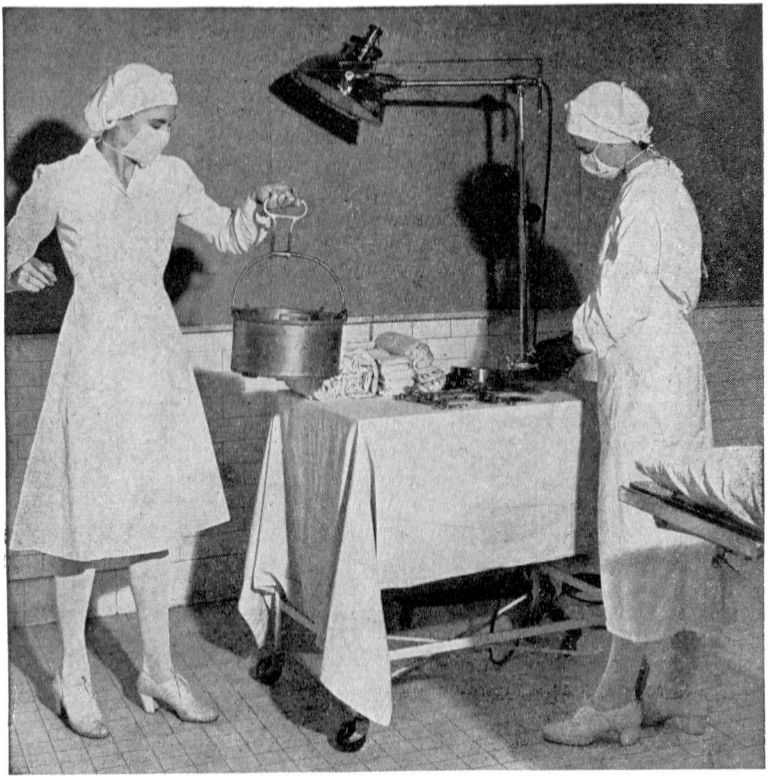

FIG. 309. Sterile nurse receiving sterile supplies and instruments from the circulating nurse. (Wilmot Castle Co., Rochester, N. Y.)

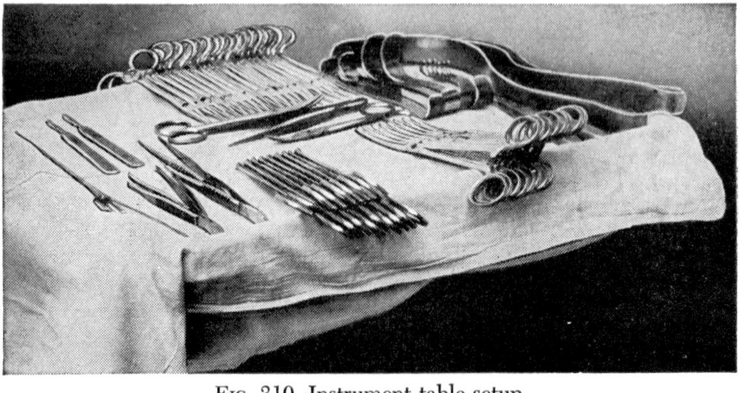

FIG. 310. Instrument table setup.

himself or will have them handed to him by one of his assistants. In general, the order in which instruments are used should be kept in mind: (1) the scalpel to make the incision; (2) artery forceps to clamp off superficial bleeding points; (3) tissue forceps to aid in further dissection, etc. Figure 310 shows one method of arranging the instrument table.

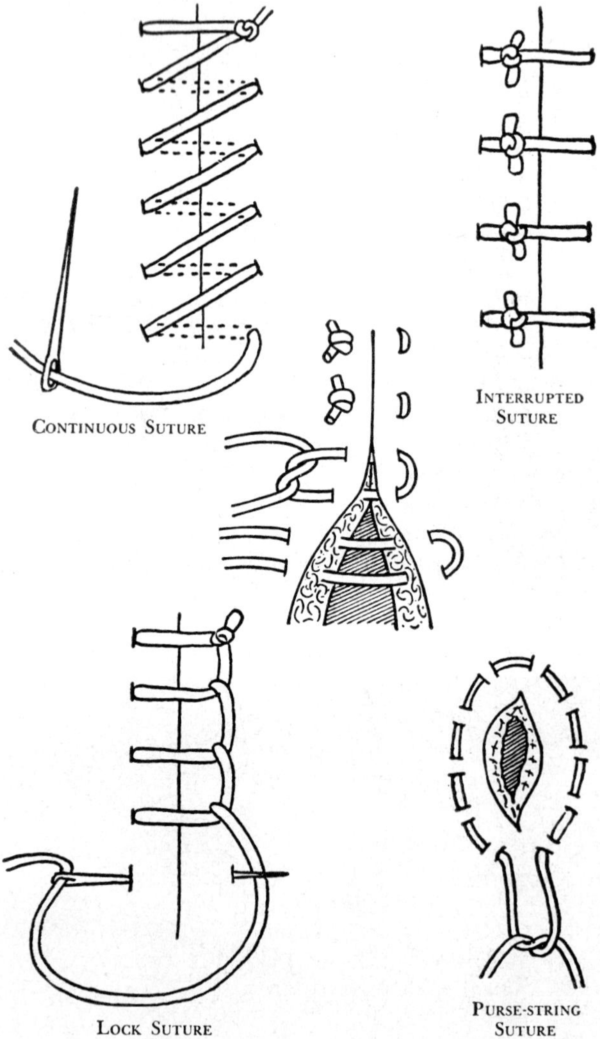

FIG. 311. Common suture stitches. (Bauer & Black, Chicago)

LIGATURES AND SUTURES

After the instruments are placed, the scrubbed nurse will select and prepare ligatures and sutures according to the needs of the operation and the preference of the surgeon.

Generally, a *ligature* (a tie) is a free piece of suture material, not threaded on a needle, and of considerable length (10 to 18 in.) or on a spool, for the purpose of tying blood vessels that have previously been clamped with an artery forceps.

A *suture*, on the other hand, is threaded on a needle and is used for sewing or suturing together the edges and the surfaces of tissue, for checking the flow of blood, fastening drainage tubes in position, etc. Sutures are either *interrupted*, each stitch tied separately, or *continuous*, the thread running in a series of stitches, only the first and last of which are tied. The length of sutures naturally varies considerably. Each depends on the character of the work

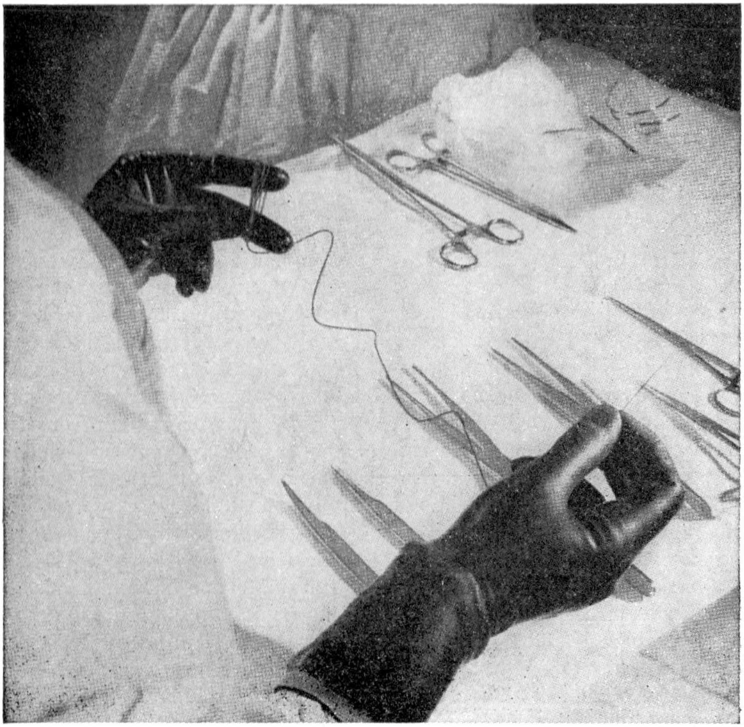

FIG. 312. Unwinding catgut sutures. Strand is gently pulled out straight with an even pull to remove kinks. (Davis & Geck, Inc., New York)

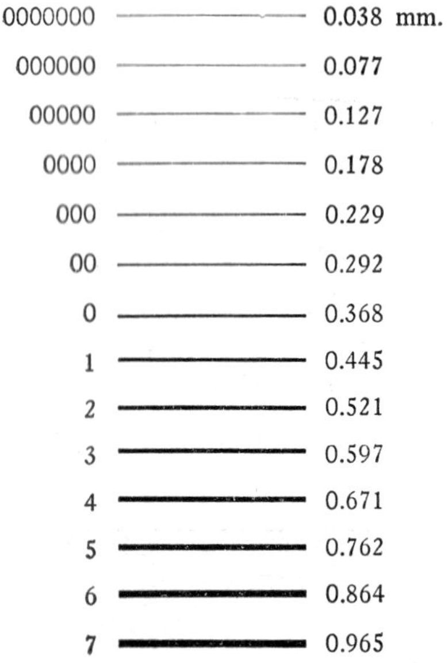

FIG. 313. U.S. Pharmacopoeia suture gauges. (Ziegler, P. F.: Text Book of Sutures, Bauer & Black, Chicago)

and the size of the operation. Deep work, in the pelvis for instance, requires a much longer suture than would be necessary in suturing in an area closer to the surface of a wound. Experience and judgment, along with the desire of the operator, must be the determining factors in details of sutures and ligatures.

Testing of suture material is usually unnecessary if it is purchased from reliable firms who gauge and test for tensile strength. However, if testing is undertaken, it must be done carefully. A length of suture material is tested by holding the ends in each hand and exerting a firm, steady pull. Any jerking will weaken it considerably. Likewise, it is injurious to handle suture material any more than is absolutely necessary, such as constantly drawing it through the fingers, etc. Sutures which have been folded in glass tubes are kinked and inconvenient to use. By a brief dip in sterile saline and gentle stretching, these kinks are easily removed by the suture nurse before the suture is handed to the surgeon. This is especially important in heavier types of catgut sutures. Prolonged soaking should be avoided because it makes the catgut rubbery and reduces its tensile strength. Spiral-wound suture material is available and is more convenient to use than a suture wound on a reel.

TYPES

Sutures and ligatures are of two main types: those which are absorbed and those which are not. Catgut, Cargile membrane and fascia lata are of the *absorbable* type, while silk, linen, cotton, nylon, wire, silkworm gut, etc., comprise the *nonabsorbable* group. For the most part, absorbable sutures are used under the skin, while the nonabsorbable kind may be used almost anywhere. The criteria of many surgeons is to select a suture material which is strong and produces the least amount of tissue reaction.

Absorbable Sutures. CATGUT is made from the submucous layer of sheep's intestine, which is cleaned, dried, twisted into threads of various sizes and prepared for use by special processes, which include innumerable inspections of gauge and tensile strength and scrupulous sterilization.

Catgut is made in different sizes.

The strands are graded according to their caliber and range from No. 0000000 (sometimes marked 7-0), the finest, to No. 4, the very coarse. The sizes in most common use are 000, 00, 0 and 1. The length of time of complete absorption of catgut in a wound is reckoned by the action of certain hardening agents. Therefore, "Type A, Plain Surgical Gut," "Type C, Medium Chromic Gut," etc., refer to different preparations of suture material which affect absorption time. Chromic catgut has been treated by a tanning process with chromic salts, and absorption is delayed for from 10 to 40 days.

Catgut is purchased in glass tubes in which a 54-inch length is wound on a reel and immersed in an antiseptic. Such tubes are sealed hermetically and are sterile on the inside. They are of two types: boilable and nonboilable, which means that the former may be autoclaved or boiled, whereas the latter type of tube must be sterilized by immersion in an antiseptic for at least 18 hours. The nonboilable tubes can be purchased in nonsterile cartons or in sterile cans (Fig. 306). If they are not sterile, the tubes must be thoroughly washed with soap and water and dried before they are placed in a recommended alcoholic solution.

Catgut tubes should not be broken until the scrubbed nurse is ready to prepare her sutures. When breaking suture tubes, a sterile cover is wrapped around the filled tube and broken in a prescribed manner (Fig. 314).

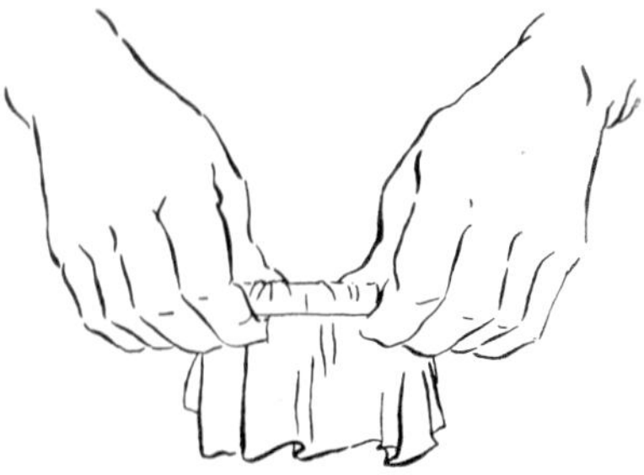

FIG. 314. When breaking suture tubes, a sterile towel or gauze is wrapped round tube to protect gloves and hands. By grasping tube by the ends and pulling against the thumbs, the tube is broken easily. (Davis & Geck, Inc., from Manual of Sutures and Ligatures.)

CARGILE MEMBRANE (insultoic membrane) is obtained from the peritoneum of the ox and is available in sheets approximately 4 by 8 inches in single or double thickness. It is prepared in tubes, as is catgut. Such membrane is used in repair processes where peritoneum has been removed; it is used also in preventing adhesions.

FASCIA LATA is prepared after it is obtained from the fibrous tissue in the thigh of an ox. It comes in strips or sheets and is used in reconstructive orthopedic surgery as well as for the repair of hernia.

Nonabsorbable Sutures. Sutures which have been placed in the skin are removed, but those which are used under the skin remain buried.

SILK THREAD is obtained from the silkworm and goes through many processes before it can be used for surgical suturing. Silk may be black, colored or white; however, black is seen more easily in tissues and is preferred. It may be twisted or braided and it comes in sizes comparable with catgut. Size range is from very fine to very coarse: A-B-C-1 to 8. It is available in sterile tubes and envelopes and can be purchased on unsterile spools which can be rewound to smaller amounts and sterilized. Metal or glass spools, rubber tubing and flat sheets of metal have been used with success in the rewinding process. Care must be taken to wind silk loosely and evenly. If wound tightly on something which expands during the sterilization process, the tensile strength of the silk will be reduced. (Silk contracts with heat.) Paraffin, bonewax and beeswax have been used to prevent disintegration of the strands of silk which in turn makes it easier to handle. When wax or lubricant is applied, it must be done evenly. Silk is best sterilized by autoclaving at 250° F. for 15 minutes. Two or three sterilizations are permitted without reducing the tensile strength significantly.

Cotton thread is available in a wide variety of sizes. It may be purchased in the dime store; hence, it has the advantage of being inexpensive and available. Special cotton thread for surgical use is available. It is made of long fiber cotton and is smoother and of greater tensile strength than is the ordinary sewing thread. Methods of sterilization and precautions to observe are the same as those mentioned with silk. Cotton should not be used after one sterilization, because it loses its strength. Hence, it is wise to sterilize individually wrapped spools or reels which can be opened and used as needed.

Pagenstecher (linen thread which has been coated with celluloid) is used for much the same purposes as silk. There are two colors, black and the natural linen shade, and a variety of sizes, usually designated as fine, medium and heavy. The first two sizes are more generally used. Sterilization is the same as for silk.

Metal Wire. Silver, bronze and copper have been used in surgery for a long time. Stainless steel and tantalum are the most popular today. Wire comes in various gauges and has the advantage of being strong and permanent and of causing little or no local reaction in the tissue in which it is placed. Steel alloy wire is relatively cheap, and it may be tied in knots almost as easily as silk and catgut. Meticulous technic is necessary so that kinks are not produced, thereby weakening the suture material. All ends must be cut close to the knot to prevent irritation. Tantalum is expensive, which seems to be its only disadvantage.

Metal Clips. These are made for use in controlling bleeding from vessels in brain, stomach and nerve surgery. A dispenser is available in which clips are harbored and dispensed. Michel clips are metal-toothed clips applied to hold skin edges in approximation. They require a special forceps for both application and removal. Clips and forceps may be sterilized by autoclaving with the instruments.

Plastic Materials. Nylon is a synthetic protein textile fiber made from coal-tar derivatives. It is obtainable in all sizes and is sterilized in the same manner as silk; however, it is much stronger and smoother than silk. Because of this latter property, knots must be tied with me-

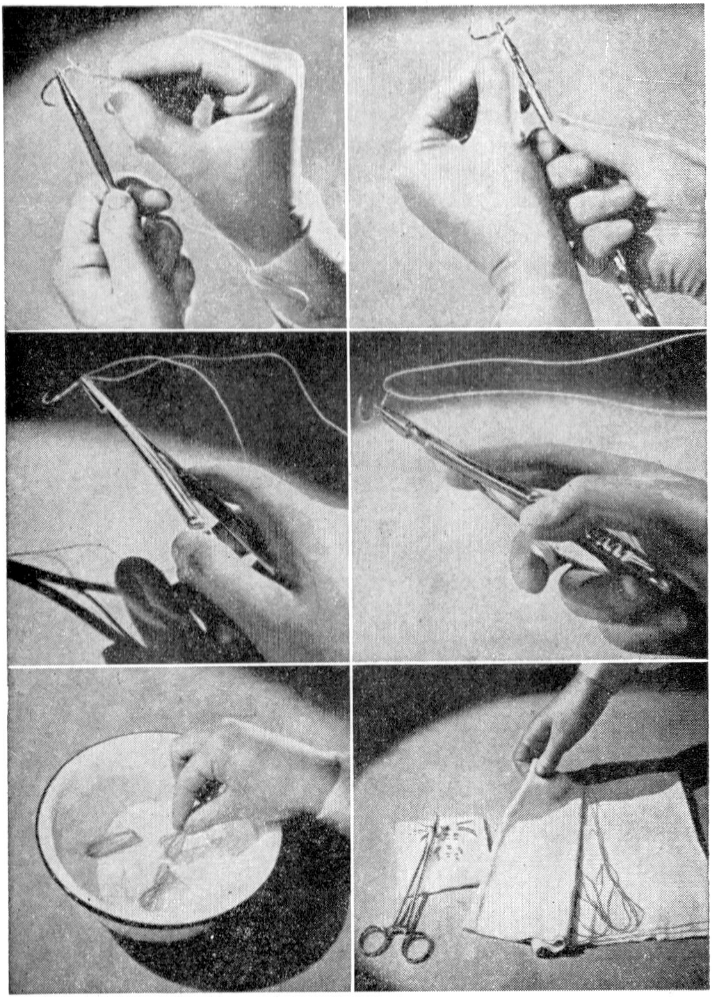

FIG. 315. Hints on handling sutures. (*Top*) Needle should be threaded from inside the curve, it is less easily unthreaded. (*Center*) Needle holder should not grasp needle close to eye, but about one-third the distance down the shaft. This prevents breaking of needle when in use. (*Bottom*) Sutures should not be soaked in water or saline, but dipped and placed between the layers of a sterile towel. (Ethicon Suture Laboratories, New Brunswick, N. J.)

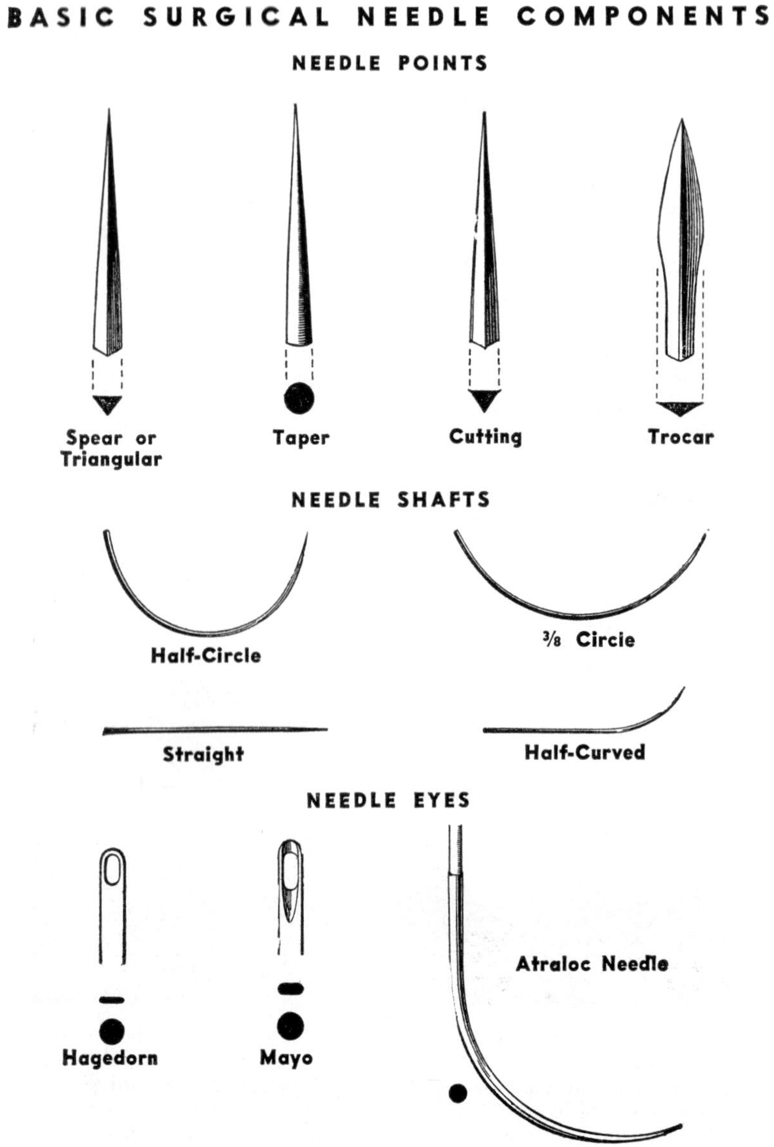

FIG. 316. (Ethicon Suture Laboratories, New Brunswick, N. J.)

ticulous technic. Nylon has good elasticity and withstands repeated sterilization.

SILKWORM GUT. This strong, smooth material is used for tension sutures, especially in the closure of abdominal wounds, or those in which there is particular strain. The strands come 10 to 12 inches in length and vary considerably in thickness. The size is identified by the terms fine, medium and heavy. Because the strands are of unequal length and of uneven diameters, this suture material is being replaced by wire, nylon and heavy silk. It can be sterilized by autoclaving. After sterilization, the gut may be stored in 70 per cent alcohol until used. Silkworm gut is exceedingly stiff and unpliable and must be soaked in hot sterile water for at least 10 minutes before use.

HORSEHAIR, obtained from the tail and mane of the horse, is a fine,

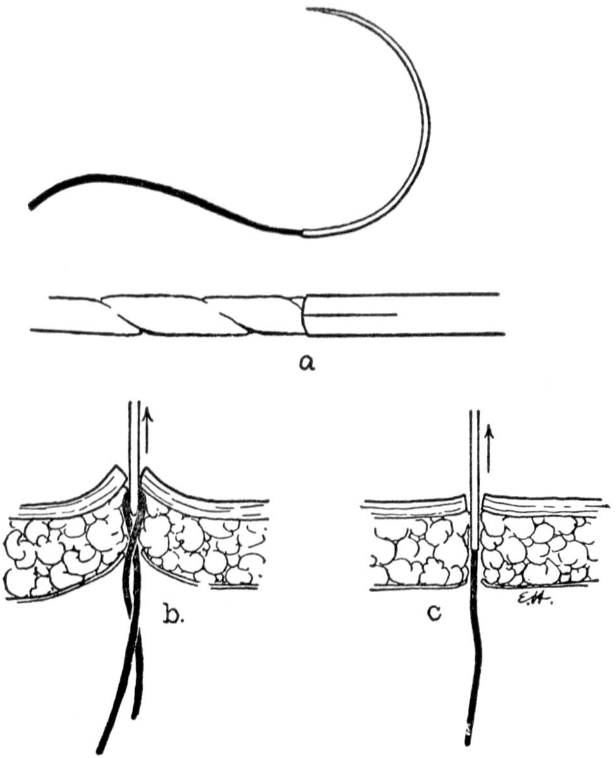

FIG. 317. Atraumatic needle and suture for intestinal sutures. Needle and suture are of same size, and, when pulled through tissue, suture fills needle hole (c). Ordinary suture and needle (b) for comparison.

pliable, elastic suture and excellent for closing small skin wounds in which there is not much tension. It may be sterilized by autoclaving and then preserved in alcohol until used. If the strands are twisted into a loose coil, it can be handled much more readily.

Suture Needles

The needles employed in surgery vary according to their use. They may be straight, full curved and half curved. Straight needles are used when the suture is to be placed at an accessible site. Curved needles are preferred, on the other hand, when the suturing is in a deep or less accessible location. Much depends, too, on the individual preference of the operator—some surgeons use a straight needle for closing a wound, while others use a curved. The same holds true for intestinal operations.

Types. Needles may be classed under two heads: cutting edge and round point. Of the cutting edge, there are three types: Hagedorn, spear point and trocar point. Cutting needles are used for the skin or any dense tissue, such as the cervix of the uterus. Round-point needles are used for operations on the intestines, the brain, the mucous membranes, nerves and such delicate structures.

Eyeless needles are popular for several reasons: (1) they do not have to be threaded; (2) they produce a minimum of tissue trauma; (3) there is less damage to the suture strand (Fig. 317).

Size. Needles come in varying sizes and caliber; usually the smallest numbers indicate the largest needles, although sometimes just the reverse of this is true, depending on the make of the needle.

Different surgeons with their individual technics use different needles. Experience and the wish of the surgeon are the only real guides as to the various uses of needles, although good judgment on the nurse's part is always a valuable asset. No intelligent nurse, for instance, would presume to hand a surgeon the same size and caliber of needle for suturing a wound of the face as she would for closing an abdominal incision. The nurse always should keep in mind the character of the work to be done and remember that dense tissues need a cutting edge, or at least a cutting point (spear or trocar), and delicate tissues are penetrated very easily and, therefore, are readily injured by large, cutting needles.

Straight needles are generally used without a needle holder, while all curved needles are used with a holder. The clamp of the holder never should come together directly on the eye of the needle. Almost invariably the needle will break if this is done.

Drainage Materials

Drainage is required to permit easy escape of pus, blood, or such fluids as otherwise might collect in wounds and delay their healing. The most common materials used for this purpose are gauze, rubber tissue and rubber tubes.

Gauze, folded in some manner to exclude any cut edges coming in contact with raw surfaces, is used where capillary drainage is desired.

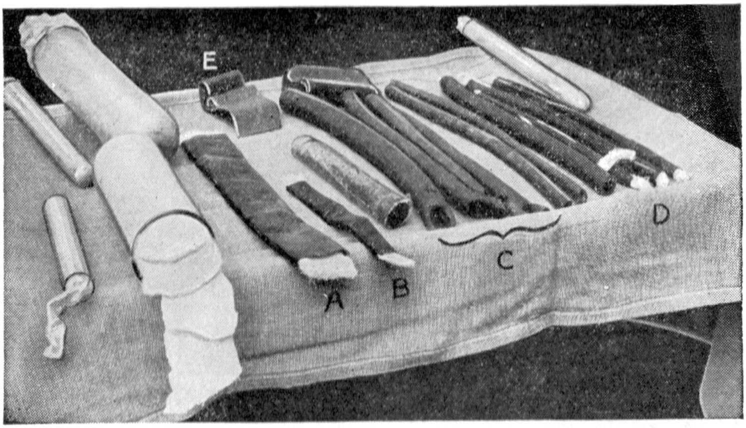

FIG. 318. Drainage materials. Gauze packed in glass tubes. (A) Cigarette drain, large size. (B) Cigarette drain, small size. (C) Fenestrated rubber tubes. (D) Split rubber tube drains with gauze wicks. (E) Rubber dam or tissue.

Bandage gauze should not be used because the sizing (starch) and the close mesh employed in its manufacture make a stiffer material and one that has less capillarity. Gauze folded in various widths may be used as packing for the control of capillary or venous hemorrhage. Gauze drains become clogged within 24 hours and are not useful after that time. When drains are required for a longer period, rubber in some form is the material of choice. Rubber tissue may be used alone or in combination with gauze. The latter is known as a "cigarette" drain. The ends of the gauze should project beyond the rubber casing to get the best results. It must be borne in mind that gauze sterilized in rubber becomes friable. Hence, the nurse should test the gauze each time before it is used, or better, the cigarette drains may be freshly prepared each time, using gauze packing and Penrose tubing which have been sterilized separately. This drain has the advantage of capillarity and at the same time does not clog or adhere to the edges of the wound. Cigarette drains are used in many instances, especially in abdominal wounds. When drainage is necessary in a small wound, rubber tissue is used.

Rubber tubes of varying size and thickness make excellent material for drainage. They should have sufficient lumen to carry secretions and should be of adequate thickness to prevent their collapse. Tubes may be split lengthwise or "fenestrated" (perforated with small holes) to permit easy flow of the fluids to be drained through the tube to the exterior. If a small gauze wick is placed within the lumen of the tube, the advantage of capillarity is added. Some of the varieties are shown in Figure 318.

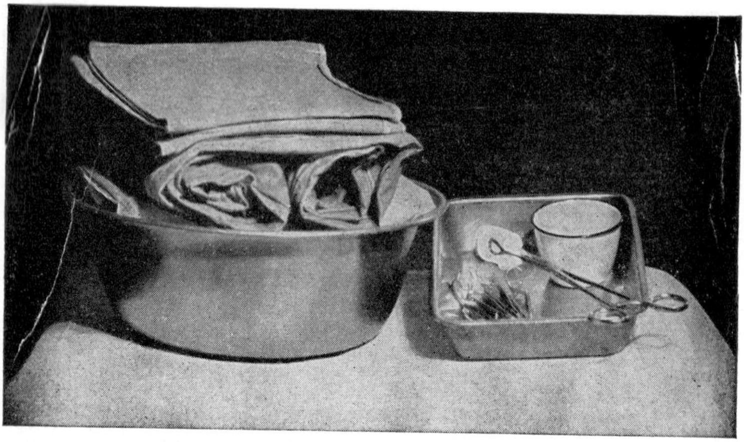

FIG. 319. Accessory table containing preliminary covers, towel clips, antiseptic cup and swab. After drapes have been applied, solution tray is removed, leaving sterile basin to be used as a hand-solution table.

IMMEDIATELY BEFORE THE OPERATION

Immediately before the patient is wheeled into the operating room, the nurse should see to it that each sterile table is covered with a sterile drape. The overhead light is turned on, and the circulating nurse assists the anesthetist and the porter in moving the patient and anesthesia equipment into the room. At this time, lights are adjusted, covers on the sterile tables are removed, footstools are placed where necessary, and the field of operation is ready to be prepared. The sheet covering the patient is withdrawn to expose the area. The surgeon or one of his assistants cleans the area with an antiseptic solution. In some instances, this is preceded by soap and water and possibly ether. The drapes are placed in such a way that the patient is completely covered, except for the site of incision. A screen over the head of the patient holds the drapes away from his face and affords working space for the anesthetist. Metal towel clips hold sterile drapes in place. Often a special table is set up with this equipment (Fig. 319).

Contamination of scrubbed personnel occurs very easily during this period of draping the patient and preparation of operative field. It is essential that the nurse be attentive as to what is sterile and what is not. This applies not only to her hands but also to her gown and sterile tables. There should be no question about sterility. For example, if there is a doubt as to whether an unsterile cover of the patient touched a sterile table, the table should be removed or the drape may be removed and replaced with a sterile one.

After preparation of the patient and application of sterile drapes, a waterproof cover of duck canvas or plastic material may be used to cover the lower part of the patient. The purpose of this is to prevent contamination from dampness penetrating the sterile covers to the unsterile area below. Many surgeons prefer to cover the waterproof material with a wet towel. This prevents instruments from slipping, even where the area is not flat. This towel can be changed if it becomes soiled.

RESPONSIBILITIES OF THE CIRCULATING NURSE DURING THE OPERATION

The circulating nurse has many responsibilities. She is at the beck and call of the scrubbed personnel and the anesthetist. Under no condition is she permitted to leave the room unless she is replaced. Some of her activities include the following:

1. Observe technic at all times to see that it is maintained. If there is a break, it must be remedied.
2. Attach the suction apparatus and check to see that it is functioning properly.
3. Keep the scrubbed nurse supplied with dressings, suture materials, etc.
4. Place buckets strategically to receive discarded sponges.
5. Retrieve instruments, etc., which accidentally fall from the table.
6. Replace saline or water in basins as necessary.
7. Check infusions.
8. Regulate temperature of the room as necessary.
9. Count, with the sterile nurse, all sponges opened for use and permit no gauze of any kind to be carried from the operating room during an abdominal operation.
10. Prepare adhesive for the wound.
11. Take care of emergency specimens.
12. Notify the floor when the patient is ready to be returned.

RESPONSIBILITIES OF T SCRUBBED NURSE

The scrubbed nurse may b sponsible for passing instrume sutures, sponges, etc., or her resp sibilities may be divided so that s is passing sutures and sponges whi a physician passes all instruments to the surgeon. In some instances, a nurse's responsibility is to wring out and pass sponges, particularly on an abdominal case.

The scrubbed "instrument" nurse soon learns that the first instrument to be used by the surgeon is the scalpel. When this is being used, the assistants must be provided with sponges and hemostats which are used to control bleeding. The scalpel blade is discarded after the skin incision is made and replaced by a fresh blade. Since the skin cannot be sterilized, the blade used on the skin is considered contaminated. The next step is to provide ligatures for tying the vessels which are clamped. If the nurse holds each end of the "tie," the surgeon is able to grasp the ligature in the middle. All ligatures must have excess threads cut after the tie is completed; therefore, an assistant must be provided with scissors. By knowing these basic steps, a nurse is soon able to anticipate the needs of the surgeon and his assistants without being told. Some surgeons use a sign language so that the nurse knows by a gesture what he would like next. By learning the various steps of different types of operations, the nurse who is alert soon becomes proficient and is a valuable aid to the surgeon.

In passing instruments, the handle or part of the instrument which one would ordinarily hold in using it,

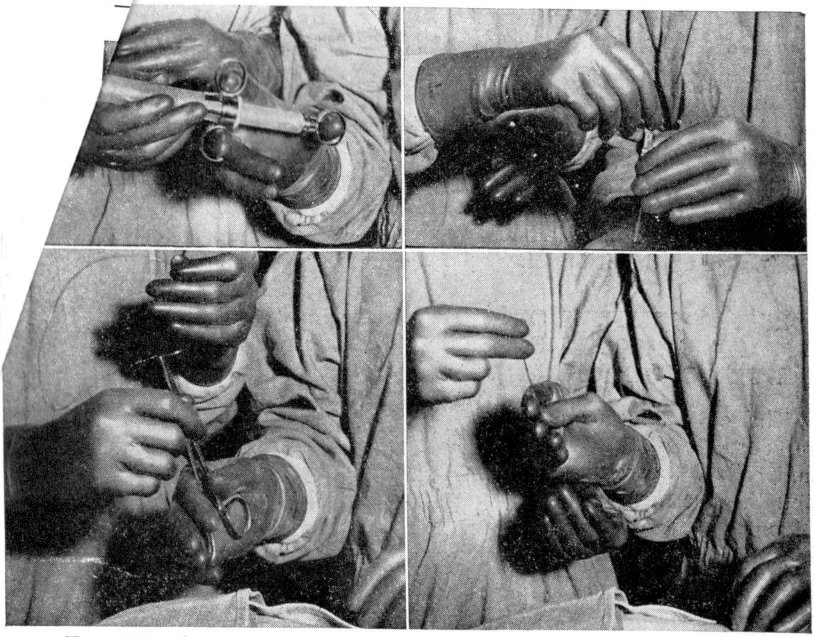

FIG. 320. The scrub nurse—technic of passing sutures and instruments.

(*Top, left*) Passing the syringe. The ring type of syringe should be passed so that the rings may be grasped easily by the surgeon in the fingers of the right hand.

(*Top, right*) Forceps to be passed by grasping the end in the fingers, the open part of the forceps down. As most surgeons are right-handed, the forceps usually are passed to the surgeon's left hand.

(*Bottom, left*) Method of passing a needle holder. Handle portion of the needle holder should be placed firmly in the right hand of the surgeon. The nurse should pass the needle holder, holding it in such a way that the surgeon may grasp it without looking. The nurse should be careful that she is not caught by the needle.

(*Bottom, right*) Passing a straight needle to the surgeon. The tip of the needle is held in the hand between the fingers and the thumb of the nurse's right hand. The eye end of the needle then is placed in the fingers of the surgeon's right hand.

should reach the surgeon's hand (Fig. 320); otherwise, he must drop it and pick it up or turn it to use. If the surgeon has good assistants his eyes need never leave the wound. Likewise, the nurse who constantly observes the progress made by the surgeon is more able to anticipate his needs. This implies that her tables should be arranged in such a way (and she should know the arrangement) that she can reach any article without having to turn her head to look for it. Obviously, this can come only with practice. The surgeon should not expect a new nurse to have this skill nor should a new nurse be placed in a situation for which she is not properly prepared and supervised.

When sutures are being used (Fig. 320), a duplicate should be kept in reserve. The end of a suture never should be wrapped around a needle holder nor should it be dragged over the instruments or drapings. A needle which has been used should be replaced in the holder as soon as the surgeon lays it down. Constant checking to see that all needles are accounted for is necessary. Suture material which is cut on the bias facilitates threading. Gloves which are clean and wet make the handling of instruments and sutures much easier than dry, sticky gloves. When an instrument has been used, it should be washed and placed in its proper position. Instrument tables and the working field on the patient never should be cluttered.

When the intestinal tract is opened, all sponges, instruments, etc., which come in contact with this area are considered contaminated for other "cleaner" parts of the wound. Hence, when this is anticipated, a drape may be placed over the working area and all supplies used can be confined to this field. When the intestine has been closed, these instruments, drapes, etc., must be removed and the gloves of the operating team must be changed.

A basin should be provided to receive any specimen. Care must be taken that cultures or other specimens are cared for properly.

In an abdominal case, the scrubbed nurse should check the counting of all sponges with the circulating nurse before she passes the suture for closure of the peritoneum.

After the skin is closed and the dressings have been applied, the scrubbed nurse collects all drapes and removes all tables from the operating room. She is personally responsible for taking care of any specimens, seeing that they are properly labeled and transported to the laboratory. Often an operation is performed wholly for the purpose of securing a piece of tissue for diagnosis. To misplace or lose a specimen may mean that a patient will have to have another operation. She should also remove needles from holders, knife blades from knife handles, etc., so that whoever is responsible for instrument cleaning is not cut accidentally. Dressings and linens which were not used do not have to be discarded. They can be repackaged later and autoclaved.

BETWEEN OPERATIONS

Every possible precaution should be taken to avoid undue haste, and at the same time as little time as possible should be lost in going from one case to another. Sufficient time must be allowed for the proper cleaning of the room and the floor. Nothing—instruments, supplies, suture material, etc.—that has been used for one case should be used for another without resterilization. Gowns and gloves, of course, must be changed between cases.

AT THE END OF THE OPERATIVE SCHEDULE

Following the day's operations, the entire operating suite must receive

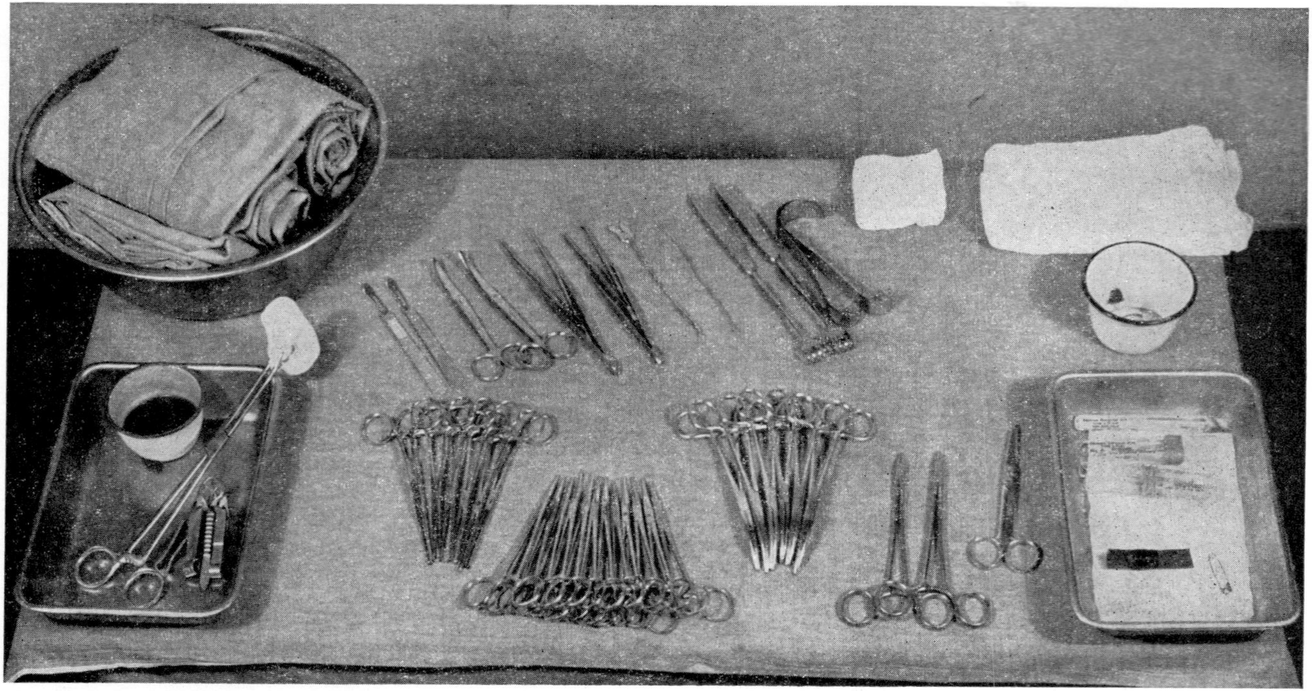

FIG. 321. Instrument table setup for simple operation, such as incision and drainage, biopsy, plastic operation and so forth. The table illustrates the basic setup. Additional instruments may be added according to the type of operation.

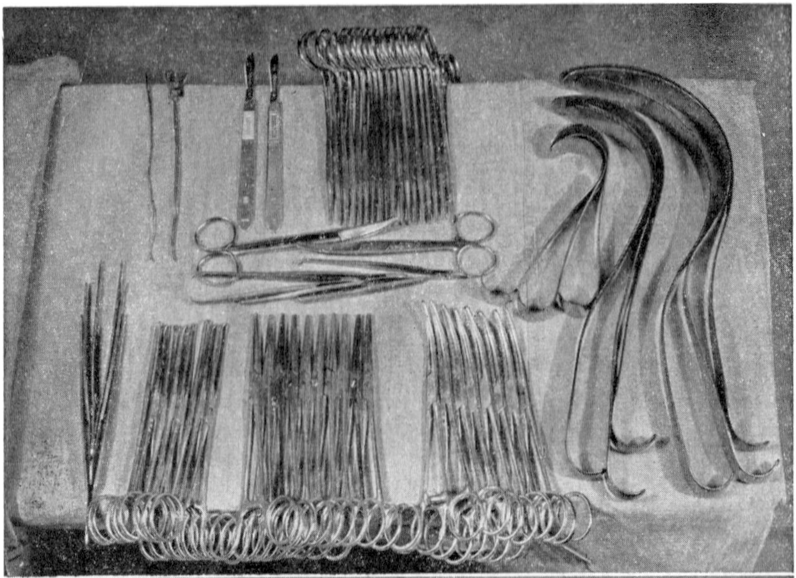

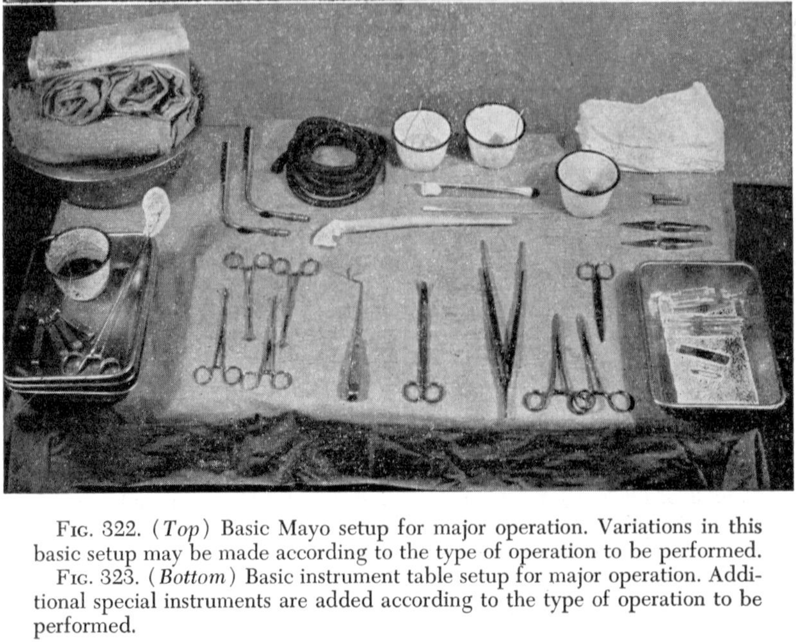

FIG. 322. (*Top*) Basic Mayo setup for major operation. Variations in this basic setup may be made according to the type of operation to be performed.

FIG. 323. (*Bottom*) Basic instrument table setup for major operation. Additional special instruments are added according to the type of operation to be performed.

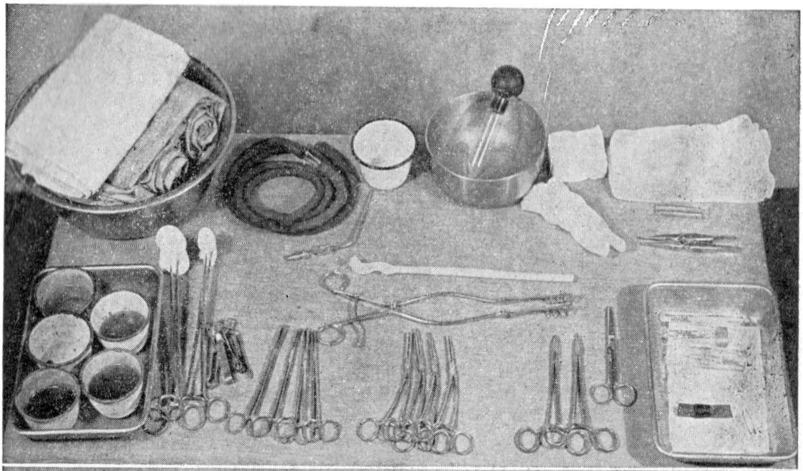

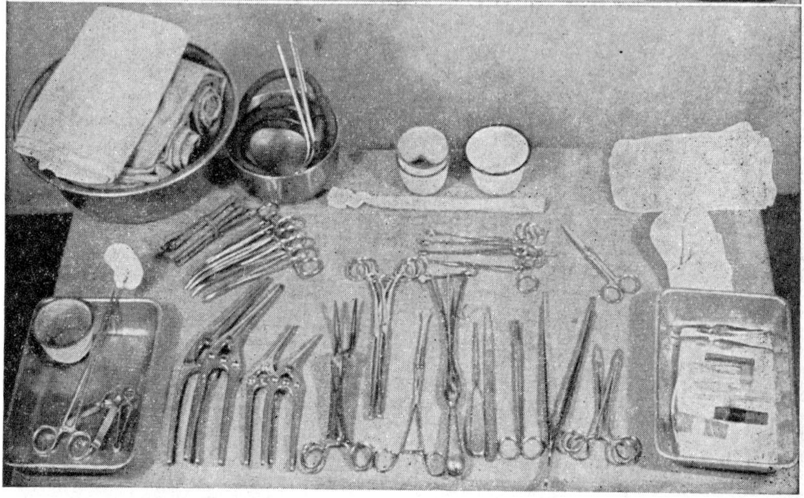

Fig. 324. (*Top*) Variation of instrument table setup for thyroidectomy. Note the special instruments used in this type of operation. Note the special thyroid retractor, the Lahey grasping forceps and the Crile muscle clamps.

Fig. 325. (*Bottom*) Variation of the instrument table setup for intestinal operations. Note the various types of intestinal clamps, anastomosis clamp, Babcock clamps and so forth. Note the cotton and silk wound on rubber tubes as spools.

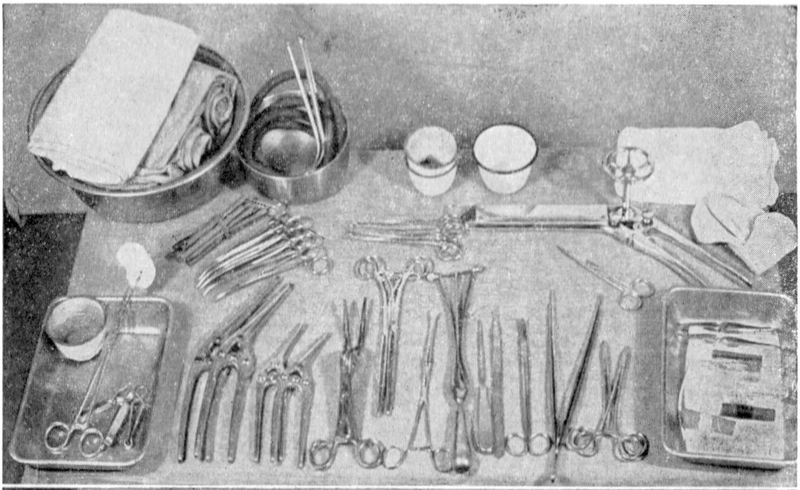

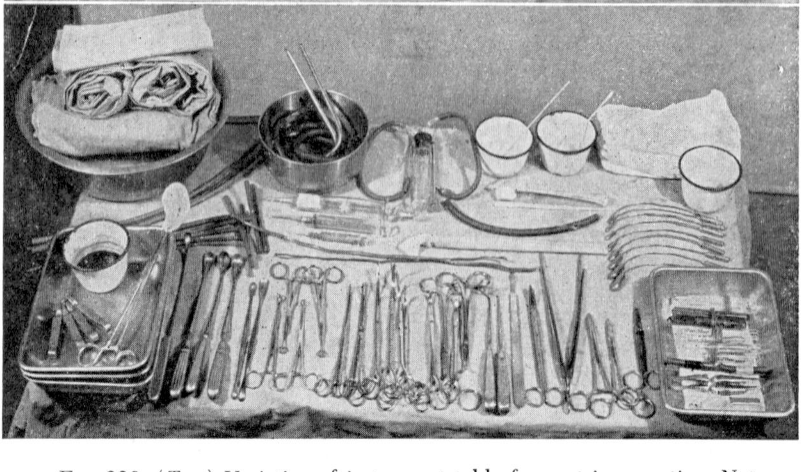

Fig. 326. (*Top*) Variation of instrument table for gastric operation. Note the intestinal clamps, anastomosis clamps, the von Petz instrument, the Babcock clamps, long forceps.

Fig. 327. (*Bottom*) Variation of instrument table for gallbladder and common duct surgery. Note the stone scoops, the various types of curved stone forceps, cystic duct clamps, the Backus dilators, malleable probes, T-tubes and catheters, syringes, gallbladder trocar and aspirating device.

a thorough cleaning, with particular attention to the operating room proper. Soiled linen must be sorted carefully to prevent valuable instruments being sent to the laundry.

Floors should be scrubbed thoroughly. All tables, stools, basin racks, etc., must be well washed to remove blood stains and any other foreign material. The operating table and pad should be washed thoroughly with soap and water.

The care of instruments, needles, gloves, etc., after use has already been taken up in detail (pp. 654-662) and will not be repeated.

All unused sterile supplies, including packages that have been opened, must be resterilized, even though the contents apparently have not been touched. When in doubt, resterilize.

Utensils and special apparatus must be cleansed and sterilized or put away, as the case may demand.. Everything that has been used during the course of the day's operations should be returned to its rightful place in condition to be used again at a moment's notice. The operating room must always be in a state of preparedness.

INSTRUMENT SETUPS

For a simple operation such as a biopsy of lymph node, suturing of a laceration, etc., the instruments, suture materials, drapes and dressings can be conveniently placed on one table (Fig. 321). Basic instruments for a simple setup are as follows:

Sponge forceps and towel clips
Scalpel
Scissors (dissecting and nurse's)
Forceps, plain and toothed
Hemostats, straight and curved
Allis forceps
Retractors
Suture needles and needles
Grooved director and/or probe

Modifications of this setup are made in terms of the type of operation and the preference of the surgeon. If the arrangement of this table is standardized, it becomes a simple matter to make minor additions for such operations as hemorrhoidectomy, minor amputations, minor plastic operations, tonsillectomy, etc. For an incision and drainage of an abscess, obviously retractors and suture equipment are unnecessary, whereas a culture tube and drainage material should be added.

For a simple abdominal procedure, such as an appendectomy or herniorrhaphy, or a larger dissecting operation such as a mastectomy or radical neck dissection, a Mayo instrument stand plus an instrument table is usually used. The Mayo stand ordinarily contains the basic instruments found in the simple setup described above. The instrument table is convenient for the specialty instruments as well as drains, suture material, dressings, etc. From such a setup as the basic Mayo stand and appendectomy instrument table, the more major procedure setups can be developed. Figures 322 and 323 show the basic abdominal tables.

Probably the most frequent modification in the Mayo setup is the variation in retractors which is necessary, depending upon the depth of the wound. In operations near the surface, shallow curved or rake retractors would be used, whereas in operations in deeper cavities, such as abdomen and chest, deeper and larger retractors are desirable.

Figures 324 to 327 illustrate several variations in the instrument table as necessary for various commonly performed operations.

SAFETY PRACTICES IN THE OPERATING ROOM

The operating room nurse has a responsibility for the safety of every patient who comes to her department. Some of the practices which are especially significant are presented.

Emergency equipment always should be available and in usable condition. This includes suction apparatus, airways, drugs, etc. No excuse is acceptable when a patient's life is lost due to negligence.

All solutions which are used in the operating room should be labeled plainly. In order that mistakes be averted, the policy of tinting solutions is helpful. There is no justification for a patient's receiving an injection of ether when the surgeon assumed that he was using procaine hydrochloride.

Although it is not the direct responsibility of the nurse to check anesthesia equipment, she must be aware of the importance of maintaining proper connections of tubing leading to gas machines, suction outlets, air under pressure, etc. For example, a wrong connection made by a well-intentioned nurse or auxiliary worker may result in a patient's receiving carbon dioxide when his precarious condition demands oxygen.

Occasionally, a needle breaks and is lost in the tissues of the patient. This may be a hollow needle which can break at the hub during an injection or it may be a suture needle. It is extremely important that such an accident be reported to the surgeon, who will initiate steps to localize and remove the foreign object.

The recovery of all instruments and sponges used during an operation is imperative. Even though the surgeon assumes the responsibility for a correct count, the nurse is in a unique position to verify such an accounting.

The possibility of fires and explosions in the operating room is always present because of the nature of materials used. In maintaining a safety program, the following points will be helpful:

1. Combustible anesthetic agents when mixed with oxygen are explosive and dangerous when ignited.
2. Many disinfecting agents are combustible and also hazardous. Noncombustible disinfecting agents which are suitable for most needs are available.
3. All possible sources of ignition should be guarded against when combustible anesthetic and disinfecting agents are being used.
4. Some clothing fabrics have the ability to become charged with static electricity and will produce sparks of sufficient energy to ignite combustible anesthetic gas mixtures. For this reason outer garments of wool, silk, and synthetic textile materials such as sharkskin, nylon, and rayon should not be worn by operating room personnel or visitors in any areas where combustible anesthetic agents are being used.
5. Woolen blankets should not be permitted in the operating room.
6. All equipment should be inspected frequently to make reasonably sure that it is in good condition and offers no hazard due to lack of repairs. This should include testing of the conductive

floors and inspection of extension cords and all portable equipment, particularly the anesthetic equipment.

7. Anesthetic apparatus, including gas cylinders, should not be draped or covered in any way which would confine or collect any leaking gas and thereby increase the fire hazard.

8. Conductive floors should be kept clean. They should not be waxed or otherwise coated with a floor dressing material which will materially increase their electrical resistance. Wax is frequently tracked onto the operating floor from other areas. Soap film due to incomplete rinsing after floor washing has been known to build up and thereby insulate the floor.

9. Conductive shoes or foot-to-floor electrical contacts should be kept clean and should not be worn outside the area for which they are intended. They should be tested on the wearer prior to each entry into a surgical event. An abrasive such as steel wool is excellent for cleaning shoes to make them sufficiently conductive.

10. All persons and equipment in the room, including the patient, should be electrically connected to prevent a potential difference of static electricity from building up between persons or objects.*

The medicolegal implications of the problems presented are obvious. Only some of the more common possibilities have been mentioned. Accidents will not occur if all personnel are well informed and alert.

* Griffin, N. L.: Preventing fires and explosions in the operating room, Am. J. Nursing **53**:812, 1953.

REFERENCES AND SUGGESTED READING

Unit Thirteen: Operative Aseptic Technic

General

Alexander, E. A.: Operating Room Technic, ed. 2, St. Louis, Mosby, 1949.

——: There's a lot to learn in the O. R., Am. J. Nursing **49**:584-586, 1949.

Alexander, F.: Maintaining a sterile field during gastro-intestinal surgery, Am. J. Nursing **52**:705-707, 1952.

Bell, H. S.: Practical nurses in the operating room, Am. J. Nursing **52**:580, 1952.

Brown, R. E., Livingstone, H. M., and Willard, Joel: Silent music soothes the surgical patient, Mod. Hosp. **72**:51-53, 1949.

Cutler, E. C., and Zollinger, Robert: Atlas of Surgical Operations, ed. 2, New York, Macmillan, 1949.

Holtzhausen, E. A.: Non-nurse assistants scrub for surgery, Am. J. Nursing **50**:482, 1950.

Lee, D. M., Collins, W. T., and Largen, T. L.: A reappraisal of absorbable glove powder, Surg., Gynec. & Obst. **95**:725-737, 1952.

McConnell, M.: Surgery on color television, Am. J. Nursing **50**:277, 1950.

Operative Procedure, ed. 9, New Brunswick, N. J., Ethicon Suture Laboratories, 1947.

Ruehlow, C. M.: Drape for instrument table, Am. J. Nursing **44**: 570-571, 1944.

Walter, C. W.: The Aseptic Treatment of Wounds, New York, Macmillan, 1948.

——: Scrubbing for surgery, Am. J. Nursing **52**:188-189, 1952.

Weise, R. D.: Operating room administration, Am. J. Nursing **48**: 94-98, 1948.

INSTRUMENTS

Hall, E. D.: Surgical Instrument Guide for Nurses, New York, Weck, 1954.

Schafer, M. K.: Fracture trays, Am. J. Nursing **45**:822-823, 1945.

RUBBER GOODS

Cook, C. B.: Surgical-glove-saving technique, Hospitals **23**:41-42, 1949.

Lehmann, E. E., and Bishop, F. W.: To process surgical gloves, Mod. Hosp. **71**:78-80, 1948.

SAFETY IN THE O. R.

Griffin, N. L.: Preventing fires and explosions in the operating room, Am. J. Nursing **53**:812, 1953.

Recommended Safe Practice for Hospital Operating Rooms, Boston, National Fire Protection Association, 1951.

STERILIZATION

Berman, P., and Beckett, J. S.: Sterilizing surgical supplies, Am. J. Nursing **52**:1212-1214, 1952.

Lehmann, E. E.: Replacing drums with packs, Am. J. Nursing **48**: 522-523, 1948.

SUTURE MATERIAL

Davis & Geck Suture Manual, New York, Davis & Geck, 1953.

Harms, M. T.: Preparation and use of cotton sutures, Am. J. Nursing **48**:651-652, 1948.

The Ethicon Book of Sutures, New Brunswick, N. J., Ethicon Suture Laboratories, 1946.

The Ethicon Manual of Surgical Knots, New Brunswick, N. J., Ethicon Suture Laboratories, 1947.

Ziegler, P. F.: Textbook on Sutures, Chicago, Bauer & Black, Div. of Kendall Co., 1944.

CENTRAL SUPPLY

Frey, T. E.: Central supply service, Am. J. Nursing **51**:119, 1951.

Norton, P. A.: Planning a central supply department, Am. J. Nursing **52**:1215-1216, 1952.

Sterilization Chart

For pressure steam (autoclave) sterilization the sterilizer should be regulated carefully so that the maximum temperature indicated by the thermometer is within the range of 250°–254° F. (121°–123° C.). Time the performance when the thermometer indicates 250° F. *For hot air sterilization* the sterilizer should be regulated, unless otherwise specified below, so that the temperature indicated by the thermometer comes within the range of 320°–325° F. (160°–163° C.). Do not time the performance until the prescribed temperature is indicated by the thermometer.

Article	Method	Time (minutes)
Bronchoscopes	See mfr's specifications	
Bone Wax	Hot air	60
Bougies	Autoclave	15
Brushes (scrub)	Autoclave	15
Catheters (woven base)	Autoclave	15
Catheters (latex)	Autoclave	15
Catheters (gum elastic)	Chemicals only	
Catheters (hard rubber)	Chemicals only	
Cellophane	Autoclave	30
Cystoscopes	Chemicals only	
Cystoscopes (Kirwin type)	Autoclave	15
Diapers	Autoclave	30
Drains (gutta percha)	Chemicals only	
Drains (rubber tubing)	Autoclave	20
Drums-Dressing (loosely packed)	Autoclave	30
Drums-Dressing (full—not compressed)	Autoclave	45
Electric Cords	Autoclave	15
Glassware (vessels inverted)	Autoclave	15
Glassware (laboratory)	Hot air	60
Gloves (rubber)	Autoclave	15
Glycerine	Hot air	60
Hard Rubber Details	Chemicals only	
Instruments (routine)	Autoclave	15
Instruments (emergency)	(270° F.) Autoclave	3
Instruments (cutting edge)	Hot air	60
Instruments (cataract knives)	Chemicals only	
Instruments (tenotomes)	Chemicals only	
Instruments (urethrotomes)	Chemicals only	
Intravenous Sets	Autoclave	30
Jars-Dressing (loosely packed)	Autoclave	30
Lamps (diagnostic)	Chemicals only	
Maternity Packs	Autoclave	30
Mattresses (hair)	(220°–230° F.) Autoclave	30
Mattresses (Foamex rubber)	Autoclave	30
Milk Formulas	(212° F.) Autoclave	30
Milk Formulas	(230° F.) Autoclave	10
Miller-Abbott Tubes	Chemicals only	
Nebulizers	Chemicals only	
Needles (suture; hypodermic)	Hot air	60
Oils—Various (small quantity)	Hot air	60
Operating Motors	See mfr's specifications	

Used by permission of the American Sterilizer Company, Erie, Pa.

STERILIZATION CHART

ARTICLE	METHOD	TIME (MINUTES)
Paraffin Gauze	Hot air	120
Petrolatum	Hot air	120
Petrolatum Gauze	Hot air	120
Plastic Materials	See mfr's specifications	
Proctoscopes	Chemicals only	
Rubber Goods (gloves)	Autoclave	15
Rubber Goods (sheeting)	Autoclave	20
Rubber Goods (tubing)	Autoclave	20
Scalpel Blades (spares, in bottles)	Autoclave	30
Sigmoidoscopes	Chemicals only	
Solutions (aqueous)		
Erlenmeyer (Pyrex) flask–2,000 ml.	Autoclave	35
Erlenmeyer (Pyrex) flask–1,000 ml.	Autoclave	25
Erlenmeyer (Pyrex) flask– 500 ml.	Autoclave	20
Erlenmeyer (Pyrex) flask– 200 ml.	Autoclave	15
Erlenmeyer (Pyrex) flask– 125 ml.	Autoclave	15
Erlenmeyer (Pyrex) flask– 50 ml.	Autoclave	13
Fenwal (Pyrex) flask–2,000 ml.	Autoclave	45
Fenwal (Pyrex) flask–1,000 ml.	Autoclave	30
Fenwal (Pyrex) flask– 500 ml.	Autoclave	25
"Square-Pak" (Pyrex) flask–1,000 ml.	Autoclave	35
Serum Bottle (Pyrex)–9,000 ml.	Autoclave	55
Milk Dilution Bottle–100 ml.	Autoclave	15
Test Tubes (18 x 150 mm.)	Autoclave	12
Test Tubes (32 x 200 mm.)	Autoclave	15
Test Tubes (38 x 200 mm.)	Autoclave	20
Sulfa Drugs (powder)	(300°–315° F.) Hot air	90
Surgical Packs	Autoclave	30
Sutures (non-boilable tubes)	Chemicals only	
Sutures (boilable tubes)	Autoclave	15
Sutures (silk; cotton; linen; nylon)	Autoclave	15
Syringes (unassembled)	Autoclave (or) Hot air	30 60
Syringes (assembled)	Hot air	60
Tongue Depressors	Autoclave	30
Transfusion Sets	Autoclave	30
Trays (all kinds)	Autoclave	30
Urethroscopes	Chemicals only	
Utensils	Autoclave	15

Used by permission of the American Sterilizer Company, Erie, Pa.

Index

Continued from front end paper

Combining Forms and Prefixes—Continued

Odont- (G) *tooth:* odontology, dentistry.
Olig- (G) *little:* oligemia, deficiency in volume of blood.
Oo- (G) *egg:* oocyte, original cell of egg.
Oophor- (G) *ovary:* oophorectomy, removal of an ovary.
Ophthalm- (G) *eye:* ophthalmometer, an instrument for measuring the eye.
Ortho- (G) *straight, normal:* orthograde, walk straight (upright).
Oss- (L) *bone:* osseous, bony.
Oste- (G) *bone:* osteitis, inflammation of a bone.
Ot- (G) *ear:* otorrhea, discharge from ear.
Ovar- (G) *ovary:* ovariorrhexis, rupture of an ovary.

Para- (G) *irregular, around, wrong:* paradenitis, inflammation of tissue in the neighborhood of a gland.
Path- (G) *disease:* pathology, science of disease.
Ped-[1] (G) *children:* pediatrician, child specialist.
Ped-[2] (L) *feet:* pedograph, imprint of the foot.
Per- (L) *through, excessively:* percutaneous, through the skin.
Peri- (G) *around, immediately around* (in contradistinction to para): periapical, surrounding apex of root of tooth.
Phil- (G) *love:* hemophilic, fond of blood (as bacteria that grows well in presence of hemoglobin).
Phleb- (G) *vein:* phlebotomy, opening of vein for bloodletting.
Phob- (G) *fear:* hydrophobic, reluctant to associate with water.
Pneum- or **Pneumon-** (G) *lung* (pneum—air): pneumococcus, organism causing lobar pneumonia.
Polio- (G) *gray:* poliomyelitis, inflammation of gray substance of spinal cord.
Poly- (G) *many:* polyarthritis, inflammation of several joints.
Post- (L) *after:* postpartum, after delivery.
Pre- (L) *before:* prenatal, occurring before birth.
Pro- (L and G) *before:* prognosis, forecast as to result of disease.
Proct- (G) *rectum:* proctectomy, surgical removal of rectum.
Pseudo- (G) *false:* pseudoangina, false angina.
Psych- (G) *soul or mind:* psychiatry, treatment of mental disorders.
Py- (G) *pus:* pyorrhea, discharge of pus.
Pyel- (G) *pelvis:* pyelitis, inflammation of pelvis of kidney.

Rach- (G) *spine:* rachicentesis, puncture into vertebral canal.
Ren- (L) *kidney:* adrenal, near the kidney.
Retro- (L) *backward:* retroversion, turned backward (usually, of uterus).
Rhin- (G) *nose:* rhinology, knowledge concerning noses.

Salping- (G) *a tube:* salpingitis, inflammation of tube.
Semi- (L) *half:* semicoma, mild coma.
Septic- (L and G) *poison:* septicemia, poisoned condition of blood.
Somat- (G) *body:* psychosomatic, having bodily symptoms of mental origin.
Sta- (G) *make stand:* stasis, stoppage of flow of fluid.
Sten- (G) *narrow:* stenosis, narrowing of duct or canal.
Sub- (L) *under:* subdiaphragmatic, under the diaphragm.
Super- (L) *above, excessively:* superacute, excessively acute.
Supra- (L) *above, upon:* suprarenal, above or upon the kidney.
Sym- or **Syn-** (G) *with, together:* symphysis, a growing together.

Tachy- (G) *fast:* tachycardia, fast-beating heart.
Tens- (L) *stretch:* extensor, a muscle extending or stretching a limb.

[1] **Ped**—from Greek *pais,* child.
[2] **Ped**—from Latin *pes,* foot.